Textbook of Geriatric Dentistry

Textbook of Geriatric Dentistry

Third edition

Edited by

Poul Holm-Pedersen
Emeritus Professor, Department of Odontology,
University of Copenhagen, Denmark

Angus W. G. Walls
Director, Edinburgh Postgraduate Dental Institute,
University of Edinburgh, UK

Jonathan A. Ship
formerly of the Bluestone Center for Clinical Research,
New York University (NYU) College of Dentistry, USA

WILEY Blackwell

This edition first published 2015 © 2015 by John Wiley & Sons Ltd.

Registered office: John Wiley & Sons, Ltd, The Atrium, Southern Gate, Chichester, West Sussex, PO19 8SQ, UK

Editorial offices: 9600 Garsington Road, Oxford, OX4 2DQ, UK
The Atrium, Southern Gate, Chichester, West Sussex, PO19 8SQ, UK
1606 Golden Aspen Drive, Suites 103 and 104, Ames, Iowa 50010, USA

For details of our global editorial offices, for customer services and for information about how to apply for permission to reuse the copyright material in this book please see our website at www.wiley.com/wiley-blackwell

Library of Congress Cataloging-in-Publication Data

Textbook of Geriatric Dentistry / edited by Poul Holm-Pedersen, Angus W.G. Walls, Jonathan A. Ship. — Third edition.
p. ; cm.
Includes bibliographical references and index.
ISBN 978-1-4051-5364-5 (cloth)
I. Holm-Pedersen, Poul, editor. II. Walls, Angus, editor. III. Ship, Jonathan, editor.
[DNLM: 1. Dental Care for Aged—methods. 2. Geriatric Dentistry–methods. 3. Aged–physiology. 4. Aged–psychology. WU 490]
RK55.A3
618.97′76—dc23
2014045934

A catalogue record for this book is available from the British Library.

Wiley also publishes its books in a variety of electronic formats. Some content that appears in print may not be available in electronic books.

1 2015

Contents

Notes on contributors, vii

Preface Third edition, 2015, xi

Preface Second edition, 1996, xiii

Preface First edition, 1986, xv

1 Demography – impact of an expanding elderly population, 1
S. Jay Olshansky

2 Biological and physiological aspects of aging, 7
João F. Passos and Thomas B.L. Kirkwood

3 Aging of bone and muscle, 17
Arnold Kahn and Poul Holm-Pedersen

4 Sensory changes and communication in the practitioner–aged patient relationship, 27
Kevin Kawamoto and H. Asuman Kiyak

5 Aging from a psychological perspective, 39
Terry Fulmer, Sheryl Strasser and Toni C. Antonucci

6 The impact of social and environmental forces on aging, 47
H. Asuman Kiyak and Nancy R. Hooyman

7 Clinical assessment of the elderly patient, 61
Elisa M. Ghezzi, Douglas B. Berkey, Richard W. Besdine and Judith A. Jones

8 Medical issues in the dental care of older adults, 81
Peter B. Lockhart and Scott Furney

9 Psychiatric disorders in old age – implications for the dental practitioner, 103
Angela R. Kamer, Mony J. de Leon and Martin J Sadowski

10 Disability in old age – the relationship with oral health, 119
Kirsten Avlund

11 Nutrition and oral health for the older person, 131
Angus W. G. Walls

12 Pharmacology and aging, 145
Elisa M. Chávez and Peter L. Jacobsen

13 Preventive oral health care for elderly people, 155
J. H. Meurman

14 Treatment planning for the geriatric patient, 165
Frederick Hains and Judith Jones

15 Caries in the older person, 181
Angus W. G. Walls and David Ricketts

16 Pathology and treatment of diseases of the pulp, 199
John Whitworth

17 Pathology and treatment of gingivitis and periodontitis in the aging individual, 211
Poul Holm-Pedersen, Frauke Müller and Niklaus P. Lang

18 Pathology and treatment of oral mucosal diseases, 225
Palle Holmstrup, Jesper Reibel and Ian C. Mackenzie

19 Salivary function and disorders in the older adult, 245
Jonathan A. Ship

20 Oral and maxillofacial surgery for the geriatric patient, 255
Michael Turner and Mark Greenwood

21 Orofacial pain in older adults, 265
Dena J. Fischer and Joel B. Epstein

22 Concepts and techniques for oral rehabilitation measures in elderly patients, 277
Niklaus P. Lang, Frauke Müller and J. Mark Thomason

23 Oral health-related quality of life, 301
Finbarr Allen and Jimmy Steele

24 Influences on older adults' use of dental services, 311
H. Asuman Kiyak

25 Oral health care programmes for homebound people, nursing home residents and elderly inpatients, 323
Ronald L. Ettinger and Jane M. Chalmers

26 Clinical management of the cognitively impaired older adult and the terminally ill older patient, 345
Jane M. Chalmers, Ronald L. Ettinger and Michael Wiseman

Index, 361

Notes on contributors

Finbarr Allen
Department of Restorative Dentistry
University College Cork
Cork
Ireland

Toni C. Antonucci
Institute for Social Research
University of Michigan
Ann Arbor, MI
USA

Kirsten Avlund
formerly of
Department of Public Health
University of Copenhagen
Copenhagen
Denmark

Douglas B. Berkey
Department of Applied Dentistry
University of Colorado School of Dental Medicine
Centennial, CO
USA

Richard W. Besdine
Center for Gerontology and Health Care Research
Brown University
Providence, RI
USA

Jane M. Chalmers
formerly of
Department of Preventive and Community Dentistry
The University of Iowa College of Dentistry
Iowa City, IA
USA

Elisa M. Chávez
University of the Pacific
Arthur A. Dugoni School of Dentistry
San Francisco, CA
USA

Joel B. Epstein
Department of Oral Medicine and Diagnostic Sciences
College of Dentistry
University of Illinois at Chicago
Chicago, IL
USA

Ronald L. Ettinger
Department of Prosthodontics and Dows Institute of Dental Research
College of Dentistry
University of Iowa
Iowa City, IA
USA

Dena J. Fischer
Department of Oral Medicine and Diagnostic Sciences
College of Dentistry
University of Illinois at Chicago
Chicago, IL
USA

Terry Fulmer
Bouve College of Health Sciences
Northeastern University
Boston, MA
USA

Scott Furney
Department of Internal Medicine
Carolinas Medical Center
Charlotte, NC
USA

Elisa M. Ghezzi
University of Michigan School of Dentistry
Ann Arbor, MI
USA

Mark Greenwood
Oral and Maxillofacial Surgery
School of Dental Sciences
Newcastle University
Newcastle upon Tyne
UK

Frederick Hains
Department of General Dentistry
Boston University Goldman School of Dental Medicine
Boston University
Boston, MA
USA

Poul Holm-Pedersen
Copenhagen Gerontological Oral Health Research Center
Department of Odontology
University of Copenhagen
Copenhagen
Denmark

Palle Holmstrup
Department of Odontology
University of Copenhagen
Copenhagen
Denmark

Nancy R. Hooyman
School of Social Work
University of Washington
Seattle, WA
USA

Peter L. Jacobsen
Department of Pathology and Medicine
University of the Pacific
Arthur A. Dugoni School of Dentistry
San Francisco, CA
USA

Judith A. Jones
Department of General Dentistry
Boston University Goldman School of Dental Medicine
Boston University
Boston, MA
USA

Arnold J. Kahn
California Pacific Medical Center Research Institute
and
Department of Cell and Tissue Biology, School of Dentistry
University of California
San Francisco, CA
USA

Angela R. Kamer
Department of Periodontology and Implant Dentistry
NYU College of Dentistry
New York, NY
USA

Kevin Kawamoto
School of Communications
College of Social Sciences
University of Hawai'i at Manoa
Honolulu, HI
USA

Thomas B.L. Kirkwood
Centre for Integrated Systems Biology of Aging and Nutrition
Henry Wellcome Laboratory for Biogerontology Research
Institute for Aging and Health
Newcastle University
Newcastle upon Tyne
UK

H. Asuman Kiyak
formerly of
School of Dentistry
Institute on Aging
University of Washington
Seattle, WA
USA

Niklaus P. Lang
School of Dental Medicine
University of Berne
Berne
Switzerland

Mony J. de Leon
Center for Brain Health
Department of Psychiatry
NYU School of Medicine
New York, NY
USA

Peter B. Lockhart
Department of Oral Medicine
Carolinas Medical Center
Charlotte, NC
USA

Ian C. Mackenzie
Centre for Cutaneous Research
Blizard Institute of Cell and Molecular Science
Barts and the London School of Medicine and Dentistry
London
UK

Jukka H. Meurman
Institute of Dentistry
University of Helsinki
Helsinki
Finland

Frauke Müller
School of Dental Medicine
University of Geneva
Geneva
Switzerland

S. Jay Olshansky
School of Public Health
University of Illinois at Chicago
Chicago, IL
USA

João F. Passos
Centre for Integrated Systems Biology of Aging and Nutrition
Henry Wellcome Laboratory for Biogerontology Research
Institute for Aging and Health
Newcastle University
Newcastle
UK

Jesper Reibel
Department of Odontology
University of Copenhagen
Copenhagen
Denmark

David N.J. Ricketts
Dundee Dental School
University of Dundee
Dundee
UK

Martin J. Sadowski
Departments of Neurology, Psychiatry and Pharmacology
NYU School of Medicine
New York, NY
USA

Jonathan A. Ship
formerly of
Bluestone Center for Clinical Research
NYU College of Dentistry
New York, NY
USA

Sheryl M. Strasser
School of Public Health
Georgia State University
Atlanta, GA
USA

Jimmy Steele
School of Dental Sciences
Newcastle University
Newcastle upon Tyne
UK

J. Mark Thomason
School of Dental Sciences
Newcastle University
Newcastle upon Tyne
UK

Michael D. Turner
Department of Oral & Maxillofacial Surgery
Jacobi Medical Center
Bronx, NY
USA

Angus W.G. Walls
Edinburgh Postgraduate Dental Institute
University of Edinburgh
Edinburgh
UK

John Whitworth
School of Dental Sciences
Newcastle University
Newcastle upon Tyne
UK

Michael Wiseman
Faculty of Dentistry
McGill University
Montreal, Quebec
Canada

Preface

Third edition, 2015

When the first edition of *Textbook of Geriatric Dentistry* was published almost 30 years ago, it was one of the first books ever on this topic; maybe it really was the very first international book addressing the topic in a broader perspective, not just "dentures for old people". The prefaces of the first and second editions of the book tell some of the history of geriatric dentistry and its development over three decades. The topics extend from basic biological, cellular, physiological, psychological and social aspects of aging, with special attention to the clinical problems of oral health care for older adults. This new edition also addresses comprehensive aspects of medical and psychosocial conditions, as well as aging in a life-course perspective, all of which have an impact on oral health care and well-being in old age. In addition, this volume includes chapters on palliative care at the end of life, pain management and long-term care.

In preparing the book it has been a privilege to work with some of the world's most distinguished scientists and clinicians. Sadly, four of our authors have passed away much too early during the production of this book: Kirsten Avlund, Jane Chalmers, Asuman Kiyak and Jonathan Ship, the latter also co-editor of this new edition. They will never see their chapters published. This book is dedicated to the memory of these authors. Their death is a great loss for their families and close friends, and for the entire community of gerontology scholars. We also want to pay a special tribute the co-editor of the two first editions of the book, Harald Löe, former Director, National Institute of Dental and Craniofacial Research (NIDCR), Bethesda, who died in 2008.

Poul Holm-Pedersen and Angus W. G. Walls
April 2015

Preface

Second edition, 1996

The first edition of *Geriatric Dentistry — A Textbook of Oral Gerontology* appeared in 1986. During the 10 years past, the demographic trends have continued to bring attention to the greying of the populations in industrialized countries. Also, in the course of the last decade, much of the scientific research – and especially that dealing with molecular biology – has provided new information on genetic governance and environmental mechanisms inherent to the life and death of the cells.

A vast number of scientific articles on the psychosocial and somatic needs of the aging macroorganism, and their clinical implications, has been published in more and more journals.

It is now time for summation and interpretation.

Thus, important objectives of this edition are to provide to the reader a comprehensive and convenient account of the complex issues of aging, to produce an assembly of the current concepts of systemic and oral disorders in the aging patient, and present the means to their solution or amelioration, with the full realization that these challenges can only be met by basic knowledge and clinical competence.

It has been said that the evolution of a profession is evidenced by the scope and quality of its literature. It is our hope that this text might be a small contribution to this principle. However, the merit of this edition, we feel, lies in the wide expanse and penetrating depth with which each of the authors approached the topics.

Poul Holm-Pedersen and Harald Löe
January 1996

Preface

First edition, 1986

Some of the world's great artists have depicted the face of old age. *Leonardo's* sketchbooks illustrate the gnarled features, the wrinkles, the compressed lips, and the sunken jaws of the elderly. Rembrandt's self-portraits similarly record in meticulous detail the lines, the changes in pigmentation, and the moles that mark the aging skin. Today we seek the cellular and molecular changes in the oral tissues that underlie these signs of age.

This search is given extra emphasis by the dramatic increase in the proportions of older people in the populations of all industrialized countries. This trend is expected to continue, with the result that the elderly as a segment of society with special abilities as well as special needs, will become increasingly prominent.

In the industrialized world the new generations of elderly will be better educated and more demanding of social and health services than past generations. Many will retain their natural teeth; only a minority will wear complete dentures. These changes in health status, in attitude and behavior, will have a significant impact on oral health needs, creating new challenges for the dental profession.

The prevention and treatment of oral and dental diseases require a thorough knowledge of the biological variables influencing disease patterns in the aging patient. The relationship between oral and general health and the effects of chronic ailments and diseases on the ability of the older patient to accept treatment must be understood if dental health care is to have a reasonable chance of success. Dentists of tomorrow will need a broader range of knowledge, clinical skills, and human understanding to recognize and treat the oral health problems of their older patients. Cognizant of these needs, special courses and programs in dentistry for the elderly are being included in many undergraduate and graduate dental school curricula.

The objective of this book is to provide a comprehensive review of the processes of aging and their relevance to the delivery of dental health care. Its target audiences are undergraduate and postgraduate students as well as practicing clinicians. The chapters cover the biological, psychological, social and medical aspects of aging, with particular attention to the clinical problems of dental care of the aging patient. The title, *Geriatric Dentistry — A Textbook of Oral Gerontology*, was chosen because the term "geriatric dentistry" is an accepted name for the discipline. However, the book is not restricted to the "geriatric patient", but addresses virtually every aspect of oral health of the elderly, including normal and pathological changes associated with aging. Therefore, the term "oral gerontology" has been adopted to reflect the interdisciplinary character of this subject and to emphasize clinical management in a broader sense. It is our hope that it will contribute to a better understanding of the many facets of dental care for the aged and that it may prove useful to clinicians, health professionals, and researchers within geriatric dentistry and related disciplines.

Pout Holm-Pedersen and Harald Löe
1986

CHAPTER 1

Demography – impact of an expanding elderly population

S. Jay Olshansky
School of Public Health, University of Illinois at Chicago, Chicago, IL, USA

Introduction

Scientists who study the demography of aging investigate trends in, and characteristics of, fertility, mortality and migration and how these components of population change influence, and are influenced by, the environments in which people live. This is a new area of scientific inquiry because aging, as a uniquely demographic phenomenon of populations, has been experienced on a large scale by only one species – humans – and even then only for the last century. Among the many social and economic changes that population aging has brought forth, one of the most important has been dramatic increases in the absolute number of people who live into older regions of the lifespan – a phenomenon that will accelerate in the coming decades.

It is important to understand the difference between population aging and individual aging. Individual aging refers to the biological changes that occur in our cells, tissues and organs with the passage of time, and it is measured demographically at the level of the individual by the duration of our lives. By contrast, population aging is characterized by shifts in the age structure of groups of people such that the relative proportion of older persons (often defined by those aged 65 and older) increases in relation to the number of people under the age of 65. The most common measures that are used to track changes in population aging across time or between population subgroups include the median age, expected remaining years of life (i.e. life expectancy) at middle and older ages and the percentage of the total population aged 65 and older.

Causes and consequences of population aging

For most of recorded history there has been a consistent (stable) pattern of fluctuating birth rates and death rates. Until about the middle of the 19th century, death rates had consistently fluctuated between peaks and troughs as a result of communicable diseases that periodically decimated populations, followed by times of relative stasis. Birth rates were extremely high during most of human history. On average, women gave birth to about seven babies during their reproductive years. Many of the children died in their first year of life from communicable diseases, but death rates were also extremely high throughout the age structure. In fact, the risk of death was so high at middle and younger ages that survival into older ages (beyond age 65) was a rare event by comparison to survival patterns observed today. Living into extreme old ages (ages 85 and older) was an extremely rare occurrence. Since birth rates have almost always exceeded death rates by a small margin throughout most of our history, the size of the human population has grown steadily for thousands of years.

If you were to count the number of people alive at all ages in a given year and plot them on a graph, what you would see is a characteristic age distribution that resembles the shape of a pyramid (see Figure 1.1). This is a common age pattern among humans and many other forms of life where there are a large number of young followed by progressively fewer middle aged and older members of the population. In a hypothetically closed population with no migration, the horizontal bars in the age pyramid reflect the number

Textbook of Geriatric Dentistry, Third Edition. Edited by Poul Holm-Pedersen, Angus W. G. Walls and Jonathan A. Ship.

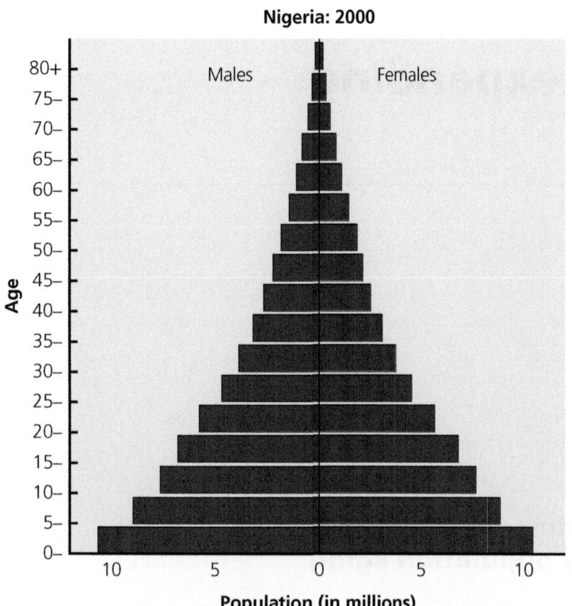

Figure 1.1 Age pyramid for humans in Nigeria in the year 2000. *Source:* United Nations, 2001.

of people surviving to each age range from an original birth cohort based on prevailing death rates. However, in an open population with migration and changing vital rates (which reflect the true nature of living conditions), the age pyramid reflects historical patterns of fertility, mortality and migration. The age pyramid is what characterized the human age distribution throughout most of our history, but this changed rapidly during the 20th century.

During the last 100 years a combination of events led to dramatic changes in the stable patterns of birth rates and death rates that had likely existed for thousands of years. Advances in public health led to the availability of clean water and refrigeration, sewage disposal and improved living and working environments. These developments combined with modern medicine to significantly reduce the transmission of, and death rate from, air- and water-borne infectious diseases. Within a single generation the environmental conditions that permitted the easy transmission of diseases that killed infants and children and women during childbirth were profoundly altered. From a biological perspective, modifications of this magnitude and importance suggest that fundamental changes in the forces of natural selection operating on the human species had occurred.

As the risk of death at younger ages declined rapidly, the high birth rates that were needed to replace the children who died from infectious diseases began to subside. Since the decline in birth rates lagged behind the decline in death rates, the result was rapid population growth during the 20th century – from one billion in 1900 to more than 6.5 billion by the turn of the 21st century. The eventual transformation of birth rates and death rates to the lower levels now observed in most developed nations is what set the stage for the demographic phenomenon of population aging.

When death rates declined at younger ages, the base of the age pyramid expanded and its apex became smaller by comparison. When the apex of an age pyramid decreases relative to its base, it may be said that a population is becoming younger. Thus, the first demographic consequence of declining early-age mortality was a younger population. However, within a single generation those saved from dying at younger ages began to reach middle and older ages, thereby altering the population's age composition by increasing the size of the middle and apex of the age pyramid relative to its base (see Figure 1.2). When death rates at younger ages stabilize at extremely low levels, as they have in all countries with high life expectancies, the base of the age pyramid then becomes sensitive only to changes in birth rates. With a stable base and a growing middle and apex, a permanent shift in the age structure occurrs from its historical pyramid shape to that of a square-like or rectilinear form. Although temporary increases in birth rates (like those observed in the post-World War II era) can slow population aging and even temporarily reverse it, the new rectilinear age structure will eventually reassert itself as the children from the larger birth cohorts survive to older ages. The transformation from stable high birth and death rates to stable low birth and death rates has led to permanent changes in the age structure of the human species.

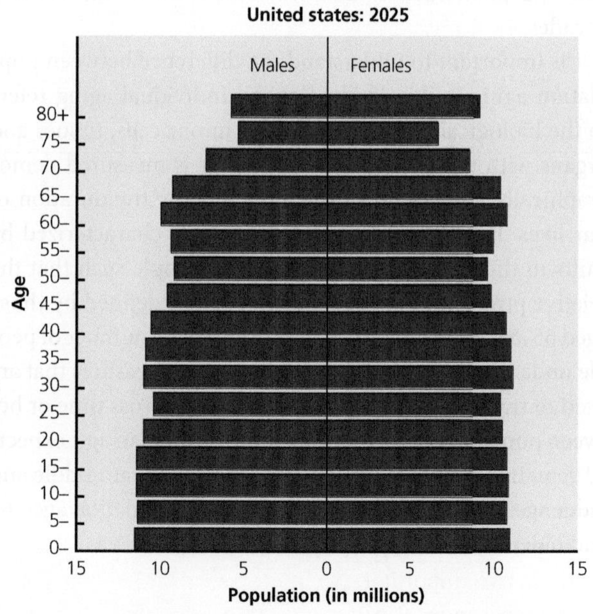

Figure 1.2 Age pyramid of the future with a shift in the historical pyramidal shape to that of a square-like or rectilinear form. *Source:* United Nations, 2001.

The social, economic and health implications associated with population aging are profound. Consider an ongoing debate in the health and demographic sciences known as the compression versus expansion of morbidity hypotheses. When death rates decline at younger ages the proportion of each birth cohort surviving past ages 65 and 85 increases rapidly. By way of example, in France the proportion of the female birth cohort of 1900 that was expected to survive to ages 65 and 85 based on death rates in that year was 39% and 3.5%, respectively. By comparison, the female birth cohort of 2000 is expected to have 90% and 50% survive past ages 65 and 85, respectively. These unprecedented patterns of survival into older ages are now common throughout the nations of the developed world, and they have led scientists to track the health of these aging pioneers and how prospective changes in death rates at older ages might influence the future health of the older population.

One school of thought argues for what has come to be known as the compression of morbidity hypothesis. With this hypothesis it is suggested that lifestyle changes and advances in medicine will continue to reduce the risk of death from fatal diseases and simultaneously lead to a postponement in the onset and age progression of the nonfatal disabling diseases. The premise of this theory is that there is a fixed biological limit to life towards which populations are headed, and as improved lifestyles successfully postpone the onset and expression of fatal diseases and nonfatal but highly disabling diseases and disorders, more people will be pushed towards their biological 'limit' to life, and morbidity and disability will be compressed into a shorter duration of time before death.

A second school of thought proposes what has come to be known as the expansion of morbidity hypothesis. The proponents of this hypothesis maintain that the forces influencing the onset and age progression of nonfatal diseases associated with senescence are mostly independent of the forces influencing the risk of death from fatal diseases. If death rates from fatal diseases continue to decline, it is hypothesized that the saved population will be exposed to a longer duration of time during which the nonfatal but highly disabling diseases and disorders of senescence have the opportunity to be expressed. In other words, the extension of life resulting from continued progress made against fatal diseases is hypothesized to eventually prolong the period of disability in old age among future cohorts of older persons.

A debate has taken place in the scientific literature regarding these two important hypotheses. Although the evidence suggests that in the 1980s several countries were experiencing an expansion of morbidity, since then there is evidence to suggest that some compression has been occurring. However, research in this area should be interpreted with caution because empirical studies addressed to this debate have focused on health transitions observed only during the recent past (since 1980). It is distinctly possible that future cohorts of older persons will be notably different in many ways from current older generations because of the high degree of selection that occurred among people living to older ages in today's world. Furthermore, it is not possible to know with any degree of certainty whether the health status of future cohorts of older persons will be better or worse than previous cohorts passing through the same ages.

Relationship between individual aging and population aging

The transformation of birth rates and death rates to currently stable low levels was caused, in part, by the same forces of declining mortality that contributed to unprecedented increases in life expectancy. During the Roman Empire life expectancy at birth was estimated to be about 28 years. By 1900 life expectancy for men and women combined had increased to 45 years in the nations with the lowest death rates at that time, but by the 21st century life expectancy at birth has risen to between 75 and 80 years. Most of the gains in life expectancy during the mortality revolution of the last century are a product of declining early age mortality, but notable reductions in middle and old age mortality have been observed in recent decades. In today's high life expectancy populations of North America, Western Europe, Scandinavia and Japan, death rates at younger ages have declined to such low levels that 98 out of every 100 babies born will live past the age of thirty.

As life expectancy continues to rise due to further expected reductions in middle and old-age mortality, survival into increasingly older regions of the lifespan by larger segments of the population is inevitable. Thus, life-extending technologies and lifestyle modification that bring forth declining death rates contribute to population aging by further expanding the apex of the age pyramid relative to its base. How much higher life expectancy can rise is a question of great interest and debate among scientists today, but one thing most can agree on for now is that population aging is an inevitable demographic phenomenon that will be accelerated by anticipated reductions in the risk of death.

Population aging and geriatric dentistry

In the last century the unprecedented aging of humanity has enabled modern populations to witness something that was rarely observed in the history of our species – old age and the diseases and disorders that accompany it, as well as the wisdom and benefits that accompany healthy survival into regions of the lifespan rarely experienced by our ancestors. At one level we have taxed our bodies to their limits, exposing our joints, muscles, bones, teeth and brains to decades more use than any previous human population. We have come to better understand the limitations of our bodies and how some components, such as neurons, muscle fibers and tooth enamel, do not replicate during the course of life. In a very important way, some components of our bodies that are critical to survival, such as muscles and neurons, represent limiting factors that will preclude a further dramatic extension of life unless it becomes possible to alter their rates of decline with age. However, we have also come to learn that there is no aging or death program for humans, which means that in many important ways it is possible to influence the way in which we age as individuals, and thus the degree to which individual aging influences population aging.

Dentistry will influence, and will be affected by, the demographic phenomenon of population aging and its antecedent causes in several ways. Population aging is defined, in part, by the extension of the lives of millions of people into their 8th, 9th and 10th decades of life who would ordinarily have never lived that long had they not been born in the modern era. As the extremely large baby boom cohorts of the post-World War II era move through the age structure and reach retirement ages, the unique health care needs of this population are going to challenge health care systems across the globe. The demand for geriatric dentistry will parallel the rising demand for all of the health care fields. It is also worth noting that younger generations might need less geriatric dentistry as they grow old since these birth cohorts were exposed to fluoridated water.

At one level, dentistry is unique in public health because it is known that, with sufficient preventive maintenance, it is possible to retain our teeth at a high level of functional performance for most of our lives. In other words, it may very well be possible that among most people, when properly maintained, teeth can outlast most other components of the human body. The same cannot be said for muscle mass and neurons, both of which are known to respond well to use, but which still experience significant functional declines no matter how hard we try to maintain them at younger ages. Furthermore, even with the loss of our natural teeth, it is possible to indefinitely maintain functionality with prosthetics. The same cannot be said for most other parts of the body.

Dentistry is also unique in its effect on population aging because primary prevention practiced in our early and middle ages can not only help to maintain oral health, such practices may also reduce the risk of a number of chronic fatal diseases throughout life – the most important among them is heart disease. Thus, the field of dentistry has the potential to reduce the risk of death at older ages, extend the duration of life, and thereby further accelerate the demographic phenomenon of population aging. However, geriatric dentistry in the 21st century will not be without its challenges. With many more people living into extreme old ages (e.g. beyond age 100) where only a small segment of the population used to survive, geriatric dentistry will face health issues associated with the systemic aging of other components of the body – most notable among them are bone density and immune surveillance.

Like many other public health fields, dentistry will be profoundly influenced by the demographic changes in the population that have already taken place and those that are forthcoming. It may very well be true that the health and aging of the entire body is visible through the lens of the mouth, so dentists have the ability to monitor the health status of their patients at a higher level of frequency than primary care physicians. Dentistry in the 21st century will maintain its position as a central component to public health and will no doubt further contribute to the extension of life and an anticipated acceleration in population aging.

Further reading

Dublin, L.I., Lotka A.J. & Spiegelman M. (1949) *Length of life: study of the life table.* Ronald Press, New York.

Finch, C.E. & Crimmins, E.M. (2004) Inflammatory Exposure and Historical Changes in Human Life-Spans, *Science*, **305**, 1736–1739.

Fries, J.F. (1989) The compression of morbidity: near or far? *The Milbank Quarterly*, **67**, 208–323.

Hayflick, L. (2000) The future of ageing. *Nature*, **408**, 267–269.

Himes, C. (2005) *Elderly Americans. Population Bulletin*. Population Reference Bureau, Washington, DC.

Kinsella, K. & Velkoff, V.A. (2001) *An Aging World: 2001*. US Census Bureau, Series P95/01-1, US Government Printing Office, Washington, DC.

Kirkwood, T.B.L. (1992) Comparative life-spans of species: Why do species have the life spans they do? *American Journal of Clinical Nutrition*, **55**, 1191S–1195S.

Kirkwood, T. & Finch, C. (2000) *Chance, Development and Ageing*. Oxford University Press, New York, NY.

Macdonell, W.R. (1913) On the expectation of life in ancient Rome, and in the provinces of Hispania and Lusitania, and Africa. *Biometrika*, **9**, 366–380.

Martin L.A. & Preston S.H. (eds) (1994) *Demography of Aging*. National Research Council, National Academy Press, Washington, DC.

McNeill, W.H. (1976) *Plagues and Peoples*. Anchor, Garden City.

Olshansky, S.J. & Ault, B. (1986) The fourth stage of the epidemiologic transition: the age of delayed degenerative diseases. *The Milbank Quarterly*, **64**, 355–391.

Olshansky, S.J., Carnes B. & Cassel C. (1993) The aging of the human species. *Scientific American*, **268**(4), 46–52.

Olshansky, S.J., Carnes, B.A. &, Butler, R. (2001) If Humans Were Built to Last. *Scientific American*, **284**(3), 50–55.

Omran, A. (1971) The Epidemiologic Transition: A Theory of the Epidemiology of Population Change. *Milbank Memorial Fund Quarterly*, **49**, 509–538.

Perls, T., Silver, M.H. & Lauerman, J.F. (2000) *Living to 100: Lessons in living to your maximum potential at any age*. Basic Books, New York, NY.

Rowe, J.W. & Kahn, R.L. (1987) Human aging: usual and successful. *Science*, **237**(4811), 143–149.

United Nations. (2001) *World population prospects: the 2000 revision*. United Nations, New York, NY.

Williams, G.C. (1957) Pleiotropy, natural selection and the evolution of senescence. *Evolution*, **11**, 398–411.

CHAPTER 2

Biological and physiological aspects of aging

João F. Passos and Thomas B.L. Kirkwood
Campus for Ageing and Vitality, Newcastle University, Institute for Ageing and Health, Newcastle University, Newcastle upon Tyne, UK

We are currently experiencing an unprecedented change in the age structure of our societies, as average life expectancy continues to increase at a staggering rate of 2 years every 10 years, which means 5 hours every day. In the developed world the fastest growing population group is the people over 80 years old. The world's population over 65 years old is currently growing at a rate of 2.4 per cent per year, which is actually faster than the global total population.

The increases in life expectancy, which began in the mid-1800s, can be explained by dramatic changes in the familial, social, economic and political organization of societies but more importantly by improvements in medicine and sanitation. These demographic changes represent a major challenge for both clinicians and scientists alike, since it becomes imperative to understand the nature of the aging process and how to deal with the medical problems of the increasing elderly population. Currently, we are beginning to understand why aging occurs and what molecular mechanisms are involved in the aging process.

The primary objective of this chapter is to elucidate the molecular mechanisms involved in the aging process and how these impact on organ physiology, in particular the oral environment.

What is aging and why does it occur?

Aging is a progressive generalized impairment of function resulting in a loss of adaptive response to stress and in a growing risk of age-associated disease. The overall sum of the changes occurring with aging increases the probability of dying within the population.

It was first noted by Gompertz (1825) that, in humans, cohort mortalities show an exponential rise with increasing chronological age [1].

Regardless of the specific mechanisms behind aging, there are three different views of its origins. One view is that aging simply occurs, and that natural selection has played no important part in its genesis. It is suggested that, like any man-made machine which inevitably decays and becomes dysfunctional with time, living organisms suffer age-dependent **wear and tear**.

Two other views propose that natural selection played a crucial role in the process. One comprises the so-called **adaptive theories** of aging, which state that aging has some sort of direct competitive advantage and that it is programmed in a similar way to development. There are several lines of evidence which show that these theories do not make sense from an evolutionary point of view. One of the main objections is that there is little evidence from natural populations that aging is a significant contributor to mortality in the wild. Data available from populations in the wild show that mortality in the early and middle periods of life is usually quite high, preventing many individuals from surviving long enough to experience aging. There are of course exceptions to the general rule, particularly in larger mammals, but it is well established that even in these cases the number of individuals reaching old age is very small. So, the argument that aging could have evolved to prevent old individuals from competing for resources with younger individuals does not stand on firm ground, as Figure 2.1 illustrates.

One of the other arguments that has been presented in support of programmed aging is that there is a clear heritable

Textbook of Geriatric Dentistry, Third Edition. Edited by Poul Holm-Pedersen, Angus W. G. Walls and Jonathan A. Ship.

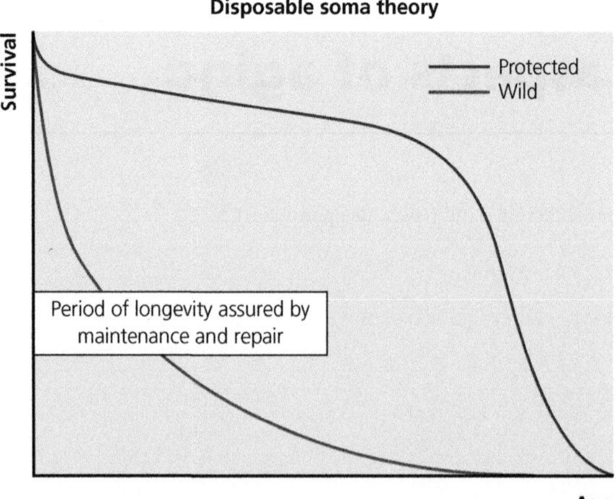

Figure 2.1 Evidence supporting the disposable soma theory of aging: the survival curve of a wild population tends to show little sign of age-associated mortality, which only becomes apparent when the population is in a protected environment.

component to human aging and also that in recent years large numbers of genes affecting longevity have been identified. For instance, in the nematode *Caenorhabditis elegans* several mutations have been identified that lead to substantial extension of the organism's lifespan [2]. However, it has also been argued that many of these genes are involved in pathways involved in resistance to stress and maintenance of these organisms. Moreover, even when the environment and genes are the same, individual nematodes show remarkable variation in terms of aging phenotypes and lifespan [3].

Another contrasting view suggests that aging is not adaptive and has evolved as an indirect consequence of natural selection. One widely accepted version of this view is the '**disposable soma theory**', which suggests that aging is a consequence of natural selection maximizing resources in maintenance of germ cells to the detriment of somatic cells, thereby allowing age-dependent damage of the latter. This view supports the idea that wear and tear does occur as we age, but that this is more a consequence of resource allocation rather than simple inevitable time-dependent decay. There is growing evidence that maintenance mechanisms fail with aging, as we shall discuss in the next section.

Aging of cells: molecular mechanisms of aging

We are now starting to understand why the decline in function associated with aging occurs. However, what the mechanisms involved are is not yet clear. Currently, several components within the cells have been identified which are particularly susceptible to 'wear and tear' and to the apparent failure of maintenance mechanisms within cells which occurs as we age.

We will now examine the various proposed molecular mechanisms which impact on the aging process.

Somatic mutation and DNA damage theories

The idea of aging being caused by a loss of ability to repair cellular components has been the basis of the concept that chromosomal abnormalities might underlie the aging process. This idea can be dated back to 1959, when Szilard postulated that lifespan might be determined by the rates of random chromosomal 'hits' which render 'all genes carried by that chromosome inactive'. He assumed that the rate of 'hits' would be constant throughout life and would lead to an age-dependent decrease in the number of functional cells. Although Szilard's notion of major chromosomal hits has not withstood detailed examination, it is reasonable to assume that processes that interfere with the integrity of somatic cell DNA will lead to a loss of function of cells.

The modifications to which DNA may be subjected can be of two types: mutations and damage. Mutations are any changes in the sequence of genomic DNA and can be of three sorts: **point mutations**, which occur when only a single DNA base pair is changed; **deletions**, which occur when DNA base pairs are deleted from the genome and **insertions**, which occur when sequences of DNA (often so-called 'transposable elements') move from one region of the genome into another. DNA damage, on the other hand, refers to any chemical alterations occurring in DNA which do not affect the polynucleotide sequence. These include pyrimidine dimers, single and double strand breaks, covalent cross-linking of DNA strands, oxidative modifications of certain nucleotides, and so on.

DNA damage is a common occurrence in mammalian cells. Measurements by various groups have indicated that in humans more than 10 000 oxidative modifications of DNA occur per cell per day [4]. If such damage remained unrepaired, one would expect that the cells would become non-functional in a very short period of time. Luckily for us, for each specific type of damage that can occur in DNA there is also an enzyme which is able to repair it. The repair ability of DNA differs between species and cell types. For instance, it has been shown that embryonic stem cells, which are undifferentiated cells able to divide without apparent limit, have better DNA repair capability than their differentiated daughters [5]. These differentiated daughter cells lose their capacity to regenerate indefinitely, mostly due to loss of telomerase activity, an enzyme able to elongate telomeres (see below).

Moreover, a correlation between lifespan of different species and the ability to repair DNA has been observed in various independent studies. In the first study made,

Hart and Setlow (1974) established primary fibroblast cultures from seven mammalian species and then irradiated them with ultraviolet light in order to generate DNA damage. Then, they measured the extent of DNA synthesis outside the S phase from the cell-cycle (unscheduled DNA synthesis), which depended on the incorporation of 3H-thymidine into DNA [6]. The results clearly showed a relationship between longevity and the extent of DNA repair. Other groups have subsequently confirmed an association between DNA repair capacity and longevity, although it must also be noted that differences in body size contribute part of this association.

Also striking, was the finding by Ames in 1994 that the extent of DNA damage products present in the urine of different species was directly proportional to the animals' oxygen consumption [7]. From these results it was concluded that oxidative damage could be a major cause of DNA damage. These results linked DNA damage to oxidative stress which we will discuss in the next section.

The oxidative stress theory of aging

With the exception of a few organisms which are adapted to live under anaerobic conditions, the majority of animals and plants require molecular oxygen in order to produce energy. Oxygen is, therefore, essential in the energy producing reactions which enable the subsistence of life as we know it. However, it is also known that exposure to higher concentrations of oxygen than the ones present in air, is toxic to animals and plants.

Different animal species consume oxygen differently and have different **respiratory quotients (RQ)**, which can be calculated as a ratio of CO_2 produced versus O_2 consumed. This quotient measures the inherent composition and utilization of carbohydrates, lipids and proteins as they are converted to energy and can be used as an indication of the metabolic rate.

In 1928 Raymond Pearl proposed that lifespan varies inversely with **basal metabolic rate** (the 'rate of living hypothesis') [8]. This was supported by the observation that animals appear to have a fixed quota of heartbeats. If the heart rate of a mouse was multiplied by its lifespan, a number would be obtained that is similar to most other mammals. This *metabolic* theory, together with others in the beginning of the 20th century, was based on the finding that an inverse relationship existed between lifespan and metabolic rate. However, no mechanistic interpretation was presented until almost 20 years later, to explain why this relation occurred.

Denham Harman was the first to associate **free radicals** with aging [9]. Free radicals are very reactive chemical species mostly derived from molecular oxygen, which have an impaired electron on the outer orbital. Previous work had shown that ionizing radiation could produce free radicals and that exposure to radiation limited lifespan. Harman established a connection between data showing that irradiation of living systems induces mutation, cancer and aging through production of free radicals and indirect data that free radicals are produced normally in living tissues.

Harman also reasoned that the most likely source of free radicals would be respiratory enzymes that utilize molecular oxygen (particularly those containing iron), the action of catalase on hydrogen peroxide and the splitting of water. However, no direct evidence at that time supported the existence of free radicals in living cells. Only 13 years later, with the discovery of a highly specialized enzyme able to convert superoxide anion in water and hydrogen peroxide (superoxide dismutase), was the importance of endogenous free radicals firmly established [10] and a role in the aging process reconsidered.

Have we acquired enough evidence to support Harman's idea? Are free radicals responsible for aging? Oxygen metabolism does lead to production of reactive oxygen species, but cells possess antioxidant defences able to eliminate them. So perhaps aging could be caused by a progressive failure in the defence system and not by pro-oxidant generation. Actually, two schools of thought exist, one that favours the rate of aging being dependent on the level of antioxidant defences and the other on the level of reactive oxygen species produced. Orr and Sohal (1994) reported the first direct evidence that increased levels of antioxidant enzymes, particularly cytosolic CuZn-superoxide dismutase (CuZn-SOD) and catalase, could together extend medium and maximum lifespan, confer greater resistance to ionizing radiation and oxidation of proteins and DNA in the fruitfly *Drosophila melanogaster*. An earlier study had already shown that *Drosophila* lacking cytosolic CuZn-SOD suffered a significant reduction of lifespan [11], supporting the importance of antioxidant defences in the aging process. There are many conflicting data concerning the way antioxidants affect lifespan. Several studies overexpressed CuZn-SOD and found no significant increase in lifespan in *Drosophila* [12, 13], while others showed lifespan extensions of 33 to 40% [14, 15]. However, recently, these latter experiments have been questioned, due to the fact that an insufficient number of control strains were used, and that controls had artificially short lifespans [16, 17]. More recently, a study was conducted where various combinations of antioxidant genes were overexpressed simultaneously in relatively long-lived *Drosophila* strains, a greater number of control strains was used, but no extension of lifespan was observed in any case [18]. This result can be seen as evidence against antioxidant defences being a limiting factor in aging, at least in lower organisms.

Studies in mice have also proved inconclusive. For instance, mice carrying a heterozygous deletion of the mitochondrial superoxide dismutase, an enzyme able to convert superoxide anion in water and hydrogen peroxide, showed indications of increased oxidative stress and high cancer incidence but not accelerated aging [19]. However, a recent study showed that targeting catalase (an antioxidant enzyme able to convert hydrogen peroxide into water) to mitochondria increased the lifespan of transgenic mice [20].

The role of mitochondria in aging

Mitochondria are the 'power houses' of aerobic eukaryotic cells and have also been implicated as having a role in the aging process. Mitochondria have two membranes: one which surrounds the entire organelle (the outer membrane) and an inner membrane possessing infoldings called cristae. Embedded in the inner membrane, mitochondria possess enzymes that together catalyse the oxidation of organic components by molecular oxygen (O_2). These oxidations are used to generate ATP, which is the major energy-carrying molecule in cells. Mitochondria produce more than 90% of the ATP that cells require for survival.

However, there is a price to pay for the utilization of oxygen and its reduction into water by electrons carried through the respiratory chain. Incomplete reduction of molecular oxygen can generate univalently reduced oxygen $O_2^{\cdot}$ or superoxide radicals, which can in turn be converted into other reactive oxygen species which damage the major cellular macromolecules such as proteins, lipids and carbohydrates.

In addition to energy production, mitochondria perform multiple functions which are essential for a cell, such as the maintenance of intracellular homeostasis of calcium ions (they act as calcium buffers). They also have a role in triggering programmed cell death (apoptosis).

Mitochondria possess their own DNA, and each mitochondrion contains several copies of this mtDNA, which is maternally inherited. MtDNA is a circular loop 16 569 base pairs long and encoding 13 proteins (which are subunits of the electron transport chain), 22 transfer RNAs and 2 ribosomal RNAs (which are necessary for protein synthesis within the mitochondria). Mutations have been shown to occur in mtDNA leading to several pathologies. Since there are several copies of mtDNA in each mitochondrion, a 'heteroplasmic' condition can exist when both mutant and wild-type mtDNA coexist in the same cell. However, a 'homoplasmic' condition exists when only wild-type or only mutant mtDNA exist in a cell. Mitochondrial pathology can occur when the level of mutant mtDNA exceeds a given threshold.

What happens to mitochondria with aging? As mentioned above, mitochondrial oxidative phosphorylation is the predominant source of energy in cells, but also the most important source of endogenous free radicals. This led to the concept that the close proximity between the sites of free radical production and mtDNA would render the latter more susceptible to damage than the nuclear genome and lead to defects in mitochondrial metabolism.

It has been reported that mtDNA mutations tend to increase with aging in several tissues of the mammalian body. Such results were first observed in post-mitotic cells such as neurons and muscle cells [21] but have since been described in highly proliferative cells such as the epithelial stem cells of the gut wall [22].

The role of mtDNA in aging is currently under intense debate. It has been found that homozygous knock-in mice expressing a proof-reading-deficient version of the nucleus-encoded catalytic subunit of mtDNA polymerase γ (PolgA) showed an extremely high level of mtDNA mutations and deletions and a significant decrease in lifespan [23]. However, even though mitochondrial function was affected, no evidence for increased oxidative stress was found in these animals [24, 25]. Most strikingly, mice that were heterozygous for PolgA function showed no significant reduction in lifespan despite a mtDNA mutation burden 30 times higher than in old wild-type animals [26]. These studies suggested that mtDNA mutation load does not limit lifespan of wild-type mice and that mtDNA mutations, even at very high levels, do not necessarily lead to increased mitochondrial ROS generation.

These data do not necessarily undermine the involvement of mitochondria in aging. Mitochondrial electron transport chain components are not solely encoded by mtDNA and about 3000 genes participate in the biogenesis of a single mitochondrion (only 1% of these are mtDNA encoded). Thus, it is possible that other factors contribute, together with mtDNA mutations, to failure of mitochondria with aging.

Cell renewal and the telomere loss theory

Another important aspect to take into account when studying cellular aging is the existence of two types of cells in an organism: those which are able to divide and those which cannot divide, the latter called post-mitotic.

As observed for instance in liver, which contains dividing cells, once a partial hepatectomy is conducted, the organ is able to regenerate itself and resume its normal size. The capacity for regeneration may play an important part in delaying the aging process, as dramatically seen in certain organisms such as *Hydra*, which appear to escape senescence by continuously regenerating their cells [27]. Weissman, a German zoologist who was the first to seriously address the problem of aging in the 19th century, obviously thought so and proposed that one of the reasons for aging would be that somatic cells had a finite lifespan [28]. This idea is now again a focus of intense interest in connection with the role played by stem cells in protection against tissue degeneration. A decline in adult stem cell function has been shown to occur during aging, likely contributing to the decline in organ homeostasis and regeneration with age.

However, most somatic cells (mitotic) do not possess the ability to regenerate indefinitely. As first observed by Hayflick and Moorfield, when fibroblasts are grown in culture they can undergo only a certain number of divisions before becoming irreversibly arrested [29]. Several mechanisms were proposed at the time to explain the phenomenon but none had greater impact than the one first proposed by Russian biologist Alexei Olovnikov. After learning about Hayflick and Moorfield's discovery in the late sixties, Olovnikov predicted that the progressive shortening of the ends of chromosomes (telomeres) might offer an explanation for finite cell division in cells grown in culture [30]. This is a striking example of scientific foresight, since it took more than 20 years to show experimentally that the amount of telomeric DNA declines with aging of human fibroblasts [31] and even more time to show that ectopic expression of the catalytic subunit of telomerase, an enzyme able to counteract telomere shortening, can lead to cell immortalization on its own [32].

Telomere shortening was proposed as a counting mechanism, which could explain two distinct observations: first, the inevitability of the 'Hayflick limit', and second, the fact that one could freeze cells at a certain population doubling (PD) and the cells would retain the memory of their PD and when thawed undergo the expected maximum number of divisions [33]. However, it has also been shown that oxidative stress impacts on telomere shortening and can accelerate the rate of aging of human fibroblasts grown in culture [34], and that alterations in mitochondrial function occurring with aging (including higher production of superoxide radical) could also impact on telomere maintenance [35]. Moreover, population studies have revealed that psychological stress, which is related with higher oxidative stress, could be responsible for the incidence of shorter telomere length in women [36]. This is again proof that the idea of a counting mechanism for telomere shortening only holds true if the influence of both intrinsic and extrinsic sources of stress is excluded.

What is the relevance of telomere shortening to aging? In various cross-sectional studies it has been found that short telomere length (in peripheral blood cells) is associated with an increased risk of various age-related diseases including myocardial infarction, atherosclerosis and Alzheimer's disease [37]. It has also been shown that telomerase-deficient mice, which have very short telomeres, cannot regenerate their liver after partial hepatectomy, suggesting that telomere length has a functional impact on organ regeneration [38]. The same appears to be true for stem cells. Mice with dysfunctional telomeres have decreased proliferation of intestinal stem cells and impaired self-renewal of haematopoietic stem cells, which can be overcome by depleting checkpoint gene p21/Cdkn1a [39].

In summary, several studies have clearly shown that telomeres have a role in stem cell function, organ regeneration and as sensors of stress and therefore play an important role in the aging process. A summary of the main molecular mechanisms involved in the aging process is presented in Figure 2.2.

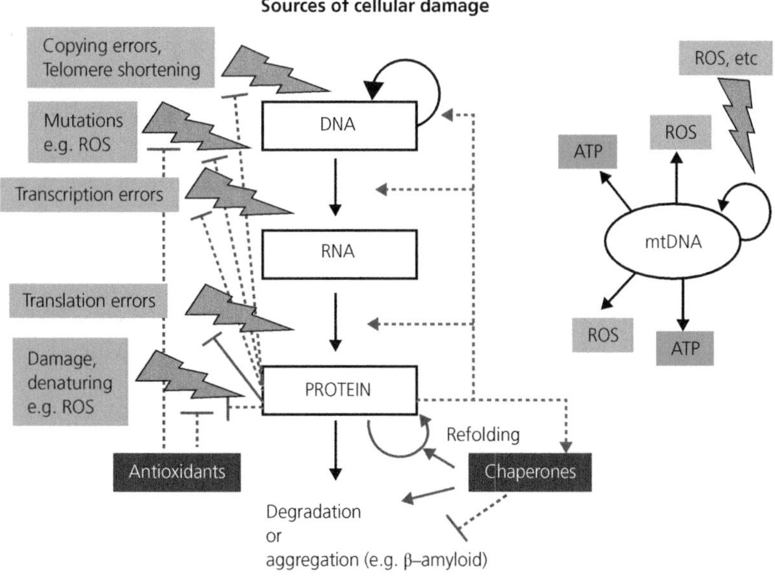

Figure 2.2 Various sources of cellular damage can lead to aging: DNA, RNA and proteins can be subjected to mutations, transcription (RNA) and translation (protein) errors and damage due to increasing reactive oxygen species (ROS) mostly produced by the mitochondria during the aging process. mtDNA can also be affected by the ROS produced by the mitochondria and affect mitochondrial function (including ATP production).

Aging of organ systems

We are now starting to understand the intrinsic processes that lead to the aging of cells, but what is the outcome in terms of tissues and organs? How does aging of cells contribute to organ failure? What major organs are affected with aging?

In the United States in 1900 the three major documented causes of death were respiratory, digestive and central nervous diseases. This had changed dramatically by 1986, when the major causes of reported deaths were cardiovascular complications, cancer and accidents [40]. So, during the 20th century the major causes of death had changed, indicating strongly that changes in the environment had a major impact.

Organ physiology and morphology alter considerably with age. It has been reported that the weight of various organs declines with age, as a consequence of cell loss. Moreover, the amount of fat in the body increases with age and the amount of water decreases. The molecular mechanisms that give rise to these changes are not completely understood. In the next section we will refer to changes occurring in the oral environment with age and also the impact of the immune system on the process. Moreover, we will try to relate these changes to specific molecular mechanisms occurring with aging.

Age-related changes occurring in the oral environment

The primary function of the digestive system is to transform food into a form that cells can use and to provide the uptake of nutrients and excretion of waste. The human mouth, or oral cavity, plays an important role in digestion by providing mechanical maceration of food by teeth. The oral environment also serves as a barrier against infection.

As we have already discussed, recent demographics indicate an unprecedented increase in the number of elderly people. Moreover, more than 66 per cent of older adults now retain their natural dentition, which differs from previous generations. Thus, it is essential to understand the mechanisms involved in the decay in the oral environment that occurs with aging and its consequences.

The teeth and oral mucosa

It is quite difficult to determine if changes occurring in teeth are actually a consequence of age, or a consequence of pathological conditions which can occur early in life and then become aggravated with age. Thus, one can define age-related changes in teeth as changes occurring only in functional, intact teeth from older individuals.

The teeth do change with time due to wear and tear, which leads to changes in the coloration and form of the teeth. The cementum becomes gradually thickened with age. Pulpal changes observed with age include a decrease in the number of cells and increase in the amount of fibrous tissue.

One of the most obvious features of aging is a reduction in size of the pulp chamber, caused by the continual secretion of dentinal matrix (physiological secondary dentinogenesis) by odontoblasts [41].

The specific molecular mechanisms behind tooth decay with aging are not yet known. One possibility is failure of the immune system with aging, to which we will refer later in this chapter. One of the problems occurring in older adults is root tooth decay, mainly due to recession of the gums, which makes the root of the teeth more exposed to bacteria.

Syndromes of accelerated aging have been associated with tooth decay. For instance, Hutchinson–Gilford progeria syndrome (HGPS), which is a rare genetic disorder resulting in phenotypes suggestive of accelerated aging, has been related to the onset of abnormal dentition. Progeria patients are unremarkable at birth, but by two years of age these patients start developing severe growth retardation which results in short stature, osteoporosis, poor muscle development and atrophy and a mean age of death at 12–15 years. The molecular mechanism causing HGPS is the loss of gene encoding for lamin A, which is part of the fibrous network underlying the nuclear envelope. Homozygous mice lacking lamin A show several of the phenotypes commonly observed in HGPS, including abnormal dentition, such as a gap between the two incisors and yellowed teeth [42].

Other mice models of accelerated aging, involving defects in both nuclear [43] and mitochondrial DNA [23], have been associated with loss of bone density and osteoporosis, which can also have an impact on dentition. So, it might be that various molecular mechanisms together contribute to failure of the processes which contribute to maintenance of dentition with age.

Another fundamental process which might influence tooth decay with age is related to age-dependent failure in the teeth's natural ability to regenerate their own damaged structures. It is now well known that teeth possess dental stem cells which are able to produce dentine-like hard structure after injury [44]. Changes in stem cell functionality could interfere with the ability of teeth to repair time-sustained damage.

Salivary glands and secretion

Another important feature of the oral environment is the ability to secrete saliva via the salivary glands. It was once claimed that changes in salivary flow rate are a normal feature of aging. If such claims were true, it would indeed pose an important health issue, since saliva plays an essential role in the maintenance of the oral environment. It helps lubrication, mucosal protection and soft tissue repair. It also contains antibacterial factors, such as imunoglobulins G and A, and has a role in digestion, remineralization of teeth and maintenance of pH. A decrease in the volume of saliva can lead to detrimental effects, such as impaired digestion of starch through salivary amylase and nutritional intake, difficulties in mastication, deglutition. Furthermore, a dry mouth could contribute to plaque.

The findings of impaired salivary flow with age have been questioned because of problems in the design of experiments in the earlier studies, which compared performance between healthy young individuals and older, debilitated individuals. If in fact, a comparison between healthy populations is conducted, no age-dependent significant changes are observed in terms of salivary flow [45]. Several cross-sectional and longitudinal studies have since supported these findings and it is now believed that salivary gland dysfunction is not a normal process of aging. However, it is believed that many of the systemic diseases, immunological disorders and also certain treatments and medications which are commonly used in geriatric populations have important effects on salivary flow.

There are data which suggest that once women reach menopause they can become vulnerable to a variety of oral problems, such as dysfunctional salivary glands, which lead to oral discomfort and burning mouth. However, different studies have obtained conflicting results and it is not known if menopause is an important factor in changes in the salivary gland function. Further information on the impact of aging on salivary flow and function can be found in Chapter 19.

In summary, the data seem to be consistent that it is not age *per se* that leads to these changes in the oral environment but external factors associated with it. One of these important external factors is the immune system which has been shown to play an important role in human aging.

Immunological changes with aging

Complex organisms are continuously prone to infection due to pathogens and parasites. As a consequence, vertebrates have evolved a defence system which is called the immune response. The consequences of failure in the immune system are well illustrated in patients suffering from AIDS, in which the human immunodeficiency virus (HIV) leads to complete depletion of an essential component of the immune system. Mortality in these patients is usually attributed to infection, such as pneumonia and prevalence of certain tumours, such as Karposi's carcinoma.

Changes in the immune system can have a major impact on the organism. Firstly it is known that infectious diseases represent the major cause of morbidity and mortality in older people [46]. These changes in the immune system can lead to detrimental effects in other organs (including the oral environment) and lead to various diseases associated with aging.

The immune response of vertebrates is able to distinguish foreign proteins from the proteins of the organism itself. This foreign material is recognized as possessing an antigen. Exposure to an antigen initiates production of an immune response that specifically recognizes the antigen and destroys it.

The immune response is comprised of two major lines of defence: one is the non-specific response (called the **innate immune response**) and the other is an acquired, specific response (called the **adaptive response**). The adaptive response is dependent on T and B lymphocytes. B cells mature in the bone marrow, while T cells mature in the thymus. The type of response mounted by the immune system is dependent on the nature of the antigen and is defined according to whether it is executed by B cells or T cells. B cells are part of the **humoral response**, which involves the secretion of antibodies. Antibodies are immunoglobulin proteins. The **cell-mediated response** is executed by T cells, whose main function is to recognize a target antigen by a specific receptor called a **T-cell receptor**.

The purpose of each type of immune response is to be able to counteract and eliminate a foreign target. In order to achieve this purpose the immune system has to be able to distinguish between what is 'self' and what is 'non-self'. If such a distinction cannot be made, then autoimmune disease can occur, in which the immune system attacks its own body. It was such a property that gave rise to one of the first immunological theories of aging; the idea that the loss of self-tolerance increases with aging, first proposed by Walford in 1969 [47].

Several lines of data support the idea that autoimmunity increases with age. It has been shown that there is an age-dependent increase in the percentage of T-cells binding to autologous antigens [48] and in the expression of autoreactive B-cells [49]. Another important mechanism in immunosenescence is a problem known as immune 'exhaustion'. The most obvious sign of immunosenescence is an increased susceptibility to infection, which is a major cause of death in the elderly.

Various studies have shown that T-cells can undergo a limited number of divisions and reach senescence. One of the mechanisms suggested for this arrest has been **telomere shortening**, which we already mentioned previously. Peripheral blood T-cells show high levels of telomerase after activation, however they decline quite rapidly in 10 PDs and are virtually undetectable at senescence [50].

The frequency of näive T-cells carrying receptors for a particular antigen is very low so that, in response to challenge, T-cell clones must rapidly undergo numerous rounds of cell division in order to produce sufficient cells to cope with the antigenic insult.

Under chronic stress (caused for instance by chronic diseases) this expansion can occur continuously and lead to immunosenescence, and this is thought to play an important role in the altered immune status in the elderly [51].

Conclusions

In this chapter we have reviewed the molecular mechanisms thought to be involved in the aging process and possible outcomes in terms of organ physiology. Concerning the oral environment, a myriad of studies has revealed changes in both teeth and salivary gland function and maintenance. Other factors, such as failure of the immune system and stem cell function, might also affect maintenance of the oral cavity.

The understanding of the specific molecular mechanisms involved in the aging process represents a major challenge to the scientific and medical community, in order to cope with the demands of an increasing elderly population.

References

1 Gompertz, B. (1825) On the nature and function expressive of the law of human mortality and on a new mode of determining life contingincies. *Philosophical Transactions of the Royal Society of London*, **115**, 513–585.

2 Kenyon, C. (2005) The Plasticity of Aging: Insights from Long-Lived Mutants. *Cell*, **120**(4), 449–460.

3 Kirkwood, T.B. & Finch, C.E. (2002) Ageing: the old worm turns more slowly. *Nature*, **419**(6909), 794–795.

4 Ames, B.N., Shigenaga, M.K. & Hagen, T.M. (1993) Oxidants, Antioxidants, and the Degenerative Diseases of Aging. *Proceedings of the National Academy of Sciences of the United States of America*, **90**(17), 7915–7922.

5 Saretzki, G., Walter, T., Atkinson, S., Passos, J.F., Bareth, B., Keith, W.N. *et al.* (2008) Down-Regulation of Multiple Stress Defence Mechanisms During Differentiation of Human Embryonic Stem Cells. *Stem Cells*, **26**(2), 455–464.

6 Hart, R.W. & Setlow, R.B. (1974) Correlation between deoxyribonucleic acid excision-repair and life-span in a number of mammalian species. *Proceedings of the National Academy of Sciences of the United States of America*, **74**(6), 2169–2173.

7 Ames, B.N. (1994) The assay of endogenous oxidative DNA damage as related to aging. In: A.K. Balin (ed), *Practical Handbook of Human Biologic Age Determination*, CRC Press, Boca Raton, FL, pp. 397–405.

8 Pearl, R. (1928) *The Rate of Living*. Alfred A. Knopf, New York, NY.

9 Harman, D. (1956) Aging: A theory based on free radical and radiation chemistry. *Journal of Gerontology*, **11**, 298–300.

10 McCord, J.M. & Fridovich, I. (1969) Superoxide dismutase. An enzymic function for erythrocuprein (hemocuprein). *Journal of Biological Chemistry*, **244**(22), 6049–6055.

11 Phillips, J.P., Campbell, S.D., Michaud, D., Charbonneau, M. & Hilliker, A.J. (1989) Null mutation of copper/zinc superoxide dismutase in Drosophila confers hypersensitivity to paraquat and reduced longevity. *Proceedings of the National Academy of Sciences of the United States of America*, **86**(8), 2761–2765.

12 Seto, N., Hayashi, S. & Tener, G. (1990) Overexpression of Cu-Zn Superoxide Dismutase in Drosophila Does not Affect Life-Span. *Proceedings of the National Academy of Sciences of the United States of America*, **87**(11), 4270–4274.

13 Reveillaud, I., Niedzwiecki, A., Bensch, K.G. & Fleming, J.E. (1991) Expression of bovine superoxide dismutase in Drosophila melanogaster augments resistance of oxidative stress. *Molecular Cell Biology*, **11**(2), 632–640.

14 Orr, W.C. & Sohal, R.S. (1994) Extension of life-span by overexpression of superoxide dismutase and catalase in Drosophila melanogaster. *Science*, **263**(5150), 1128–1130.

15 Parkes, T.L., Elia, A.J., Dickinson, D., Hilliker, A.J., Phillips, J.P. & Boulianne, G.L. (1998) Extension of Drosophila lifespan by overexpression of human SOD1 in motorneurons. *Nature Genetics*, **19**(2), 171–174.

16 Tower, J. (1996) Aging mechanisms in fruit files. *BioEssays*, **18**(10), 799–807.

17 Sohal, R.S., Mockett, R.J. & Orr, W.C. (2002) Mechanisms of aging: an appraisal of the oxidative stress hypothesis. *Free Radical Biology and Medicine*, **33**(5), 575–586.

18 Orr, W.C., Mockett, R.J., Benes, J.J. & Sohal, R.S. (2003) Effects of overexpression of copper-zinc and manganese superoxide dismutases, catalase, and thioredoxin reductase genes on longevity in Drosophila melanogaster. *Journal of Biological Chemistry*, **278**(29), 26418–26422.

19 Van Remmen, H., Ikeno, Y., Hamilton, M., Pahlavani, M., Wolf, N., Thorpe, S.R. *et al.* (2003) Life-long reduction in MnSOD activity results in increased DNA damage and higher incidence of cancer but does not accelerate aging. *Physiological Genomics*, **16**(1), 29–37.

20 Schriner, S.E., Linford, N.J., Martin, G.M., Treuting, P., Ogburn, C.E., Emond, M., *et al.* (2005) Extension of Murine Life Span by Overexpression of Catalase Targeted to Mitochondria. *Science*, **308**(5730), 1909–1911.

21 Cottrell, D.A. & Turnbull, D.M. (2000) Mitochondria and ageing. *Current Opinion in Clinical Nutrition and Metabolic Care*, **3**(6), 473–478.

22 Taylor, R.W., Barron, M.J., Borthwick, G.M., Gospel, A., Chinnery, P.F., Samuels, D.C. *et al.* (2003) Mitochondrial DNA mutations in human colonic crypt stem cells. *Journal of Clinical Investigation*, **112**(9), 1351–1360.

23 Trifunovic, A., Wredenberg, A., Falkenberg, M., Spelbrink, J.N., Rovio, A.T., Bruder, C.E. *et al.* (2004) Premature ageing in mice expressing defective mitochondrial DNA polymerase. *Nature*, **429**(6990), 417–423.

24 Kujoth, G.C., Hiona, A., Pugh, T.D., Someya, S., Panzer, K., Wohlgemuth, S.E. *et al.* (2005) Mitochondrial DNA Mutations,

Oxidative Stress, and Apoptosis in Mammalian Aging. *Science*, **309**(5733), 481–484.
25 Trifunovic, A., Hansson, A., Wredenberg, A., Rovio, A.T., Dufour, E., Khvorostov, I. *et al.* (2005) Somatic mtDNA mutations cause aging phenotypes without affecting reactive oxygen species production. *Proceedings of the National Academy of Sciences of the United States of America*, **102**(50), 17993–17998.
26 Vermulst, M., Bielas, J.H., Kujoth, G.C., Ladiges, W.C., Rabinovitch, P.S., Prolla, T.A. *et al.* (2007) Mitochondrial point mutations do not limit the natural lifespan of mice. *Nature Genetics*, **39**(4), 540–543.
27 Martinez, D.E. (1998) Mortality Patterns Suggest Lack of Senescence in Hydra. *Experimental Gerontology*, **33**(3), 217–225.
28 Kirkwood, T. & Cremer, T. (1982) Cytogerontology Since 1881: A Reappraisal of August Weissmann and a Review of Modern Progress. *Human Genetics*, **60**, 101–121.
29 Hayflick, L. & Moorhead, P.S. (1961) The serial cultivation of human diploid cell strains. *Experimental Cell Research*, **25**, 585–621.
30 Olovnikov, A.M. (1996) Telomeres, telomerase, and aging: Origin of the theory. *Experimental Gerontology*, **31**(4), 443–448.
31 Harley, C.B., Futcher, A.B. & Greider, C.W. (1990) Telomeres shorten during ageing of human fibroblasts. *Nature*, **345**(6274), 458–460.
32 Bodnar, A.G., Ouellette, M., Frolkis, M., Holt, S.E., Chiu, C.P., Morin, G.B. *et al.* (1998) Extension of life-span by introduction of telomerase into normal human cells. *Science*, **279**(5349), 349–352.
33 Hayflick, L. (2000) The illusion of cell immortality. *British Journal of Cancer*, **83**(7), 841–846.
34 von Zglinicki, T., Saretzki, G., Docke, W. & Lotze, C. (1995) Mild Hyperoxia Shortens Telomeres and Inhibits Proliferation of Fibroblasts: A Model for Senescence? *Experimental Cell Research*, **220**(1), 186–193.
35 Passos, J.F., Saretzki, G., Ahmed, S., Nelson, G., Richter, T., Peters, H. *et al.* (2007) Mitochondrial Dysfunction Accounts for the Stochastic Heterogeneity In Telomere-Dependent Senescence. *PLoS Biology*, **5**(5), e110.
36 Epel, E.S., Blackburn, E.H., Lin, J., Dhabhar, F.S., Adler, N.E., Morrow, J.D. *et al.* (2004) From the Cover: Accelerated telomere shortening in response to life stress. *Proceedings of the National Academy of Sciences of the United States of America*, **101**(49), 17312–17315.
37 von Zglinicki, T. & Martin-Ruiz, C.M. (2005) Telomeres as Biomarkers for Ageing and Age-Related Diseases. *Current Molecular Medicinei*, **5**, 197–203.
38 Satyanarayana, A., Wiemann, S.U., Buer, J., Lauber, J., Dittmar, K.E., Wüstefeld, T. *et al.* (2003) Telomere shortening impairs organ regeneration by inhibiting cell cycle re-entry of a subpopulation of cells. *EMBO Journal*, **22**(15), 4003–4013.
39 Choudhury, A.R., Ju, Z., Djojosubroto, M.W., Schienke, A., Lechel, A., Schaetzlein, S. *et al.* (2007) Cdkn1a deletion improves stem cell function and lifespan of mice with dysfunctional telomeres without accelerating cancer formation. *Nature Genetics*, **39**(1), 99–105.
40 Arking, R. (1998) *Biology of Aging*. Sinauer Associates, Inc., Sunderland, MA.
41 Solheim, T. (1992) Amount of secondary dentin as an indicator of age. *Scandinavian Journal of Dental Research*, **100**(4), 193–199.
42 Mounkes, L.C., Kozlov, S., Hernandez, L., Sullivan, T. & Stewart, C.L. (2003) A progeroid syndrome in mice is caused by defects in A-type lamins. *Nature*, **423**(6937), 298–301.
43 de Boer, J., Andressoo, J.O., de Wit, J., Huijmans, J., Beems, R.B., van Steeg, H. *et al.* (2002) Premature Aging in Mice Deficient in DNA Repair and Transcription. *Science*, **296**(5571), 1276–1279.
44 Yen, A. & Sharpe, P. (2008) Stem cells and tooth tissue engineering. *Cell and Tissue Research*, **331**, 359–372.
45 Baum, B.J. (1981) Evaluation of stimulated parotid saliva flow rate in different age groups. *Journal Dental Research*, **60**(7), 1292–1296.
46 Gee, W.M. (1993) Causes of death in a hospitalized geriatric population: an autopsy study of 3000 patients. *Virchows Archiv A: Pathological Anatomy and Histopathology*, **423**(5), 343–349.
47 Walford, R.L. (1969) *Immunologic Theory of Ageing*. Munksgaard, Copenhagen.
48 Charreire, J. & Bach, J.F. (1975) Binding of autologous erythrocytes to immature T-cells. *Proceedings of the National Academy of Sciences of the United States of America*, **72**(8), 3201–3205.
49 Goidl, E.A., Michelis, M.A., Siskind, G.W. & Weksler, M.E. (1981) Effect of age on the induction of autoantibodies. *Clinical and Experimental Immunology*, **44**(1), 24–30.
50 Bodnar, A.G., Kim, N.W., Effros, R.B. & Chiu, C.-P. (1996) Mechanism of Telomerase Induction during T Cell Activation. *Experimental Cell Research*, **228**(1), 58–64.
51 Mazzatti, D.J., White, A., Forsey, R.J., Powell, J.R. & Pawelec, G. (2007) Gene expression changes in long-term culture of T-cell clones: genomic effects of chronic antigenic stress in aging and immunosenescence. *Aging Cell*, **6**(2), 155–163.

CHAPTER 3
Aging of bone and muscle

Arnold Kahn[1,2] and Poul Holm-Pedersen[3]

[1]University of California San Francisco, San Francisco Coordinating Center, California Pacific Medical Center, San Francisco, CA, USA
[2]Buck Institute for Aging Research, Novato, CA, USA
[3]Copenhagen Gerontological Oral Health Research Center, Department of Odonotology, University of Copenhagen, Denmark

Summary

Among the inevitable consequences of aging in humans and probably all vertebrates are the loss of bone (osteopenia), bone mineral density (BMD) and muscle (sarcopenia). These tissue losses are accompanied by increased fragility and fracture risk in bone and a marked decline in contractile strength (e.g. in hand grip and walking speed) in muscle. Together, the senescent changes in these two tissues are among the important defining features of the phenotype of 'frailty'.

The loss of bone and muscle, however, is not a uniform process but shows substantial variation from individual to individual and from one anatomical region to another. For example, age-related osteopenia is more pronounced in bones of the lower extremities than those of the upper body and is less evident in calvaria than long bones. The loss of muscle follows a similar regional and individual-to-individual specificity. In the mandible, the most fully investigated component of the aging orofacial skeleton, bone loss does occur but often for reasons other than, or in addition to, senescent change; reasons that include edentulism, local infection, systemic disease (e.g. diabetes) and lifestyle factors like smoking. Similarly, sarcopenia in the masseter muscle, the major muscle defining bite-strength, does occur but the fundamental nature of the muscle, in terms of fiber type composition and innervation (trigeminal versus motor neurons of the spinal cord), differs from that found in skeletal muscle as does the pattern of tissue loss.

The degree and rate of musculoskeletal tissue decline can vary as a function of many different extrinsic and intrinsic factors including diet, disease, medications, hormone levels, clinical interventions and exercise. For bones of the dental arch, not only do they respond to changes in mechanical loading (occlusal force; force generated by orthodontic appliances) but also to periodontal disease and the loss of teeth. In general, and certainly in the absence of disease, regular exercise (notably in the postcranial skeleton) and resistance/weight training can significantly mitigate if not eliminate the age-related loss of bone and muscle tissue even, in the latter instance, in the very elderly.

Given the large number of potential and actual contributing factors that affect the aging musculoskeletal system, and the complex manner in which they interact, it is difficult to highlight individual 'factors' or physiological circumstances of special importance. However, there are several that arguably do merit particular attention. These are oestrogen deficiency, hypovitaminosis D and calcium deficiency and glucocorticoid excess. Oestrogen deficiency is the key hormonal change associated with menopause and is responsible for the rapid bone loss seen in postmenopausal women and perhaps also the primary osteopenia/osteoporosis that occurs in aging men. Low vitamin D levels and calcium deficiency are very common in the elderly and contribute both directly and indirectly (in part via parathyroid hormone; PTH) to bone loss and muscle weakness. Excess glucocorticoids are associated with Cushing's disease and much more frequently with their common use as therapeutic agents in a range of inflammatory and immune disorders. Among other things, glucocorticoids accelerate bone loss and increase muscle weakness. Fortunately, there are interventions that are effective in combating osteopenia. These include dietary supplementation with calcium and vitamin D, oestrogen replacement (used with caution for reasons related to potential increases in cancer and cardiovascular disease risk), bisphophonates (alendronate/Fosamax) and selective oestrogen receptor modulators or SERMs. SERMs, e.g. raloxifene,

Textbook of Geriatric Dentistry, Third Edition. Edited by Poul Holm-Pedersen, Angus W. G. Walls and Jonathan A. Ship.

are drugs that act like oestrogen on some tissues but block the action of the hormone on other tissues.

Bone loss in aging

Bone mass inevitably declines with age but the loss does not occur uniformly either with regard to anatomical location or rate. In general, bone mass peaks at ages in the mid-20s and begins to decline by the early or mid-30s. In women, there is an acceleration in bone loss associated with menopause that continues for about 5–7 years before returning to slower rates of decline. Men also lose bone with age but, in the absence of a relatively abrupt hormonal shift equating to menopause, the decline is generally more uniform and gradual, ultimately broadly resembling the pattern of osteopenia seen in women past the immediate postmenopausal period. What is important about the loss of bone is that it, along with increasing age, contributes significantly to the risk of fracture; fractures often accompanied by increased morbidity and mortality.

Defining osteopenia and osteoporosis

Fundamentally, osteopenia and osteoporosis are terms used to describe the loss of bone. In both cases, the 'gold' standard for determining and describing the degree of loss is dual X-ray absorptiometry or DXA (sometimes also abbreviated DEXA). DXA provides information on bone mineral density (BMD), most often in values (a T-score) that relate the density level of the patient to the mean BMD of individuals at age 25. Persons are described as osteopenic if they have a BMD 1 to 2.5 SD (standard deviations) below that of the younger control group; they are classified as osteoporotic if the deviation is greater than −2.5 SD. A person with low BMD and an existing bone fracture not related to trauma (a 'frailty' fracture) may be described as having 'severe' or 'established' osteoporosis.

Aside from DXA values, there are still other ways in which osteoporosis has been classified. *Primary* osteoporosis is a term used to describe a major loss of bone (BMD) (with or without a fracture) that is *not* the result of some disorder/disease or exogenous factor known to promote bone loss, e.g. glucocorticoid excess, alcoholism or diabetes. *Secondary* osteoporosis is the condition of major bone loss that *can* be attributed to a disease/disorder or exogenous factor. Finally, osteoporosis can be also be categorized with reference to age and, in the case of women, whether or not menopause has occurred. By these criteria, *Type I* or postmenopausal osteoporosis is the condition which is associated with postmenopausal women age 55–75. *Type II* or age-related ('senile') osteoporosis is found in both men and women older than age 70 and is characterized, in both sexes, by a slower rate of bone loss than that observed immediately after menopause. Based on the loss in bone density criteria (using DXA), the prevalence of women with *osteopenia* in United States was ~22 million in 2002 and is projected to reach >30 million by 2020. The numbers for *osteoporosis* are ~7.8 million and 10.5 million respectively.

Bone mineral density is not the only characteristic of bone that contributes to fracture risk; bone macro- and micro-architectural changes, micro-fractures and bone remodelling (particularly sites of resorption) also play important roles. Thus, another, more pathophysiologically appropriate way of thinking about bone relative to osteoporotic fracture is in terms of 'quality', a term that encompasses all of these factors, plus loss in BMD, that collectively contribute to establishing the relative risk of fracture (see Seeman and Delmas [1]). On this basis, osteoporosis would be a disorder characterized by compromised bone strength predisposing to an increased risk of fracture.

Bone remodelling

To understand those changes in bone structure and mechanical function that result in osteopenia and osteoporosis, it is first necessary to understand the fundamentals of bone remodelling. In the present context, remodelling refers to the turnover of bone that occurs throughout life that, unlike the modifications that take place in bone in response to changes in mechanical loading or force, *does not* affect the overall shape of bone. This kind of 'steady-state' remodelling activity involves the localized, coordinated interaction between the osteoblasts that synthesize new bone matrix and multinucleate osteoclasts that resorb or dissolve the matrix. Collectively, this focused ensemble of resorbing and forming activity is referred to as a 'bone multicellular unit'.

Ideally, the 'reciprocity' between formation and resorption is in approximate balance, so that there is little if any net change in the amount of bone. However, with advancing age and particularly in the absence of oestrogen (e.g. in postmenopausal or ovariectomized women) there is a shift in equilibrium such that resorption exceeds formation resulting, over time, in a significant loss of bone mass and trabecular structure, and an increased risk of fracture. Circumstances that increase bone loss, including environmental factors and certain diseases (e.g. smoking, diabetes, use of glucocorticoids) and naturally occurring events like menopause, ultimately act by altering the remodelling cycle in favour of osteoclast activity and bone loss.

Most interventions aimed at restoring balance and minimizing or reversing bone loss do so by diminishing osteoclast formation and resorptive activity, e.g. with bisphosphonates, oestrogen, or SERMs, reducing the rate of remodelling (high remodelling rates equating with increased bone fragility [2]), or stimulating osteoblast activity, e.g. PTH. As with many mediators of cellular function, target cells and tissues respond differently to PTH depending on the concentration at which it is used and its mode of delivery. In this instance, the hormone promotes bone formation at low concentration or when provided intermittently, and stimulates bone resorption at high concentrations.

Molecular mediators of remodelling

While it is beyond the scope of this chapter to provide detailed coverage of the molecular mediators of bone remodelling, in recent years there have been some remarkable advances in this area which merit attention. For example, osteoclast proliferation and differentiation are controlled, in part, by two effector substances produced by osteoblasts, bone lining cells and bone marrow stromal cells; RANKL (nuclear factor kappa B ligand) and M-CSF (macrophage-colony stimulating factor). M-CSF binds to its receptor on progenitor cells, c-fms, and promotes the expansion of the osteoclast progenitor pool; RANKL binds to its receptor (RANK) on the osteoclast precursor and initiates osteoclast differentiation. The bone lining (stromal) cells also produce osteoprotegerin (OPG) a negative regulator of osteoclast expansion and activity. This latter molecule, which is member of the tumour necrosis factor receptor family, serves as a decoy receptor for RANKL, meaning that one means of increasing resorptive activity is to diminish the synthesis of OPG thus allowing for increased RANKL and RANK interaction (Figure 3.1)[3].

If RANK, RANKL and OPG are fundamental in regulating osteoclast formation and function, it follows that other effector substances known to enhance bone resorption (e.g. cytokines, hormones) might also work by controlling these basic components (Figure 3.1). Thus, for example, prostaglandin E_2, a potent stimulator of resorptive activity, appears to act by both increasing RANKL expression in osteoblasts and stromal cells, and potentiating RANK signalling (and differentiation) in osteoclast precursors (Figure 3.1). Similarly, tumour necrosis factor (TNF-a) and interleukins 1 and 6 (IL-1; IL-6) stimulate bone resorption by increasing RANKL expression at the same time, somewhat surprisingly given their ability to curtail RANKL function, enhancing OPG expression as well. Finally, in postmenopausal or ovariectomized women, oestrogen deficiency appears to increase bone resorption and bone loss by allowing for increased synthesis of M-CSF and an array of resorption-stimulating cytokines including IL-1, IL-6 and TNF-a [4, 5].

Mineral metabolism and bone

Among the most important systemic factors influencing bone remodelling and bone health are vitamin D, calcium and PTH. These factors constitute the key components of a network of interactions involving a number of organs that ultimately form a complex feedback loop that controls circulating levels of calcium. In the process of controlling calcium levels, both bone formation and resorption can be affected. Thus, the most active form of vitamin D, 1,25-$(OH)_2$cholecalciferol (or calcitriol), is formed by the sequential addition, in the liver and kidney, of hydroxyl groups to the vitamin D precursor (7-dehydrocholesterol)

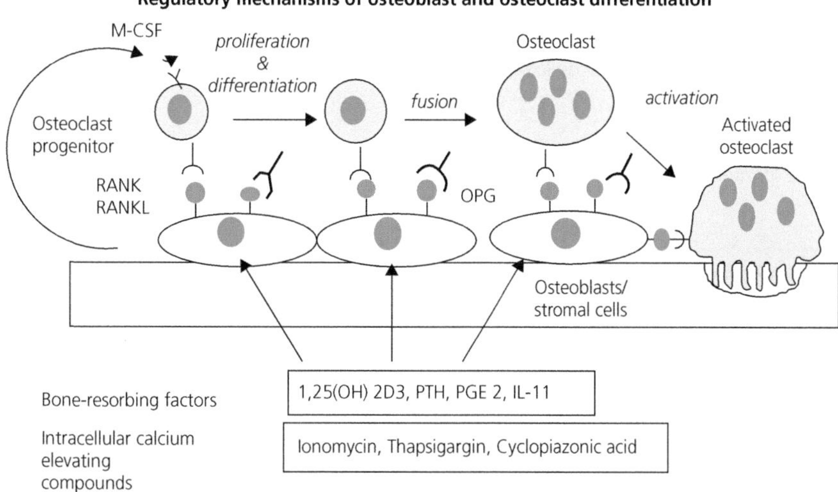

Figure 3.1 The regulation of osteoclast development and function by local and systemic regulatory molecules. *Source:* Katagiri and Takahashi, 2002 [3].

produced in skin. Cacitriol stimulates the absorption of dietary calcium in the small intestine resulting in increased circulating levels of calcium, thereby providing a mineral essential for bone growth and bone maintenance. However, under a number of circumstances including but not limited to low levels of vitamin D, vitamin D resistance and suboptimal levels of dietary calcium, serum calcium levels fall, triggering an increase in PTH production. PTH acts to increase blood calcium levels by decreasing calcium excretion, increasing calcitriol synthesis in the kidney and stimulating bone resorption. Recall that osteoporosis is ultimately the result of an imbalance between bone formation and bone resorption. Additional PTH further shifts the balance in the direction of bone loss (Figure 3.2). Vitamin D deficiency, especially with inadequate calcium, also increases the rate of remodelling; a change that contributes to increased bone fragility.

Hypovitaminosis D is common in the old whether such individuals still reside in the community or are living in an extended care facility. There are multiple possible reasons for this deficiency including inadequate dietary calcium intake, reduced biosynthesis of the vitamin D precursor 7-dehydrocholesterol and diminished synthesis of calcitriol in the kidney. These factors, plus the resultant secondary hyperparathyroidism, contribute to bone loss and fracture; problems made more acute in postmenopausal women where the oestrogen stimulation of gut calcium absorption is also reduced. This latter, oestrogen deficiency-related, reduction in calcium absorption further exacerbates the problem by creating circumstances (reduced serum calcium levels) that promote secondary hyperparathyroidism and bone loss [6].

It is very important to note that bone is not the only tissue that is affected by vitamin D deficiency. Many cell types and tissues express the vitamin D receptor indicating that multiple biological functions are likely to be altered in a vitamin D deficient or resistant state [7]. Among receptor-positive cells and tissues are nerve and muscle. It is not surprising, therefore, that severe vitamin D deficiency (osteomalacia) is characterized, in part, by skeletal pain and muscle weakness resulting in altered balance and difficulty in executing simple physical tasks (e.g. ascending stairs). Lower, subclinical levels of the deficiency also correlate with reduced muscle function, notably in the proximal lower limb and more broadly with neuromuscular deficits that may increase the likelihood of falling [7, 8]. The losses of muscle mass and strength (sarcopenia) in the elderly are discussed more fully later in this chapter.

Osteopenia and osteoporosis in men

Even though men do not experience menopause, they are subject to the osteopenia associated with aging, which, when it reaches a sufficient magnitude, results in osteoporosis. Using criteria similar to that developed for women, osteoporosis in men is defined as a reduction in BMD equal to −2.5 SD of the DXA value for healthy young men. On

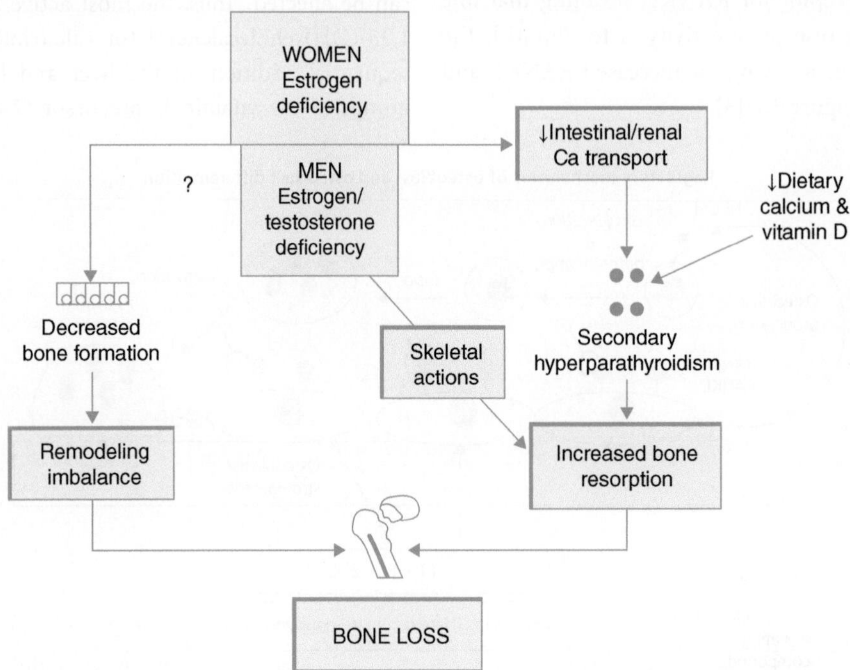

Figure 3.2 Additional PTH further shifts the balance in the direction of bone loss. *Source:* Bone Health and Osteoporosis. Reproduced from Office of the Surgeon General (US), 2004 [26].

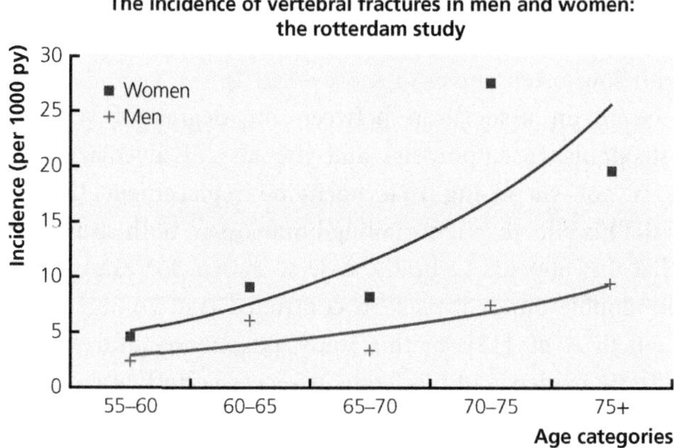

Figure 3.3 The incidence of vertebral fracture as a function of age in men and women. *Source:* Van Der Klift *et al.*, 2002 [27]. Reproduced with permission of John Wiley & Sons Ltd.

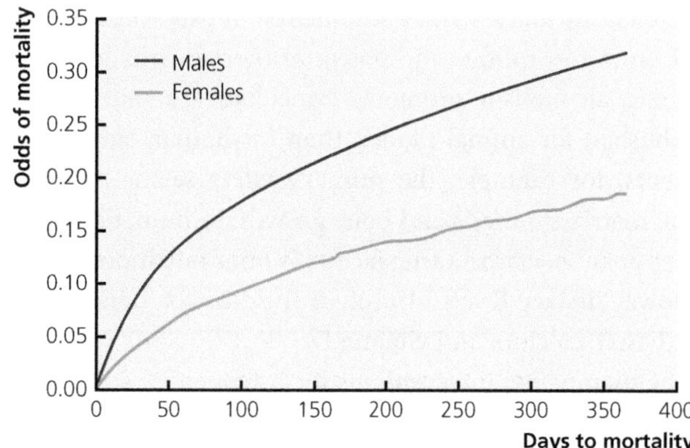

Figure 3.5 Twelve-month survival analysis for hip fracture patients by gender (age 65+). *Source:* Bass *et al.*, 2007 [29]. Reproduced with permission of Elsevier.

this basis and using lower levels of BMD loss to define osteopenia (−1 to -2.5 SD), the prevalence for osteoporosis in Caucasian and Asian men in the US, according to one study, is 6% and osteopenia 47%. These frequencies are less for African-American and Hispanic men; a distinction almost certainly due to the higher initial values in BMD in the latter groups. As with women, the age-related loss in BMD is associated with an increased risk of fracture with a conspicuous increase in occurrence observed about a decade later in men than women [9] (Figure 3.3).

This differential in the age of onset and lower incidence of fractures in men is related to the absence of menopause, differences in the type of bone lost (trabecular in men versus cortical in women) and greater initial peak bone mass.

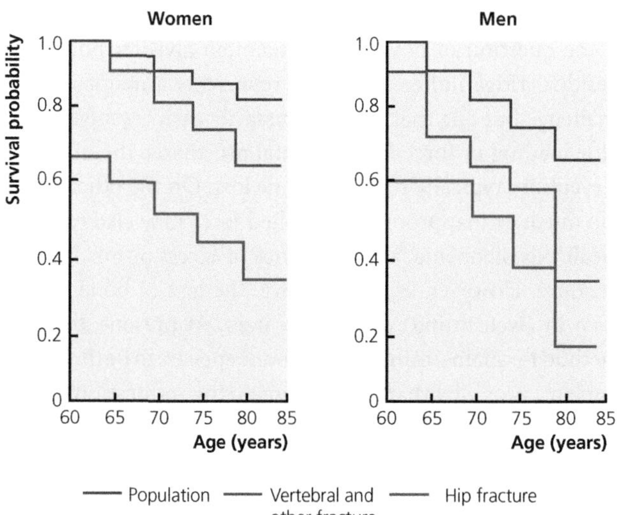

Figure 3.4 Cumulative survival probability after fracture. Survival is reduced after any type of fracture, vertebral or non-vertebral, more so in men than women. *Source:* Center *et al.*, 1999 [28]. Reproduced with permission of Elsevier.

However, the morbidity and mortality associated with hip fracture are substantially greater in men over 75 than in older, postmenopausal women (Figures 3.4 and 3.5). The reason for this difference has not been fully resolved but likely includes older age at time of fracture and any of a number of possible comorbidities, e.g. cancer, diabetes.

'Primary osteoporosis' is the diagnosis in approximately 50–60% of cases of major bone loss in men of advanced age. If it occurs in men younger than 65–70 years, it is usually attributed to factors unknown that are believed to act independently of, or in addition to, age (a circumstance also referred to as 'idiopathic osteoporosis'). While the pathophysiology of primary osteoporosis remains to be fully understood, it is likely that the decrease in sex steroid hormone production, higher levels of steroid hormone binding globulin and changes in hormone sensitivity play essential roles. Of interest, it is diminished oestrogen rather than testosterone that may be the critical factor. (Testosterone is converted to oestrogen by the enzyme aromatase.) Oestrogen acts to maintain if not increase osteoblast activity and to suppress osteoclast function, thereby favouring bone formation. In the absence of the oestrogen, the reverse would be true and resorption would dominate.

'Secondary osteoporosis' accounts for 40 to 50% of the cases of severe bone loss in men of all age. While a large number of possible causes have been identified, the three major etiologies for secondary osteoporosis are alcohol abuse, glucocorticoid excess (e.g. from Cushing's syndrome or chronic glucocorticoid therapy) and hypogonadism. The loss of bone due to hypogonadism is almost certainly related to low or absent levels of sex steroids, particularly oestrogen, needed to maintain bone forming activity and curtail excessive bone resorption. Excess glucocorticoid promotes osteopenia by suppressing sex steroid production (effectively creating a hypogonadal state), resulting in a suppression of osteoblast formation and a stimulation of osteoclastogenesis and bone resorption. The potential mechanisms by which chronic alcoholism promotes bone loss are much better established for animal models than for human subjects. In rodents, for example, the primary effect seems to be on bone matrix synthesis and bone growth. In humans, among other possible contributing factors is poor nutrition, leading to lower dietary levels of protein (needed for bone matrix synthesis), calcium and vitamin D.

The therapeutic interventions for osteopenic/osteoporotic men include, as for osteoporotic women, calcium and vitamin D supplementation, exercise and the use of bisphosphonates (e.g. alendronate and risedronate) or PTH as teripeptide (recombinant human PTH 1-34). The latter may be particularly useful in individuals at high risk of fracture (see Bonnick [9]).

Bone loss in the craniofacial skeleton

With the notable exceptions of the mandible and to a lesser extent the maxilla, age-related bone loss has been little studied in the craniofacial skeleton. The focus on the mandible and maxilla is understandable, given the prominence of these bones in mastication and facial appearance. However, because of edentulism and periodontal disease, two commonly encountered conditions that can independently cause bone loss, the mandible and maxilla have also proved to be complex situations in which to investigate the osteopenia associated with aging. Tooth loss results in localized bone loss, in part because it eliminates a source of mechanical loading (force) and perhaps stem cells and growth factors (in the periodontium) important in maintaining bone mass, particularly in the alveolar bone that surrounds the tooth roots. Periodontal disease has a similar consequence because as a bacterial infection it is a source of inflammatory cytokines (e.g. prostaglandin, interleukins) that stimulate osteoclastic activity and bone resorption.

Nonetheless, the consensus of most studies is that there is a naturally occurring, age-related loss of alveolar bone that occurs independently of edentulism and periodontal disease. Moreover, there appears to be a positive association between osteoporosis in the postcranial skeleton and the osteopenia that occurs in the alveolus [10]. Illustrative of the latter are the findings of Wactawski-Wende *et al.* [11] who compared the risk (odds ratio; OR) of loss of alveolar bone with the severity of loss in bone mineral density elsewhere in the body. The data show that the greater the systemic osteoporosis the higher the risk of alveolar bone loss. For example, after adjustment for various co-factors including age, weight, hormone use and education, the OR for alveolar crest bone loss for an osteoporotic woman (T score <-2.5) age 70 years or older is about 3.6. This compares to an OR value of '1' set for controls ('normal' women) with a T score >-1 or ~ 2.7 for women with 'low' osteoporosis (T score -1 to 2).

Given an association between the degree of systemic osteopenia (osteoporosis) and the loss of alveolar bone, it is not surprising that hormone replacement therapy (HRT) is effective in curtailing bone loss in both situations. That this appears to be the case is shown, for example, in the double-blinded, placebo controlled trial conducted by Civitelli *et al.* [12]. In this study, postmenopausal women with no evidence of moderate or severe periodontal disease were treated with conjugated oestrogen (alone or in combination with medroxyprogesterone) or given placebo, and followed for three years. Alveolar crest height and alveolar bone density were determined from bitewing radiographs; postcranial bone density from DEXA. The data showed that HRT increased alveolar bone mass and perhaps height in parallel with increases in postcranial bone density in the femur. Indeed, the increases occurring at one site correlated with those observed at the other.

As noted above, even though oral bone loss occurs for most individuals as part of the aging process, the loss of teeth remains a very important factor in determining the extent and location of oral osteopenia. In the worst-case scenario, tooth loss-related bone loss may be so extensive that it makes restoration of effective masticatory function extremely difficult. Following the loss of teeth, there is an accelerated resorption of residual alveolar bone that lasts for several months followed by a slower rate of localized ostepenia that may continue for many years, even in the presence of dentures. The loss in the mandible is about four times greater than that observed in the maxilla [13–15].

The question of how best to maintain alveolar bone (the 'residual ridge') after tooth loss represents a major clinical challenge but one that is not necessarily easily resolved. Too little loading or force from a dental prosthesis, the usual intervention, typically results in bone loss. On the other hand, too much or inappropriately applied force may also result in localized osteopenia, a consequence of excess or misdirected pressure. However, as noted above, the loss of bone occurs even in (well fitting) denture wearers. At present, the best method for maintaining alveolar bone appears to be the dental implant, provided that the accompanying restoration allows for balanced occlusal loading on mastication and that subsequent care controls periodontal disease at the implant site.

Sarcopenia

Muscle, like bone, undergoes marked, senescent changes with age. In addition to the loss in mass (sarcopenia), there is also a loss in strength; an important if not key component in the phenotype of 'frailty' seen in many elderly individuals and a major factor in the increased risk of falling and bone fracture observed in such individuals. The loss of muscle tissue in both men and women appears to begin in the third decade of life, and becomes clearly evident at the end of the fifth decade. When tracked as a function of whole body mass, the loss progresses in a curvilinear fashion after age 45–50 [16].

By this measure, at least, the rate of muscle loss accelerates with advancing years. In addition, although men at all ages have a larger muscle mass than women, they appear to lose muscle more rapidly than women. Relatively speaking, the muscles of the lower body experience more sarcopenia than those associated with the upper appendicular skeleton; a change that undoubtedly contributes to the losses observed in mobility and balance. An illustration of the age-related loss in major muscle mass in the lower leg (thigh) is shown in the CT image in Figure 3.6.

As a physiological and clinical outcome, it is the loss of strength rather than the sarcopenia, *per se*, that is most important, even though the two parameters of age-related muscle change are closely correlated. In general, by the seventh and eight decades of life, both men and women exhibit 20–40% less muscle strength than their younger counterparts; a loss that is even greater in the very elderly. The rates of loss, as calculated in longitudinal studies, appears to be in the range of 1–3% per year (10% per decade).

The age-related loss in skeletal muscle mass is a function of a reduction both in fiber size and number. In skeletal muscle, these changes primarily affect type II myofibers. Type II myofibers are the 'fast' responding muscle cells responsible for generating short bursts of contractile activity. In contrast, Type I myofibers, which are associated with sustained muscle contraction, increase as a proportion of the whole, at least in the vastus lateralis part of the quadriceps muscle [17]. A similar differential occurs in fiber area where it is the type II fiber that atrophies with age. Of interest, while type II fiber atrophy correlates strongly with the loss in muscle strength, changes 'upstream' of the myofiber are also occurring that contribute to fiber atrophy, e.g. loss of motor neurons and motor neuron innervation (neurons provide trophic hormones necessary to develop and maintain muscle myofibers), decreased physical activity, diminished caloric and protein intake and the reduced availability of certain hormones, including oestrogen growth hormone and IGF-1[17, 18]. It should be noted, however, that there are exceptions to the pattern of skeletal sarcopenia observed in the general population. For example, in male master runners (age range from 40–88 years), the declines in leg strength and change in muscle fiber type composition expected in the fifth or sixth decades of life are not observed until the eighth decade, indicating that chronic endurance training can delay significant changes in muscle structure and function. The same kind of exception holds true for master weight lifters when compared to healthy controls (age range, 40–87 years). Even though there is an age-related loss in muscle power and strength in both groups, lifters begin with greater strength and remain stronger over time [19].

Loss of cardiac and smooth muscle

As with skeletal muscle, cardiac muscle also undergoes changes with age and, in general, it is of a similar type. Cardiomyocytes are lost with age, albeit at a slower rate in women than men. There is also a lengthening of the

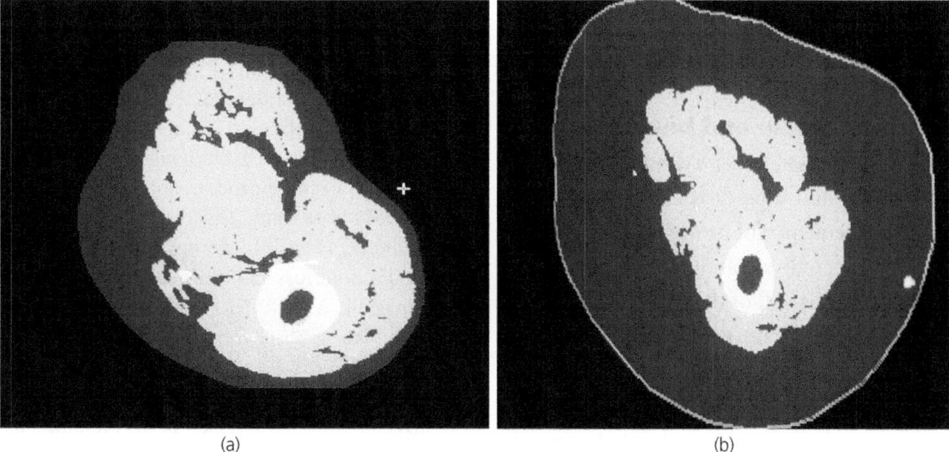

Figure 3.6 a) CT scan of a thigh muscle of a healthy young adult. The thigh bone is white. The muscle area (yellow) is not indicative of sarcopenia. http://www.ars.usda.gov/is/AR/archive/may05/. b) CT scan of a thigh muscle of a sedentary older adult. The thigh bone is white. The greatly reduced muscle area (yellow) indicates sarcopenia. *Source:* USDA Agricultural Research Magazine, May 2005 (53:5), p. 16.

contraction and relaxation cycle and a decline in cardiac power and reserve under conditions of stress [20]. The situation with smooth muscle is less clear, in part because it seems to have been less well studied. Age-related thickening (hypertrophy) of the smooth muscle layer in blood vessels and intestine has been reported along with increased muscle tone and changes in the collagen (increased cross-linking) and elastin components (reduced in amount and more fragmented) of the extracellular matrix. All of these changes contribute to increased vascular resistance. Interestingly, habitual aerobic exercise not only protects against senescent changes in skeletal muscle, it also does so for intestinal (smooth) and cardiac muscle, at least in mice [21].

Sarcopenia in the jaw musculature

It is difficult to directly compare age-related changes in jaw muscles with the changes observed elsewhere in the body. In large measure, this is because of the presence of myosin heavy chains (MyHCs) normally seen only in developing cardiomyocytes and, perhaps more important, the presence of hybrid fibers that contain more than one type of MyHC and exhibit intermediate contractile properties [22, 23]. Moreover, there are other structural differences. While the aging jaw musculature (e.g. the masseter), like muscles elsewhere in body, shows a reduction in the cross-sectional area, the pattern of fiber type change differs from that seen in typical skeletal muscle. Specifically, the loss in masticatory muscle is related to a decline in the proportion (and size) of type I fibers and a gain in the number of type II fibers; a pattern opposite to that seen in skeletal myofibers in the trunk and limbs. (The exception to this may be the digastric muscle that shows changes in fiber composition similar to that of other skeletal muscles [24]). Functionally, there are also changes. Jaw muscle contraction time is increased with age along with the latency period, and the number and amplitude of reflex responses is reduced [22, 23].

Immobilization and muscle and bone loss

One of the most easily demonstrated and dramatic situations that leads to both muscle and bone loss is immobilization. The latter can be the consequence of prolonged bed rest, exposure to zero gravity, of paralysis and the placement of a fractured limb in a plaster cast. All of these examples strongly emphasize the importance of 'use' (contraction, loading) in the maintenance of bone and muscle structure and function. They also suggest the possibility of a common mechanism or, if not, perhaps a cause-and-effect relationship between sarcopenia and osteopenia. If, for example, bone maintenance is dependent upon muscle contractile activity, then a diminution in the latter would result in a loss of bone. This kind of dependent relationship was suggested, for example, from the results of a study of the 'muscle-bone unit' during the pubertal growth spurt of boys and girls. Using a surrogate of muscle force, viz., lean body mass, the data showed that increases in the latter (muscle) precede increases in bone mineral content by several or more months [25].

References

1 Seeman, E. & Delmas, P.D. (2006) Bone quality – the material and structural basis of bone strength and fragility. *New England Journal of Medicine*, **354**, 2250–2261.

2 Heaney, R.P. (2007) Bone health. *American Journal of Clinical Nutrition*, **85**, 300S–303S.

3 Katagiri, T. & Takahashi, N. (2002) Regulatory mechanisms of osteoblast and osteoclast differentiation. *Oral Diseases*, **8**, 147–159.

4 Lerner, U.H. (2006) Inflammation-induced bone remodeling in periodontal disease and the influence of post-menopausal osteoporosis. *Journal of Dental Research*, **85**, 596–607.

5 Lerner, U.H. (2006) Bone remodeling in post-menopausal osteoporosis. *Journal of Dental Research*, **85**, 584–595.

6 Riggs, B.L. (2003) Role of the vitamin D-endocrine system in the pathophysiology of postmenopausal osteoporosis. *Journal of Cellular Biochemistry*, **88**, 209–215.

7 Campbell, P.M. & Allain, T.J. (2006) Muscle strength and vitamin D in older people. *Gerontology*, **52**, 335–338.

8 Allain, T.J. & Dhesi, J. (2003) Hypovitaminosis D in older adults. *Gerontology*, **49**, 273–278.

9 Bonnick, S.L. (2006) Osteoporosis in men and women. *Clinical Cornerstone*, **8**, 28–39.

10 Jeffcoat, M. (2005) The association between osteoporosis and oral bone loss. *Journal of Periodontology*, **76**(Suppl 11), 2125–2132.

11 Wactawski-Wende, J., Hausmann, E., Hovey, K., Trevisan, M., Grossi, S. & Genco, R.J. (2005) The association between osteoporosis and alveolar crestal height in postmenopausal women. *Journal of Periodontology*, **76**(Suppl 11), 2116–2124.

12 Civitelli, R., Pilgram, T.K., Dotson, M., Muckerman, J., Lewandowski, N., Amamento-Villareal, R., Yokoyama-Crothers, N., Kardaris, E.E., Hauser, J., Cohen, S. & Hildebolt, C.F. (2002) Alveolar and postcranial bone density in post-menopausal women receiving hormone/estrogen replacement therapy: a randomized, double-blind, placebo-controlled trial. *Archives of Internal Medicine*, **162**, 1409–1415.

13 Bodic, F., Hamel, L., Lerouxel, E., Baslé, M.F. & Chappard, D. (2005) Bone loss and teeth. *Joint, Bone, Spine*, **72**, 215–221.

14 Kingsmill, V.J. (1999) Post-extraction remodeling of the adult mandible. *Critical Reviews in Oral Biology & Medicine*, **10**, 384–404.

15 Wyatt, C.C. (1998) The effect of prosthodontic treatment on alveolar bone loss: a review of the literature. *Journal of Prosthetic Dentistry*, **80**, 362–366.

16 Janssen, I., Heymsfield, S.B., Wang, Z.M. & Ross, R. (2000) Skeletal muscle mass and distribution in 468 men and women aged 18-88 yr. *Journal of Applied Physiology*, **89**, 81–88.

17 Larsson, L., Grimby, G. & Karlsson, J. (1979) Muscle strength and speed of movement in relation to age and muscle morphology. *Journal of Applied Physiology*, **46**, 451–456.

18 Doherty, T.J. (2003) Invited review: Aging and sarcopenia. *Journal of Applied Physiology*, **95**, 1717–1727.

19 Pearson, S.J., Young, A., Macaluso, A., Devito, G., Nimmo, M.A., Cobbold, M. *et al.* (2002) Muscle function in elite master weightlifters. *Medicine & Science in Sports & Exercise*, **34**, 1199–1206.

20 Goldspink, D.F. (2005) Aging and activity: their effects on the functional reserve capacities of the heart and vascular smooth and skeletal muscles. *Ergonomics*, **48**, 1334–1351.

21 Rosa, E.F., Silva, A.C., Ihara, S.S., Mora, O.A., Aboulafia, J. & Nouailhetas, V.L. (2005) Habitual exercise program protects murine intestinal, skeletal, and cardiac muscles against aging. *Journal of Applied Physiology*, **99**, 1569–1575.

22 Korfage, J.A., Koolstra, J.H., Langenbach, G.E. & van Eijden, T.M. (2005) Fiber-type composition of the human jaw muscles – (part 1) origin and functional significance of fiber-type diversity. *Journal of Dental Research*, **84**, 774–783.

23 Korfage, J.A., Koolstra, J.H, Langenbach, G.E. & van Eijden, T.M. (2005) Fiber-type composition of the human jaw muscles – (part 2) role of hybrid fibers and factors responsible for inter-individual variation. *Journal of Dental Research*, **84**, 784–793.

24 Monemi, M., Thornell, L. & Eriksson, P. (1999) Diverse changes in fibre type composition of the human lateral pterygoid and digastrics muscles during aging. *Journal of the Neurological Sciences*, **171**, 38–48.

25 Rauch, F., Bailey, D.A., Baxter-Jones, A., Mirwald, R. & Faulkner, R. (2004) The 'muscle-bone unit' during pubertal growth spurt. *Bone*, **34**, 771–775.

26 Office of the Surgeon General (US). (2004) Diseases of Bone, In: *Bone Health and Osteoporosis: A Report of the Surgeon General*, Ch. 3, Office of the Surgeon General (US), Rockville, MD.

27 Van Der Klift, M., De Laet, C.E.D.H., Mccloskey, E.V., Hofman, A. & Pols, H.A.P. (2002), The Incidence of Vertebral Fractures in Men and Women: The Rotterdam Study. *Journal of Bone Mineral Research*, **17**, 1051–1056. doi: 10.1359/jbmr.2002.17.6.1051.

28 Center, J.R., Nguyen, T.V., Schneider, D., *et al.* (1999) Mortality after all major types of osteoporotic fracture in men and women: an observational study. *Lancet*, **353**, 878–882.

29 Bass, E., French, D.D., Bradham, D.D. & Rubenstein, L. Z. (2007). Risk-Adjusted Mortality Rates in Elderly Veterans with Hip Fractures. *Annals of Epidemiology*, **17**, 514–519.

CHAPTER 4

Sensory changes and communication in the practitioner–aged patient relationship

Kevin Kawamoto[1] **and H. Asuman Kiyak**[†2]
[1]School of Communications, College of Social Sciences, University of Hawai'i at Manoa, Honolulu, Hawaii USA
[2]School of Dentistry, Institute on Aging, University of Washington, WA, USA

This chapter aims to help dental professionals adapt their communication styles to meet the needs of a growing older population that is experiencing *normal* changes in its sensory and cognitive abilities, as well as elders who are coping with Alzheimer's disease and other dementias. Therefore we will focus on age-related and pathological changes in the communication senses – vision and hearing – that affect older adults' ability to communicate effectively with the dental practitioner. Normal aging also affects memory and learning skills, which can compound the impact of declining vision and hearing. Elders with dementia experience even more problems in the clinical setting. Following a discussion of these changes and their implications for enhancing patient–provider communication, we will address age-related changes in sensory functions that affect the oral environment – taste, smell, and proprioception. We will also consider the implications of these issues for managing older dental patients with significant impairments in these areas. It is also imperative for dentists and hygienists to become sensitized to the cultural and historical factors that influence the oral health habits and dental beliefs of the current cohort of older adults, practices and beliefs that are often inconsistent with new scientific evidence. This is especially true for older adults with an irregular dental care history.

How important is it to understand communication processes in dentistry? More precisely, how important is it to practise good communication skills with older adults? Any dentist who has spent hours explaining a treatment procedure and its risks and alternatives to an 80-year-old patient, only to have the patient return two weeks later and ask what the dentist is planning to do to him or her, and why; or worse yet, to return after the procedure has been completed and complain that it was more painful and costly than he or she expected, knows that failures in communication often occur with older patients. We can conclude that communication problems have occurred in this case. But is this a problem with the sender, the receiver or the message? Furthermore, are there situational demands on the clinician and the patient that impede the effective transmission of the message and its understanding and acceptance by the patient?

[†]Author is deceased.

The importance of dental communication

Successful communication strategies can significantly improve the likelihood of obtaining a thorough and accurate medical and dental history and allow the dental practitioner to provide the most appropriate treatment in accordance with the patient's needs and wants and personal resources. Effective communication can also prevent errors in the patient's comprehension of home care and future dental needs. With the increased emphasis on preventive dentistry today, dental professionals are increasingly aware of the importance of establishing rapport with patients and understanding what motivates them to maintain good home care, to seek regular preventive appointments, and to avoid emergency visits to the dental office. Indeed, it is becoming more and more evident that the successful dental provider today is not necessarily the one who is most technically competent, since most patients cannot judge such skills, but the one who has good communication skills and can establish rapport with patients. If the dentist does not perceive a message

Textbook of Geriatric Dentistry, Third Edition. Edited by Poul Holm-Pedersen, Angus W. G. Walls and Jonathan A. Ship.

of distress from the patient, the patient may experience mistrust and anger toward the dentist, and may even avoid further treatment by this dentist. This may be a particular problem with some older patients who grew up in an era of deference to the health care provider and who are reluctant to express their concerns or any distress, for fear of sounding 'ungrateful' or 'critical'. Other elderly patients are unable to articulate their concerns and dental problems because of sensory or cognitive decline, especially those with dementia.

Elements of communication

Communication is the process of transmitting, perceiving and interpreting information through verbal and nonverbal channels. Both the sender and receiver of a particular message must possess certain skills, including verbal skills in expressing oneself with the correct semantic and symbolic language, and the corresponding ability to perceive and correctly interpret the semantics and nuances of a given message. The receiver must also possess reasonably intact auditory and visual receptors to receive the message, as well as adequate cognitive capability to interpret the direct and indirect meanings of the incoming message.

Theories of interpersonal communication can help dental professionals develop effective communication strategies when interacting with older patients. As the name implies, interpersonal communication refers to the process between at least two individuals. Conventional theories of interpersonal communication are usually predicated on a model that illustrates:

1 the encoding and sending of a message;
2 the receiving and decoding of a message;
3 the potential for 'noise' to distort the intended message between sender and receiver;
4 feedback, the verbal or nonverbal response to a message that can alert the sender to

whether the message was received as intended (see Figure 4.1).

This representation of the interpersonal communication process, based on the information transmission model of communication by Shannon and Weaver, has been refined over the years by communication scholars. It is presented

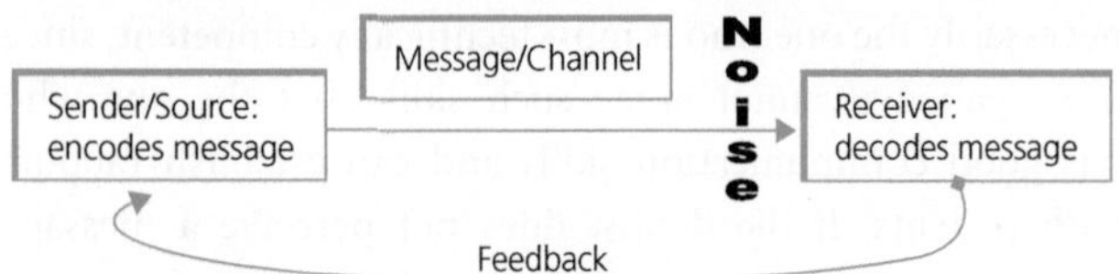

Figure 4.1 Basic model of interpersonal communication. Based on the Shannon–Weaver model of information transmission, 1949.

here because of its simplicity and ease of applicability to a wide range of communication situations.

The goal of effective communication is to ensure that the sender's message reaches the receiver and is decoded properly (i.e. that the message received is what the sender intended). However, many things can interfere with that message being received and decoded properly, or being received at all. These barriers to effective communication are referred to as 'noise'. In the broader sense, noise is anything that interferes with a message getting across from the sender to receiver. It could be a disability, such as the receiver being hard of hearing and thus missing part of the spoken message. It could also be because the receiver is suffering from so much stress and anxiety that s/he is unable to concentrate on the message; or that the sender is inarticulate, so his/her spoken words cannot be clearly understood; or that the receiver is not familiar with the cultural nuances and communication patterns of the sender and is unable to 'read between the lines', decipher metaphors or interpret idiomatic expressions. Noise can also be environmental, such as a room that is too cold, too 'busy' or overstimulating. Distracting, unpleasant or unwanted sounds - such as a loud conversation in an adjacent operatory - can interfere with the clear transmission of a message, especially for patients who have difficulty concentrating. In the following section, we will consider the role of declining vision, hearing, learning and memory skills on creating such noise.

Sensory changes with aging

A significant barrier to successful communication with older patients is the normal, age-related decline in sensory processes. Probably in no other area of gerontology is the clinical and research evidence so conclusive. As we get older, we cannot see, hear, touch, taste or smell as well as we did when we were young. The decline in most sensory modalities starts relatively early. We reach our optimum capacities in our 20s, maintain this peak for a few years and gradually decline. The rate of decline varies among the senses and among individuals. For example, visual accommodation declines for most people after age 45, whereas olfactory function is often maintained into the 70s. Because these changes are gradual, we adapt and use compensatory mechanisms as each sensory mode declines. We rely on other, still-intact systems, stand closer to people and objects we want to hear or see, use nonverbal cues such as touch and different body orientations and use bifocals and hearing aids. However, internal and external compensatory mechanisms are more difficult if the decline in any one system is severe or if multiple sensory channels deteriorate concurrently. Over time, decrements in the primary senses of vision and hearing can impair communication so drastically that they affect an older person's social life. Specific changes with age in the visual and auditory systems are described in this section, followed by several recommendations for improving communication with older people who are experiencing significant declines in these senses.

Changes in visual function

Most age-related changes in vision that affect the day-to-day functioning of the older person are attributable to structural changes in the cornea, lens and rods and cones in the retina. However, these changes are aggravated by alterations in the central nervous system that block the neurotransmission of stimuli from the sensory organs. Changes in the visual pathways of the brain and the visual cortex may be responsible for the observed age-related decline in visual sensation and perception.

Accommodation, or the ability to focus from near to far, declines with age. In fact, we begin to experience this problem in the middle years. Many adults start using prescription lenses for the first time at ages 45–55 specifically for reading and close-up work. Others must adjust to bifocals or new forms of transition lenses and contact lenses. Furthermore, because of differential rates of hardening in different parts of the lens, there is uneven refraction of the light that reaches the lens. This results in a serious problem of glare for many older people, especially in settings with uneven distribution of light (for example, the dental light or a large window facing the dental chair) or the glare from glossy surfaces such as highly polished floors.

Another age-related change in the lens that affects visual functioning is its increased opacity. The lenses of a young child's eyes are quite transparent. With aging, they become more opaque, so that less light reaches the retina. In extreme cases, one or both lenses may become so opaque that no light can reach the retina, producing the condition of *cataracts* (this is *not* a normal change with aging but it is the leading cause of blindness worldwide and results in the most common type of surgery performed on older adults). In most older people, however, the opacity is significant enough to produce functional problems at low light levels but not severe enough to be labeled a cataract. Problems with low light vision increase linearly from age 30 to 70. Older people may need up to three times as much light as do younger people to function effectively in their environment.

Colour, depth and distance perception also deteriorate with aging. Because of increasing yellowing of the lens, combined with changes in visual and neural pathways, older adults have more difficulty with colour discrimination, particularly in the blue–green end of the colour spectrum. These two colours tend to fade and become gray. Boundaries become blurred and contours are dimmed when colours in a similar wavelength range are used together. With respect to depth and distance perception, the loss of convergence of images formed in the two eyes results in a rapid decline in the ability to judge distances and depths after age 75. This is particularly true in low light situations and in the absence of orienting cues, such as stairs with no colour distinctions at the edge or ramps with varying slopes.

Another age-related change in visual function is difficulty adapting from light to dark. This is due to the diminished supply of oxygen to the retina and slower shifts from rods to cones, the cells in the retina that are responsible for scotopia (night vision) and photopia (day vision), respectively. Older people require more time to adjust from a brightly lit setting to a dimly lit one, such as entering a dental office directly from the outside.

Some older adults experience diseases of the eye such as age-related macular degeneration (AMD), glaucoma and cataracts. These conditions can significantly impair the older person's ability to accomplish activities of daily living, increase the risk of falls and fractures, and result in isolation if the older person feels anxious about leaving the safe confines of their familiar home environment. These diseases are not common but increase with age. In fact, when all types of visual impairments are considered, their prevalence increases from 55 per 1000 people at age 55–64, to 225 per 1000 among those 85 and older.

Changes in auditory function

Although vision is important for negotiating the physical environment, hearing is vital for communication. Because hearing is closely associated with speech, its loss disrupts a person's understanding of others and even the recognition of one's own speech. An older person who is experiencing hearing loss learns to make changes in behaviour and social interactions, so as to reduce the detrimental social impact of hearing loss. Unlike younger persons who are hearing-impaired from birth or early childhood, an older person who gradually loses hearing acuity in late life rarely learns sign language to compensate for this loss.

The most common cause of auditory deficiencies in old age is *presbycusis* or progressive bilateral sensorineural loss of the ability to hear high-frequency and low-volume sounds. Unlike vision, which can deteriorate more rapidly in one eye than the other, hearing loss generally occurs in both ears at the same time but not necessarily to the same extent. The ability to hear high frequency sounds declines linearly from age 20 to 70 and accelerates over time, such that about one-quarter of adults 65–74 are estimated to have some loss of hearing, increasing to more than one-third of those over 75 and half of those 85 and older. Even mild presbycusis can cause problems with comprehending speech, which occurs between 300 to 2000 Hz. In particular, they may have difficulty in distinguishing among the sibilants, high frequency consonant phonemes such as *s, f, sh, t, th, k,* and *p*.

Tinnitus is another problem that can impair hearing in old age. This is a high-pitched ringing in one or both ears that is particularly acute at night or in quiet surroundings. The incidence increases from 3% for young adults to 9% for middle-aged people and 11% among those age 65–74. Individuals who have been exposed to high-volume and high-frequency noise throughout their lives (e.g. city dwellers and factory workers) are at greater risk of tinnitus than those from rural, low-noise environments. Women generally experience less tinnitus or presbycusis than men. Tinnitus cannot be cured but people suffering from it can generally learn to manage it or try alternative treatments such as acupuncture.

To some extent, the older person with a high-frequency hearing loss may compensate for this problem by raising the volume of the information to be heard; this is the principle behind hearing aid design. One of the difficulties with this approach, however, is the concomitant increase in the volume of background noise. Another compensatory mechanism is to isolate the stimulus from background noise or at least to eliminate it as much as possible. This would be particularly useful in the dental office, where background noise can be extremely disruptive for the aged patient.

Memory and learning in old age

Learning and memory are two cognitive processes that must be considered together. That is, learning is assumed to have occurred when an individual is able to accurately retrieve information from his or her memory store. Conversely, if an individual cannot retrieve information from memory, it is assumed that the learning process has been inadequate. Thus, learning is the process by which new information (verbal or nonverbal) or skills are *encoded* or put into one's memory. Memory is the process of retrieving or recalling the information that was *stored* in the past. Although several types of memory have been identified, communication problems often occur because of changes in *primary* (or *working*) *memory* and *secondary* (or *long-term*) *memory*. Primary (also referred to as short-term or working) memory is a temporary stage of holding, processing and organizing information. Working memory is critical for our ability to process new information. We all experience situations where we hear or read a bit of information such as a phone number or someone's name; we use that name or number immediately, then forget it. In fact, most adults can recall 7 ± 2 pieces of information (e.g. digits, letters, words) for 60 seconds or less. In order for information to be stored in our secondary or long-term memory, it must first be rehearsed or 'processed' actively. This is why primary memory is often described as a form of 'working memory' that decides what information should be attended to and what can be ignored. This new material is generally lost if there is no opportunity to rehearse it, or we are distracted while trying to retain it for the 60 seconds that it lasts in primary memory.

Aging has little impact on the storage capacity of primary memory, but the encoding process which occurs in primary memory declines. This requires some organization or elaboration of the information received. Older adults are less likely than young people to process information in this manner. Indeed, some researchers argue that aging leads to a decline in 'attentional resources' or mental energy to organize and elaborate newly acquired information in order to retain it in secondary memory. Once the information is processed, the individual cannot transfer it rapidly to secondary memory. As a result, when more new information enters the system, there is interference from the previous material that is still incompletely processed. This is especially true when the two sets of information differ only slightly; one example related to oral hygiene is the case where brushing instructions given by a hygienist today may differ slightly but in a significant manner from that given earlier by another hygienist. *Perceptual noise* is a related phenomenon that may explain the greater distractibility of older adults. In this case, the older person cannot suppress information in secondary memory (i.e. previous oral hygiene techniques) that interferes with learning another task (new oral hygiene procedures being taught by the hygienist).

Perceptual speed is the time required to recognize a stimulus and respond to it; this also declines with aging, primarily because of slower reaction time and sensory processing ability. Accordingly, older people have more problems holding information in their working memory while receiving new stimuli through sensory memory (known as 'simultaneity'). This is compounded by the possibility that it takes more effort for older people to ignore irrelevant stimuli and complete the primary to secondary memory transfer. For this reason, older people need a slower pace of instruction and more time to process information before further material is presented.

Secondary memory is the part of our memory store where we retain everything we have learned throughout our lives; unlike primary memory, it has an unlimited capacity.

However, older people need more time to transfer new information to secondary memory as well as a more relaxed environment for learning. Unfortunately, the dental environment often does not provide such an opportunity. Time constraints on the busy dentist or hygienist and numerous distractions, such as the noise from nearby operatories, phone calls, or interruptions by staff or other patients, make it difficult for the older patient to concentrate on the new information that the clinician is trying to convey. The problem is compounded if the older person perceives the new material as irrelevant or unfamiliar or confusing. These problems, as well as age-related decline in the ability to organize new information in secondary memory, can be overcome by helping the older learner to structure the information. In dentistry, this may take the form of an outline of the dental procedures to be undertaken, either chronologically or in order of costs or time involved. Home care instructions may also be structured in terms of what the patient should do first, second, and so on. This provides the older person with a method of storing information in secondary memory; more importantly, it allows easier retrieval from memory when it is time to perform oral hygiene at home (e.g. 'First apply fluoride toothpaste on a soft toothbrush. Next, brush for two full minutes.'). Written instructions should also be structured in this manner and provided to both the elder and caregivers.

Implications of sensory and cognitive declines for the dental practitioner

What are the implications of these normal, age-related changes in sensory and cognitive decline for the dental care provider? This section first recommends communication techniques to compensate for age-related declines in vision and hearing, and then discusses strategies for communicating with elders who are experiencing problems with learning and memory.

Compensating for visual and auditory decline

The recommendations below are intended to aid in the reception of communication by the aged patient. They focus on vision and hearing problems, as well as losses in the cognitive domain:

1. When written materials are prepared for older patients (for example, home care instructions, an appointment calendar, recommended treatment), **use bold, large print**. This is a simple but effective way to assist the older person's visual function. Nevertheless, it is surprising how often health information intended for an elderly audience is written in small, illegible type or even handwritten. Available computer graphics programs make it relatively easy for any dental practice to print their materials in large, block letters.

2. Use **contrasting colours** for written messages. Again, a graphics program and a colour printer allow the use of multiple colours and printing on paper with a contrasting colour. For example, dark blue letters against a pale yellow background work especially well. Even if black letters are used, the material can be effective if the colour contrasts are strong (e.g. avoid duplicate copies that are dull or faded). The use of blue–green–purple together in any printed material should be avoided.

3. When speaking with older patients, one can aid their use of compensatory mechanisms by **facing the patient directly and maintaining eye contact**. This permits older people who have severe hearing loss to read lips, if they have that skill, and to block out extraneous sounds. The words 'let' and 'left', for example, may *sound* the same to a person who is hearing impaired, but the mouth and lip formation when pronouncing these two words are sufficiently different, and that visual cue may be all the patient needs to make the distinction. Direct eye contact also aids in orienting the individual with poor visual function.

4. **Standing closer to older patients** may also aid their reception of information through auditory and visual channels. However, the dental professional must be sensitive to cultural differences in this area, because some elders may react negatively to the invasion of their personal space. On the other hand, the nature of dental treatment requires close contact between the patient and dentist or hygienist. As a result, even older people who have a greater need for physical distance between themselves and others may be more willing to allow the dental practitioner to intrude in their personal space. Similarly, one must be cautious in the use of touch. Many health practitioners have found that **increased touching** can aid in communicating with older patients who have sensory impairments. It allows interpersonal barriers to be reduced and increases empathy between the speaker and the listener, but it may create discomfort for some older people. However, to the extent that both the patient and the dental provider are comfortable with tactile contact during discussions, this is recommended.

5. The pattern and volume of speech should also be considered. Thus, it will aid the older person's comprehension if dental professionals **speak more slowly and clearly, but without exaggerating each syllable**. Speaking more distinctly reduces the possibility of the older listener losing parts of speech or confusing some consonant phonemes such as *k, p, s, sh, t,* and *th*. It would also be helpful to avoid using homonyms together in one sentence so that the older

listener will be less likely to confuse words. **Raising one's voice slightly** may be helpful, but there is no need to shout!

6. Finally, it would help to **speak with older patients and, if appropriate, with their caregivers or family members in a quiet, unhurried environment**. The private office is a better setting in which to discuss the patient's health history and dental complaints, and to discuss treatment options than is the waiting room or the dental operatory. The private office generally has less background noise, fewer distracting conversations that can divert patients' attention, and allows greater privacy for older people to express their thoughts in confidence. It is also important to **avoid physical barriers such as a desk between the patient and dentist**. These objects increase the physical distance between the listener and speaker, and create a psychological barrier that makes it difficult for older patients who are unfamiliar with dental environments to express their concerns to the dentist.

Compensating for cognitive decline

It should be clear by now that normal aging does not make us severely forgetful or unable to learn. Our memory does, however, become more susceptible to stimulus overload and perceptual noise. We experience more problems in sorting disorganized or meaningless information and material that must be manipulated before it can be stored. With age, we also experience more problems in handling a large amount of new material at one time. Learning requires more time, and the information needs to be repeated to be stored in long-term memory. Thus, we are less effective learners in old age if information is presented rapidly, exposed briefly and interrupted frequently.

Older patients can certainly learn new techniques in preventive dentistry and home care. They should be fully informed about the proposed treatment plan. However, based on the description of age-related cognitive changes presented above, the dental team may benefit from some of the recommendations listed below. This can help reduce potential problems of patient dissatisfaction, non-compliance and frustration due to misunderstandings between the dental team and older patients.

1. Discuss examination findings and treatment recommendations in a **quiet, relaxed setting with no background noise**. As described in the section above for assisting elders with hearing loss, the dentist's office is much more conducive to such discussions than the operatory. One background noise often overlooked by people working in any setting is the 'canned music' that plays continuously and may seem innocuous to staff but may be disruptive to the older person trying to focus on new information from the dentist or hygienist.

2. **Structure the message** so that it is presented chronologically or in a step-by-step manner (for example: 'Remove your dentures at night, brush them with a medium toothbrush or denture brush, place the dentures in a cup of warm water overnight and rinse your mouth.'). Dental treatment planning may be explained best by procedure and sequence (e.g. 'We will first extract the two molars from your upper right side. After this area has healed, we will design a partial denture to replace these teeth. Next we will repair your lower denture, about 4 weeks from now.'). This oral information should be accompanied by a brief, typed form that provides the same information and a calendar with appointment dates and times marked.

3. **Take more time** to listen to the complaints or concerns of older patients, to discuss dental procedures and to repeat the message. It is essential to allow more time to explain dental procedures to older patients. This should include time for clarifying technical terms, for allowing the patient to ask questions at each step and even for asking the patient to recount specific points. This method of *active inquiry* has proven successful in the classroom; unfortunately it is rarely used in the clinical setting.

4. **Do not present too much information at once**. In an attempt to reduce information overload, dental providers must avoid the tendency to give all home care instructions and procedures in one visit. The older patient has a greater chance of retaining the information in secondary memory if the technique of *successive approximations* is used. With this approach, one can explain in one visit the recommended procedures for home care of partial dentures, followed by a description of caring for natural teeth at the next visit. At a subsequent visit, one can review dietary habits and counsel the patient on nutritional needs. Family members and caregivers can also be given this information to assist the older patient with newly acquired oral health information.

5. Finally, it helps to **use multiple modes of communication**. Information presented in a written format and reviewed orally with the patient is retained longer than either talking to patients or giving them a written message 'to read when you get home'. Instead of an appointment card, the patient could be given a calendar for the month where scheduled appointments are highlighted. In addition to words, symbols to represent the type of appointment (e.g. a denture to represent an appointment for a denture adjustment; a toothbrush to symbolize a cleaning appointment) could be used. This type of 'redundancy' in providing multiple modes of information can be a highly effective method to improve communication with older adults. Littlejohn writes: 'Redundancy compensates for

noise. As noise distorts, masks, or replaces signals, redundancy allows the receiver to correct or fill in missing data'. One example in the dental setting occurs when a clinician is treating a patient with severe short-term memory problems. The dental provider may need to calmly respond to repeated questions about aspects of a procedure that have been explained more than once already, or may need to be attuned to nonverbal feedback from a patient who clearly is confused or anxious because s/he has forgotten what was explained ten minutes ago. Redundancy in a calm, compassionate manner can provide the reassurance older patients need in order to feel comfortable and oriented to their surroundings, especially during a long procedure.

Box 4.1 summarizes these recommended communication strategies for elders who are experiencing sensory and cognitive declines.

Box 4.1 Compensating for sensory and cognitive decline in older patients.

A. **Compensating for vision problems:**
 1) Use bold, large print for written text.
 2) Use contrasting colours for written messages.
 3) When speaking in person, face the patient directly and maintain eye contact.
 4) Stand closer to older patients.
 5) Use touch as a way to reduce the distance.

B. **Compensating for auditory decline:**
 1) Speak more slowly and clearly, but without exaggerating each syllable.
 2) Raise voice slightly but without shouting.
 3) Speak with older patients and their caregivers in a quiet, relaxed setting.
 4) Avoid physical barriers between the patient and dentist.

C. **Compensating for cognitive decline:**
 1) Structure the message.
 2) Take more time with older patients.
 3) Do not present too much information at once.

D. **Compensating for sensory and cognitive decline:**
 Use multiple channels of communication and multiple modes of presentation.

Dental professionals who are aware of the many potential causes of noise can try to minimize, mitigate or eliminate them when communicating with older patients who are experiencing problems with vision, hearing and cognitive functions. Ascertaining whether a patient has difficulties with hearing, attention, a history of dental anxiety, cognitive impairments and other deficits can help the clinician improve communication strategies. Information about a patient's communication difficulties can be obtained from patients themselves, from relatives, caregivers and patient histories.

Nonverbal communication

Nonverbal communication is used by both the sender and receiver of messages. It includes facial expression, eye contact, gaze, body posture, physical distance and touch. Both innate and learned facial expressions are useful in conveying human emotions, including fear, anxiety and pain. Changes in body posture, such as increased rigidity of the body, clenching of the fists and flexing, tensing or tapping the feet or palms are also signs of anxiety, tension and pain. These nonverbal messages are often ignored by a dentist or hygienist who is focused on completing a procedure. Moreover, sometimes the patient's verbal and nonverbal communication may contradict each other. For example, patients may be successful in masking their emotions and/or denying pain when the clinician *does* detect nonverbal cues of pain or anxiety in the patient's face. This is especially true among today's older cohort, who grew up in an era when emotional expression was unacceptable and a sign of poor self-control. This means that dental providers must be acutely aware of any nonverbal cues and ask their older patients who seem to be masking their emotions throughout the course of treatment how they are feeling.

A number of evidence-based studies reaffirm the importance of using nonverbal communication to establish a good relationship with patients. Researchers who videotaped 181 nursing encounters with older adult patients observed six nonverbal behaviours: (1) patient-directed eye-gaze, (2) affirmative head nodding, (3) smiling, (4) forward leaning, (5) affective touch and (6) instrumental touch. The researchers found that 'with the exception of instrumental touch, these nonverbal behaviours are important in establishing a good relationship with the patient'.

Attentiveness to a patient's nonverbal cues can also alert clinicians to signs of pain when the patient is not able to express pain through language. Blomqvist and Hallberg found that nurses could perceive patients' pain by watching, listening and noticing – especially when the patient was not able to express pain verbally. Paralinguistic communications such as verbal agitation or confused talk, grimaces with mouth, motor aggressiveness and restlessness were observed among those with cognitive impairment. Interestingly, some patients reported that their reluctance to discuss their pain with a nurse was related to the personality of that nurse, which suggests the importance of health care professionals establishing a good relationship with their patients using both verbal and nonverbal communication. When interacting with patients who have cognitive or physical impairments, the dental professional's awareness of such intricacies of human communication can be a considerable asset to the patient and the dental practice as a whole.

Communicating with elders who have dementia

The challenges of communicating with someone who has dementia (including Alzheimer's disease, which comprises the majority of dementia cases) have been vividly depicted in video documentaries (e.g. 'Complaints of a Dutiful Daughter' and 'Quick Brown Fox: An Alzheimer's Story') as well as feature films ('Iris' and 'Away from Her'). These portrayals show older adults gradually losing their capacity for memory – beginning with their short-term memory – and becoming more confused and more dependent on their caregivers for activities of daily living.

Dementia is a cluster or group of symptoms that results in a loss of mental functioning that was achieved during the normal development of the individual through the life cycle. Symptoms of dementia include memory loss, difficulty performing familiar tasks, problems with language, disorientation to time and place, poor or decreased judgment, problems with abstract thinking, misplacing things, changes in moods or behaviour, changes in personality, and loss of initiative. There are different types of dementia, and not all patients will present with the same symptoms. Even patients who have the same type of dementia, such as Alzheimer's disease, may present very differently from one another due to a variety of factors. For example, some patients with highly developed social skills may be better able to mask their symptoms and may appear to have no cognitive impairments in the disease's early stages. Patients in these early stages may appear normal during their clinic examination but have difficulty with follow-through at home due to memory and organizational deficits.

Dental professionals may find it useful to know what kinds of language problems they may encounter with patients who have dementia. Box 4.2 lists some of the more common ones, including anomia, aphasia and echolalia. Because people use language to communicate a wide range of things – how they feel, what they want, what they think, what they see and so forth – when language fails to achieve its intended purpose, nonverbal communication can often be used to convey and detect meaning, to express emotions and to offer comfort. Clinicians must be especially attuned to both verbal and nonverbal feedback with dementia patients. Problematic or troubling behaviours may be an indication of pain, discomfort, confusion, side effects of medications, infection, fatigue, as well as overstimulation in an unfamiliar environment.

Box 4.2 Verbal communication disorders associated with dementia.

Anomia	problems in finding the correct words, often resulting in incomplete sentences, distractibility, the use of pseudo words and abnormal conversational patterns.
Agnosia	loss of ability to recognize objects, people, sounds, smells or shapes.
Amnesia	total or partial loss of memory.
Aphasia	loss of language ability.
Attention-deficit	impaired ability to focus and concentrate for an extended period.
Echolalia	repetitious vocalizations.

The dental professional's own body language, volume and tone of voice, diction, gestures and eye contact may be just as important as his or her spoken words in helping to increase a patient's comfort and comprehension. Dementia patients may not fully understand language as well as they once did, but they are probably still capable of 'feeling' another person's emotions, be they anger, frustration, compassion, patience or understanding. Imagine being in a foreign country and not understanding the language spoken by the people there. A helpful, compassionate person in that country does not need to speak your language to convey the warmth and care they feel towards you.

Communicating with caregivers of elders with dementia

When treating older adults with dementia, it is important to involve their caregivers in the patient's dental care. Caregivers can be family members or unrelated to the patient, paid or non-paid, and may work with the patient at home or in an institutional setting. There are an estimated 43.5 million family caregivers of adults 50 and older in the United States. The vast majority of long-term care to older adults is provided by families in the elder's own home or other community-based settings, not in nursing homes. While some of the patients seen in a dental practice will live in an institutional setting, many more are likely to be assisted by family members, friends and neighbours.

Caregivers can be the dental professional's ally in dental care of a patient with dementia. The caregiver can provide information to the dental practitioner about the different medications an elder is taking; can be involved in helping the elder keep appointments and providing transportation; and can help the elder practise good oral hygiene at home. However, dental practitioners should remember to address the patient directly, even if the caregiver is physically present and in close proximity. As in other health care interactions, these patients should not be talked about as if they were not there.

Dental practitioners should also be aware that caregivers may be experiencing a considerable amount of stress due to their caregiving responsibilities. It is important not to unnecessarily overload the caregiver with too many additional responsibilities. Enlist the caregiver as a partner in the elder's overall health care regimen, using the 'tell, show, do' teaching technique of explaining an activity in words to the patient and caregiver, demonstrating the activity for them, and then having the patient do it, in some cases with the caregiver's assistance.

Clinicians who work with older patients may find themselves on the frontlines of noticing a patient's cognitive declines, possibly even before family members (especially if the patient's closest kin live far away). When older patients suddenly start repeatedly missing appointments or exhibit other problematic behaviours or personality changes, dental professionals may need to contact a close family member to share their concerns. These behaviours may not be due to dementia, but they are signs that the patient's health status needs to be assessed or more closely monitored. For this and other reasons, it is important that key contacts for the patient are kept up to date and that any medical changes since the previous dental appointment be duly noted.

Cultural differences and cultural competence

Another relevant aspect of nonverbal communication with older patients is cultural variation in facial and body expressions. For example, individuals from different cultures often differ in their comfortable speaking positions (e.g. avoiding or seeking eye contact, speaking in an equal or superior position relative to the other) and physical distance during a conversation. Touch is a nonverbal form of communication that is more readily accepted by people from some cultures than from others. Note, for example, how people from southern Europe and South America are, in general, more likely than people from northern Europe to touch each other on the arm or shoulder as they speak. Gender and religious issues are also important when communicating with persons of the opposite sex in some cultures. Although some gerontologists have promoted the value of touching in communicating with older people who have severe vision and hearing deficits, the clinician should be aware of the preferences of a specific older patient before assuming that all elders appreciate being touched during social interactions.

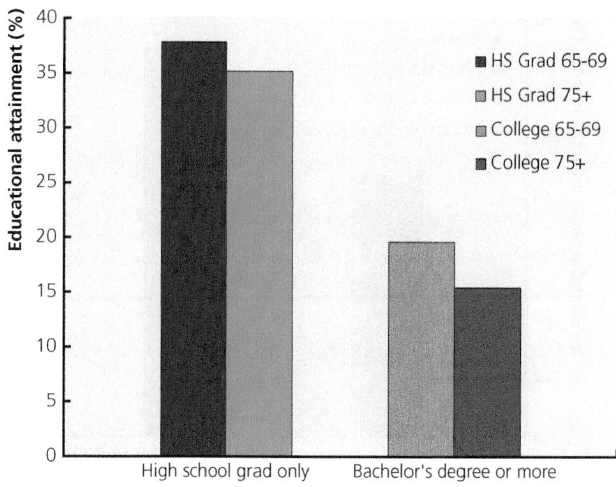

Figure 4.2 Educational attainment by age cohort.

Another cultural barrier that is more likely with today's cohort of older people, and perhaps less so in the future, is lower educational achievement than among younger adults. As shown in Figure 4.2, the proportion of adults age 75 years and older who have completed high school and college is considerably lower than among their peers age 65–69 years. Educational achievement is even lower for many elders who have immigrated or are refugees from developing countries; many may have only completed primary school. These differences highlight the importance of communicating at a simpler level with the old-old (i.e. age 75 and older) and with many immigrant elders. This is particularly true in dentistry, where technology has resulted in rapid advances in materials, equipment and procedures, so that for elders who are episodic users of dental services, the modern dental office may seem intimidating and unfamiliar. Many dental terms that seem like part of everyday language to an educated younger adult may be totally indecipherable to a less educated older person.

Experience with the dental care system

It is important to recognize that the cohort aged 65 years and older grew up in an era when preventive dentistry and regular dental visits for checkups and cleanings were rare. Most dentists before the 1960s did not emphasize preventive visits or rigorous home care. Dental visits were made for emergency treatment, often precipitated by pain. This generally led to extractions rather than heroic attempts to save the teeth.

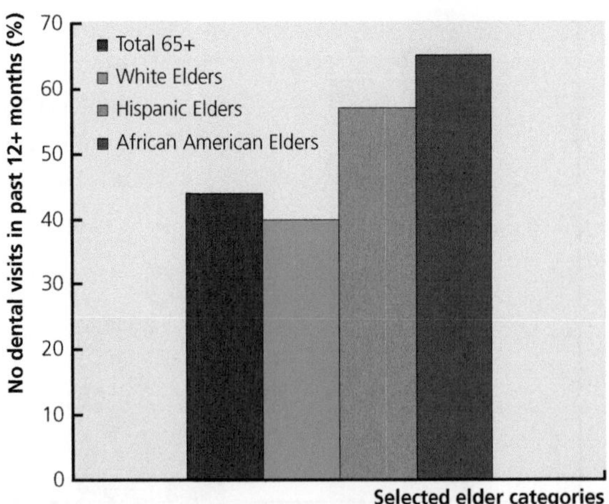

Figure 4.3 Differences in utilization of dental services.

Even today, many older people do not seek dental care unless it is for an emergency. As shown in Figure 4.3, the 2004 USA National Health Interview Survey found that older persons are not regular users of professional dental services. Older adults from ethnic minority backgrounds are even less likely than whites to seek dental care. Differences between poor and non-poor elders are even more striking; 32% versus 67% report making preventive dental visits, respectively. The reason given most often by elderly non-users for not seeking dental care is a perceived lack of need, and the attitude that dental care is not important in the later years.

Hence, it is even more important for dentists to emphasize prevention and the need to maintain all viable remaining natural teeth with their older patients. The challenge for most dentists is to empathize with older patients who ask why they should make numerous dental visits and spend their limited finances to retain so few teeth. This reflects a dental value system far different from today's younger generation that is willing to invest not only in preventive dental care, but also orthodontic treatment, whitening procedures and replacement procedures for missing teeth (e.g. bridges, implants). An open-minded approach on the part of the dentist is crucial in such situations. The dentist must recognize these cohort and educational differences in elderly patients and learn to communicate the inherent benefits of natural teeth over complete dentures or a completely edentulous mouth.

Age-related changes in oral-sensory functions

Normal, age-related changes in oral-sensory functions – taste, smell and proprioception – may influence older adults' abilities to taste, smell and enjoy foods. In some cases these changes are attributable to chronic diseases and the medications used to treat them. Although age-related sensory changes are gradual, continued dissatisfaction with the smell and taste of food may result in malnutrition among elders who no longer enjoy eating and therefore reduce their dietary intake or make unsafe food choices (e.g. by increasing sugar and salt content).

It was once thought that age brought dramatic decreases in the number of taste buds on the tongue, that this loss of receptor elements led to functional loss experienced as a dulling of taste sensations and that these changes accounted for older people's reduced enjoyment of food. Subsequent studies, however, have challenged each link in this chain of reasoning. Aging does not result in a significant loss of taste buds or in the number of papillae on the tongue. The experience of '*dysgeusia*', or distortion of normal taste sensation, that some older adults complain about is mostly attributable to some systemic diseases and many of the medications used to treat them. The problem is aggravated by a reduction in saliva, also caused by some medications and radiation for head and neck cancers. Saliva plays a critical role in taste, by making food more soluble and carrying the taste stimulus to the taste buds. Reduced salivary flow can also impair taste function, especially impairing sour taste recognition thresholds. Environmental pollutants such as airborne chemicals and metallic particles have also been implicated in taste perception and gustatory function.

Although older adults' taste function does not undergo a general decline in strength, it demonstrates specific changes. For example, while the relationship between taste intensity and stimulus strength is age-stable, judgments of taste intensity become less reliable with age. Older adults have more difficulty than younger people in discriminating between varying intensities of a flavour (tested by increasing or decreasing the level of bitterness of coffee, sweetness of tea, etc.). These differences have been observed across age groups, from teens to people in their eighties. It is also important to note that there is tremendous variation within the same age groups; in studies where the average taste performance of older individuals is poorer, some perform as well as, or better than, many younger persons.

Appreciation of food does not depend on taste alone. The sense of smell clearly is involved. Sensitivity to airborne stimuli plays a key role in the smell and taste of foods. Older people perceive airborne stimuli as less intense than younger persons, and do less well on odour detection and identification. External factors such as smoking and medications contribute to these differences, but even after accounting for these factors, age differences persist. When parallel assessments are made in the same individual, age-related declines for smell are greater than for taste. Researchers have found that peak performance in smell identification occurs during ages 30–50, then declines by age 70, so that by age 80 more than half experience major olfactory impairment. One way to improve older adults' enjoyment of eating is to enhance the elements that add flavour and aroma, such as herbs and spices. Adding even a tablespoon of herbs or olive oil to food can dramatically improve its enjoyment by making the olfactory and flavour chemicals more available to the taste buds without increasing fat or sugar content significantly. Adding colour to food can also enhance its perceived flavour. These additions can also help elders to sharpen their sensitivity to tastes and odours, improve the palatability and intake of food, increase their salivary flow and ultimately enhance their quality of life. Researchers have found that enhancing flavour to intensify its taste and odour by making the flavour of existing foods more intense (e.g. increasing the flavour of roast beef, ham, or cheese) can improve older adults' satisfaction and food intake. Finally, tactile and proprioceptive stimulation to the brain can decline with aging due to diminished neural activity in the sensory receptors in and around muscles, and under the skin. Older adults with proprioceptor decline may lack the ability to sense the movement of their tongue and thus have difficulty controlling its movement. They may also have problems sensing the location of their limbs. These problems with controlling tongue and limb movement can be an obstacle to home care and dental procedures, especially if proprioceptor decline impairs balance. This is an important consideration when older patients are transferring in and out of the dental chairs, or even when the chair is being tilted into different positions. By warning the older patient *before* making any adjustments in chair position (e.g. 'I am going to lower the back of your seat now'), one can prevent a startle response and reduce adaptation problems.

Conclusions

This chapter has focused on the impact of age-related changes in vision, hearing, memory and learning on communicating with older dental patients. We have emphasized the need for dental professionals to improve their communication skills with older adults who are experiencing these normal declines, as well as those who have dementia. Communication entails listening as well as speaking. In listening to aged patients with diverse challenges to their communication abilities, the dental team must be sensitive to the elder's concerns with costs, pain, time involved and sometimes their embarrassment about their inadequate home care that may have resulted in extensive decay and periodontal destruction.

Even such seemingly simple issues as transportation to the dental office may be a problem for older adults. They may not feel comfortable telling the dental care provider or the office receptionist that they cannot make it for repeated appointments because they must rely on friends or family to drive them, or because they cannot afford multiple taxi rides. It is not unusual to have a cancellation or no-show in such cases, if the patient feels compelled to accept an appointment time that is convenient for the dental office but impossible for the elder to find a ride. It is incumbent upon the dental team to ask the older patient when is a good time and day to come in for a dental appointment, and empathize with the patient's social and psychological circumstances. By being sensitive to and responding to the patient's concerns, the dental practitioner can go a long way in establishing rapport with the older patient, and thereby make it more likely that the patient will return for preventive visits and will practise the recommendations for home care and treatment options made by the dental provider.

Changes in taste and smell, as well as in proprioception, can also affect older adults' oral health behaviours and the ability to treat them in the dental chair. It is important to assess the reasons for these problems and make necessary adjustments if external factors such as smoking and medications are involved. Such understanding can help with effective communication with older adults. Such awareness is part of good dentistry and provides an important service to a growing segment of the older patient population. Many of the strategies mentioned in this chapter can be incorporated into everyday practice with patients regardless of their age, impairments or health status. Good communication skills in general are part of good people skills and can greatly enhance the oral health of older adults.

Further reading

Alzheimer's Association. (2005) *10 warning signs of Alzheimer's disease fact sheet.* http://www.alz.org.

Blomqvist, K. & Hallberg, I.R. (2001) Recognising pain in older adults living in sheltered accommodation: The views of nurses and older adults. *International Journal of Nursing Studies*, **38**, 305–318.

Caris-Verhallen, W.M.C.M., Kerkstra, A. & Bensing, J.M. (1999) Nonverbal behaviour in nurse-elderly patient communication. *Journal of Advanced Nursing*, **29**(4), 808–818.

Clem, R. (1996) Speech and hearing deficits associated with Alzheimer's disease. In: R.L. Dippel & J.T. Hutton (eds), *Caring for the Alzheimer patient*, 3rd edn, Prometheus Books, Amherst, NY.

Family Caregiver Alliance, National Center on Caregiving (2015) Selected caregiver statistics. Retrieved from https://caregiver.org/selected-caregiver-statistics.

Gilbert, G.H., Duncan, R.P., Heft, M.W. & Coward, R.T. (1997) Dental health attitudes among dentate black and white adults. *Medical Care*, **35**, 255–271.

Hooyman, N.R. & Kiyak, H.A. (2008) *Social gerontology: A multidisciplinary perspective*, 8th edn, Allyn & Bacon, Boston, MA.

Littlejohn, S.W. (2001) *Theories of human communication*, 7th edn, Wadsworth, Thomson Learning, Belmont, CA.

Schiffman, S.S. (2000) Intensification of sensory properties of foods for the elderly. *Journal of Nutrition*, **130**, 927S–930S.

Schiffman, S.S. (1997) Taste and smell losses in normal aging and disease. *JAMA*, **278**(16), 1357–1362.

Schoenborn, C.A., Vickerie, J.L. & Powell-Griner, E. (2006) Health characteristics of adults 55 years and over: U.S. 2000-2003. *Advance Data from Vital and Health Statistics*. No. 370, NCHS, Hyattsville, MD.

Shannon, C. & Weaver, W. (1949) *The mathematical theory of communication*. University of Illinois Press, Urbana, IL.

Spielman, A.I. & Ship, J.A. (2004) Taste and smell. In: T.S. Miles, B. Nauntofte & P. Svensson (eds), *Clinical Oral Physiology*, Ch. 2, Quintessence Publishing Co., Ltd, Copenhagen.

Stuen, C. Older adults with age-related sensory loss. In: B. Berkman (ed), *Handbook of social work in health and aging*. Oxford, New York, 2006.

Zacks, R.T., Hasher, L. & Li, K.Z.H. (2000) Human memory. In: F.I.M. Craik & T.A. Salthouse (eds), *The handbook of aging and cognition*, 2nd edn, Erlbaum, Mahway, NJ.

CHAPTER 5

Aging from a psychological perspective

Terry Fulmer[1], Sheryl Strasser[2] and Toni C. Antonucci[3]
[1]Bouve College of Health Sciences, Northeastern University, Boston, MA, USA
[2]School of Public Health, Georgia State University, Atlanta, GA, USA
[3]Life Course Development Program of the Institute for Social Research, University of Michigan, Ann Arbor, MI, USA

Background

Demographic changes have rapidly increased the number of older people, an increase which will both continue and accelerate as the 'baby boomers' reach retirement age. By 2050 the number of people over 65 will rise by 135% and those over 85 by 401%. These demographic changes also mark significant cohort differences in that people reaching older adulthood are healthier, better educated and will live longer than ever before.

Whereas development was at one time considered complete by age 16, it is now recognized that development is a lifelong process and that transitions from middle to late adulthood are both considerable and important. Whether the focus is on retirement, health or functional change, the aging process has significant psychological implications. This chapter focuses on the psychological aspects of aging and the scientific research to date that can inform appropriate health care practice. As individuals live longer, psychologists continue to explore the unique ways individuals in late adulthood think, feel and behave. The psychology of aging is an important emerging specialty in which knowledge is accumulating at a rapid rate. In this chapter, prominent psychological concepts of aging that have emerged over the past 50 years will be reviewed with an emphasis on the most recent and pertinent findings. The goal is to provide basic information on the major psychological themes related to aging so that oral health clinicians can better appreciate the life span, family and developmental context within which all older people should be viewed. We consider how continuity and change in cognitive function, personality and stress might influence and inform interactions with, and health care for, older adults.

> "Chronological age has been a traditional variable for organizing research and theory. Nevertheless, it has become increasingly understood to be an index of aging-related change but not necessarily a cause or source of theoretical explanations. – James Birren
>
> Reproduced from Schaie and Willis, 2011.

In general, psychology can be defined as the study of an individual's mental processes and how those processes influence behaviour [1]. The challenge that exists among researchers dedicated to the study of psychological aging processes is how to define parameters of aging, and how to better understand the underlying mechanisms that contribute to the wide variability in aging.

Historical overview

In 1959, James E. Birren, a pioneer in integrating psychological aging research with the biological and social sciences, published the first edition of the *Handbook of Aging and the Individual*. The publication of Birren's work marked a significant new era in the arena of aging research, as the psychology of aging was previously an obscure research domain. By the late 1960s, clear distinctions between children and adults were being observed by psychologists. However, few researchers focused on the unique characteristics and changes exhibited by older adults. Most notably, the work of Lewin and Werner emphasized developmental trends associated with chronological age versus specific behavioural patterns [2].

With the growing appreciation of the developmental perspective, the lifespan theoretical approach emerged in

Textbook of Geriatric Dentistry, Third Edition. Edited by Poul Holm-Pedersen, Angus W. G. Walls and Jonathan A. Ship.

the 1970s and 1980s. The work of psychologists such as Riegel, Salkind and Baltes popularized theories based on the proposition that both internal factors, such as genetics and intellect, as well as external forces, including social, environmental and cultural interactions, played a role in developmental processes [3–5]. Researchers began documenting that ecological influences – biological, interpersonal and broad cultural determinants – affected patterns of psychological aging among older adults and biopsychosocial models emerged.

The lifespan and life course perspectives

The lifespan perspective emphasizes the individual's growth and development over time. Some argue that this development consists of distinct phases or stages of individual development such as skill-attainment and mastery while others view this as a continuous, cumulative experience. The life course approach, a complementary but more sociological view of change, focuses on group changes over time and age, thus considering both the familial and social context within which the individual develops. In the 1920s, Freud's psychoanalytic theory surmised that personality traits and character structure were developed in childhood and were rigid by adulthood [6]. Later, Jung argued that older adults could realize new potential late in life [7] but it was Erikson who expanded and detailed this perspective. He specified multiple levels of adult development stages including several in early- and mid-adulthood as well as generativity and ego integrity as the optimal final stages achieved only late in life [8]. Over time, psychoanalytic paradigms, built upon the views of Freud, Jung and Erikson, have transitioned from being overwhelmingly negative and associated with loss and despair, to a lifespan perspective where one's character can become more refined and accepting during the maturation process [9].

Longevity significantly increased during the last century because of improved public health and fewer infant deaths. This increased longevity, coupled with a decrease in the number of children being born, changed the age distribution of the country. This has major political and social implications. The United States federal government established the National Institute on Aging in 1975 marking a national commitment to understanding and advancing the psychology of aging [1] and simultaneously international interest grew. While the average American's lifespan considerably increased, this was not accompanied by an improved quality of life. In 1975 Dr Robert Butler, the first director of the National Institute on Aging, published his Pulitzer Prize winning book *Why Survive: Being Old in America*, which deftly built an evidence-based description of how socially, medically, politically and culturally, United States policies for safeguarding the dignity of older adults were failing miserably [10]. In 2002 after reviewing the evidence from the 25 years since he wrote the book, he sadly reiterated these points, noting that we had made very little, if any, progress improving the quality of life of older Americans.

The life course and lifespan perspectives of human development have broadened the scope of aging research to emphasize the importance of an interdisciplinary approach. Of special interest is the newly evolving field of developmental science which has both encouraged an interdisciplinary approach and helped create sub-specializations within developmental psychology. The psychology of aging now represents a substantial research and practice domain that is highly distinguished as a unique area of concentration. This research can be useful to clinicians as they seek to hone their skills as health care providers to older people. While health care providers recognize the importance of understanding their patients, of taking a broader perspective on their patients' life choices and decisions, and on the benefits of continuity of care, traditional training has not included detailed study of the aging individual. Awareness of those characteristics and changes most common among older people will have the rewarding effect of improving both the care and satisfaction of the patient [2].The life span perspective has served as the basis for research integration and practice while improving interdisciplinarity among health care professionals. The ultimate result of better knowledge about the patient will be better care choices, thus maximizing patient treatment success.

Psychologists have studied how older people feel about growing older through both individual and cohort designs. While some individuals view retirement as a period of loss many, especially those with good health and sufficient financial resources, see retirement as a rite of passage into older adulthood – a period filled with increased freedom to pursue personal interests and nurture creative tendencies and enhanced time spent with family. At best this period is seen as a time for enjoying one's own agenda at a self-determined pace [3]. Interestingly, some research has shown this to be also true among socio-economically disadvantaged people. For those whose adult work life has been a time of uncertain and erratic income, retirement can also mark positive changes as one becomes eligible for Medicare, perhaps the best or only health care insurance ever enjoyed by the individual.

In addition, although one's social security (and perhaps small pension) might be small, it is steady, consistent and reliable and thus may be a significant improvement over their active work life income.

At the same time, research clearly indicates that as individuals age, concerns about health and disability prove to be the greatest threat to their well-being [11]. Interestingly, older people usually do not fear death but rather are concerned about achieving death with dignity and not becoming a burden to family members or others they care about [12, 4].

Psychological research on aging examines both individual and cohort effects. With increased life expectancy, several cohorts of older people now co-exist. For example, 'Baby Boomers' differ from those born during the World War II era and have been exposed to specific social and political influences that have shaped their attitudes and behaviours. Their early life experiences are significantly different and these differences are likely to affect their old age. For example, World War II babies may have experienced medical, nutritional and social deprivations which continue to manifest in their old age. On the other hand, the Baby Boomers were born into a time of affluence and growth, advantages that appear to be following them through to their old age. They had childhoods marked by good nutrition, medical care, the latest in preventive health activities. As older people, they continue to benefit from these early advantages as well as better education, better adult living conditions and more proactive views of health and aging. Research findings indicate that more positive self-perceptions of aging are associated with the practice of preventive health behaviours [13, 14]. This is an important point for oral health care professionals to note: with cohort change, oral health practices and subsequent expectations for maintaining oral health throughout retirement are now different. Furthermore, clinicians have an opportunity to influence oral health care prevention practices for better health in old age.

Ageism

Most industrial counties are now youth-oriented societies. While some older adults find growing old to be a very positive experience, negative stereotyping and treating people unfairly because they are advanced in age – or ageism – is pervasive. Ageism has been fuelled by both social and institutional forces [10, 15]. For example, the media frequently depict older adults negatively. Continued growth and development among older adults is rarely portrayed in the media and even worse, older adults are usually absent from media representation altogether or portrayed as feeble and forgetful. Health care professionals often treat older people differentially, assuming they are incompetent, ignorant and/or unable to understand their own health care. Unfortunately, most clinical and professional programmes lack specialized training and education regarding aging populations [16, 17]. With increased knowledge about the usual changes of aging, health care providers can improve the care they provide and the health of their patients. Interviews with older adults indicate that they often experience negative stereotyping which can have extensive consequences including higher rates of depression.

Cognitive processes and aging

Language skills, the ability to remember personal histories and instructions, decision-making and understanding contextual meaning of everyday situations can be generally described as cognitive or intellectual functioning. Older people are often concerned about their cognitive abilities as they age. A great deal of research has addressed the question of changes in cognitive functioning. In general, older adults tend to retain much of their cognitive abilities well into advanced old age. One exception is processing speed, which demonstrates a steady decline with age. Older adults have often been found to be equally able to process and accurately evaluate information but they do so at a slower rate of speed than younger people. This has direct implications for health care providers. When working with dental patients, an oral health care provider must be cognizant of what can be reasonably discussed and understood by the individual. Among older adults, practitioners must exercise caution when estimating intellectual capacity because what might be construed as intellectual limitations or the inability to understand complex information may in reality simply be a need for greater information-processing time. Older adults often require more time to reflect on information provided and decisions to be made. The general cognitive dimensions most closely examined in light of advancing age, which are covered in this section of the chapter, include intellect, memory and decision-making.

Intellectual function

The intellect, broadly defined as one's ability to learn and acquire new knowledge, was believed to diminish from early adulthood onward, especially in relation to learning, remembering, making rational decisions and effectively managing life's daily flow of events [18]. Cross-sectional and longitudinal research have now shown that people retain much of their intellectual functioning with age, especially when healthy. While there is substantial scientific evidence to suggest that intellectual functioning demonstrates intrapersonal stability over the life course, there is also evidence indicating that intellectual functioning is highly influenced by outside factors [19]. Psychological research offers considerable insight into the mitigating factors affecting learning that help explain stability and decline in old age.

Factors that have been found to be significantly associated with intellectual changes can be classified as internal and external. To illustrate, individual personality differences (internal) have been identified as contributing factors in intellectual performance variance among aging individuals. Specifically, older adults who maintain more flexible attitudes, who are more confident in their abilities and who maintain interest in social interactions tend to have less acute intellectual decline [1]. Similarly, social or external characteristics such as educational attainment, socioeconomic status, marital status and involvement with stimulating social or work environments have also been linked to higher intellectual performance [20]. Another critical variable associated with intellectual performance is health status. Those older adults with declines in biological capacity, regardless of the independent passage of time, have a corresponding cognitive performance decline [21].

Intellectual change and diminished capacity in old age have varied patterns. Clinicians should evaluate each patient as an individual in assessing self-care capacity. Using a variety of cognitive engagement approaches, oral health care professionals can gain a better sense of the person's strengths and weaknesses of understanding/processing the clinical context of their care, their chief complaint and oral health care needs. As with any patient, practitioners will enhance patient interactions by taking time to ensure that elderly patients understand treatment plans and oral health care instructions.

Memory

Psychological research has sought to compare how memory is lost or preserved among aging populations. As with intellectual functioning, memory is an umbrella term that encompasses a wide range of functions that are uniquely measured. In the most basic definition, explicit memory is understood as an awareness to try to remember. 'A theory of implicit memory is presented that describes it as a form of general plasticity within processing networks that adaptively improve function via experience' [22]. Cognitive psychologists now delineate different aspects of memory and have documented few age-related deficits in primary memory, with age-related differences in procedural and semantic memory depending on the demand characteristics of the specific situation. Research also suggests that aging is associated with declines in episodic memory [23].

This is critical to overall health care since one's inability to remember either in the long- or short-term may hinder the health care provider–patient interaction. Older adults show disproportionate declines in explicit memory for association relative to item information. However, the source of these declines is still uncertain [24]. One explanatory model for this impairment links a slowing of learning with a consequential slowing of the ability to remember. However, just as with intellectual assessment, health care providers must be cautioned that memory assessments may not adequately measure an older adult's ability to recall and retrieve information. Timing and social response biases have become critical elements. In line with previous comments concerning processing speed, there is considerable scientific evidence to indicate that older adults fare poorer than young adults on speed-based memory tests [25]. What is not clear, however, is how the two groups differ in terms of implicit memory performance, when accuracy and depth of detail are ultimately measured. While older adults may have slower reaction times and recall scores on psychological tests assessing short-term memory and speed as compared with younger adults, older adults tend to outperform their younger counterparts in higher order intellectual functioning, such as applied experience and long-term memory exercises [26].

Decision-making and reasoning with age

Another category of cognitive research has been concerned with *executive functioning* abilities, or concentration on how memory relates to decision-making, goal-setting and the ability to organize, prioritize and control one's thoughts and behaviours [27]. Psychologists are focusing research attention on understanding how aging adults' mental capacity requirements factor into health care preferences. Evidence indicates that aging adults' decisions and influencing values regarding the intensity of health care treatment remain stable over time [28]. This is important information for oral health care professionals who must appreciate that an aging patient's preferences for more or less invasive clinical treatment options are likely to remain unchanged (in the absence of major medical conditions in later life) despite popular beliefs to the contrary.

If decision-making and reasoning appear to be compromised in any given patient, it is essential that oral health care providers make an effort to determine whether this cognitive impairment is due to pathophysiological or mental status changes or stress. Psychologists have made gains in

Table 5.1 Thematic approaches to personality and adjustment in the aging process

CHANGEABILITY OF TRAITS--	TYPOLOGIES--	AGING PATTERNS:
Stable versus Shifting with age	–Integrated versus Isolated –Resistant versus Conforming	Ranging from optimal to impaired

understanding how specific impairment of one's executive function is associated with degenerative disease processes [29]. Further, there has been sound progress in understanding precursors to intensifying cognitive impairment. Psychological researchers have examined the ecological influences that may also contribute to cognitive stability or deterioration later in life. Research examining every day cognitive functioning among older people indicates that older people can show signs of impairment when stressed [30]. Many older people are uncomfortable with authority figures (including the medical profession), and have significant concerns about their own health and the associated health care costs. Therefore, it is likely that any interaction with a health care professional is cause for stress thus compromising the older patient's reasoning and decision-making ability.

Personality and adjustment

Personality can be defined as patterns of cognition, emotion and behavioural tendencies. Psychologists generally agree that personality consists of both trait (stable) and state (transient) characteristics. Theories of personality have covered a broad spectrum from promoting personality traits as genetically-determined and unchanging to the assumption that personality is shaped entirely by unpredictable environmental influences in all phases of life. A middle ground is now more generally accepted. The purpose of this section is to provide general knowledge relative to what is known about personality and its association with cognitive aging outcomes, and present clinical implications of this knowledge.

Constancy and change

Historically, personality has been examined within the life span perspective by identifying individuals exhibiting specific personality traits, observing their behavioural patterns and then measuring specific outcomes. In the case of aging, focus has been on cognition and health outcomes. While much of the research on personality has concentrated on the early years, researchers have increasingly addressed stability and change in personality characteristics in adulthood and aging. Research has addressed the question of whether personality traits remain consistent throughout the lifespan or if environmental factors can influence changes in one's personality later in life. Three major themes of personality and adjustment to life circumstances can be found in the scientific literature [31] and are summarized in Table 5.1.

There is no one psychological theory of aging that can describe all facets of personality, yet three basic research trajectories have been delineated: (1) longitudinal changes of traits, (2) typologies and (3) aging patterns. Trait theorists assume that traits remain stable, while state theories assume that they fluctuate. Table 5.2 presents personality traits that have been found to change and remain stable throughout all developmental stages of life.

Trait researchers have found that people with pessimistic personality traits experience more drastic cognitive decline in advanced stages of life. In terms of prominence, introversion, conformity, rigidity, caution and depression are exhibited more frequently among older people [32] although cohort differences and life span stability suggest that these may not be universal characteristics of older people. Criticism surrounding the typology and pattern perspectives is that they are constructed in such a way that a 'normative' aging process is implied, which passively implies that alternative aging patterns are divergent.

Stress and coping

As noted above, stress can impair functioning. With age, there are many factors that can induce stress. For example, disruption in one's personal environment introduces stress. The extent to which one can effectively deal with events as they arise is critical, for stress can lead to a cascade of negative events leading to decline at multiple levels including overall well-being [33, 34, 1]. Any life event can introduce stress. Regardless of whether the stress is negative (distress) caused by tragic life events, or positive (eustress), a person must confront his or her aroused emotions. If an individual is able to manage emotions in a way that does not cause harm to self or others, and effectively addresses the issue at

Table 5.2 State and trait personality characteristics by degree of constancy and changeability

Constant traits	Changing/flexible traits
Social energy	Self-confidence
Anxious/mellowness	Self-regulation
Depressive	Tolerance

hand, it is called positive coping or adaptation. However, when a person turns to destructive, negative means (whether propelled by, or in an attempt to dispel his or her emotions), it is referred to as maladaptation. A great deal of research has examined the effect of stressful life events, but researchers have also shown that minor events, known as daily hassles, can also have a cumulative significant negative effect on people [35; 33].

Coping mechanisms in old age

The way older adults react to sudden changes in emotions presented by stressors is highly dependent upon personality traits and is likely to be consistent with their previous life time patterns. Older people have been shown to exhibit two distinct coping patterns. On the one hand, older people have been shown to cope more maturely than younger adults, thought to be based upon wisdom garnered through experience. On the other hand, some older adults seem to be less able to cope with stress, an effect thought to be associated with age-related negative changes [34]. While it is plausible to assume that over time positive coping strategies are learned and developed, it must also be recognized that others may not benefit from such positive learning experiences and may be less likely to have developed a repertoire of adaptive coping strategies.

Research evidence has been accumulating indicating that an individual's response to stress – whether major life events or minor daily hassles that have a cumulative effect over time – can be linked to dysfunction and/or illness. 'Chronic job and financial strains, depression, inadequate coping, and maladaptive trait dispositions are significant risk indicators for periodontal attachment loss. Adequate coping and adaptive trait dispositions, evidenced as high problem-focused coping and low anxiety/depression trait, may reduce the stress-associated odds' [36]. Likewise, evidence indicates that positive coping and emotions lead to more effective adaptation and recovery [37]. Oral health care providers who take time to assess stress management behaviours among their older patients maximize the potential for successful early intervention, which could lead to improved health for older adults.

Conclusion

Aging is an inevitable process that is inseparable from the internal fabric of individuals as well as their environmental context. Given the aging of most countries, it is important for oral health care professionals to avoid negative stereotyping in the form of underestimating the abilities of older adults or treating them in a condescending manner. Psychological aging proves to be a highly individual experience, which can create a challenge for oral health care providers. While it is more common for professionals to recognize the declines in older adult cognitive functioning, it is important to emphasize the stability, adaptability and strengths that are often present in advanced age. The recognition that aging is not universally experienced as negative is a positive step for oral health care professionals and will enable the full potential of older adults and their oral health care to be realized.

Insights for clinicians

- Oral health treatment planning for the elderly will undoubtedly be affected by psychological factors.
- Understanding psychological changes that occur with aging can assist oral health care providers in more effectively meeting elderly patients' needs.
- Changes in aging patients' intellect, memory, personality and ability to adapt to stress may influence elderly patients' oral health care service decisions.
- Various perceptions on aging offer useful insights on how oral health care professionals can improve their interactions with elderly patients.
- By recognizing variability of aging among older patients, oral health care providers can avoid making presumptions about individual cognitive functioning and perceptions relative to advancing age.

References

1 Schaie, K. W. & Willis, S.L. (eds) (2011). *Handbook of the Psychology of Aging*, 7th edn, Academic Press, San Diego, CA.

2 Daaleman, T. & Elder G.H. Jr. (2007). Family Medicine and the Life Course Paradigm. *Journal of the American Board of Family Medicine*, **20**(1), 85–92.

3 Binder, P. & Nielsen G.H. (2005). Balancing Losses and growth: A relational perspective on identity formation in the second half of life. *Journal of American Academy of Psychoanal Dyn Psychiatry*, **33**(3), 431–451.

4 De Vries, B., Bluck, S. & Birren, J.E. (1993). The Understanding of death and dying in a life-span perspective. *The Gerontologist*, **33**(3), 366–372.

5 Fernandex-Ballesteros, R. (2006). GeroPsychology: An Applied field for the 21st Century. *European Psychologist*, **11**(3), 312–323.

6 Freud, S. (1959). *Thoughts for the times on war and death 1919*. Basic Books Inc, New York, NY.

7 Jung, C. (1954). *The Development of Personality*. Pantheon Books, New York, NY.

8 Erikson, E. (1976). Reflection of Dr. Borg's life cycle. *Daedalus*, **105**(2), 1–28.

9 Mann, C. (1985). Aging-A Developmental reality ignored by psychoanalytic theory. *Journal of the American Academy of Psychoanalysis and Dynamic Psychiatry*, **13**, 481–487.

10 Butler, R. (1975). *Why Survive? Being Old in America.* Harper Torchbooks, New York, NY.

11 Nord, E., Johansen, R. (2014). Concerns for severity in priority setting in health care: A review of trade-off data in preference studies and implications for societal willingness to pay for a QALY. *Health Policy,* **116**(2-3), 281–288.

12 De Raedt, R., Koster, E.H.W., & Ryckewaert, R. (2013). Aging and Attentional Bias for Death related and General Threat-related Information: Less Avoidance in Older as Compared With Middle-Aged Adults. *The Journals of Gerontology Series B: Psychological Sciences and Social Sciences,* **68**(1), 41–48. doi: 10.1093/geronb/gbs047

13 Levy, B.a.M.L. (2004). Preventive Health Behaviors Influenced by Self-Perceptions of Aging. *Preventive Medicine,* **39**(3), 625–629.

14 Meisner, B. A. (2012). A Meta-Analysis of Positive and Negative Age Stereotype Priming Effects on Behavior Among Older Adults. *The Journals of Gerontology Series B: Psychological Sciences and Social Sciences,* **67B**(1), 13–17. doi: 10.1093/geronb/gbr062

15 Gruman, G. (1978). Cultural Origins of Present Day "Ageism" : The Modernization of the Life Cycle In: S. Spicker, K. Woodward & D. Van Tassel (eds), *Aging and the Elderly,* Humanities Press, Atlantic Highlands, NJ.

16 Bardach, S.H. & Rowles, G.D. (2012). Geriatric Education in the Health Professions: Are We Making Progress? *The Gerontologist,* **52**(5), 607–618. doi: 10.1093/geront/gns006

17 Mentes, J.C. & Perez, G.A. (2013). The John A. Hartford Foundation Hartford Gerontological Nursing Leaders: Improving Care for Older Adults Across the Health Care Continuum. *Clinical Nursing Research,* **22**(4), 399–401. doi: 10.1177/1054773813501732

18 Palmore, E.B. (1999). *Ageism Negative and Positive,* Springer Publishing Company, New York, NY.

19 Kaup, A.R., Mirzakhanian, H., Jeste, D.V. & Eyler, L.T. (2011). A Review of the Brain Structure Correlates of Successful Cognitive Aging. *Journal of Neuropsychiatry and Clinical Neurosciences,* **23**(1), 6–15.

20 Yu, F., Ryan, L.H., Schaie, K.W., Willis, S.L. & Kolanowski, A. (2009). Factors associated with cognition in adults: the Seattle Longitudinal Study. *Res. Nursing Health,* **32**(5), 540–550.

21 MacDonald, S.W.S., De Carlo, C.A. & Dixon, R.A. (2011). Linking biological and cognitive aging: toward improving characterizations of development time. *Journals of Gerontology, Series B: Psychological Sciences and Social Sciences,* **66B**(Suppl.1), i59–i70.

22 Reber, P.J. (2013). The Neural basis of implicit learning and memory: A review of neuropsychological and neuroimaging research. *Neuropsychologica,* **51**(10), 2026–2042.

23 Head, D.R.K., Kennedy, K.M. & Raz N. (2008). Neuroanatomical and cognitive mediators of age-related differences in episodic memory. *Neuropsychology,* **22**(4), 491–507.

24 Dew, I.G.K. (2010). Differential age effects for implicit and explicit conceptual associate memory. *Psychology and Aging,* **25**(4), 911–921.

25 Hess, T.M. & Hinson, J.T. (2006). Age-related variation in the influences of aging stereotypes on memory in adulthood. *Psychology and Aging,* **21**(3), 621–625.

26 Saloman, G.G.T. (1987). Skill may not be enough: The role of mindfulness in learning and transfer. *International Journal of Educational Research,* **11**, 623–637.

27 Ettenhofer, M.L., Hambrick, D.Z. & Abeles, N. (2006). Reliability and stability of executive functioning in older adults. *Neuropsychology,* **20**(5), 607–613.

28 Martin, V.C. & Roberto, K.A. (2006). Assessing the stability of values and health care preferences of older adults. *Journal of Gerontology,* **32**(11), 23–31.

29 LG, N. (2006). Memory processes, aging, cognitive decline, and neurodegenerative diseases. *European Psychologist,* **11**(4), 304–311.

30 Willis, S.L., Tennstedt, S.L., Marsiske, M., Ball, K., Elias, J., Koepke, K.M. *et al.* (2006). Long-term effects of cognitive training on everyday functional outcomes in older adults. *JAMA,* **296**(23), 2805–2814.

31 Roberts, B.W., Walton, K.E. & Viechtbauer, W. (2006). Patterns of mean-level change in personality traits across the life course: a meta-analysis of longitudinal studies. *Psychological Bulletin,* **132**(1), 1–25.

32 Small, B.J., Hertzog, C., Hultsch, D.F. & Dixon, R.A. (2003). Victoria Longitudinal Study. Stability and change in adult personality over 6 years: findings from the Victoria longitudinal Study. *Journals of Gerontology, Series B: Psychological Sciences and Social Sciences,* **58**(3), 166–176.

33 Neupert, S.D., Almeida, D.M., Mroczek, D.K. & Spiro, A. (2006). Daily stressors and memory failures in a naturalistic setting: findings from the VA Normative Aging Study. *Psychology and Aging,* **21**(2), 424–429.

34 Pearlin, LI, Schieman, S., Fazio, E.M. & Meersman, S.C. (2005). Stress, health, and the life course:some conceptual perspectives. *Journal of Health and Social Behavior,* **46**(2), 205–219.

35 Aldwin, C.M., Jeong, Y.-J., Igarashi, H., & Spiro Iii, A. (2014). Do hassles and uplifts change with age? Longitudinal findings from the VA Normative Aging Study. *Psychology and Aging,* **29**(1), 57–71. doi: 10.1037/a0035042

36 Ng, S.K.S. & Keung Leung, W. (2006). A community study on the relationship between stress, coping, affective dispositions and periodontal attachment loss. *Community Dentistry and Oral Epidemiology,* **34**(4), 252–266.

37 Ong, A.D., Bergeman, C.S., Bisconti, T.L. & Wallace, K.A. (2006). Psychological resilience, positive emotions and successful adaptation to stress in later life. *Journal of Personality and Social Psychology,* **91**(4), 730–749.

CHAPTER 6

The impact of social and environmental forces on aging*

H. Asuman Kiyak†[1] and Nancy R. Hooyman[2]

[1] Institute on Aging, University of Washington, Seattle, WA, USA
[2] School of Social Work, University of Washington, Seattle, WA, USA

Introduction

Throughout life, people are in dynamic interaction with their social and physical environments. The availability and extent of one's social network and physical resources significantly affect one's quality of life. If individuals are encouraged to participate in the larger social structure they will maintain a broader perspective on their roles in society and what they may contribute to it. Furthermore, the desire to contribute to and to explore the environment around oneself is an integral part of human existence. It is important for dental professionals to recognize the centrality of social supports in their older patients' lives, change in social roles with aging and the availability of community resources for older adults who may need additional assistance, especially for those who choose to remain independent in the community, or to 'age in place'. In this chapter, we examine the impact of social networks, social supports and the extent of one's integration into the larger community on well-being, as well as changing social roles associated with aging in diverse cultures and how people cope with these changes. We also focus on community resources and the impact of community on an individual's aging process. Many of the studies that have examined these issues were conducted in the United States, but they have universal relevance to older adults and to the process of aging worldwide.

* H. Asuman Kiyak & N. Hooyman (adapted from pages 53–58, 221, 222, 334–341, 352, 365–367, 474–475, 477–478, 501–503, 511–517, 433–437, 453–459), *Social Gerontology: A Multidisciplinary Perspective*, © 2008, 2005, 2002, 1999, 1996. Pearson Education, Inc., Boston, MA, USA. Reproduced by permission of Pearson Education, Inc.

† Author is deceased.

Older adults in the community

The availability of resources for older adults who live independently in the community, but who need help with their activities of daily living, may affect the ability of dentists to provide services for this population. For example, how easy is it for older dental patients to make frequent visits to the dental office if they no longer drive? If the dental professional recognizes symptoms of poor nutrition or dementia in an older patient, are there community resources to which these elders can be referred? These issues become more complex for older persons who choose to **age in place**, or to live independently in their own homes rather than relocating to a retirement community or to a long-term care facility, even when they can no longer maintain their homes or manage their activities of daily living. The desire to remain in one's own home actually *increases* with age; a 2005 survey by AARP revealed that 89 per cent of respondents age 50 and older agreed with the statement, 'I would like to stay in my own home and never move'. The rate of agreement increased from 84 per cent of respondents 50–64, to 95 per cent of those 75 and older [1]. Although living in one's own home offers control over a familiar environment and access to neighbours who may be able to help the older person, it also creates hazards for those whose health and functional abilities are deteriorating. An increasing number of services may be required, but may not always be available, for those who seek to age in place with multiple chronic diseases and dementia and who lack a strong social network. The concept of **elder-friendly communities** is important to recognize when

Textbook of Geriatric Dentistry, Third Edition. Edited by Poul Holm-Pedersen, Angus W. G. Walls and Jonathan A. Ship.

providing health care to older persons. We can define these as communities that:

1 address the basic needs of older adults for safe neighbourhoods, affordable housing and adequate nutrition;
2 optimize physical and mental health by providing access to social and health services, preventive and health promotion activities, chronic disease management and end-of-life care;
3 maximize autonomy for frail and disabled elders by providing transportation and other services that allow them to remain at home but also to access necessary services;
4 promote social and civic engagement, including opportunities for the older person to find employment, to volunteer and to interact with a diverse social network [2, 3].

In the following sections of this chapter, we discuss how communities can become elder-friendly with the availability of social supports, opportunities for family and civic engagement, and the strengthening of community resources. Cross-cultural and cross-national variations in these elements of elder-friendly communities are also examined.

The importance of social networks and social support

Social networks and the availability of social supports are a critical basis for psychological and physical well-being at any age, but the need for them may increase with age-associated changes in social roles as employee, parent or partner. Such needs also exist for older adults who age in place while their neighbourhood changes. A common myth is that many older adults are lonely and isolated from family and friends. Contrary to this misperception, even older people who appear isolated generally are able to turn to an informal network, whether for information, financial advice, emotional reassurance or concrete services. **Social networks** encompass interrelationships among individuals which affect the flow of resources and opportunities. Families, friends, neighbours and acquaintances, such as postal carriers and grocery clerks, can be powerful antidotes to some of the negative social consequences of the aging process. Elders can draw on these informal networks as a source of **social support** that may be informational, emotional or instrumental (e.g. assistance with tasks of daily living). Older adults first turn to informal networks for support and move to formal relationships only when necessary, typically when they live alone [4]. **Social integration**, which encompasses both social networks and support, refers to the degree to which an individual is involved with others in the larger social structure and community. This concept captures the degree of emotional closeness, the availability of support when needed and the perception of oneself as an individual actively engaged in social exchanges, such as civic engagement. The social structure shapes the individual, but the individual may also affect his or her social structure [4–6]. Both social support and social integration take account of (1) the specific types of assistance exchanged within social networks; (2) the frequency of contact with others; (3) how a person assesses the adequacy of supportive exchanges; and (4) anticipated support or the belief that help is available if needed. Social integration, however, tends to emphasize both giving and receiving support and assistance, and thus takes account of interdependence across generations. As we will see in the next section on cultural variations in social support, most older adults try to maintain **reciprocity** – being able to help others who help them – in their social interactions. Even frail elders who require personal care from their families may still contribute through financial assistance or child care. The meaningful role of helping others also benefits the helper and is associated with positive effect, self-esteem, a sense of purpose, life satisfaction and physical and mental health. As is true across the life course, older adults give support to others because of a sense of purpose, altruism, social norms, maintenance of a lifelong pattern of helping or investing in members of the social network as a way to build social capital [7–12].

The centrality of strong social supports for physical and mental well-being is well documented. One study found that older adults with limited social support had a 3.6 greater risk of mortality within the next 5 years than those with extensive social support [13]. Elders' ability to provide social support to others enhances their perceptions of the availability of support, which is in turn generally linked to good physical and mental health. Face-to-face interactions and size of informal networks are also found to be associated with better cognitive functioning [4, 14–18]. Social support can mediate the effects of adversity and other negative life circumstances, such as retirement, widowhood, illness or relocation [19–21].

Alternatively, loss of social support through divorce, widowhood or deaths of other loved ones can contribute to health problems. For example, older adults who live alone and are not tied into informal networks are more likely to use formal services and to relocate to a long-term care facility. Their self-reported well-being tends to be lower. Similarly, extreme social isolation may be conducive to a higher risk of disability, poor recovery from illness and earlier death [4, 22–24]. The Lubben Social Network Scale, a widely used measure to assess social integration and to screen for social isolation among community-dwelling elders, has been used with culturally diverse elders and in many countries. Low scores on this scale – indicating social isolation – have been correlated with a wide range of health problems [25].

The extent to which networks vary with age is not clear-cut. Although some studies have identified a decline in friendship networks, other have found that changes occur primarily in network composition (e.g. less contact with couples, more with informal helpers), or in the role played by this network (e.g. increased need for instrumental support) [26–28]. In fact, elders who are active in retirement communities and voluntary associations may actually expand and diversify their networks. A process of social selection may occur whereby healthy people are more likely to have supportive social relationships precisely because they are healthy. Conversely, poor health status may hinder them from initiating or sustaining social relationships [29]. In some cases, negative interactions with one's informal networks, such as conflictual relationships, can adversely affect physical and mental health. Other types of negative interactions may result from an inconsistency with an older person's needs and competence level, such as disappointment that one's children are not doing enough to help after the elder's hospitalization or family members being overprotective of the older adult [30, 31].

Social supports and family relations in traditional cultures

Cross-cultural research also highlights the importance of social supports. With economic and social development, many traditional societies have had to develop new ways to address the role of their older members and their positions in their families and communities. For example, the rising standard of living in China has benefited many young adults, who often migrate to urban areas for job opportunities. This has resulted in a concentration of older adults in rural areas, where 65 per cent of China's general population and 76 per cent of its older adults reside [32]. This pattern of migration by younger workers to urban areas also occurs in other Asian countries such as the Philippines, Indonesia and Thailand, resulting in sharp declines in three-generational co-residence [33–35]. The loss of this long-held tradition of intergenerational living may significantly affect the older adult who is left behind. A recent survey in a rural region of China compared elders living in three-generational households or with grandchildren in 'skipped generation' households (i.e. where grandparents were caring for grandchildren after the parents had relocated to urban areas for employment) with elders who lived alone or with a spouse. Those in traditional multigenerational households reported greater life satisfaction and less depression than their counterparts in single-generation households. Stronger emotional ties with and financial assistance from their adult children mitigated the negative effects of living alone on elders' well-being [36].

In response to these population and economic demands, China has increased its publicly funded housing and government-funded welfare institutions for older adults, not just for childless elders as in the past. There has also been an emergence of a private residential-care-facility industry and community-based services in response to the anticipated growth of the older population (24 per cent by 2050) [37, 38]. A more radical approach to caring for a growing older population has emerged in Singapore. In 1997 the government opened a special court where older persons can bring legal claims against their children for not providing assistance in their old age.

Despite significant changes resulting from modernization in older adults' status and family relations in traditional societies, strong cultural values have been observed in mitigating the negative effects of modernization on older people. This is illustrated in modern, industrialized and urban Japanese society. Confucian values of filial piety and ancestor worship have helped to maintain older persons' relatively high status and integration in family life, as well as their leadership in national politics. Traditional values of reciprocity and lifelong indebtedness to one's parents are a major reason for continued three-generational households in Japan. The modernization of Japanese society has resulted in increased economic demands on the nuclear family. Although almost half of working-age Japanese women today are employed outside the home, they are still expected to provide care for aging parents and parents-in-law. Unprecedented numbers of older people in Japan have increased the societal costs of maintaining older members, and have created dilemmas for younger family members who are responsible for their support. Therefore, it is not surprising that the majority of respondents to a survey by the Japanese Ministry of Health and Welfare (57.3 per cent) viewed the aging population as a serious problem, and 68 per cent thought that the birth rate in Japan should be encouraged to grow [39].

Nevertheless, the majority of middle-aged persons in Japan still believe that care of older parents is the children's responsibility. Indeed, negligence toward one's parents is a source of great public shame in Japan. The Japanese government provides incentives for home care by families; they can receive subsidies to remodel their homes in order to accommodate joint households, as well as a tax credit for providing elder parent care [40]. For these reasons, the proportion of older parents living in multigenerational households, although declining, is still higher than in any other industrialized nation. In 2005, 47 per cent of people over age 65 lived with their children and grandchildren, but this was a decline from 1980, when 70 per cent of older households were multigenerational. The percentage of parents living with children is declining as a result of urbanization, industrialization, the growing number of employed women and the declining number of children since 1950. This was projected to drop even further by 2010, to 42 per cent [39, 41]. Meanwhile, the number of households consisting of only the older couple has increased. In 2005 they comprised 15 per cent of older households, compared with 8 per cent in 1980 [41–44]. The number of nursing homes and long-stay hospitals in Japan has also grown, but more community-based options are needed. All these trends suggest that traditional customs of caring for aging parents in adult children's homes in Japan are rapidly changing. Urban–rural differences in family expectations are demonstrated by the fact that 25 per cent of people age 75 and older in Tokyo live alone, compared with 15 per cent in rural regions. Despite the growth of long-term care facilities, institutionalization in any form is still viewed as abandonment by many older Japanese. As a result, most elder care still takes place in private homes. Because of public concerns about long-term care needs for its growing population of oldest-old, the Japanese Diet passed the Public Long Term Care Insurance Act in 1997 [43]. This national policy guarantees comprehensive long-term care for all Japanese persons aged 65 or older, and for those age 40 to 64 who may require long-term care. Funding is provided by a combination of mandatory insurance premiums paid by older persons and taxes that will be paid to federal, prefecture and municipal governments. Users of this service must also co-pay 10 per cent of all incurred expenses.

A strong belief in **filial piety** – a sense of reverence and deference toward elders – also plays a dominant role in family attitudes and government policies regarding care for aging parents in Korea, where the number of people 65 and older has increased threefold in the past 25 years. Surveys of young Koreans reveal that more than 90 per cent believe that adult children must care for their older parents, and in fact 90 per cent of older adults cite family as their primary source of support. These values are supported by the high proportion of people aged 65 and older – 65 per cent – who live with their adult children, even in urbanized areas like Seoul. In particular, daughters-in-law are expected to provide most of the day-to-day care for their aging parents-in-law. The government of Korea promotes family-based caregiving by sponsoring a 'Respect for Elders Day' and a 'Respect for Elders Week', as well as prizes to honour outstanding examples of filial piety. These initiatives help reduce Koreans' expectations from the government, although changing demographics today have placed a greater burden on families, with average family size down to 3.0 and with 46 per cent of all married women in Korea working outside the home [45–49]. Other Asian countries where filial piety has been maintained, despite changing work and family patterns, are Singapore, Thailand and the Philippines, where approximately 90 per cent, 70 per cent, and 67 per cent of women 60 and older, respectively, live with their adult children [42]. Filial piety in these Asian countries generally supersedes modern social and economic demands.

In some cultures, respect towards intact elders may be promoted, but a subtle acceptance of benign neglect may result in the demise of older persons who are physically and/or cognitively impaired. An ethnographic analysis of Niue, an independent Polynesian island, revealed significant discrepancies between the status of older people who were in good health and had important social and political functions and those who were too frail to care for themselves. Although medical services are free on Niue, families and neighbours did not summon visiting doctors and public health nurses, even for infected sores, painful joints and other treatable conditions in these frail elders. The basic needs of cognitively impaired elders were even more frequently ignored. This may stem from values of reciprocity. Like other societies where reciprocity is crucial for intergenerational exchanges, the frail elders of Niue can no longer contribute to the group's well-being. Therefore, such neglect may be seen as a way of merely hastening the inevitable death of weaker members of that society [50, 51].

Knowledge as the basis of older people's power has been challenged as traditional societies become more urbanized or assimilated into the majority culture, which also has implications for elder well-being. Over the course of the 20th century, American Indian elders lost their roles as mentors and counsellors to younger tribal members. Their knowledge of tribal customs and stories, language, agricultural skills and folk medicine was no longer valued as family structures changed and people migrated away from the reservation [52]. Among some cultural groups, however, including many American Indian tribes, a relatively recent revival of interest and pride in native identity and religion has been occurring, thus raising the esteem of elders who possess ritual knowledge. For example, they are often the only ones who know the words and steps for many traditional songs and dances. Knowledge of the group's culture, particularly its arts and handicrafts, native songs and epics, has enhanced the social status of older persons in these societies. Furthermore, the traditions of reverence for old age and wisdom remain strong, overriding the impact of modernization on older people's roles. The timing of such a revival is critical, however. A similar revival among Plains Indians did not have comparable positive consequences for the tribe's older members who were no longer expert in traditional ways. The growing desire for ethnic or tribal identity among many Native Americans, which has led to a conscious restoration of old forms, illustrates that modernization does not automatically erode the status of elders. Similarly, the search for one's heritage or roots has led to increased contacts between younger generations seeking this information from older persons who often are a great repository of family histories [53].

Patterns of intergenerational assistance

Generally, families establish a pattern of reciprocal support between older and younger members that continues throughout an individual's lifetime. Indeed, the dramatic growth of three and four generation families, as a result of increased life expectancy, means that such reciprocity is often multigenerational. Those with more valued resources (e.g. money or good health) typically assist those with less. Assistance that is exchanged can be concrete such as financial, but also emotional and social. At various points, older parents provide substantial support, especially financial assistance, to their children, grandchildren and increasingly great grandchildren. Regardless of socioeconomic status, most **intergenerational transfers** of resources, especially of knowledge and financial support, go from parent to child. Contrary to stereotypes, most adult children who assist their parents are not motivated by the expectation of an inheritance [7, 54]. In some instances, parents continue to provide care to adult children beyond normative expectations of 'launching' one's children to be more independent. For example, parental care remains a central role late in life for parents of adult children who are developmentally or physically disabled or chronically mentally ill. Yet many such parental caregivers are facing their own age-related limits in functional ability, energy and financial resources which can affect their caregiving ability. Another example of how older adults continue to care for younger generations is the growing number of grandparents who are primary caregivers to their grandchildren because their adult children are unable or unwilling to provide care. This is an important consideration for dental professionals who must increasingly be sensitive to the need to communicate with custodial grandparents rather than the parents about their grandchildren's oral health.

Interventions to improve social supports

Recognizing the importance of peer-group interactions for well-being, many American communities are making efforts to strengthen existing informal or formal social supports, or to create new ones if networks are nonexistent. The aim of such interventions is to alter the environment to be supportive of older people. They can be categorized as personal network building, volunteer linking, mutual help networks and neighbourhood and community development. Despite an extensive literature on the benefits of social supports, evidence is limited about how – and how well – social support interventions work [55]. Personal network building aims to strengthen existing ties, often through natural helpers – non-family members the elder can turn to because of their concern, interest and innate understanding. Such natural helpers can provide emotional support, assist with problem-solving, offer concrete services and act as advocates. Neighbours often perform natural helping roles and may strengthen these activities through organized block programmes and block watches. Service workers, often referred to as gatekeepers, can fulfil natural helping functions because of the visibility of their positions and the regularity of their interactions with the older person. For example, postal alert systems, whereby postal carriers observe whether an older person is taking in the mail each day, build upon routine everyday interactions. Pharmacists, religious leaders, bus drivers, local merchants and managers of housing for older people are frequently in situations to provide companionship, advice and referrals. Religious or faith-based institutions may also serve to strengthen and build personal networks, in some cases providing a surrogate family for older people. Through intergenerational programmes, members of religious institutions can provide help with housework, home repair, transportation, and meal preparation, as well as psychological assurance. At the same time, older members may take on many leadership and teaching roles within the church, synagogue or mosque, thereby enhancing their sense of belonging and self-worth. In many private and public programmes, volunteers can help elders develop new networks or expand their existing social supports. For example, volunteers provide chore services in older people's homes, offer peer counselling and senior centre outreach activities and serve as Friendly Visitors.

The Internet and interactive television provide new opportunities for network building with peers and across generations by providing access to online support groups and chat rooms, referral links and informational support and email for those with access to such information technology.

Internet websites, such as Third Age, have emerged as a means to build virtual community connections and reduce social isolation. Chat rooms, for example, are modelled upon community members' interests and needs; they can be altered by the changing will of the community. Older people may be drawn to such virtual communities as a way to readily connect with other people without leaving their home. Creating an electronic community, however, is obviously limited to those older people who have finances to access computers and the interest in mastering the Internet. Nevertheless, with the growing availability of networked computers at local libraries, senior centres and community centres, many elders who cannot afford their own computer or online service may benefit from such services at no cost. Although the efficacy of 'computer support' is not known, it holds promise for elders with debilitating illnesses that present physical barriers to attending support groups, for rural and other isolated populations and for those who desire anonymity.

Another approach aims to create or promote the supportive capacities of mutual help networks, especially through joint problem-solving and reciprocal exchange of resources. Mutual help efforts may occur spontaneously, as neighbours watch out for each other, or may be facilitated by professionals. They may also be formed on the basis of neighbourhood ties or around shared problems, such as widow-to-widow programmes, and support groups for caregivers of family members with chronic impairments. Interacting with peers who share experiences may reduce feelings of being alone and expand problem-solving capacities, but may also inadvertently increase stress when groups lack a professional facilitator and participants share primarily negative or widely varying experiences. Support that does not meet the recipients' needs or is perceived as critical or dismissive of problems can aggravate the problem. Overall, the kind of support, who provides it and the context in which support is provided all play a role in determining whether interventions are perceived as beneficial [55, 56].

Neighbourhood and community building is another approach that attempts to enhance a community's elder-friendly qualities, and may involve social action through lobbying and legislative activities. They aim to build upon the strengths and resources of local communities and many include an intergenerational component. Neighbourhood-based intergenerational helping networks are used to connect the formal service system to provide personal care services to frail elders. Similarly, social supports can buffer the effects of neighbourhood stressors such as crime or traffic congestion for older adults [57].

Role changes and productivity in old age

In this section we will discuss how social roles often change with aging, especially if the older adult retires. Productivity is typically thought of as paid work. In fact, two theories of social aging, disengagement and role theory, focus on the losses associated with withdrawal from the employment role. Many older adults, however, are productive without being employed or engaged in obligatory activities, and there is little empirical evidence for the concept of disengagement or withdrawal from roles. Productivity is broader than paid work; it includes any paid or unpaid activity that produces goods and services for the benefit of society, such as household tasks, child care, help to family and friends and voluntarism. There are a myriad of ways in which older adults contribute to their families, neighbourhoods, communities and society, as well as the reciprocity that elders may experience through such contributions. Older adults are viewed individually and collectively as a resource to meet their own and society's needs. Engagement in such productive activity, particularly the concept of civic engagement, is assumed to have a positive influence on older adults' mental and physical well-being [58–60].

Productivity is not the same as 'staying busy', since a contemplative elder may nevertheless be contributing to his or her own or others' well-being. This broad definition recognizes that even a homebound, chronically disabled elder may be productive by teaching family and friends about how to age with dignity, placing phone calls to check up on other neighbours, reading to a young child, listening to a grieving friend, or providing support, encouragement and life lessons to a confused adolescent. The older woman who prefers to spend hours working alone in her garden may be contributing to the 'common good' by creating beauty for neighbours to enjoy, even though she may not view herself as contributing directly to the community. Regardless of our life circumstances, there is a universal human need to be useful to society, and reaching out and giving to others can be a powerful antidote to loneliness, isolation and depression.

Older adults represent an underutilized asset in most societies. They bring the resilience and hardiness of survivors, and the wisdom of life experience and lessons learned. As such, they are a civic treasure that can provide leadership in community and religious organizations, volunteer formally or informally, and influence decision-making and legislative processes. What is critical is for older adults to be able to exercise choice over how they spend their time. Public resources are then needed to support such choices, including those to contribute to families, neighbours and communities. Although the concept of productive aging may have an implicit assumption that older adults *should* be productive and exert pressures on them to engage in activities that they would prefer not to undertake, the greater danger appears to be that our society has provided limited opportunities for older adults to be engaged and make contributions. Older adults need opportunities to choose and adjust their behaviour and aspirations to maintain a sense of competence in a changing environment. Accordingly, changes are needed in public policy and societal institutions to enhance older adults' contributions to others and to provide meaningful roles in old age [61, 62].

Retirement as a time of productivity

With increased longevity and changing work patterns, retirement may define a third or more of the life course and be as much an expected phase as having a family, completing school or working outside the home. Men in particular, but increasingly women among younger cohorts, develop age-related expectations about the rhythm of their careers – when to start working, when to be at the peak of their careers and when to retire – and they typically assess whether they are 'on time' according to these socially defined schedules.

In many developed countries, the value placed on work and paid productivity shapes how individuals approach employment and retirement. Those over age 65 were socialized to a traditional view of hard work, job loyalty and occupational stability. Current demographic trends and social policies mean that values and expectations about work and retirement are changing, as many of the young-old exit and re-enter the workforce through partial employment or new careers. As individuals live longer, a smaller proportion of their lifetime is devoted to paid employment, even though the number of years worked is longer.

Early gerontological studies emphasized the negative impacts of retirement as a life crisis due to loss [63–65]. More recent research has identified the positive effects of retirement on life satisfaction and health, especially during the first few years postretirement. Although measures of physical and psychological health may decline slightly after 6 to 7 years of retirement, most retirees still report good health and overall life satisfaction. While a major transition, the majority of retirees experience minimal stress and report being relatively satisfied with their life circumstances [66]. Activities other than paid work that provide autonomy, a sense of control and the chance to learn new things are all related to retirement satisfaction. On the other hand, activities that involve less problem-solving and complexity and are not fulfilling, have been associated with distress and depression in retirement [67, 68].

Retirement does not *cause* poor physical or mental health, as is commonly assumed [69, 70]. Although functional health does deteriorate after retirement for some, for others it improves because they are no longer subject to stressful, unhealthy or high risk work conditions. Contrary to stereotypes about retirement's negative health effects, people who die shortly after retiring were probably in poor health *before* they retired. In fact, deteriorating health is more likely to cause retirement than vice versa. The misconception that people become ill and die as a consequence of retirement undoubtedly persists on the basis of findings from cross-sectional data, as well as reports of isolated instances of such deaths. In addition, the traditional American ideology that life's meaning is derived from paid work may reinforce the stereotype that retirement has primarily negative consequences. Retirees may also be motivated to exaggerate their health limitations to justify their retirement. In fact, health status is interconnected with other factors, such as the normative acceptability of not working and the desire for a retirement lifestyle [71].

Personal and social characteristics that contribute to satisfaction in retirement include:

- perception of daily activities as useful;
- internal locus of control;
- a sense of having chosen the timing of retirement;
- living in a suitable environment;
- access to an adequate social support system of friends and neighbours.

Consistent with continuity theory, preretirement self-esteem and identity influence postretirement self-esteem. Individuals whose primary source of meaning was not employment and who have weaker work values adjust to a satisfying routine more readily than do those with strong work ethics who did not develop leisure activities when employed. Conversely, retirees who do not adjust well typically have poor health, inadequate family finances, marital problems and difficulties making transitions across the life course. Those who retire early because of poor health or lack of job opportunities or who are experiencing other stressful events in their life are less satisfied with being retired. *Occupational status,* which is frequently associated with educational level, is also an important predictor of retirement satisfaction; not surprisingly, lower-status workers have more health and financial problems and therefore less satisfaction than higher-level white-collar workers. The more meaningful work characteristics of higher-status occupations may 'spill over' to a variety of satisfying non-work pursuits throughout life. These are conducive to more social contacts and structured opportunities during retirement. For example, a college professor may have a work and social routine that is more readily transferable to retirement than that of a construction worker. Differences between retirees in upper- and lower-status occupations do not develop with retirement, but rather reflect variations in social and personal resources throughout the life course.

Since retirement is a process, preparation and planning for productive roles in old age are important for transitioning to retirement. Comprehensive preparation, an orientation towards the future and a belief in one's ability to adapt to change are associated with a generally positive retirement experience [69, 72]. In addition, occupations that demand more complex thinking, decision making and intellectual challenge (e.g. professional positions such as dentistry) may better prepare people for retirement decision-making and planning. Additionally, if non-work interests and skills are not developed prior to retirement, cultivating them later is generally difficult [67, 73].

Comprehensive retirement planning programmes that address social activities, financial resources, health promoting behaviours and family relationships are one way of encouraging a positive transition. Unfortunately, such programmes are not widespread. Even when they exist, they may be underutilized, in part because of the human tendency to deny that one is getting old. When baby boomers in the USA were asked about retirement in a national survey, only 13 per cent were economically secure and looking forward to retirement and the leisure they believe they had earned. In contrast, 32 per cent were 'strugglers' and 'anxious', primarily women who feared retirement as a time of financial hardship and worried about health care costs [74].

Leisure roles in old age

The term "leisure" evokes different reactions in people. For some, it signifies wasting time. For others, it is only the frenzied pursuit of 'leisure activities' on the weekend that sustains them through the work week. Leisure can be defined as any activity characterized by the absence of obligation that is inherently satisfying. Free time alone is not necessarily leisure. Instead, the critical variable is how a person defines tasks and situations to bring intrinsic meaning. Accordingly, leisure implies feeling free and satisfied. Individuals who do not experience such feelings may still be at 'work' rather than at 'leisure'. People's reactions to the concept of leisure are clearly influenced by cultural values attached to paid work and a mistrust of non-work time. Because of American values of productivity and hard work – especially among the current generation of older persons – many older adults have not experienced satisfying non-work activities at earlier phases in their lives. Societal values are changing, however, with more legitimacy given to non-work activities across the life course, as evidenced by the growing number of classes and businesses focused on leisure. For low-income or ethnic minority elders however leisure may be a meaningless concept if they have to continue working to survive, face higher rates of functional disability or lack resources for enjoying recreational activities. The following patterns of meaningful non-paid activity among older individuals are identified in the literature on productive aging:

- Most activity changes are gradual, reflecting a consistency and a narrowing of the repertoire of activities as people age.
- Compared to younger people, older adults are more likely to engage in solitary and sedentary pursuits, such as watching television, visiting with family and friends and reading.
- The time spent on personal care, sleep and rest, 'doing nothing in particular', hobbies and shopping take up a larger fraction of older adults' days than among younger and middle-aged individuals [74, 75].

When judged by younger persons or by middle-class standards, these essential and universal activities may be viewed as 'boring and nonproductive'. Yet the ability to perform these more mundane activities – personal care, cooking, doing errands, puttering around the house or garden or sitting in quiet reflection – can be critical to maintaining older people's competence, self-esteem and life satisfaction, especially among the oldest-old. Furthermore, these routines may represent realistic adjustments to declining energy levels and incomes. Such routine leisure pursuits, consistent with the broader concept of productive aging, may thus reflect rational choices about ways to cope that are congruent with environmental changes and may also enhance quality of life.

The major benefits of leisure activities appear to be maintaining ties with others (e.g. social support) and providing new sources of personal meaning and competence. Not surprisingly, leisure activities are associated with a positive identity and self-concept among older people. Accordingly, activities that result in a sense of being valued and contributing to society are found to be positively related to life satisfaction and mental well-being in retirement [76]. This relationship does not mean, however, that leisure activity itself creates well-being, since older people who are active also tend to be healthier and of higher socioeconomic status. The quality of interactions with others in non-work activities may be more salient for well-being than the number or frequency of interactions.

Voluntary associations and the volunteer role in old age

Voluntary association membership is often presumed to be a 'good' leisure activity, with positive effects on physical and mental health. These benefits appear to be associated with having a sense of control and social engagement [77, 78]. For example, participation in a formal community-based cultural programme was found to have positive effects on overall health, doctor visits, prescription use, loneliness and morale among older participants, whose mean age was 80 [79, 80]. In general, older people tend to be more involved in voluntary organizations than younger people, although membership in faith-based organizations is the only type that actually increases with age [74]. Membership is most closely tied to social class and varies among cultures. When socioeconomic status is taken into account, older adults show considerable stability in their general level of voluntary association participation from middle age until their 60s [81]. Similar to most retirement activities, characteristics that influence voluntary association membership include age, gender, ethnic minority status, prior activities and memberships, health and socioeconomic status. Older women are more active in voluntary associations than older men, perhaps because of their multiple roles at earlier phases of the life course. In the USA, older African Americans have higher rates of organizational membership than older white people or elders of other ethnic origin. Nevertheless, for both black people and white people, membership is most frequent among those with better health and higher income and education levels. Some ethnic minority differences exist among older Americans in the types of associations joined. Older African Americans are especially likely to belong to church-related groups and social and recreational clubs; older white people frequently are members of nationality organizations and senior citizen groups. Latinos participate in fraternal and service-oriented organizations, mutual aid societies and 'hometown' clubs.

Older persons who are active in community organizations such as senior centres derive a variety of benefits. In general, activity level is positively associated with well-being, physical health, functional and cognitive status, and increases participants' well-being, although its benefits and protective effects may differ by gender [76, 82, 83]. Socializing is a primary reward for participation in voluntary associations and aids in achieving active or healthy aging. Because these organizations are typically age-graded, people interact with others who are similar in age and interests. These interactions often result in friendships, support, a sense of belonging, mutual exchanges of resources and collective activity. Consistent with the broader concept of productivity, voluntary associations can also serve to maintain the social integration of older people, countering losses in roles and in interactions with others. Older people in voluntary organizations are found to have a sense of well-being and higher morale, although this may be attributed to their higher levels of health, income and education. When these other characteristics are taken into account, organizational membership is not necessarily related to overall life satisfaction [81]. The most satisfied members of organizations are those who become involved in order to have new experiences, achieve something, be creative and help others. Such members, in turn, participate actively through planning and leadership. Overall, voluntary association membership appears to be most satisfying when it provides opportunities for active, intense involvement and significant leadership roles.

Rates of voluntarism are highest among adults at midlife, and tend to decline after age 45, often associated with work or family roles and thus with having more rather than fewer obligations and commitments [74]. It may also reflect that younger adults are likely to volunteer in ways that will benefit their children. The rate of volunteering among older adults is lower than adults as a whole [84]. When volunteering is redefined to include informal contributions (e.g. helping neighbours), however, more middle-aged and older adults report some type of formal volunteerism and informal voluntary contributions [85]. Furthermore, older adults who serve in volunteer roles invest more hours than do younger volunteers. This suggests that, once engaged, elders are often reliable and committed [86, 87].

Contrary to the assumptions of activity theory, the desire to replace lost roles (e.g. employee or spouse) is not a primary motivator for older volunteers. Instead, older people are more likely to volunteer if they are married, well educated, involved in other organizations and employed part-time [88]. For most retirees, volunteering is apparently not a work substitute, although it may protect them from any negative effects of retirement. Most elders want roles that fully engage their capacities and interests and in ways that are meaningful to them and to their communities [61, 62].

Benefits of volunteering

Volunteer programmes serve two major social benefits; they provide individuals with meaningful social roles that enhance their well-being and they furnish organizations with experienced, reliable workers at minimal cost. Volunteering is increasingly viewed as a central component of active aging and elder-friendly communities [89]. Older volunteers generally experience psychological and health benefits These benefits include greater life satisfaction, better self-rated health, a sense of accomplishment and feelings of usefulness and physical and mental well-being, including lower rates of functional disability and depression [76, 82, 88, 90]. There is some evidence that continuous volunteering across the life course fosters higher levels of psychological well-being by buffering against losses in psychological well-being in the face of declining functional health [91]. In fact, volunteering has been found to have a protective effect on mortality, especially for those who are socially isolated. This may occur when volunteering provides older adults who lack other major sources of role identity with an opportunity to develop more meaning and purpose in their lives [82, 91]. Other factors such as self-identity, role strain and meaningfulness, also may underlie the curvilinear relationship found between volunteering and mortality [92].

Adapting to role changes in the later years

A critical personality feature in the later years, which has profound implications for social support, is an individual's ability to adapt to major changes in life circumstances, health and social status and in social roles. **Adaptation** includes a range of behaviours such as coping, goal-setting, problem-solving and other attempts to maintain psychological homeostasis [93]. Given older people's numerous experiences with life events, role loss and environmental changes, it would appear that adaptation to role changes should occur with relative ease. Indeed, in one sense, an individual who has reached age 75 or 80 has proved to be the most adaptable of his or her generation, since the ultimate proof of adaptation is survival. Older people continue to face challenges to their well-being in the form of personal and family illness, age-related declines in sensory and physiological functions and changes in their social and physical environments. To the extent that older people are capable of using coping skills that were effective in youth and middle age, they will continue to adapt to change successfully. At the same time, however, there is some research evidence that adopting new coping styles may help older adults cope with new life events that differ from their experiences in middle age and that being wedded to past ways of coping may be ineffective.

Coping is the manner in which a person responds to stress. It includes cognitive, emotional and behavioural responses made in the face of internally and externally created events. People are generally conscious of how they have coped in a particular situation and, if asked, can describe specific coping responses to a given stressor. Coping strategies may be described as 'planful behaviour' in response to a stressful situation. Some forms of coping are aimed not at resolving the problem but at providing psychological escape. Coping reactions generally serve two functions: one is *problem-focused* coping to solve a problem that has produced stress for the individual, and the other is *emotion-focused* coping to reduce the emotional and physiological discomfort that accompanies the stressful situation [94, 95].

In some cases, an individual may focus only on solving the problem *or* on dealing with the emotional distress that it creates. Such reactions tend to be incomplete and do not resolve both the emotional and functional impact of the situation. Coping must fulfil both emotion-regulating and problem-solving functions in order to alleviate stress. The question of whether coping styles change with age has been explored by researchers focused on specific challenges such as caregiving for a frail partner, or on different types of problems (e.g. retirement versus death of a loved one) or on general styles of appraising coping with diverse challenges [96]. Both age and gender differences have been found in the use of internalizing versus outwardly expressing emotions in stressful conditions; older women prefer the former and men the latter [97]. The extent to which life events are generated by the individual (e.g. deciding to retire) or are externally created with no choice by the person who experiences the event (e.g. being forced to take early retirement) can disrupt one's coping style, regardless of age. Nevertheless, uncontrollable events can often propel the older person towards further growth and development [98].

Community resources

Community resources are central to helping older people cope with changes in their social and physical environments, especially those who choose to age in place in their own homes rather than move to retirement communities or to long-term care facilities.

These formal support systems may be provided by agencies of the local and national government, by non-profit private organizations and by religious groups. The services provided by these agencies include social interaction with peers in senior centres, telephone or in-person information and assistance, hot meals, health screening, help with legal and financial matters, home maintenance and, in some locations, professional counselling. Most of these agencies have formal services as their focus, not emotional support. As noted in our discussion of social support, older people must continue to rely on themselves or on family members, friends, or a confidant for this type of support.

The size and social structure of a particular community plays a significant role in the availability and accessibility of services for older persons, and establishes norms regarding their roles in the community. Thus, for example, a large city may be more likely to provide diverse and multiple social services for its older citizens, but the anonymity of urban life may create a challenge for them to learn what services are available. Access to services may also be difficult for homebound elders, unless services are brought to the home or available by phone or on the Internet. On the other hand, rural areas generally have fewer services designed for older people and access is also difficult. The social isolation of older adults in urban areas is often discussed in the gerontological literature, but older persons on farms and in rural communities may be more isolated, unless family and friends reside nearby. Perhaps the ideal living environment for older people is a medium-sized community (10 000–30 000 residents). Such small towns are more likely to have the critical mass of older residents to justify the establishment of social and health services to benefit this population. Distances tend to be shorter and informal information networks may be more available, providing greater access to services and reducing the likelihood of isolation among frail and vulnerable elders.

There is little research that promotes one type of community over another for the older population. However, an emerging concept in the physical environment for older adults is that of **elder-friendly** or **livable communities**. This concept examines the needs and preferences of older adults at the community level. Researchers who have studied older adults' perspectives have defined elder-friendly communities as:

- addressing basic needs such as safe neighbourhoods and affordable housing;
- optimizing physical and mental health by providing access to social and health services, preventive and health promotion activities;
- promoting social and civic engagement, including opportunities for employment and volunteering;
- maximizing independence for frail and disabled elders by providing accessible public transportation and resources to help them remain at home [3, 99].

As noted above, growing numbers of communities across the United States are attempting to promote both formal and informal social supports, including opportunities for civic engagement or giving back to the community. To determine if communities fulfil these elder-friendly criteria, surveys of older residents in diverse areas have been conducted. A 2005 national survey of 1000 adults age 50 and older by the American Association for Retired Persons (AARP) found that the availability of community services such as dependable transportation, nearby grocery stores and pharmacies, hospitals and affordable housing affected residents' satisfaction with their community. Urban dwellers were more likely to report satisfaction than those in suburbs where these services were less available. Dissatisfied residents were also more likely to feel isolated and disengaged from their neighbours and the larger community. Findings from such surveys are useful for guiding city officials and leaders in the aging network to improve housing, services and employment and volunteering opportunities for older citizens [1, 3, 99–101]. If the physical and social environment offers opportunities for older persons to participate as active members, reciprocate in providing services to their peers and to younger generations in the community and receive needed services, older persons will experience greater life satisfaction and an easier transition to old age.

References

1 AARP. (2006) *The state of 50+ America 2006*. AARP Public Policy Institute, Washington, DC.

2 Advantage Age Initiative. Advantage age communities. New York: Visiting Nurse Service of New York, 2007. Accessed March 2007 from http//www.vnsay.org/advantage.html.

3 Hanson, D., Emlet, C.A. (2006) Assessing a community's elder friendliness. *Family & Community Health*, **29**, 266–278.

4 Moren-Cross, J. & Lin, N. (2006) Social networks and health. In: R. Binstock & L. George (eds), *Handbook of aging and the social sciences*, 6th edn, Academic Press, New York, NY.

5 Antonucci, T.C., Sherman, A.M. & Akiyama, H. (1996) Social networks, support and integration. In: I.J. Birren (ed), *Encyclopedia of gerontology*, vol. **2**, Academic Press, New York, NY.

6 Berkman, L.F. (2000) Social support, social networks, social cohesion, and health. *Social Work in Health Care*, **31**, 3–14.

7 Boaz, R.F., Hu, J. & Ye, Y. (1999) The transfer of resources from middle-aged children to functionally limited elderly parents: Providing time, giving money, sharing space. *The Gerontologist*, **39**, 648–657.

8 Keyes, C.L. (2002) The exchange of emotional support with age and its relationship with emotional well-being by age. *Journal of Gerontology: Psychological Sciences*, **57B**, 518–525.

9 Krause, N. & Shaw, B. (2000) Giving social support to others, socioeconomic status and changes in self-esteem in late life. *Journal of Gerontology*, **55B**, S323–S333.

10 Kawachi, I. & Berkman, L.F. (2001) Social ties and mental health. *Journal of Urban Health: Bulletin of the New York Academy of Medicine*, **78**, 458–467.

11 Morrow-Howell, N., Sherraden, M., Hinterlong, J. & Rozario, P.A. (2001) *The productive engagement of older adults: Impact on later life well-being*, Longer Life Foundation, St. Louis.

12 Uchino, B.N. (2004) *Social support and physical health: Understanding the health consequences of relationships*, Yale University Press, New Haven, CT.

13 Blazer, D. "How do you feel about . . . ? Self-perceptions of health and health outcomes in late life. Kleemeier Award

lecture delivered at Annual Meeting of the Gerontological Society of America, Nov. 2006, Dallas, TX.

14 Cohen, S., Gottlieb, B.H. & Underwood, L.G. (2001) Social relationships and health: Challenges for measurement and intervention. *Advances in Mind–Body Medicine*, **17**, 129–141.

15 Eng, P.M., Rimm, E.B., Fitzmaurice, G. & Kawachi, I. (2002) Social ties and change in social ties in relation to subsequent total and cause-specific mortality and coronary heart disease incidence in men. *American Journal of Epidemiology*, **155**, 700–709.

16 Holtzman, R.E., Rebok, G.W., Saczynski, J.S., Kouzis, A.C., Doyle, K.W. & Eatoon, W.W. (2004) Social network characteristics and cognition in middle-aged older adults. *Journal of Gerontology: Psychological Sciences*, **58B**, P278–P283.

17 Liang, J., Krause, N. & Bennett, J. (2001) Is giving better than receiving? *Psychology and Aging*, **16**, 511–523.

18 Seeman, T.E., Singer, B.H., Ryff, C.D., Love, G.D. & Levy-Storms, L. (2002) Social relationships, gender and allostatic load across two age cohorts. *Psychosomatic Medicine*, **64**, 395–406.

19 Cohen, S. (2004) Social relationships and health. *American Psychologist*, **59**, 676–684.

20 DuPertuis, L.L., Aldwin, C.M. & Basse, R. (2001) Does the source of support matter for different health outcomes? *Journal of Aging and Health*, **13**, 494–510.

21 Everard, K.M., Lach, H.W., Fisher, E.B. & Baum, M.C. (2000) Relationship of activity and social support to the functional heatlh of older adults. *Journal of Gerontology: Social Sciences*, **55B**, S208–S212.

22 Findlay, R.A. (2003) Interventions to reduce social isolation among older people: Where is the evidence? *Ageing & Society*, **23**, 647–658.

23 Lyyra, T.M. & Heikinnen, R.L. (2006) Perceived social support and mortality in older people. *Journal of Gerontology: Social Sciences*, **61B**, S147–S153.

24 National Research Council. (2001) *New horizons in health: An integrative approach*, National Academy Press, Washington, DC.

25 Lubben, J., Blozik, E., Gillman, C., Iliffe, S., Kruse, W., Beck, J. *et al.* (2006) Performance of an abbreviated version of the Lubben Social Network Scale among three European community-dwelling older adult populations. *The Gerontologist*, **46**, 505–513.

26 Cantor, M. (1994) Family caregiving: Social care. In: *Family caregiving: Agenda for the future*. American Society on Aging, San Francisco, CA.

27 Kalmijn, M. (2003) Shared friendship networks and the life course: Analysis of survey data on married and cohabitating couples. *Social Networks*, **25**, 232–249.

28 Van Tilburg, T. (1998) Losing and gaining in old age: Changes in personal network size and social support in a four-year longitudinal study. *Journal of Gerontology: Social Sciences*, **53B**, S313–S323.

29 Wetherington, E., Moen, P., Glasgow, N. & Pillemer, K. (2000) Multiple roles, social integration, and health. In: P. Moon, K. Pillemer, E. Wetherington & N. Glasgow (eds), *Social integration in the second half of life*, Johns Hopkins University Press, Baltimore, MD.

30 Krause, N. (2004) Stressors in highly valued roles, meaning in life and the physical health status of older adults. *Journal of Gerontology: Social Sciences*, **59B**, S87–S117.

31 Krause, N. (2006) Church-based social support and mortality. *Journal of Gerontology: Social Sciences*, **61B**, S140–S146.

32 United Nations. (2006) *World population aging 1950-2050*, Department of Economic & Social Affairs: Population Division.

33 Joseph, A.E. & Phillips, D.R. (1999) Aging in rural China: Impacts of increasing diversity in family and community resources. *Journal of Cross-Cultural Gerontology*, **14**, 153–158.

34 Knodel, J. & Ofstedal, M.B. (2002) Patterns and determinants of living arrangements. In: A.I. Hermalin (ed), *Well-being of the elderly in Asia: A four-country comparative study*, University of Michigan Press, Ann Arbor, MI.

35 Zhang, H. (2004) Living alone and the rural elderly: Strategy and agency in post-Mao rural China. In: C. Ikels (ed), *Filial piety: Practice and discourse in contemporary East Asia*, Stanford University Press, Palo Alto, CA.

36 Silverstein, M., Cong, Z. & Li, S. (2006) Intergenerational transfers and living arrangements of older people in rural China. *Journal of Gerontology: Social Sciences*, **61B**, S256–S266.

37 Kaneda, T. China's concern over population aging and health. Accessed October 2006 from http://www.prb.org.

38 Zhan, H.J., Liu, G., Guan, X. & Bai, H.G. (2006) Recent developments in institutional elder care in China: Changing concepts and attitudes. *Journal of Aging & Social Policy*, **18**, 85–108.

39 National Institute of Population and Social Security Research. Housing with seniors: 1975-2010. Accessed October 2006 from http://www.jinjapan.org/insight/html/focus10/page08.html.

40 Maeda, D. & Shimizu, Y. (1992) Family support for elderly people in Japan. In: H. Kendig, A. Hashimoto & L. Coppard (eds) *Family support for the elderly: The international experience*, Oxford University Press, Oxford.

41 National Institute on Aging. (2011) Global health and aging. Accessed February 2015 from http://www.nia.nih.gov/sites/default/files/global_health_and_aging.pdf.

42 Kinsella, K. & Velkoff, V.A. (2001) *An aging world: 2001. US Census Bureau Series*. US Government Printing Office, Washington, DC, 95/01-1.

43 Maeda, D. (1998) *Recent policy of long-term care in Japan*. Paper presented at meetings of the American Public Health Association, Washington, DC.

44 Morioka, K. (1996) Generational relations and their changes as they affect the status of older people in Japan. In: T. Harevan (ed), *Aging and generational relations*, Aldine de Gruyter, New York.

45 Kim, K.H. (1998) A study of determinants of elderly people's co-residence living patterns. *Journal of the Korea Gerontological Society*, **18**, 107–122.

46 Levande, D.I., Herrick, J.M. & Sung, K.T. (2000) Eldercare in the United States and South Korea. *Journal of Family Issues*, **21**, 632–651.

47 Sung, K.T. (1998) An exploration of actions of filial piety. *Journal of Aging Studies*, **12**, 369–386.

48 Sung, K.T. (2000) Respect for elders: Myths and realities in East Asia. *Journal of Aging & Identity*, **5**, 197–205.

49 Sung, K.T. (2001) Family support for the elderly in Korea: Continuity, change, future directions and cross-cultural concerns. *Journal of Aging & Social Policy*, **12**, 65–77.

50 Barker, J.C. (1997) Between humans and ghosts: The decrepit elderly in Polynesian society. In: J. Sokolovsky (ed), *The cultural context of aging*, Bergin & Garvey, Westport, CT.

51 Glascock, A.P. (1997) When is killing acceptable? The moral dilemma surrounding assisted suicide in America and other societies. In: J. Sokolovsky (ed), *The cultural context of aging*, Bergin & Garvey, Westport, CT.

52 Baldridge, D. (2001) Indian elders: Family traditions in crisis. *American Behavioral Scientist*, **44**, 1515–1527.

53 Keith, J. (1990) Age in social and cultural context: Anthropological perspectives. In: R. Binstock & L. George (eds), *Handbook of aging and the social sciences*, 3rd edn, Academic Press, New York, NY.

54 Silverstein, M., Conroy, S.J., Wang, H., Giarrusso, R. & Bengtson V. (2002) Reciprocity in parent-child relations over the adult life course. *Journal of Gerontology: Social Sciences*, **57B**, S3–S13.

55 Hogan, B., Linden, W. & Najarian, B. (2002) Social support interventions: Do they work? *Clinical Psychology Review*, **22**, 381–440.

56 Davison, K.P., Pennebaker, J.W & Dickerson, S.W. (2000) Who talks: The social psychology of illness support groups. *American Psychologist*, **55**, 205–217.

57 Schieman, S. & Meersman, S. (2004) Neighborhood problems and health among older adults. *Journal of Gerontology: Social Sciences*, **59B**, S89–S97.

58 American Society on Aging. Atlantic philanthropies support ASA's new project to promote civic engagement. ASA Connections. Accessed December 2005 from http://www.asaaging.org/asaconnection/05mar/top.cfm.

59 Gerontological Society of America. Press release: The GSA announces initiative on civic engagement in older Americans. Accessed December 2005 from http://www.geron.org/press/engagement.htm.

60 Hinterlong, J., Morrow-Howell, N. & Sherraden, M. (2001) Productive aging: Principles and perspectives. In: N. Morrow-Howell, J. Hinterlong & M. Sherraden (eds), *Productive aging: Concepts and challenges*. Johns Hopkins University Press, Baltimore, MD.

61 Freedman, M. (2001) Structural lead: Building new institutions for an aging America. In: N. Morrow-Howell, J. Hinterlong & M. Sherraden (eds), *Productive aging: Concepts and challenges*. Johns Hopkins University Press, Baltimore, MD.

62 Freedman, M. (2002) Civic windfall? Realizing the promise in an aging America. *Generations*, **26**, 86–89.

63 Atchley, R.C. (1976) *The sociology of retirement*, Wiley/Schenkman, New York, NY.

64 Atchley, R.C. (1983) *Aging: Continuity or change*, Wadsworth, Belmont, CA.

65 Streib. G. & Schneider, C.J. (1971) *Retirement in American society: Impact and process*, Cornell University Press, Ithaca, NY.

66 Witt, V.G. (1998) *Life satisfaction in late adulthood: Role transitions and social integration*. American Sociological Association.

67 Drentea, P. (1999) *The best or worst years of our lives? The effects of retirement and activity characteristics on well-being. Dissertation Abstracts International*, **60**, 1771A.

68 Moen, P. (1999) *Retirement and well-being: Does community participation replace paid work?* American Sociological Association.

69 Moen, P. (2001) The gendered life course. In: R. Binstock & L. George (eds), *Handbook of aging and the social sciences*, 5th edn, Academic Press, San Diego, CA.

70 Moen, P., Kim, J. & Hofmeister, H. (2001) Couples' work status transitions and marriage quality in late midlife. *Social Psychology Quarterly*, **64**, 55–71.

71 Mutchler, J.E., Burr, J.A., Massagli, M.P. & Pienta, A. (1999) Work transitions and health in later life. *Journal of Gerontology: Social Sciences*, **54B**, S252–261.

72 Ekerdt, D.J., Kosloski, L. & DeViney, S. (2000) The normative anticipation of retirement by older workers. *Research on Aging*, **22**, 3–22.

73 McLaughlin, D.K. & Jensen, C. (2000) Work history and U.S. elders' transitions into poverty. *The Gerontologist*, **40**, 469–479.

74 Prisuta, R. (2004) *Enhancing volunteerism among aging baby boomers. Reinventing aging: Baby boomers and civic engagement*. Harvard School of Public Health, Center for Health Communication, Boston, MA.

75 Johnson, R. & Schaner, S. (2005) *Value of unpaid activities by older Americans tops $160 billion per year*. Brief No. 4, The Urban Institute. Perspectives on Productive Aging, Washington, DC.

76 Menec, V. (2003) The relation between everyday activities and successful aging: A 6-year longitudinal study. *Journal of Gerontology: Social Sciences*, **58B**, S74–S82.

77 Newson, R. & Kemps, E. (2005) General lifestyle activities as a predictor of current cognition and cognitive change in older adults: A cross-sectional and longitudinal examination. *Journal of Gerontology: Psychological Sciences*, **60B**, P113–P120.

78 Verghese, J., Lipton, R., Katz, M., Hall, C., Derby, C., Kuslansky, G. *et al.* (2003) Leisure activities and the risk of dementia in the elderly. *New England Journal of Medicine*, **348**, 2508–2516.

79 Cohen, G.D. (2005) *The mature mind: The positive power of the aging brain*. Avon Books, New York, NY.

80 Cohen, G.C., Perlstein, S., Chapline, J., Kelly, J., Firth, K. & Simmens, S. (2006) The impact of professionally conducted cultural programs on the physical health, mental health and social functioning of older adults. *The Gerontologist*, **46**, 726–734.

81 Cutler, S.J. & Hendricks, J. (2000) Age differences in voluntary association memberships: Fact or artifact. *Journal of Gerontology: Social Sciences*, **55B**, S98–S107.

82 Greenfield, E. & Marks, N. (2004) Formal volunteering as a protective factor for older adults' psychological well-being. *Journal of Gerontology: Social Sciences*, **59B**, S258–S264.

83 Van Willigen, M. (2000) Differential benefits of volunteering across the life course. *Journal of Gerontology: Social Sciences*, **55B**, S308–S319.

84 Corporation for National and Community Service. (2006) *Key volunteer statistics*. CNCS, Washington, DC.

85 AARP. (2003) *Enhancing volunteerism among aging boomers*. AARP, Washington, DC.

86 Independent Sector. (2002) *Giving and volunteering in the United States, 2001*. Independent Sector, Washington, DC.
87 Peter Hart Research Associates. (2002) *Older Americans and volunteerism*. Peter Hart Research Associates, New York, NY.
88 Morrow-Howell, N., Hinterlong, J., Rozario, P. & Tang, F. (2003) The effects of volunteering on the well-being of older adults, *Journal of Gerontology: Social Sciences*, **58B**, S137–S146.
89 O'Neill, G. & Lindberg, B. (2007) Civic engagement in an older America. Gerontological Society of America. Accessed Feb. 2007 from www.agingsociety.org/agingsociety.
90 Musick, M.A. & Wilson, J. (2003) Volunteering and depression: The role of psychological and social resources in different age groups. *Social Science & Medicine*, **56**, 259–269.
91 Greenfield, E. & Marks, N. (2007) Continuous participation in voluntary groups as a protective factor for the psychological well-being of adults who develop functional limitations. *Journal of Gerontology: Social Sciences*, **62B**, S60–S68.
92 Shmotkin, D., Blumbstein, T. & Modan, B. (2003) Beyond keeping active: Concomitants of being a volunteer in old-old age. *Psychology of Aging*, **18**, 602–607.
93 Ruth, J.E. & Coleman, P. (1996) Personality and aging: Coping and management of the self in later life. In: J.E. Birren & K.W. Schaie (eds), *Handbook of the psychology of aging*, 4th edn, Academic Press, San Diego, CA.
94 Lazarus, R.S. (1999) *Stress and emotion: A new synthesis*. Springer, New York, NY.
95 Lazarus, R.S. & Folkman, S. (1984) *Stress, appraisal and coping*. Springer, New York, NY.
96 Ryff, C.D., Kwan, C.M.L. & Singer, B.H. (2001) Personality and aging: Flourishing agendas and future challenges. In: J.E. Birren & K.W. Schaie (eds), *Handbook of the psychology of aging*, 5th edn, Academic Press, San Diego, CA.
97 Diehl, M., Coyle, N. & Labouvie-Vief, G. (1996) Age and sex differences in strategies of coping and defense across the life span. *Psychology of Aging*, **11**, 127–139.
98 Diehl, M. (1999) Self-development in adulthood and aging: The role of critical life events. In: C.D. Ryff & V.W. Marshall (eds), The self and society in aging processes. Springer, New York, NY.
99 Austin, C., Flux, D. & Ghali, L. (2001) A place to call home: Final report of the elder friendly communities project. Calgary, Alberta, 2001. Accessed January 2007 from http://www.elderfriendlycommunities.org/A-place-to-call-home.pdf
100 Feldman, P.H. & Oberlink, M.R. (2003) The AdvantAge initiative: Developing community indicators to promote the health and well-being of older people. *Family & Community Health*, **26**, 268–274.
101 Kochera, A. & Bright, K. (Winter 2005–2006) Livable communities for older people. *Generations*, **29**, 32–36.

CHAPTER 7

Clinical assessment of the elderly patient

Elisa M. Ghezzi[1], Douglas B. Berkey[2], Richard W. Besdine[3] and Judith A. Jones[4]

[1]University of Michigan, School of Dentistry, USA
[2]University of Colorado, School of Dental Medicine, USA
[3]Brown University, USA
[4]Department of General Dentistry, Boston University, USA

Introduction

The provision of excellent oral health care to an increasingly aging population requires effective approaches to patient evaluation. Dentists are working with an ever larger number of frail or functionally dependent older adults, many of whom present with extensive medical problems, take multiple medications and have complicated psychosocial issues that can significantly affect the prognosis of dental intervention. Thus it is critical that dentists take a consistent and systematic approach to patient assessment. Competency demands that clinical assessment should be the keystone in geriatric dental practice. A comprehensive, effective assessment allows the provider an understanding of the patient that transcends a specific chief complaint or diagnosis.

This chapter addresses principles useful in the comprehensive evaluation of older people and discusses the perspectives and techniques helpful in obtaining a thorough patient history as well as performing a detailed clinical examination. The contents of this chapter address general medical concepts; specific oral and dental components of assessment are also discussed.

Principles of geriatric medicine

'Old people are sick because they are sick, not because they are old.'
Sir Ferguson Anderson, famous Scottish Geriatrician

Dental corollary: 'Old people have lost all their teeth because they had dental disease, not because they are old.
L.C. Niessen, personal communication

Certain fundamental principles provide the foundation for the competent practice of geriatric medicine and dentistry (Box 7.1). Essential among them is the need to separate disease from age. Sir Ferguson Anderson, a noted Scottish geriatrician, said it best (see above). The importance of separating disease from age-related changes cannot be overemphasized.

Box 7.1 Principles of geriatric medicine.[a]

- Age-related changes
- Disease-related changes
- Interactions of age and disease
- Disease chronicity
- Atypical presentation of disease
- Multiple pathology
- Multiple medications
- Functional loss

[a]Personal communication: John Rowe and Richard Besdine, Harvard Division on Aging, ~1983.

Age-related physiological changes occur over the lifespan; e.g. decrease in kidney function (glomerular filtration rate or GFR), vital capacity and cardiac index. This is to be differentiated from disease-related changes; e.g. anaemia. At times, the age- and disease-related changes are additive; geriatricians coined the term *homeostenosis* to describe the process whereby the body's normal, redundant homeostatic mechanisms are compromised by age-related changes. The combination of aging plus disease puts substantial stress on even the best-maintained oral environment.

Disease-related changes reflect disease processes. Anaemia results from underlying pathological processes; e.g. iron, folate or vitamin B_{12} deficiency, rather than old age.

Textbook of Geriatric Dentistry, Third Edition. Edited by Poul Holm-Pedersen, Angus W. G. Walls and Jonathan A. Ship.

Curvature of the spine is the result of osteoporosis, rather than age, *per se*. Similarly, periodontal diseases and caries are due to disease processes, not age. While some diseases may be more common with advancing age, they are signs of, or are, actual disease processes and need to be recognized as such.

Interactions of age and disease are varied. Age can decrease the likelihood of diseases, like multiple sclerosis and lupus erythematosis, which are more common in early middle and middle age. Age can have no influence on disease. For example, haematocrit does not change with age, so changes in haematocrit are from disease processes rather than age. Age can also increase the likelihood of disease, for example Parkinsonism and dementias. Age-related changes can also mimic disease. For example, abnormalities of glucose tolerance tests are more common among elders. Age changes can also equal disease. Examples of this are the benign prostatic hypertrophy that occurs in men and the hormonal changes that occur with menopause in women. Finally, age can modify the presentation of disease, as in hyperthyroidism and acute myocardial infarction.

Disease chronicity: the prevalence of chronic disease, defined as any condition lasting more than three months [1], is directly proportional to age. Seventy-four per cent of those over 65 years of age in the United States have at least one chronic disease; 38% have two or more [2]. By age 75+, only 18% of elders have no chronic medical problems and half have two or more [2]. Some individuals grow old with chronic illnesses acquired in earlier years. However, for many, chronic disease first appears late in life and interacts with age-related changes to accelerate loss of organ reserve. The most frequent chronic diseases among those aged 65–74 years old in the United States are: hypertension (50%), arthritis (47%), heart disease (27%), cancer (19%), coronary heart disease (19%) and diabetes (19%) (Table 7.1) [3].

Table 7.1 Common chronic impairments and habits in persons age 65+ years (USA, 2005)[a]

Chronic conditions	65–74 years (%)	75+ years (%)
Hypertension	49.6	54.8
Arthritis	46.8	54.2
Chronic joint symptoms	45.1	48.2
Heart disease	26.8	36.6
Cancer (any)	19.1	24.7
Diabetes mellitus	19.1	15.6
Coronary heart disease	19.0	25.4
Sinusitis	14.6	12.8
Ulcers	11.4	13.3
Stroke	6.2	12.5

[a]Reference [3].

Table 7.2 Common chronic impairments and habits in persons age 65+ years (USA, 2005)[a]

Chronic impairments	65–74 years (%)	75+ years (%)
Hearing	30.4	48.1
Vision	13.2	22.0
Edentulous	30.4	48.1
Physical difficulties[b]	29.8	46.7
Current smokers	11.1	5.8
Former smokers	40.4	38.4
Current drinkers	47.3	37.9
Former drinkers	25.0	26.5

[a]Reference [3].
[b]Percentage with any physical difficulty that is very difficult or cannot be done at all.

Hearing, vision, tooth loss and physical disabilities are the most common chronic impairments in persons aged 65 years and older in the United States (Table 7.2). Alcohol use is a common habit, but few elders continue to smoke in old age (Table 7.2) [3].

The high prevalence of chronic disease among older people is a major determinant of health care use and costs. As the elderly population increases, chronic disease will continue to dominate our health care environment and to produce higher rates of disability (Table 7.2). Successful chronic disease management requires sensitive and accurate assessment of functional status at baseline, and regularly thereafter, with efforts concentrating on management, functional improvement and postponing deterioration. A large percentage of all health care resources in the United States are devoted to chronic conditions [4]; at the same time, medical spending for elders varies widely [2]. Out of pocket costs for elders increase with advancing age and increase dramatically toward the end of life [2].

Atypical presentation of disease: certain diseases can also present atypically in the elderly. Flu or pneumonia can present as people just not 'feeling themselves'. Myocardial infarction can present without chest pain. Anaemia can present as fainting or a fall. A serious infection can present without fever. Thus the importance of a thorough evaluation in the elderly cannot be overstated.

Multiple pathology, or the clustering of diseases and problems in one person, is a common characteristic of illness in old age, putting elderly patients at risk for functional decline due to late disease detection. Moreover, one disease or symptom may mask others. Numerous concurrent problems in an older person can devastate health and functional status. An early study of people in the community over age 65 years in Scotland found nearly 3.5 (mean) major problems in each individual [5]. Among elderly patients being admitted to hospitals, an average of six pathological conditions was discovered per person [6]. Several studies documented the frequency and intensity of multiple pathology in older people [7, 8]. Furthermore, a nursing home survey in the United States identified the most common problems coexisting in elderly residents in long-term care (Box 7.2) [9].

Box 7.2 Common coexisting conditions in the institutionalized elderly.[a]

- Congestive heart failure
- Depression
- Dementia
- Chronic renal failure
- Angina pectoris
- Osteoarthritis
- Osteoporosis
- Gait disorder
- Urinary incontinence
- Vascular insufficiency
- Constipation
- Diabetes
- Sensory deficits
- Sleep disturbance
- Adverse drug reactions
- Anaemia

[a]Reference [9].

Multiple pathology threatens older patients in several ways. First, unidentified problems are likely to influence one another and cause harm through disease–disease interactions. These interactions are especially common and dangerous in frail elderly patients, in whom major functional losses can become permanent in spite of eventual detection and treatment of the multiple causative problems. For example, an 84-year-old woman living independently in the community has the following problems: trouble walking due to a painful knee, difficulty chewing foods, visual impairment, urinary urgency and mild diet-controlled diabetes. Over the course of several days, she becomes lethargic after discontinuing eating due to mouth pain, develops a fever and, on her way to the bathroom at night, leaks urine on the floor. She slips and falls, fractures her osteoporotic hip and in the hospital is found to have bacteraemia from oral flora. Hyperosmolar dehydration due to diabetes is out of control, hip fracture and sepsis are all initially treated successfully, but a postoperative myocardial infarction is followed by mural thrombus and a devastating dominant hemisphere embolic stroke. After 7 weeks in the hospital, she is discharged to a nursing home. Her community problem list of (1) degenerative osteoarthritis of the knee with slow gait, (2) atrophic vaginitis, (3) osteoporosis, (4) cataracts, (5) periodontal disease, (6) Type II diabetes mellitus and (7) coronary insufficiency had never been assembled or considered by her physician, who thought of her as 'one of my old women'. Her poor oral hygiene had not been managed, nor had her painful and dysfunctional mastication due to periodontal disease been considered as a risk factor for dehydration, malnutrition or bacteraemia. Her gait had never been evaluated, either for primary treatment of the underlying arthritis or for support with a cane. Her cataracts had not been evaluated for surgery, her vaginitis had not been identified or treated with oestrogens for comfort or reduction of urinary urgency and her osteoporosis had not been considered for treatment. The late diagnosis of treatable if not curable problems whose interaction and neglect have ultimately produced permanent functional deficits is a preventable part of geriatric care. It is not farfetched to consider that appropriate and timely oral health care could have prevented sepsis, exacerbation of diabetes, the episode of incontinence with fall, hip fracture, postoperative heart attack, stroke and the loss of independent living.

Second, undetected problems can interact with diagnostic evaluation or treatment of a known problem and produce iatrogenic harm (for example, disease–treatment interaction). An 80-year-old man with congestive heart failure who presents at the hospital is started on potent diuretics, with immediate reduction in shortness of breath and improved physical findings. His poorly fitting dentures, mild diabetes, prostatic hypertrophy and gait disorder of early Parkinsonism are not considered. The rapid diuresis and fluid shifts result in further loosening of his upper denture, which falls out during eating and breaks. He is then anxious and less able to eat. Dehydration, initiated by the diuretic, is exacerbated by reduced oral intake. The diuretic also overwhelms his already compromised prostatic urethra and produces retention with overflow incontinence. Blood sugar and uric acid rise into symptomatic ranges. Confused and unsteady, he falls and suffers a subdural haematoma and is not discovered on his bathroom floor for two days. The final outcome is a predictably catastrophic result of ignoring his (1) dentures, (2) diabetes, (3) hyperuricemia, (4) prostatism and (5) gait difficulty in the haste to treat his heart failure. Careful consideration of all coexisting problems before initiating treatment for one is a cardinal rule of geriatric care.

The length of the problem list increases with age and rises to more than 10 or even 20 in the oldest and most frail, especially in the nursing home. When all problems are not identified and carefully considered, disease–disease and disease–treatment adverse interactions are common.

In older patients, a domino effect of interacting problems and interventions can create an irreversible chain of functional losses and can lead to infirmity, dependence and, if uninterrupted, eventually to death.

Polypharmacy: the management of chronic diseases is more often than not through the chronic use of medications. However, elders often get into difficulty due to drug–drug, drug–disease and drug–food interactions. Previously well elders on new medications can present as slow, confused, somnolent or even delirious. It is therefore of the utmost importance to update medication lists at every appointment. Similarly critical is to ask about non-prescription drugs, which can potentiate or interact with the prescription ones, as well as have adverse effects of their own.

Enquiring about a patient's current medications can also serve as an important assessment tool in itself. Current medications can tell a provider about the severity or even the presence of a previously unknown disease state. A patient who can tell you the name, dose and reason why they are taking each drug is qualitatively different and, at a minimum, has a higher level of health literacy than one who takes a blue pill in the morning and two yellow ones each night. Finally, it is important to ask patients whether they take their medications as directed, for at least two reasons. Firstly, if they are not, their medical problems may be less under control than they should be. Secondly, this will give you an indication of how compliant a patient will be with treatment, oral hygiene instructions and medications you may prescribe.

Functional loss is the final common pathway for many problems in older people. Functional impairment means a decreased ability to meet one's own needs. Central are assessment of activities of daily living (ADL) [10], including bathing, mobility, eating, toileting, dressing and grooming/hygiene; and assessment of instrumental activities of daily living (IADL), including housekeeping, cooking, shopping, banking, laundry, telephone use, managing medications and driving or using public transportation. The ability to maintain good oral hygiene is a part of ADL. In addition, objective assessments of cognition and behaviour and of social, economic and emotional state are required to document the health-related functioning of older people, including the capacity of the individual to maintain good oral hygiene.

When older adults are ill, the first sign of a new problem or reactivated chronic disease is rarely a single, specific complaint that helps to localize the organ system or tissue in which the disease occurs. Instead, one or more non-specific problems appear which themselves are manifestations of impaired function [11].

These problems quickly impair independence in previously self-sufficient elderly people without necessarily producing the usual clinical signs or symptoms of disease. Thus, falling, confusion, urinary incontinence, fainting, dizziness and loss of appetite/weight are frequently the first manifestations of disease in an older person, regardless of the organ system or tissue in which disease occurs (Box 7.3). These non-specific manifestations of disease occurring anywhere in the body have been called the geriatric syndromes. Their importance cannot be overemphasized; they demand prompt and comprehensive evaluation. A common theme among the syndromes is that aging in and of itself causes diminution in reserve capacity of the organs and organ systems, so that superimposed disease often results in unusual manifestations, called the syndromes. It is the progressive restriction of the ability to maintain homeostasis (called homeostenosis by some geriatricians) that produces weak links that fail first under the stress of illness; this phenomenon is a basic principle of the interaction of disease with biological aging [12]. Deterioration of function and loss of independence in older adults are early and subtle signs of active disease; rapid and thorough clinical evaluation is the appropriate response.

Box 7.3 Functional presentations of illness.

- Stopping eating or drinking
- Falling
- Urinary incontinence
- Dizziness
- Acute confusion
- New onset dementia or worsening of previously mild dementia
- Weight loss
- Failure to thrive
- Fatigue

Relationship of function and disease: a major component of clinical education is mastering the signs and symptoms associated with specific pathological conditions. Since disease and functional loss both increase with age, it is often assumed that the length of an older person's problem list predicts functional disability. But a long problem list does not necessarily produce major loss of function; independent older people often have shockingly long lists of serious problems. Individuals with short or even single-item problem lists may be severely disabled.

Patient behaviour

When illness occurs, the behaviour of the patient is influenced by social, cultural, psychological and biological phenomena [13], including the perceived severity of illness, disruption of daily life, denying or minimizing symptoms, previous experiences with care and the availability of care [12]. Since aging additionally influences health and illness behaviour, it is helpful to consider the impact of aging on illness behaviour and learn its clinical implications [14].

Perceived severity of illness: although personal perception of health problems depends on many issues (e.g. biological health, personality, previous experience with disease and its treatment), peer group healthiness can also influence one's assessment of clinical phenomena and seeking of treatment. The healthy 90-year-old living independently in an apartment building with friends who are equally vigorous and active is more likely to take seriously a new systemic or oral symptom or disabling condition than her sister living in a nursing home, where the norm is dependence and disability.

Normalization, the tendency to overestimate one's own state of health, is common among older adults. This is important because older people who minimize the extent of disease are at risk for negative outcomes if they do not report symptoms and subsequently get no treatment. Older people who overestimate their healthiness may attribute perceived change in feeling or function to a transient or external occurrence rather than to disease. Lack of perceived need greatly influences the utilization of health services. For example, falls may be attributed to a warped floor or poor lighting or to the stiffness of arthritis or the poor vision that 'happens to all us old people'. Older people also tend to underestimate the severity of a problem even when they do acknowledge the presence of illness. Oral cancerous lesions may be dismissed as harmless mouth sores. Chest pain may be attributed to muscle strain or rheumatism rather than to heart disease and getting lost in a familiar environment may be blamed on failing vision.

Previous interactions with clinicians who ignored complaints can also make older people dismiss symptoms and thus cause delay in seeking care. The common misconception that disability and functional decline are a part of normal aging results in ignoring of symptoms and delay in the treatment of potentially improvable conditions. Notable mouth dryness, for example, may be falsely attributed to increased age alone instead of a symptom of polypharmacy or Sjögren's disease.

Underreporting of symptoms/disease: the symptoms of serious but often treatable general and oral diseases are frequently under-reported, although they are more common in older people. In one study in the United States [15], nearly 90% of older individuals had experienced symptoms in the previous 30 days but only 30% had sought care or advice from their doctors. Nearly 90% named a relative when asked whom they would consult about illness and fewer than 10% named a health professional. In another study, less than 1% of 2000 symptoms among older people were reported to any health professional [16]. Of 20 potentially serious symptoms, more than half were not reported to a health professional. Health care professionals should assume an aggressive role in eliciting useful symptom information from the patient.

It appears that older people perceive discomfort and disability adequately but are generally unlikely to report symptoms and thus do not receive evaluation, diagnosis and treatment until late in illness progression. A common explanation for non-reporting is the societal belief that aging, in itself, causes loss of independence and physical problems. This 'ageist' view makes it likely that older people experiencing the same symptoms that bring middle-aged patients to the doctor will not seek care, will silently suffer as disease progresses and will be burdened with the functional losses of untreated illness. Although declines in several biological functions accompany normal human aging, these declines are slow and modest; and the functional impact of these declines is further ameliorated by the decades over which they occur and by physiological reserve. Major functional decline occurring abruptly in an older adult is caused by disease, not aging; diagnostic evaluation is the appropriate clinical response. In addition to ageism, depression or dementia also can disrupt accurate reporting of symptoms.

Underreporting of symptoms by older people seems to contradict the common ageist perception by clinicians of frequent hypochondriasis in old age. Not only are older people less often hypochondriacal than the middle-aged, but when the older persons do complain, important disease is more often found at the root of the complaint [17].

Patient assessment

Careful evaluation of an older person may require modification and supplementation of the usual clinical examination administered to younger patients. Components of the medical and oral history, clinical examination, the physical environment and communication techniques require special attention.

Medical examination and assessment

Dentists treating the elderly must complete a written and oral medical health assessment. The written health assessment must be standardized so as not to omit any important issues. However, a verbal review of pertinent medical history, medications, allergies, social history, habits and review of systems is essential as it will often elicit medical and functional problems not identified in the written history.

Principles of history taking

A good way to take a medical history is to sit at eye level, in a quiet room facing the patient. Because elders may be sensitive to glare, do not back light (i.e. DO NOT sit with a bright light behind your face) as the patient may need visual clues or to read your lips to understand what you are saying. Speak slowly, clearly, with lower tone not an increase in volume (unless necessary). Recording an adequate history is essential; if necessary, you can assist with the written history. Asking a patient if they can read the small type is often less intimidating than asking if they can read.

Communication techniques for the clinical assessment of the older patient

Whether obtaining medical or oral history, the manner in which the information is gathered can improve its accuracy and usefulness. Communication issues for older adults as well as effective communication techniques are discussed in detail in Chapter 4. It is vitally important to build good communication ties between the patient and provider in order to establish a trusting relationship. The patient should be encouraged to discuss not only the chief complaint but also any other possible symptoms, feelings and fears.

The physical environment for assessment may need to be modified due to medical, behavioural and sensory challenges of older people. Sensory impairment, physical discomfort and communication difficulty require an individualized approach to every patient, regardless of age; however general principles of approach are useful for health professionals caring for older patients (see Chapter 4).

Begin the interview with reassurance and introduce yourself to establish a friendly relationship. Older people can often be comforted by a gentle touch on the hand or arm during conversation. The location of the interview should be free of noise to allow communication and prevent distraction, especially for the many older patients with hearing impairments (Table 7.2). As not all older people are hard of hearing, it is best to ask about hearing at the outset rather than to shout unnecessarily. Words should be spoken clearly, directly facing and level with the patient to allow lip reading and other visual clues. Speaking louder is helpful and necessary to communicate with a hearing-impaired older person. The voice should be increased in the lower frequency range rather than the high range, since presbycusis (the most common hearing impairment) causes hearing loss of high frequencies. As presbycusis causes poor perception of consonants, in addition to speaking louder, exaggerated consonant articulation also helps. Most relevant, ask whether the patient has a hearing aid, whether it works and whether it has been brought along. A reminder about bringing a hearing aid or any other prosthetic to the office before the visit is most critical to effective communication.

Low vision is a problem for 10% of persons aged 55–84, increasing to 22% in those over 85 years of age and 26% of nursing home residents [18]. Age-related changes in vision are attributed to low accommodation, loss of low contrast acuity, diminished colour discrimination, and reduction in the attentional visual field, as well as increased difficulty with dark adaptation and sensitivity to glare. Common diseases that can impair vision include age-related macular degeneration, cataracts, glaucoma and diabetic retinopathy. Since visual impairment is common in older people, adequate lighting is important for safety, perception of health care instructions and emotional comfort for the patient. Shadows can make a room dangerous for older patients; very bright light, especially from above, can be painful following cataract extraction without lens implantation. Because aging eyes accommodate less efficiently, the interviewer should avoid positioning himself or herself in front of a brightly lit background. As with the hearing aid, glasses should be brought to and worn at health care encounters.

Safety and comfort require that equipment used in the examination be selected for older people's needs. Chairs of adequate height to allow easy sitting and arising are essential. Since the patients are years and often decades older than their dentists, formal address such as Mr, Miss, Mrs or Ms should be used *unless* the patient indicates a preference for first names. An exception would be in patients with dementia, who often best respond to their first names.

Components of a comprehensive medical examination and assessment

Patient assessment should be initiated the moment the patient arrives at the dental clinic. The practitioner should note a first impression of the patient. The patient's physical appearance, nutritional state, gait, posture, attitude and behaviour may provide important clues during the assessment and diagnosis process.

It has been said that the patient will try to tell us the diagnosis if we only listen. Yet gathering an adequate history from older people is more complex and time-consuming, not only because they have had more time to accumulate disease, but also because disease is more common in aged people. In addition, more aspects of everyday life become relevant to health care in old age and must be discussed. Besides the patient interview and previous records, friends, family members and other health professionals who have participated in the care of the patient might be contacted as part of the history. Although family members can make important contributions to the history, reliance on the family or allowing them to dominate the evaluation interferes with the assessment of the patient's view of the problem and with the clinician's perception of cognition and emotion. Intellectual impairment, mild or severe, is not a reason to skip the history. Demented patients are often able to describe their symptoms and changes with therapy. The patient should be seen alone first unless there is outright refusal. Only after the patient is interviewed should the family join or be seen separately. A well-intentioned family member should not control the patient's visit.

The medical assessment of the elderly patient extends beyond the determination of medical health status and includes evaluation of cognitive, affective, functional, environmental, social, economic and spiritual status (Figure 7.1) [19].

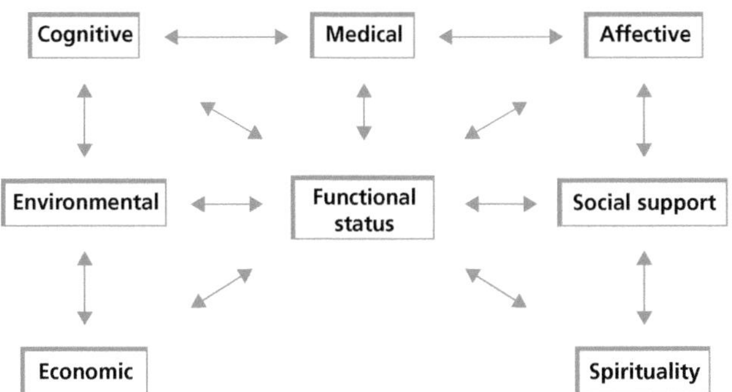

Figure 7.1 Interacting dimensions of geriatric assessment. From: Reuben, D.B., Principles of Geriatric Assessment, 1999 [19]. *Source:* Hazzard *et al.*, 1999. Reproduced with permission of McGraw-Hill.

Box 7.4 Essential elements of the geriatric medical assessment.

- Patient identification
- Chief complaint
- Dental history
- History of present illness
- Past medical history
- Review of systems
- Medications
- Allergies
- Diet history
- Social history
- Habits
- Physical examination
- Vital signs
- Laboratory assessment
- Cognitive/mental status
- Functional asessment

The essential elements of the geriatric medical assessment include the following (Box 7.4).

(a) ID (identification) – a brief description of the patient, e.g. a 77-year-old man with hypertension, osteoporosis and chronic obstructive pulmonary disease.

(b) Chief complaint and dental history – in the patient's own words, why they are coming to the dentist. Careful attention should be given to accurately understanding the patient's perceived needs and priorities for care. Because numerous health complaints go unreported, specific closed-ended interview strategies should be followed [20]. Questions should be directed towards the specific reason for the dental visit, the previous history of dental utilization, the reasons for the last visit, the existence of previous radiographs or other dental records and any barriers to receiving comprehensive oral health care (such as finances or fear and anxiety). Enquiry about previous dental visits should elucidate a past experience of: (1) fainting; (2) allergic reactions; (3) abnormal bleeding; or (4) other complications during or following dental or oral treatment. Specific enquiries should elicit oral symptom experience (Box 7.5).

(c) History of present illness – the story behind why they are coming, for instance how often they have pain, what precipitates it and how severe is it, on a scale of one to ten?

(d) Past medical history and review of systems – before any procedure is performed, essential medical data must be gathered. Little *et al.* [21] have identified essential information:

1) under the present care of a physician;
2) previous hospitalizations;

3) current medications (both prescription and over-the-counter);
4) allergies;
5) heart disease, heart murmur, high blood pressure or a history of rheumatic fever;
6) diabetes;
7) tuberculosis or other lung diseases;
8) hepatitis or other liver diseases;
9) kidney disease; and
10) bleeding disorders or blood disorders.

Box 7.5 Oral symptom enquiries.

All patients	Dentate	Edentate
General mouth discomfort	Tooth pain or sensitivity	Denture slippage
Mouth sores or growths	Grinding or clenching	Denture discomfort
Mouth dryness	Food entrapment	Food under denture
Bad breath	Cavities	Phonetic problems
Temporomandibular joint pain or clicking	Broken teeth	
Altered taste	Tooth mobility or flaring	
Chewing problems	Bleeding gums	
Neck swellings or pain		
Swallowing problems		

Because many older adults do not remember or provide accurate health history information, additional questions helpful in determining the diagnosis of undiagnosed cardiovascular and/or pulmonary disease might include: (1) history of chest pain, shortness of breath, fatigue; (2) ankle oedema; (3) dizziness or fainting; and (4) using more than two pillows to sleep.

Emphasis should be placed on expanding the typical medical history. For example, information on significant weight loss or gain may relate to nutritional status, cancer, diabetes mellitus, depression and dementia, drug-induced anorexia or thyrotoxicosis. Additional information should include antibiotic prophylaxis concerns (for example, heart valve replacement and prosthetic devices), history of chemotherapy or radiotherapy, cortisone usage, chronic obstructive pulmonary disease (bronchitis and emphysema), nervousness, thyroid disease, jaw joint pain, seizures, oral ulcerations, osteoarthritis and rheumatoid arthritis. Finally, any chronic or recurring psychiatric conditions (including anxiety and nervousness), as well as the 3 D's: delirium (altered consciousness), depression (changes in mood) and dementia (cognitive impairment) should be elicited.

When conducting broad-based health assessment of the older adult patient, the dentist should identify areas that need clarification from a physician, dental specialist, additional caregivers or other significant health care professionals. A multiple-copy consultation request form can be used for this purpose.

At every recall visit the dentist must do the following: (1) ascertain if the patient has undergone any surgeries, ER visits or hospital admissions since the last visit; (2) update the medical history to see if any changes have occurred since the last visit; and (3) update the list of medications to determine if any changes have occurred since the last visit.

(e) Medications – all current prescribed and over-the-counter medications and their effects on elderly patients should be listed. In a national study of drug use and purchase in Sweden, conducted between July and December 2005, drug use increased with increased age, and only 6% of all men and 5% of all women age 75+ did not purchase any drugs. Among this same age group, 7% of men and 6% of women purchased only one drug, 27% of men and 23% of women purchased 2–4 different drugs, 39% of men and women purchased 5–9 drugs and 21% of men and 27% of women purchased 10 or more different medications [22]. Recall that medications can indicate disease severity, the patient's level of awareness, elicit information omitted in history and give an indication of the dental IQ and the level of patient compliance.

Drug lists are often available in dental and medical records, yet believing them to be accurate and complete can be especially dangerous for older people. Drugs may be duplicated when the patient visits multiple physicians not known to one another, and treatment may be neglected if we assume that all medicines listed are still being taken. The most reliable medication lists come from physically inspecting and enquiring about all drugs in the patient's possession. The patient and family should be asked to bring all medicines for inventory. All prescription and over-the-counter drug containers should be inspected, and the patient should be asked which are taken for what symptoms and at what intervals. Discrepancies are common at any age, but occur more often and with more adverse consequences in older patients.

The dentist should pay particular attention to identifying adverse drug reactions that may impact dental and oral interventions (Box 7.6).

The dentist may use several important resources to aid in comprehending the significant, yet complex medical and dental issues associated with drugs. References might include the *Drug Facts and Comparisons* [23], the *Physician's Desk Reference* [24] or corresponding drug manuals. Online computer drug programs and hand-held databases are also available and might include Epocrates and PDR.net.

Box 7.6 Selected signs of adverse drug reactions.

- Dry mouth
- Sialorrhoea
- Bleeding
- Orthostatic hypotension
- Allergies
- Lowered stress tolerance
- Oral soft tissue lesions
- Movement disorders
- Mental disorders
- Altered host resistance

(f) Allergies – find out about medications and foods.

(g) Diet history – relevant for most older individuals, especially when disease management includes food restriction or diet alteration. Such a diet could interfere with nutrition or increase the risk factors for oral diseases.

(h) Social history – social and family history must include information not usually collected from younger individuals. Socioeconomic status, health care expenditures, insurance coverage, drugs (for example, current and past use of coffee, alcohol, cigarettes, recreational drugs, etc.), and relationships with friends and family play a major role in the overall well-being and mental health of older people and have been shown to correlate with better outcomes [25]. Resources in the neighbourhood and home, including friends, family and clergy, determine what kind and intensity of activities can be managed in the community, including assistance with oral hygiene activities.

Social history and supports are critical to understanding frail elders. It is important to ascertain the elder's level of social support. You need to know whether the elder comes alone, and, if not, who brings the elder to the dentist. You need to learn about the adequacy of patient's access to needed personal and medical services.

(i) Physical examination – the increased burden of disease in older patients consumes more time for adequate history and examination, yet less time is typically allocated to older patients in clinical encounters [26]. Physical examination requires special attention in older patients, but professionals should not feel that a great deal more must be done and time spent in examining the patient. Some components, however, do require special attention, and certain findings mean something different in older people.

(j) Vital signs – it is important to record a baseline blood pressure for all patients. Hypertension affects a large number of older adults (more than 50%), and blood pressure screening usually provides important data for risk management. If there are abnormal findings or postural hypotension is suspected, blood pressure measurements can be done after the patient has been lying quietly for at least 10 minutes and then standing for at least 3 minutes, to determine if postural hypotension exists [27]. Note should be made of whether the patient becomes symptomatic or not upon standing, and any blood pressure or pulse change should likewise be recorded.

The dentist should record and carefully consider elevated blood pressure readings. In persons with elevated blood pressure, it is recommended that 2–3 additional readings separated by several minutes be averaged and accepted as baseline [21]. Systolic blood pressure (SBP) greater than 140 mm Hg and diastolic blood pressure (DBP) greater than 90 mm Hg generally should be referred for evaluation. When SBP is over 180 mm Hg or DBP is over 110 mm Hg dental care should be deferred and the patient should be referred immediately for treatment.

Additional consultations should be sought when other atypical vital signs are noted: (1) pulse rate less than 60 or greater than 100; (2) irregular pulse rhythm; (3) more than five premature ventricular contractions per minute; (4) respiration rate more than 20 per minute; and (5) in instances of suspected acute infection, temperature readings less than 36 °C (96.8 °F) or greater than 37 °C (98.6° F). Because, however, infections in elderly people often present with less fever than in young people, septic older patients are occasionally without fever. Therefore, clinical suspicion about infection should be high for ill older patients, regardless of recorded temperature. In addition, since older people are particularly vulnerable to accidental hypothermia, temperature readings less than 36 °C (96.8 °F) or 'low-normal' temperature recordings should be verified with appropriate low-reading thermometers. If disease presentation suggests or is consistent with hypothermia, a low-reading thermometer should be used whether the screening temperature is normal or not.

(k) Laboratory assessment – should be performed if the medical history and review of systems reveal medical conditions that need assessment prior to certain treatments. An example would be an elder on Coumadin (Warfarin Sodium) for atrial fibrillation. A CBC, platelet count and INR would be appropriate prior to oral surgery in such an individual.

(l) Cognitive/mental status – affective and organic mental disorders occur frequently in older adults. Nearly 20% of those older than 75 years of age have some degree of clinically detectable impairment of cognitive function. Severe depression is evident in 20% of elders age 85 and over, compared with 15% in persons 84 or younger. Mental status is therefore another important component of the assessment [2]. The classic signs and symptoms of depression include sadness, decreased appetite or weight loss, difficulty concentrating, guilt, loss of interest in those things previously important, changes in sleep patterns, loss of energy, change in psychomotor behaviour (degree of arousal) and suicidal thoughts or actions. Many older adults, however, present with a less dramatic level of actual sadness and may appear to have cognitive blunting (especially memory deficits); differentiation from dementia is therefore important [28]. Depression may also be the first manifestation of Alzheimer's disease, as well as a wide variety of physical illnesses (e.g. cardiovascular disease, cancer), and may also be the primary cause of somatic complaints, including oral discomfort. When dementia is screened for, deficits in memory, judgment, intellect, orientation and possibly a flat affect are warning signs. Mental status testing may be helpful in assessing older individuals. The Mini-Mental State Examination (MMSE), which utilizes a 30 point scale, is widely used (Table 7.3) [29, 30]. Scores under 20 indicate moderate to severe dementia.

(m) Functional assessment – should include evaluation of the patient's basic ADL [10] and IADL. As indicated earlier (Table 7.2), half of persons age 75+ and 30% of 65–74 years have extreme difficulty or cannot perform one or more physical activities [3]. Dental providers need to know whether their patients can walk, transfer, eat, dress, bathe, toilet and groom themselves. Of critical importance to oral health is the patient's manual dexterity. Similarly critical are whether the patient manages their own finances, arranges transportation on their own or depends on others for these essential activities.

Oral examination and assessment

A comprehensive oral assessment includes a detailed oral health history, evaluation of any prostheses and conducting a meticulous clinical evaluation of extraoral, perioral and intraoral structures and conditions. Although methods may vary among individual practitioners, a consistent approach should be used from one patient to the next to assure completeness.

Patients should also be queried on their compliance with preventive oral health behaviour (e.g. brushing, flossing, use of fluoridated toothpaste, fluoride mouth rinse), as well as their ability to chew (with or without removable prostheses, and if they currently use them), taste and swallow. Finally, it is helpful to know how satisfied patients are with their smiles and if they would like to improve their oral aesthetics.

Extraoral clinical examination

When the dental history interview is completed, the next general step in the assessment process is a detailed extraoral clinical examination of the head and neck.

Facial form

Examine: symmetry and size of eyes, nose, mouth and ears; facial profile of maxilla and mandible; skin colour; swellings (unilateral or bilateral).

Considerations: Light skin colour may suggest susceptibility to skin cancer; unilateral swelling may represent a

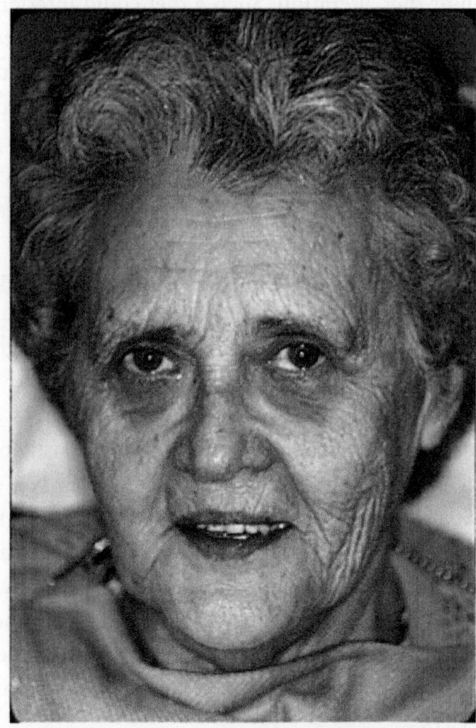

Figure 7.2 Assess facial symmetry to identify swelling of any structures.

Table 7.3 The Mini-Mental State Examination (MMSE)[a]

POINTS	SCORE	TASK
		Orientation
5	( )	Ask the patient: What is the (year) (season) (month) (day) (date)? Score one point for each correct answer.
5	( )	Ask the patient: Where are we? (country) (state) (county) (city) (location)? Score one point for each correct answer.
		Registration
3	( )	Name three objects: APPLE, BOOK, COAT. Then ask the patient to name all three objects. Score one point for each correct answer. Then repeat the items back to the patient until s/he can correctly repeat them back. Record the number of trials: ______
		Attention and calculation
5	( )	Have the patient count backwards from 100 by 7's (100, 93, 86, 79, 72). Have the patient stop after five answers. Score one point for each correct answer. Alternatively, ask the patient to spell "WORLD" backwards. Score one point for each correctly placed letter. Record the patient's spelling: ____________
		Recall
3	( )	Ask the patient to recall the three objects in 'Registration' above. Score one point for each correct answer.
		Language
2	( )	Point to a pencil and a watch, and ask the patient to name them. Score one point for each correct answer.
1	( )	Ask the patient to repeat the phrase, 'No ifs, ands, or buts'. Score one point if performed correctly.
3	( )	Ask the patient to follow a three-stage command: 'Pick up the paper in your right hand, fold it in half, and put it on the floor.' Score one point for each instruction followed correctly.
1	( )	Ask the patient to read and obey the following: 'CLOSE YOUR EYES'. Show the patient the stimulus card. Score one point if performed correctly.
1	( )	On a separate page, ask the patient to write a sentence. Score one point if performed correctly.
1	( )	Ask the patient to copy the design of intersecting pentagons. Score one point if performed correctly. 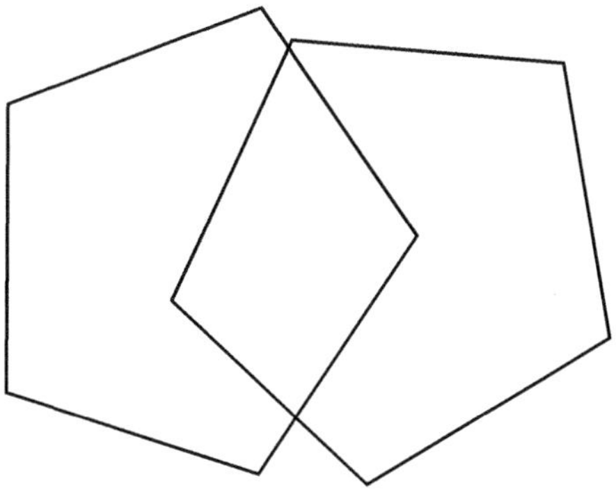
30	( )	**TOTAL**

[a]Reference [29].

cellulitis or salivary gland tumour; bilateral swelling could implicate Sjögren's syndrome, masseter muscle hypertrophy or cherubism. Asymmetry of the neck may represent a benign or malignant tumor (e.g. lymphoma).

Skin

Examine: pigmentation; colour; texture; elasticity; presence of oedema; nodules; ulcerations; scars; or other surface aberrations.

Considerations: bluish-black pigmentation may represent bruising; yellow or red pigmentation could imply jaundice or vascular lesions, respectively; texture changes can be a result of wear and tear or altered thyroid status; dehydration may cause elasticity loss. Systemic diseases may induce petechiae, cyanosis, flushing, pallor and eruptions.

Hands

Examine: size, shape, flexibility, movement.

Considerations: disfigurement of joints and digits due to rheumatoid and osteoarthritis inhibiting ability to provide adequate oral hygiene independently, swelling of joints and tissues. Lack of mobility may be a manifestation of a CVA (cerebrovascular accident or stroke).

Hair

Examine: colour; texture; and distribution.

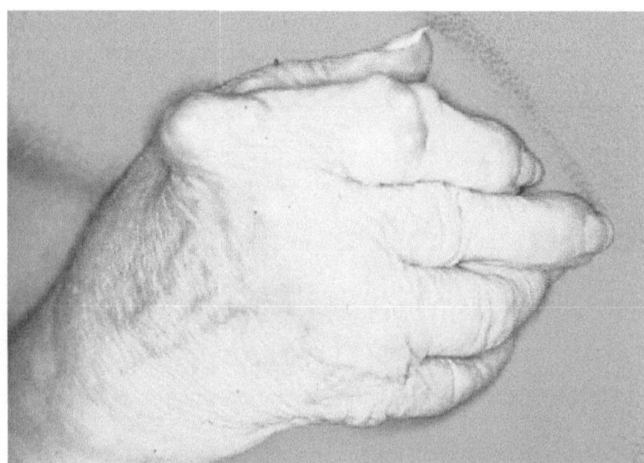

Figure 7.3 Severe arthritis makes oral hygiene and denture insertion difficult.

Considerations: systemic diseases may alter hair colour and texture; watch for sudden hair loss.

Eyes

Examine: sclera; lens; size and characteristics of eyes and lids; conjunctiva.

Considerations: red sclera/allergy and yellow sclera/jaundice; opacities in the lens suggest poor patient vision; exophthalmos and redness or ulcerations of conjunctival surfaces may represent signs of systemic disease.

Ears

Examine: anatomy and palpation.

Considerations: anomalies may suggest mastoiditis; referred mandibular molar pain; myofacial pain dysfunction syndrome.

Lymph nodes

Examine: size, tenderness and mobility. Use bimanual technique.

Considerations: preauricular or postauricular lymphadenopathy may suggest infections of scalp, eyes or temporal or frontal areas. Submental, submandibular or cervical nodes portend oral or pharyngeal infections, autoimmune diseases or tumours (benign or malignant).

Temporomandibular joint and muscles of mastication

Examine: tenderness, joint sounds, maximum opening distance and jaw movements. *Considerations*: pain, crepitus, clicking, trismus or deviations when opening or closing may suggest muscle dysfunction, internal joint inflammation or derangements, neoplasm, trauma, arthritis, dislocation, ankylosis or arthrosis.

Parotid gland

Examine: anatomy and surface characteristics. Milk gland to evaluate clarity, consistency and amount of secretion.

Considerations: enlargement, nodules and pain.

Sinuses

Examine: palpation and percussion testing.

Considerations: sinusitis and referred maxillary molar and premolar pain.

Neck

Examine: visual inspection and palpation.

Considerations: thyroid enlargement; jugular vein distension, use of accessory muscles of respiration; lymphadenopathy, forceful pulsations (hypertension or thyrotoxicosis); and expansile pulse (aneurysm).

Breath

Examine: halitosis.

Considerations: poor hygiene, periodontal disease, caries, chronic sinusitis, acute necrotizing gingivostomatitis (ANUG), hairy or coated tongue, systemic diseases (diabetes, uraemia, upper respiratory disease) and external factors (alcohol, drugs, garlic).

Intraoral and perioral soft and hard tissue examination

Soft tissue and dry mouth evaluation

The lips and corners of the mouth are usually examined first for mucosal changes (ulcers, erythroplakia, leukoplakia, exophytic lesions), areas of swelling or enlargement and evidence of actinic cheilitis (degenerative changes, especially in the vermilion of the lower lip) (Figure 7.4). The corners of the mouth may present with inflammation and redness, a crusty appearance or fissures characteristic of

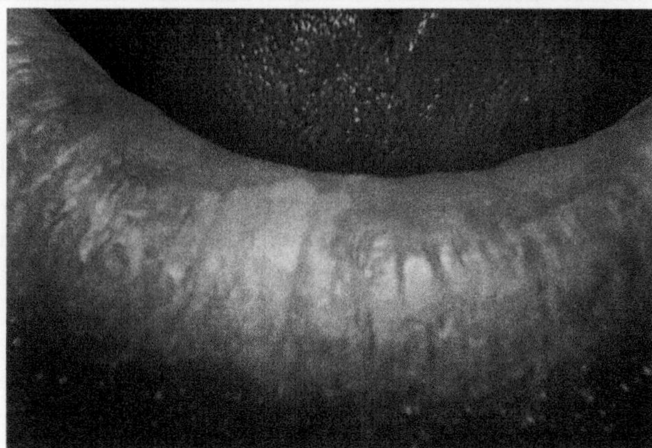

Figure 7.4 Actinic cheilitis (solar cheilitis) on lower lip.

angular cheilitis (often associated with nutritional deficiencies, vertical dimension loss, extension of oral bacterial or fungal infections, drooling, and local habits). Herpes simplex, squamous cell carcinomas, trauma, chancres and systemic pigmentation associated with Addison's disease and Peutz–Jeghers syndrome are all atypical findings.

Areas of tenderness and induration should be identified by palpation of the buccal mucosa and mucobuccal folds. Assessment of lesions, colour and salivary duct openings opposite the second maxillary premolar (Stensen's duct) is necessary. Long-term use of corticosteroids, antibiotics and cytotoxic agents may be associated with the presence of opportunistic *Candida albicans* infection. These lesions are typically soft, white and slightly elevated non-fixed plaques (Figure 7.5) but may also be areas of erythroplakia. A culture should be taken to determine the causative agent if doubt exists. Radiating white striae characteristically surrounding painful, eroded, variable-sized areas are indicative of erosive lichen planus, which may be secondarily infected with *Candida*.

The dorsal, ventral and lateral surfaces of the tongue (which is handled with a gauze square) should be closely inspected for atypical size, colour, papillae, coatings, lesions and tremors or movements. The floor of the mouth and contiguous structures should also be examined and palpated. The most frequent sites of oral cancer in the United States population (representing more than half of intraoral carcinomas) are the lateral border and base of the tongue.

Mouth dryness should also be noted when the tongue and adjacent structures are examined (see also Chapter 19). Older adults frequently present with either acute or chronic salivary flow reduction. Look for pooling of saliva in the floor of the mouth. It is easy to identify whether this is absent or present during the course of the examination. Generalized dryness and a red, pale or atrophic tissue appearance, as well as a fissured or inflamed tongue devoid of papillae may signal a dry mouth. The patient, besides describing a possible dry or burning sensation, may have difficulty with eating, tasting, speaking and the use of dentures. Mucosal infections may also be apparent, as well as multiple carious lesions, which are usually found at the gingival margins. Clinical assessment of function may be aided by palpating or 'milking' the major salivary glands. The quantity and quality, such as pus, viscosity and casts, should be observed at duct entrances (Wharton's and Stensen's). Patients with gland hypofunction may not have the same subjective complaints predictive of dry mouth. The dentist can ask specific questions to help identify the patients with salivary problems (Box 7.7) [31].

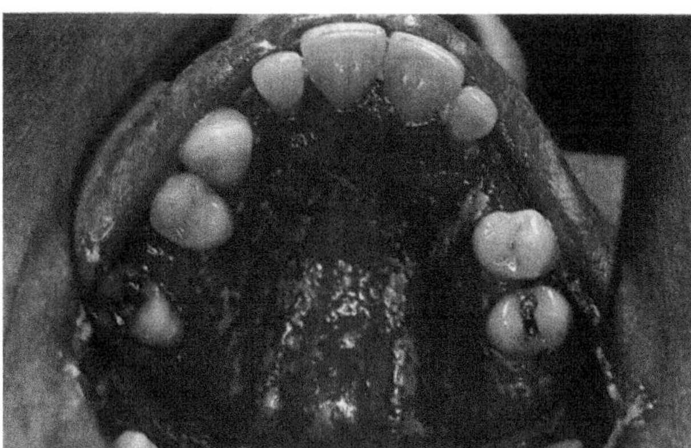

Figure 7.5 Acute pseudomembraneus candidiasis on palate.

Box 7.7 Questions to identify salivary problems.[a]

1 Do you have difficulty swallowing food?
2 Are fluids necessary to help you swallow dry food?
3 Is your mouth dry when eating?
4 Does it seem as if the amount of saliva in your mouth is too little most of the time?

[a]Reference [31].

Medication use is the most common cause of mouth dryness in this age group. Additional causes may be radiotherapy, dehydration, emotional stress, salivary gland infection or malignancy, surgery, diabetes, anaemia, avitaminosis and collagen vascular diseases (for example, Sjögren's syndrome).

Both the soft and hard palate should be palpated and examined for lesions and symmetry. Erythema should be noted on all tissues covered by removable prostheses. Denture stomatitis may be indicated by either an erythematous granular or a smooth appearance. The strength of motion of the soft palate should also be evaluated. Documentation of the size, shape (e.g. pedunculated), colour, consistency, contour, surface, bleeding, pain and three-dimensional location of all oral lesions should be made.

Depressing the tongue with a mirror or tongue blade allows for better visualization of the oropharynx. Exudate, colour, masses and the gag reflex should be ascertained. There should be no enlargement or inflammation of the palatine tonsils.

Tooth structure loss, caries and restorations

Attrition (occlusal wear) (Figure 7.6), erosion and abrasion (nonocclusal frictional factors) and resultant tooth structure loss are very prevalent in older adults. Approximately 75%

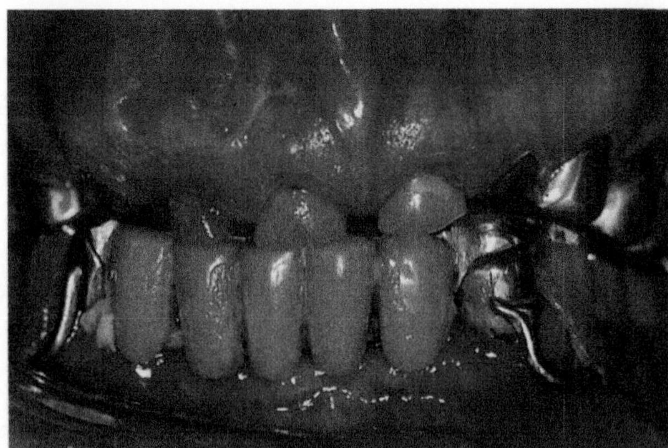

Figure 7.6 Severe attrition.

of the examined elderly people living in a community-based study had at least one tooth that had all the incisal or occlusal enamel lost to attrition, and 4% had at least one tooth worn down to the gingiva [32]. Abrasion had resulted in notable loss of tooth structure in 30% of the participants. Tooth fractures, significant areas of abrasion and attrition, as well as chemically-induced tooth loss (erosion) should be noted during the examination. In order to control and minimize tooth structure loss, occlusal problems and dysfunction of the temporomandibular joint, the precipitating factors should be determined and efforts made to control their etiology.

Both coronal and root caries are prevalent in older adults (Figure 7.7; see Chapter 15). The Iowa Study showed that 77% of the dentate subjects presented with a new coronal or root caries lesion in 3 years [33]. Factors influencing this high rate included malaligned and shifting teeth, faulty restorations, recession of gingival tissues, mouth dryness, medications, poor oral hygiene, change in diet and partial denture design or clasps. Identification of these carious lesions is accomplished by careful clinical and radiographic examination. Frank lesion (gross cavitation) diagnosis is generally quite easy. However, in the absence of radiographic confirmation, incipient lesions at proximal surfaces not accessible to direct visual-tactile examination are more difficult to identify. An active caries process cannot be confirmed by the presence of only pigmentation or stain.

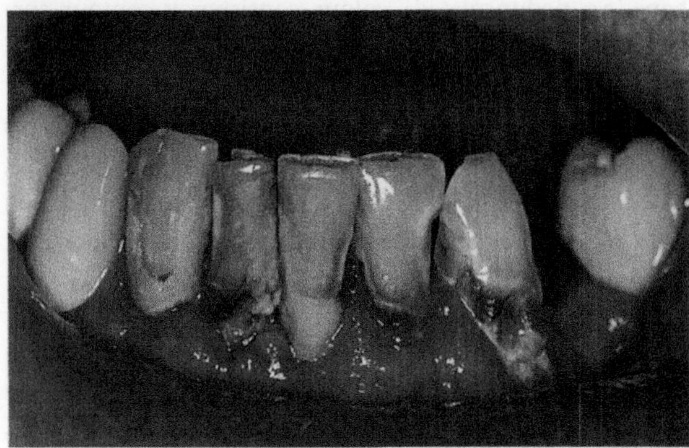

Figure 7.7 Active coronal and root caries in mandibular anterior teeth.

Coronal pit-and-fissure lesions should be recorded when the explorer catches in the grooves and when the catch is accompanied by softness at the area base and adjacent enamel or opacity indicative of demineralization or undermining. Evidence of softness, which is obtained by scraping the enamel with an explorer, should be recorded on smooth surface lesions, in addition to visual inspection of demineralization (white lesion or decalcification). A discontinuity of enamel with explorer-confirmed softness should be identified for proximal surfaces. Anterior proximal lesions can be detected by transillumination. Failing restorations (restorations with marginal defects or fractures that may or may not be associated with caries) and nonrestored surfaces are fairly equal causes for coronal and interproximal lesions.

Root caries is usually found on virgin root surfaces exposed by gingival recession, but may also appear adjacent to previous restorations. Buccal and proximal surfaces are the most common sites for root caries lesions, which generally develop coronally to the current gingival margin. The gingival pocket is the site of only a few lesions. These subgingival root caries lesions may be located proximate to marginal gingival inflammation. They may initially appear as small, round lesions that spread laterally and coalesce to form a collar around the tooth. These lesions undermine the enamel by creating a ledge but do not directly affect the outer enamel. Enamel fracture is facilitated by more advanced lesions, which gives the impression that the caries developed both in the root and coronal portion of the tooth. Such lesions are often found under moderate to heavy accumulations of plaque and much less frequently under calculus deposits.

The diagnostic criteria for defining and characterizing active versus arrested root caries lesions are discussed in Chapter 15. When potential root carious lesions are evaluated, modification of the standard approach to coronal caries detection should be considered. Cementum seems to present the tactile sensation of yielding to the explorer tip under firm pressure because it is less dense than enamel. To distinguish carious from sound cementum, it is necessary to feel for greater comparative softness associated with the lesion, as well as easy explorer removal with no withdrawal resistance or sticking. All root surfaces should be examined carefully. Vertical bitewing radiographs may be helpful in identifying interproximal root surface lesions, but not buccal or lingual surface root surface lesions.

The periodontium

Severe periodontal disease in dentate elderly people is probably less common than might be presumed [34]. Conservative long-term periodontal management can maintain teeth with appreciable loss of the supporting tissues (see Chapter 17). Several parameters must be considered and recorded in a thorough periodontal examination. These include the location and degree of gingival bleeding and inflammation, and associated plaque and calculus build-up (slight, moderate or heavy). The relative positioning of opposing and proximal teeth, as well as inadequate proximal contact and marginal ridge relationships, should be examined and charted. These areas can be identified by impaction of food. All remaining teeth should be charted using 6–8 periodontal probings per tooth for pocketing as well as recession (Figure 7.8) to calculate periodontal attachment loss. The anterior teeth mobility may be tested by placing the handles of the dental mirror on both the lingual and labial surfaces to transmit alternate directional force. Vertical displacement is elicited by pressure on the occlusal or incisal surface. A large sickle scaler can be used to exert directional force to assess posterior teeth.

Bone loss with bifurcation or trifurcation involvement with multirooted teeth should also be recorded. Classifications are: (a) Incipient – slight bone loss; (b) Class 1 – definite bone loss; (c) Class 2 – moderate to severe bone loss extending deeply under the tooth; and (d) Class 3 – through and through, i.e. very severe bone loss extending from one furcation entrance to another.

Periapical and bitewing radiography is used to determine the level of supporting bone. The lamina dura (a thin radiopaque line) that surrounds the roots of the teeth should be closely inspected. Periodontal disease may be implied by a lack of continuity. Traumatic occlusion may be indicated by a widening of the periodontal ligament space at the apex and contralateral side. Wide periodontal spaces suggest mobile teeth. If bone levels are more than 1.5 mm apical to the cemento-enamel junction, a diagnosis of horizontal bone loss can be made. A specific periodontal diagnosis (such as normal, gingivitis or periodontitis: early, moderate or advanced; localized or generalized) should be recorded for each tooth. In addition, serous, purulent or bloody discharge from periodontal pockets upon palpation should be noted. Buccal or lingual swelling and additional evidence of periodontal abscess formation, should also be recorded.

Alveolar ridge

Extensive alveolar bone changes are common in partially or fully edentulous elderly people. The mandibular alveolar crest height loss can approach 1 cm (Figure 7.9). The dentist should determine and record alveolar ridge characteristics, including the shape, size, alveolar mucosa integrity, tuberosities, interarch distance and the degree of bony resorption associated with tooth loss. The necessary surgical intervention may be determined from this information, and the future soft- and hard-tissue changes and prosthesis prognosis may be predicted (see Chapter 22).

Occlusion

There should be a clinical and laboratory component to the occlusal examination. During opening and closing of the mouth, deviations and deflections associated with maxillary and mandibular midlines should be checked. The maximum opening can be measured with a Boley gauge or a plastic prosthodontic ruler (40–60 mm is the normal range). The Boley gauge can also measure overbite (maxillary and mandibular incisor vertical overlap), overjet (maxillary and mandibular incisor horizontal overlap) and intraocclusal distance (the difference between the vertical dimension of rest position and the vertical dimension of maximum

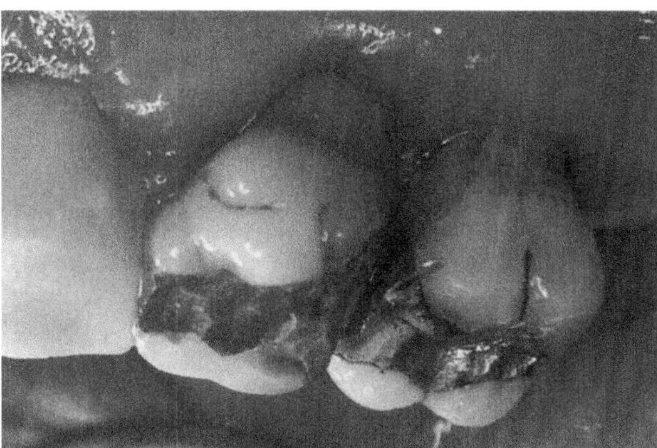

Figure 7.8 Maxillary molar lingual recession contributing to moderate to severe periodontal attachment loss.

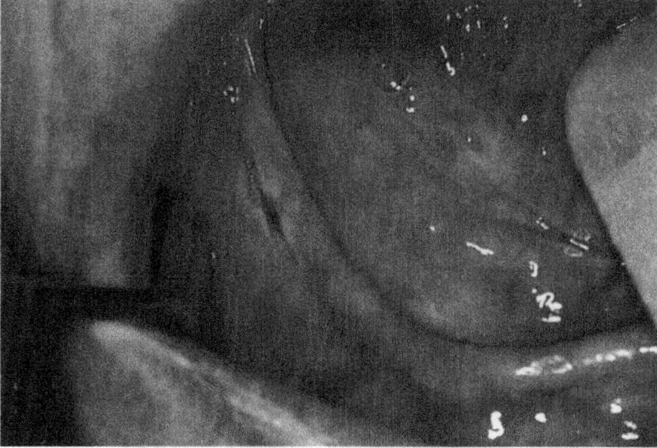

Figure 7.9 Atrophic mandibular posterior ridge with evidence of leukoplakia caused by chronic trauma.

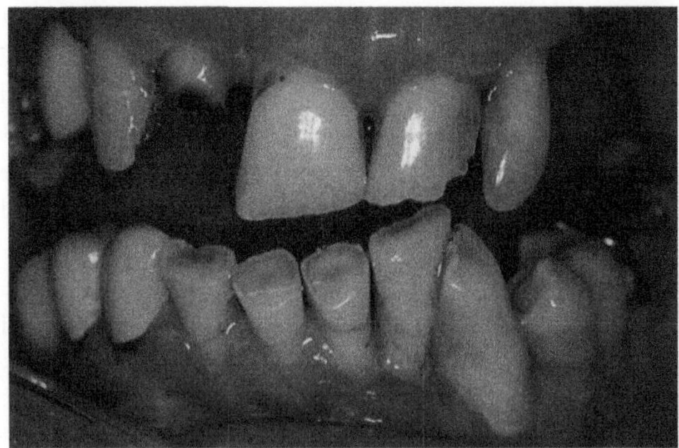

Figure 7.10 Malaligned occlusion and fractured teeth in an older adult.

intercuspation). In adults, normal spacing can vary from 0 to 11 mm, but 2–3 mm is adequate for proper function. Notations should also be made of anterior and posterior crossbites, end-to-end relationships, open bites, Angle's molar relationship classification (Class 1 – normal, Class 2 – disto-occlusion and Class 3 – mesio-occlusion) and discrepancies between the centric relation and centric occlusion. Dysfunctional occlusion can be identified by (1) tooth mobility and migration; (2) pain in the temporomandibular joint, periodontium or tooth; (3) alterations in the lamina dura; (4) widening of the periodontal membrane space; and (5) atypical occlusal wear (Figure 7.10). These clinical findings suggest problems but do not strongly predict actual chewing impairment. Asking whether the patient can chew apples or hard rolls may help to quantify chewing deficits.

Mounted diagnostic casts can be used when appropriate to more closely study the size, shape and position of the teeth, occlusal facets and supporting tissue structures. Wear patterns, deflecting contacts and tooth-to-arch relationships not obvious during clinical examination can be ascertained using a face-bow transfer and an adjustable articulator.

Diagnostic aids

Radiographic evaluation is one of the more important diagnostic tools in oral assessment (Box 7.8). Radiographs are invaluable in identifying caries, periapical lesions, periodontal disease and intraosseous lesions when coupled with clinical examination and case history. Radiographs also aid in evaluating the sinus, preprosthetic assessment, identification of trauma and detection of other abnormalities. It may be difficult to recognize recurrent or secondary caries in older adults because radiopaque restorations may mask new lesions. Proper vertical angulation is necessary to obtain diagnostic radiographs. A cupped-out or notched-out appearance of an ill-defined radio-lucency may identify root caries. Cervical burnout may occasionally be misinterpreted as cemental caries, and precise clinical examination is necessary if in doubt. The radiographic display of the pulp is important in identifying calcifications, evidence of resorption, periapical lesions (Figure 7.11) and diminished chamber size. Evidence of chronic periodontal disease (alveolar bone resorption on the distal and mesial surfaces) and occlusal trauma (periodontal ligament space thickening) may also be visualized radiographically.

Box 7.8 Assessment tools for oral examination.

Caries	Periodontal disease	Oral pathology
Visual: pigmentation; stain; caries indicator solution	Visual: recession; bone loss	Visual: size; shape; colour; pain, bleeding, 3D location
Explorer examination	Palpation: tooth mobility	Palpation
Radiographs	Periodontal probing	Oral exfoliative cytology
Transillumination	Radiographs	Biopsy: excisional; incisional; fine needle aspiration; toluidine blue staining
Pulp testing: thermal; electric	Laboratory testing: microbiological bacterial and inflammatory marker tests (e.g. CRP, IL1β, TNFα)	Oral candidiasis cultures
Laboratory testing: microbiological caries activity tests (bacterial) Salivary flow evaluation		

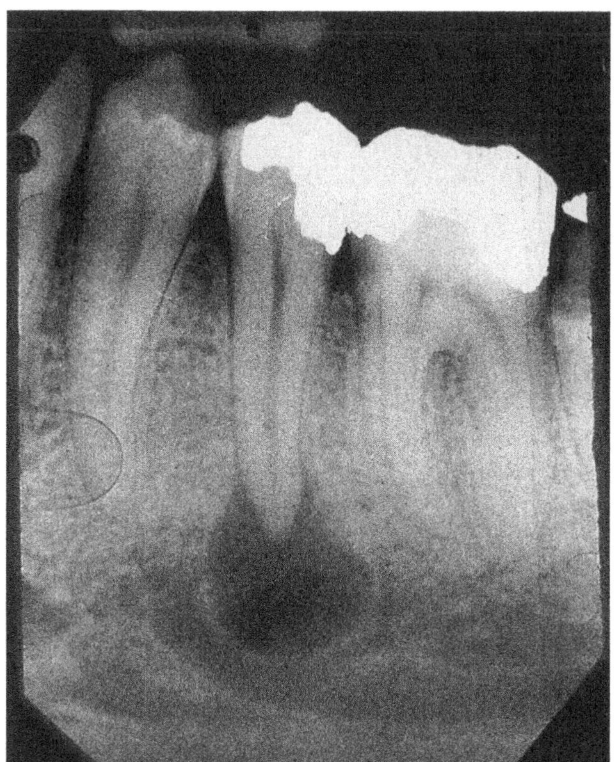

Figure 7.11 Radiograph of lower left second premolar demonstrating significant periapical pathology.

There are several recommendations for effective radiographic assessment [35]. Radiographs cannot replace a complete clinical examination, including patient history. Radiographs should be individualized and based on high-yield selection criteria, including previous periodontal or endodontic therapy, the presence of implants, clinical evidence of periodontal disease or deep carious lesions, a history of pain or trauma, swelling, tooth mobility, a deep or large restoration and the presence of other intraoral findings such as salivary hypofunction. When evaluating restorative, periodontal and endodontic needs, panoramic radiographs are usually less effective than intraoral films. Panoramic radiographs, however, play a very important role in the examination for pathological conditions that are not visible clinically or with intraoral radiographs. A current panograph (within 6 months) should be considered by the dentist prior to the fabrication of complete dentures. For dentate patients, the initial examination usually requires a comprehensive set of radiographs (bitewing and periapical radiographs). Full-mouth intraoral radiographs or a panoramic radiograph are usually indicated for the edentate patient. Dentate recall patients at lower risk (no caries within past 2 to 3 years and no periodontitis) should have posterior bitewings at 2- to 3-year intervals, whereas patients with high caries risk need them every 12 to 18 months. In areas where clinical periodontal signs are present, periodontal recall patients should have individualized examination using periapical and/or bitewing radiographs.

Pulp assessment is necessary when patients complain of pain, when radiographs display periapical radiolucencies and when there is soft-tissue swelling or fistulas (see also Chapter 16). It is also required when the tooth is discoloured and prior to crown preparation or the abutment designation of fixed or removable prostheses. Percussion sensitivity usually suggests an acute apical lesion, but may also signal a chronic pathological condition. Hot and cold thermal testing can aid in the diagnosis of pulpalgia, both moderate and advanced. Thermal testing is of little help in diagnosing periapical problems. Electric pulp testing is probably the most effective method of determining pulp vitality in younger patients. However, for elderly people, the positive and negative predictive value of pulp testing (likelihood that the tooth is vital when it tests positively and likelihood that the tooth is nonvital when it tests negatively) is not as consistent. Due to sclerosed pulp chambers, older adults may have vital teeth that respond negatively when tested. Measurement may also be made difficult by teeth with full-coverage restorations and large restorations. The dentist must use several different examinations, tests and radiographs to achieve an accurate diagnosis.

Laboratory testing is an additional method of assessing older patients. Some laboratory tests can be performed in the dental office while others require referral to a laboratory or physician. Laboratory tests, stemming from chairside recognition of systemic and local pathological processes, can provide valuable information for the dentist in making a diagnosis. These tests include microbiological testing (direct examination of oral specimens, throat cultures, antibiotic sensitivity tests, caries activity tests, oral candidiasis cultures and root canal and root apex cultures); blood tests, including blood sugar, serology, haematology, blood chemistry and immunohaematology; urinalysis to test for renal diseases, diabetes mellitus and hyperthyroidism; contact allergy testing; oral exfoliative cytology; and oral biopsy, excisional and incisional with aspiration.

Biopsy is the most accurate method of diagnosing soft-tissue lesions. If the dentist is not comfortable performing the biopsy, the patient may be referred to a dentist who is more familiar with soft tissue biopsies (e.g. oral medicine specialist, oral pathologist, oral and maxillofacial surgeon). Excisional biopsy is the best method for relatively small, well-defined lesions, although oral pathologists do not need a large specimen for accurate diagnosis. Multiple incisional biopsies may be indicated for larger or diffuse lesions. Oral exfoliative cytology, fine needle aspiration (FNA), brush biopsy, vital dyes and stains (toluidine blue), chemiluminescence, fibre-optic transillumination and direct optical fluorescence may also be used for diagnostic reasons.

Prosthetic evaluation

A careful evaluation should be made in situations where missing teeth require restoration for optimum function. Decisions on when and how to restore edentulous areas should be made after careful examinations of the maxilla and mandible and their existing skeletal and dental relationships. Impressions and mounted study models are essential to this assessment, as are the appropriate radiographs (including CT scans if implants are considered). (For more detail, see Chapter 14 on treatment planning.)

When existing prostheses are present, they should be carefully evaluated. Patient speech patterns should be noted initially. Inadequately articulated 's' sounds as well as clicks and whistles may denote several problems: significant soft/hard tissue changes that have occurred since the prosthesis was fabricated, impaired oral-muscular function or an improperly fabricated denture [36]. The aesthetic appearance of the dentures should also be examined. When the prosthesis is removed, evaluate for: (1) denture defects (cracks, missing teeth, worn teeth or denture base); (2) denture adhesive usage; (3) the presence of denture identification; and (4) the presence of food debris, plaque or calculus. Clinical examination for potential prosthesis-related pathology is also important. This includes angular cheilitis, denture stomatitis, traumatic ulcers, inflammatory and peripheral hyperplasia, severe alveolar ridge resorption and movable fibrotic tissue (epulis fissuratum).

When the prosthesis is reinserted, the functional aspects of the denture should be assessed. They include: (1) stability (resistance to pressure applied in a horizontal direction); (2) retention (resistance to pressure applied in a vertical direction); (3) the vertical dimension of occlusion (the amount of interocclusal distance available); (4) occlusal contacts; (5) peripheral border extensions; and (6) the relative positioning of maxillary and/or mandibular prostheses (Figure 7.12).

Patient perception is also very important. Queries should be made regarding satisfaction with denture aesthetics, function and comfort as well as any desire for receiving additional prosthodontic treatment to address deficiencies. It is conceivable that important mitigating factors (for example, the patient's perceived needs, severe residual ridge resorption, severe impairments, mouth dryness) may overrule treatment for objective prosthesis deficiencies.

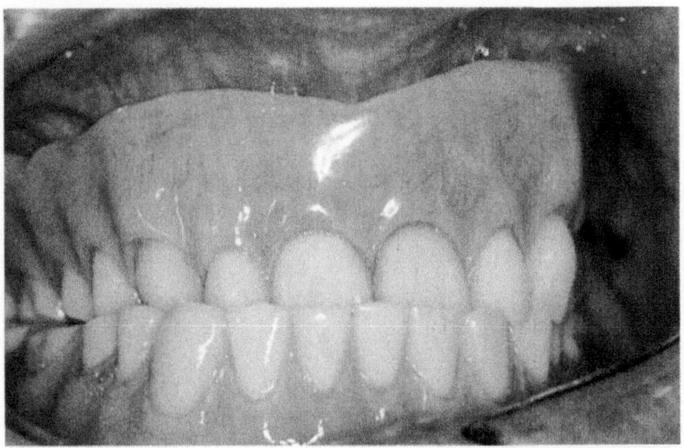

Figure 7.12 Severely worn prostheses with subsequent dysfunctional shift in mandibular position.

Differential

The differential is a list of diagnoses for the patient either based upon the information collected, or suspected, and that requires further evaluation. The differential directs the clinician to Plan (below).

Plan

The plan, directed by the differential, outlines what additional (if necessary) tests and consultations are required. The plan also lists all treatments performed at that visit. The treatment plan developed from the assessment information should include both short and long term goals. Consideration should be given to the patient's desires, function, aesthetics, finances, removal of infection and oral and systemic risk factors for further oral disease. Continual refinement of the treatment plan occurs as accurate diagnoses are established, information organized and goals prioritized to fit the patient's needs and desires. A complete discussion of treatment planning is in Chapter 14.

Conclusion

Thorough assessment has been described as the keystone of geriatric medicine and dentistry. The dentist must determine which factors directly influence the physical, psychosocial and dental health outcomes associated with older adults. Dental examination strategies should identify objective clinical signs and subjective patient perceptions, as well as other important prognostic factors affecting potential treatment approaches. The diseases and conditions mentioned here, as well as approaches to their prevention and treatment, are reviewed comprehensively in the subsequent chapters.

References

1 Jack, S.S. & Ries, P.W. (eds) (1981) National Center for Health Statistics, Public Health Service. Current estimates from the National Health Interview Survey, United States, 1979. *Vital and Health Statistics Series 10*, No. 136, DHHS Pub. No. (PHS) 81-1564. US Government Printing Office, Washington, DC.

2 National Institute on Aging, National Institute of Health. (2007) *Growing old in America: The health and retirement study*. US Department of Health and Human Services. NIH Publication No. 07-5757.

3 Pleis, J.R. & Lethbridge-Çejku, M. (2006) Summary health statistics for U.S. adults: National health interview survey, 2005. National Center for Health Statistics, *Vital Health Statistics*, Series 10 (Number 232).

4 Cluff, L.F. (1964) Chronic disease, function and quality of care. *Journal of Chronic Diseases*, **34**, 299–304.

5 Williamson, J., Stokoe, I.H., Gray, S., Fisher, M., Smith, A., Mcghee, A. *et al.* (1964) Old people at home: their unreported needs. *Lancet*, **283**, 1117–1120.

6 Wilson, L.A., Lawson, I.R. & Brass, W. (1962) Multiple disorders in the elderly: a clinical and statistical study. *Lancet*, **280**, 841–843.

7 Guralnik, J.M., LaCroix, A.Z., Everett, D.F. & Kovar, M.G. (1989) Aging in the eighties: the prevalence of comorbidity and its association with disability. *Advance Data from Vital and Health Statistics*, No. 170. National Center for Health Statistics, Hyattsville, MD.

8 Fried, L.P. & Wallace, R.B. (1992) The complexity of chronic illness in the elderly: from clinic to community. In: R.B. Wallace & R.F. Woolson (ed) *Methodologic issues in the epidemiologic study of the elderly*. pp. 10–19, Oxford University Press, New York, NY.

9 Besdine, R.W. (1988) Clinical approach to the elderly patient. In: J.W. Rowe & R.W. Besdine (eds), *Geriatric medicine*. pp. 23–36, 2nd edn, Little, Brown & Company, Boston, MA.

10 Katz, S., Ford, A., Moskowitz, R., Jackson, B. & Jaffe, M.W. Studies of illness in the aged. The index of ADL: A standardized measure of biological and psychosocial function. *JAMA*, **185**, 914–919.

11 Besdine, R.W. (1980) Geriatric medicine: an overview. *Annual Review of Gerontology & Geriatrics*, **1**, 135–153.

12 Besdine, R.W., Levkoff, S.E. & Wetle, T. (1984) Health and illness behaviors in elder veterans. In: T. Wetle & J.W. Rowe (eds), *Older veterans: linking VA and community resources*. pp. 1–33, Harvard University Press Cambridge, MA.

13 Mechanic, D. (1978) *Medical sociology*, 2nd edn, Free Press, New York, NY.

14 Levkoff, S.E., Cleary, P.D., Wetle, T. & Besdine, R.W. (1988) Illness behavior in the aged: implications for clinicians. *Journal of the American Geriatric Society*, **36**, 622–629.

15 Shanas, E. (1962) *The health of older people*. Harvard University Press, Cambridge, MA.

16 Brody, E.M. (1985) Tomorrow and tomorrow and tomorrow: toward squaring the suffering curve. In: C.M. Gaitz, G. Niederehe & N.L. Wilson (eds) *Aging 2000: our health care destiny*. pp. 371–380, Vol. **II**, Springer-Verlag, New York.

17 Stenback, A., Kumpulainen, M. & Vauhkonen, M.L. (1978) Illness and health behavior in septuagenarians. *Journal of Gerontology*, **33**, 57–61.

18 Watson, G.R. (2003) Assessment and Rehabilitation of Older Adults with Low Vision. In: W.R. Hazzard, *et al.* (eds), *Principles of Geriatric Medicine and Gerontology*, pp. 1223–1237, Ch. 95, 5th edn, McGraw-Hill, New York, NY. ISBN: 0-07-140216-0.

19 Reuben, D.B. (1999) Principles of Geriatric Assessment. In: W.R. Hazzard *et al.* (eds) *Principles of Geriatric Medicine and Gerontology*, p. 467, Part 2, Ch. 33, 4th edn, McGraw-Hill: New York, NY.

20 Berkey, D.B. & Holtzman, J.M. (1987) Oral health. In: R. Ham (ed) *Geriatric medicine annual 1987*. pp. 222–236, Medical Economics Books, Oradell, NJ.

21 Little, J.W., Falace, D.A., Miller, C.S. & Rhodus, N.L. (2007) *Dental management of the medically compromised patient*, 7th edn, Mosby, St. Louis, MO.

22 Wettermark, B., Hammar, N., MichaelFored, C., Leimanis, A., Otterblad Olausson, P., Bergman U. *et al.* (2007) The new Swedish Prescribed Drug Register-opportunities for pharmacoepidemiological research and experience from the first six months. *Pharmacoepidemiology and Drug Safety*, **16**, 726–735.

23 Lippincott Williams and Wilkins (2007) *Drug facts and comparisons 2008*, 62nd edn, Lippincott Williams and Wilkins, St. Louis, MO.

24 Thomson Healthcare (2007) *Physician's desk reference 2008*, 62nd edn, Thomson Healthcare, Montvale, NJ.

25 Berkman, L.F. (1986) Social networks, support, and health: taking the next step forward. *American Journal of Epidemiology*, **123**, 559–562.

26 Keeler, E.B., Solomon, D.H., Beck, J.C., Mendenhall, R.C. & Kane, R.L. (1982) Effect of patient age on duration of medical encounters with physicians. *Medical Care*, **20**, 1101–1108.

27 Lipsitz, L.A. (1989) Orthostatic hypotension in the elderly. *New England Journal of Medicine*, **321**, 952–957.

28 Ham, R. (1987) Alzheimer's and the family. In: R. Ham (ed) *Geriatric medicine annual 1987*. pp. 73–103, Medical Economics Books, Oradell, NJ.

29 Folstein, M.F., Folstein, S.F. & McHugh, P.R. (1975) "Mini-Mental State": a practical method for grading the cognitive state of patients for clinicians. *Journal of Psychiatric Research*, **12**, 189–198.

30 Anthony, J.C., LeResche, L., Niaz, U., van Korff, M.R. & Folstein, M.F. (1982) Limits of the "Mini-Mental State" as a screening test for dementia and delirium among hospital patients. *Psychological Medicine*, **12**, 397–408.

31 Fox, P.C., Bush, K.A. & Baum, B.J. (1987) Subjective reports of xerostomia and objective measures of salivary gland performance. *Journal of the American Dental Association*, **115**, 581–584.

32 Beck, J.D. & Hunt, R.J. (1985) Oral health status in the United States: problems of special patients. *Journal of Dental Education*, **49**, 407–425.

33 Hand, J.S., Hunt, R.J. & Beck, J.D. (1988) Coronal and root caries in older Iowans: 36-month incidence. *Gerodontics*, **4**, 136–139.
34 Hunt, R.J. (1986) Periodontal treatment needs in an elderly population in Iowa. *Gerodontics*, **2**, 24–27.
35 Kantor, M.L., Zeichner, S.J., Valachovic, R.W. & Reiskin, A.B. (1989) Efficacy of dental radiographic practices: options for image receptors, examination selection, and patient selection. *Journal of the American Dental Association*, **119**, 259–268.
36 Gordon, S.R. & Jahnigen, D.W. (1983) Oral assessment of the edentulous elderly patient. *Journal of the American Geriatric Society*, **31**, 797–801.

CHAPTER 8

Medical issues in the dental care of older adults

Peter B. Lockhart[1] and Scott Furney[2]
[1]Department of Oral Medicine, Carolinas Medical Center, Charlotte, NC
[2]Department of Internal Medicine, Carolinas Medical Center, Charlotte, NC

The elderly patient

The status of the maxillofacial and oral-pharngeal tissues can have a significant impact on systemic health and overall well-being in the elderly patient. It is unusual to find an older patient without any evidence of oral disease, and every effect should be made to prevent and treat caries and periodontal disease, except in certain circumstances when the risk/benefit ratio does not justify dental care. Although the link between oral and systemic disease (e.g. atherosclerosis) is controversial and unresolved, we can assume that elderly patients are at greater risk from acute and chronic oral infection due to multiple medications and medical disorders, more compromised immune function, age-related impaired renal, liver and cardiovascular function, and a greater likelihood of life threatening illnesses such as infective endocarditis. Therefore, it is incumbent on the dentist providing care to the elderly patient to conduct an appropriate medical history and review of systems, and to have an understanding of common medical problems that influence the delivery of oral health care services.

The medical history

Introduction

The goal of the medical history is to obtain sufficient information from the patient and other sources (e.g. medical records, family) to ensure that the nature and manner of dental care delivery is appropriate (Box 8.1). The vast majority of medical urgencies or emergencies in the dental office are avoided by understanding the patient's medical status and its implications for appropriate dental care.

Box 8.1 Points for taking a medical history.

- Remember that the patient and/or family might not understand the need for an accurate medical history in the dental setting and this needs to be explained.
- Be persistent but patient.
- If you need to use an interpreter, try to use a professional health care interpreter and not members of the patient's family.
- If you need to gain consent for intellectually impaired patients, make sure that the person whose consent you gain (parent/guardian) has the legal authority to provide consent.

History taking

There is an art to eliciting accurate information from patients and it requires practice and attention to detail. Once this is accomplished, there may be gaps that necessitate contacting the patients' medical provider(s) for additional information and discussion. This will help establish the medical risk for different levels of dental procedures, and the need for additional precautions such as antibiotic prophylaxis, sedation or adjustment of medications.

Elements of the history

There is a time-honoured content and format for history taking and it includes the following elements.

Past medical history

Hospitalizations: dates, reason(s) for admission, and outcomes.
Operations: dates, reason(s) for surgery and findings.
Allergies: drugs, foods, latex.

Textbook of Geriatric Dentistry, Third Edition. Edited by Poul Holm-Pedersen, Angus W. G. Walls and Jonathan A. Ship.

Medications: drugs of particular concern include
- immunosuppressives (e.g. steroids, cancer chemotherapy, organ antirejection drugs).
- antibiotics, antifungals, antivirals.
- anticoagulants (e.g. warfarin, antiplatelet drugs).

Helpful questions include:
- 'Are you being treated by your doctor for any medical conditions?' Ascertain how stable or severe the condition is and the extent to which it interferes with daily living activities.
- 'Have you been treated in the past, or are you currently being treated for ... ' (key medical conditions that have importance for the dental setting).

Specific questioning about hospitalizations, operations, allergies and current medications will elicit most medical history of consequence to dental practice and it can be used to supplement the standard health questionnaires.

Review of systems

The following is a list of points that would be covered for a complete review of systems. Although generally unnecessary in the outpatient setting, it can be used to obtain significant additional information not elicited in the past medical history. A positive ('Yes') response should be probed in depth and significant negatives ('No') should also be noted.

General: weight loss or gain; anorexia; general health throughout life; strength and energy; fever; chills; or night sweats.

Cardiovascular: palpitations; chest pain and radiation; history of myocardial infarction; orthopnoea (number of pillows); hypertension; oedema; phlebitis; murmur; exercise tolerance; cardiac valve prosthesis; or history of endocarditis.

Respiratory: cough (type); haemoptysis; dyspnea; wheezing; pneumonia; asthma; seasonal allergies; bronchitis; or emphysema.

Neurological: loss of smell; taste or vision; muscle weakness or wasting; muscle stiffness; paraesthesia or anaesthesias; lack of coordination; tremors; seizures; syncope; fatigue; aphasias; memory changes; or paralysis.

Psychiatric/emotional: general mood; problems with 'nerves'; bruxism/clenching; insomnia; or medications.

Endocrine: hot/cold intolerance; voice change; polydypsia; polyuria; polyphagia.

Gastrointestinal: appetite; food intolerance; abdominal pains; nausea or vomiting; haematemesis; hepatitis; jaundice; spleen or liver problems; alcohol abuse; or ulcers.

Genitourinary: urinary tract infections; incontinence.

Musculoskeletal: trauma; fractures; arthritis; inflamed joints; arthralgias; myalgias; muscle weakness; limitation of motion; or joint prosthesis.

Dermatological: pigmentation changes; jaundice; lesions; or biopsies.

Head, eyes, ears, nose, throat (HEENT):
- Head: headache; fainting; nausea or vomiting; vertigo; dizziness; pains in head or face; or trauma.
- Eyes: vision; glasses; diplopia; blurring; pain; dryness; burning; or photophobia.
- Ears: decreased hearing or deafness; pain.
- Nose: epistaxis; stuffiness; hay fever; colds; or change in sense of smell or taste.
- Mouth and throat: pain; sore throat; dental pain; dental hygiene history; bleeding or painful gums; sore areas or lesions of the mouth; bad taste; loose teeth; halitosis; dysphagia; temporomandibular joint (TMJ) dysfunction; trismus; voice changes; neck stiffness; nodes or lumps; or trauma.

Haematological: increased bruising; bleeding problems; lumps; or anaemia.

Family history

Find out what illnesses grandparents, parents, siblings and children have/had. If any of these relatives are dead, at what age did they die and from what? Ask about family history of tuberculosis, diabetes, heart disease, hypertension, allergies, bleeding problems, jaundice.

Social history

The social history includes the patient's (former) occupation; marital status; children.

Common medical problems in the elderly with consequences for oral health care delivery

I. Allergy

A. Overview

Allergies are of particular importance in dentistry for several reasons, most importantly because a life-threatening reaction (i.e. anaphylaxis) can occur within seconds of exposure to some allergens.

B. Dental management considerations

Patients should be asked about sensitivity to medications, drugs, foods or materials such as latex, especially those drugs that might be used in the course of dental treatment (e.g. antibiotics, codeine, aspirin-containing compounds). In addition, patients should be questioned about a history of asthma or hay fever and if they have a family history of atopy since there is a greater likelihood that the patient will also have allergies.

The first step is to determine the nature of the allergy, to include: the drug and dosage given and other medication(s) taken at the same time to exclude drug interactions. Ask about: the time sequence, that is, how soon after the injection/ingestion/exposure did the response occur?; the reaction (e.g. syncope, tachycardia, peripheral vasodilitation, loss of consciousness, breathing difficulty or rash); and the therapy (e.g. drugs administered and the response to them). You should also record the name(s) of the clinician(s) involved.

After you have determined the nature of the allergy and differentiated it from other drug-related side effects, such as syncope, GI upset and overdose, specific consideration must be given to the following:

1 Allergy to local anaesthetics must be qualified. Although syncope (vasovagal) is not uncommon following anaesthetic injections, lidocaine allergy is extremely rare, or related to another component of the anaesthetic carpule (e.g. a preservative).
2 Although many reactions to drugs and foods are not true allergies, patients should not be challenged with a substance identified as a possible allergen in a non-hospital, uncontrolled setting without personnel with appropriate training in resuscitation, drugs and equipment.
3 In cases of documented or suspected allergy, patients should be referred to an appropriate clinician (clinical immunologist or allergist) for testing and/or desensitization.

II. Bleeding disorders

A. Overview

There are a wide variety of bleeding disorders that are common in the elderly. Although clinically significant oral bleeding is rare, it can occurr with patients with haematological disorders or those taking certain medications. The medical history is critical to identifying the potential for a bleeding disorder and determining the risk of invasive dental procedures. The history will help to determine if the bleeding disorder is the result of an inherited (congenital) or an acquired (from disease or drugs) problem. For example, ask about:

- Prolonged bleeding after an invasive procedure (e.g. tooth extraction). Determine the origin; that is, was it from local factors (e.g. spitting following a tooth extraction) or a systemic cause (medication or disease).
- Liver, renal or bone marrow disease, or underlying malignancy, any of which can result in a coagulopathy.
- Anticoagulant medications (e.g. warfarin, aspirin and other anti-platelet drugs).
- Use of herbal supplements (e.g. Garlic, Ginko, Ginseng), especially when used in combination with anticoagulants.
- Spontaneous oral bleeding is rare in the absence of at least minor trauma and is almost always from the gingival crevice or periodontal pocket.
- Unexplained bleeding, bruising or petechial rash, which could indicate coagulopathy or thrombocytopaenia.

Laboratory testing for a systemic origin of oral bleeding involves familiarity with a limited number of coagulation tests. The major tests are:

- Prothrombin time (PT)/international normalized ratio (INR): measures extrinsic pathway factors and it is most often used to monitor anticoagulation with warfarin. It is also a useful determinant of the potential for bleeding from liver disease. Although somewhat controversial, all but the most invasive of dental procedures, to include a limited number of extractions, can be accomplished safely with an INR of less than 3.5.
- Activated partial thromboplastin time (APTT): measures the intrinsic pathway factors. This is most often used to monitor the anticoagulant impact from intravenous heparin, invariably given to hospitalized patients for a limited time frame.
- Platelet count: quantitative measure of platelets; under 40000 per microliter raises a significant concern for oral bleeding from invasive dental procedures.
- The bleeding time test is often recommended to determine platelet function but this test has little (if any) value in dental practice since it is influenced by multiple other factors (e.g. skin thickness, vascular integrity).

  Keep in mind that the range of acceptable test result numbers (e.g. INR) underestimate the likelihood of bleeding in patients with more than one coagulopathy. For example, a patient on warfarin and with an INR of 2.5, who also has significant liver disease, is at significantly greater risk of oral bleeding.

B. Specific coagulopathies of interest to dentistry

Haemophilia A (factor VIII deficiency), Haemophilia B (factor IX deficiency), Haemophilia C (factor XI deficiency), and von Willebrand's disease are invariably diagnosed before individuals reach adulthood, and won't be discussed in this chapter.

Thrombocytopaenia is a more common disorder and indicates a platelet count under 100 000 per microliter. It can be congenital, acquired or idiopathic, and adverse drug reactions are a common cause. Bleeding from thrombocytopaenia usually occurs with platelet counts below 50 000 per microliter, and spontaneous bleeding can occur with counts below about 20 000 per microliter. With proper precautions at the time of surgery (e.g. haemostatic agents, sutures), prolonged bleeding is unusual following routine restorative and surgical procedures (e.g. extractions). Platelet counts below 20 000 might require preoperative platelet transfusion for invasive dental procedures and should be discussed with the patient's haematologist.

C. Common medications that predispose to bleeding

1. Aspirin

Patients often do not think of aspirin as a medication. Many elderly patients are taking aspirin for prolonged periods for prevention of coronary ischaemic events, as well as for their anti-inflammatory activity. Avoid aspirin and other non-steroidals in patients with bleeding disorders or those taking other anticoagulants. Although there is a non-evidence-based tradition of discontinuing aspirin about 5 days prior to elective surgical procedures, there are recent data that suggest this is unnecessary for routine dental care (including routine tooth extraction). The potential harm (e.g. stroke, heart attack) from discontinuing anticoagulants in general for dental procedures far outweighs any potential benefit such as limiting prolonged oral bleeding.

2. Warfarin (Coumadin)

This drug is generally used for atrial fibrillation, atherosclerotic vascular disease, postmyocardial infarction (MI), post cerebrovascular accident (CVA), deep venous thrombosis (DVT), pulmonary embolism (PE), or prosthetic heart valves or grafts. It is usually taken orally for long-term anticoagulation therapy. Prolongation of PT/INR test results persists for 3–4 days after the last dose. With careful surgical technique and the use of local measures, routine oral surgery, scaling and restorative procedures can usually be performed with an INR <3.5–4.0. The risk of a thromboembolic event with discontinuation of warfarin therapy is invariably greater than the risk of significant oral bleeding from a dental procedure. However, until more is known, the use of regional blocks (e.g. inferior alveolar) should be undertaken with caution.

3. Heparin and low-molecular-weight heparin(s)

These drugs are generally used parenterally in hospitalized patients as short-term treatment for conditions such as a pulmonary embolus or deep venous thrombosis and for immediate anticoagulation therapy. They are not fibrinolytic and remain active 5–6 hours after the last i.v. dose of heparin, or 24hours after the last subcutaneous dose of low-molecular-weight heparin.

4. Dabigatran (Pradaxa®) and novel anticoagulants

Dabigatran is an orally active direct thrombin inhibitor approved in the USA for prevention of stroke in non-valvular atrial fibrillation and other indications outside the USA. Although the anticoagulant effect can be monitored with aPTT or ecarin clotting test, routine monitoring is not required. Caution in dosing with renal insufficiency is necessary as the drug is renally excreted. Other direct thrombin inhibitors and oral agents targeting factor Xa, approved in Europe and Canada, are likely to be approved soon in the USA. The indications for these agents are similar to warfarin, and these agents should not be discontinued prior to dental procedures without discussion with the treating physician.

5. Clopidogrel (Plavix®)

This antiplatelet agent is used to prevent atherosclerotic events in patients with a history of myocardial infarction or cerebrovascular accident. Normalization of platelet aggregation occurs 5–7 days after discontinuation. This drug is particularly common for patients with coronary stents and it must never be stopped for routine dental procedures, and never for more invasive procedures without discussion and approval from the prescribing physician.

6. Drug interactions

Broad-spectrum antibiotics may interfere with the intestinal flora and mucosal absorption of some medications. Corticosteroids, some antifungals, oral hypoglycemic agents and cimetidine can all predispose to bleeding.

D. Dental management considerations

- In some cases the patient's physician should be consulted prior to invasive procedures, depending on the comfort level of the treating dentist. For example, patients with more than one coagulopathy (e.g. liver disease from alcoholism and warfarin) or those maintained with a high INR value (>3.5) may need adjustment for invasive dental procedures. In some situations, (e.g. multiple coagulopathies) replacement therapy might be required for some anaesthetic blocks, scaling, use of rubber dam clamps and all surgical procedures. In the vast majority of clinical scenarios there is no need to adjust the dental management beyond the usual local haemostatic measures at the time of the procedure.
- Haemostatic measures include primary closure of the wound when possible. Absorbable gelatin packing in the socket following an extraction may be desirable, along with extra sutures, if appropriate. A full liquid or soft diet following multiple dental extractions will help to avoid postoperative bleeding and loss of a clot.
- Careful oral disease prevention with routine dental office evaluation, fluoride use, strict oral hygiene and diet control should be stressed to minimize the need for invasive dental care in the future.
- Give written and verbal instructions to caregivers on postoperative haemostasis and on the absolute need to maintain fluid intake, particularly in the hot summer months.

III. Cancer

A. Overview

Cancer patients may have received any combination of surgery, chemotherapy or radiotherapy, and there are both overlapping and individual considerations for each of these treatment modalities. In addition to the type of cancer thereapy, the patient's overall medical status is of major concern. Problems that are of significance to the dentist are primarily related to radiation and/or chemotherapy.

B. Radiation therapy

Although radiation therapy (RT) for most cancers (e.g. prostate, lung, breast) has little or no discernible effect on the oral cavity or the provision of dental care, RT for the management of head and neck cancer has a high incidence of oral sequelae. For this and other reasons, the patient's medical history and plans for cancer therapy are critically important in the prevention of oral problems during and following medical therapy. This involves a review of the patient's medical record and often a discussion with the treating physician(s). Dental treatment planning and management considerations are dependent on several factors that must be considered, in particular before invasive procedures. As always, the overall evaluation begins with the patient history (Box 8.2).

Box 8.2 Significant elements in the history for the patient who has received head and neck radiotherapy.

- Date of cancer diagnosis.
- Tumour location, histology (grade).
- Overall tumour staging (from T, N, M staging) and the patient's overall prognosis, often measured in likelihood of 1, 5 or 10 year survival.
- Previous therapy (e.g. RT, chemotherapy, surgery or a combination) and plans for cancer chemotherapy prior to, during or after RT.
- RT dose, field(s) and nature of the RT. The anatomic structures receiving the primary dose; the total dose to each region; and use of fractionation (i.e. multiple RT sessions per day); and external beam radiation versus interstitial implant (brachytherapy).
- Past dental history. For example, caries incidence, xerostomia, ability to eat, taste, swallow (solids versus liquids) and oral pain.
- Risk/benefit of maintaining each remaining tooth. Mandibular teeth, especially molars, present a greater risk for osteoradionecrosis if extracted immediately before, during or at any time after RT. Depending on factors such as oral hygiene history, teeth with >4mm pockets should be considered for extraction before RT begins, especially mandibular teeth if the mandible is in the RT portal.
- The anticipated status of the major salivary glands following radiotherapy, that is, the percent loss of salivary flow from each of the glands, to include consideration for qualitative changes in saliva.
- The location and degree of existing odontogenic disease and the potential for infection (i.e. periodontal, pericoronitis, caries) during and following RT and for the rest of the patients' life.

1. Clinical and radiographic examination of the head and neck cancer patient who is planned for/is undergoing RT

- The size and proximity of the malignant tumour to oral structures, if visible.
- The status of the soft tissues of the mouth and a careful examination for xerostomia, mucositis, mucosal breakdown, exposed alveolar bone, evidence of bacterial (e.g. periodontal) or fungal infection.
- Teeth: examine the mouth and radiographs for the number, mobility, state of repair, caries (especially cervical areas), percussion sensitivity, malalignment. Although is some overlap in information, both a panoramic film and full mouth series are highly desirable.
- Trismus or limited jaw mobility.

2. Oral sequelae of head and neck radiotherapy

(a) *Mucositis*, or inflammation of the mucous membranes, results from a complicated, and as yet poorly understood, combination of events that results in thinning of the mucosa. Inflammation is usually a short-term but potentially serious problem that can interrupt the schedule for RT and potentially limit the total dose. Not infrequently, there is localized or a more generalized breakdown of the mucosa, resulting in ulceration, with an increased risk of bacteraemia and secondary infection (e.g. fungal). The management of mucositis depends on the location, extent, duration and symptomatology. If it is mild to moderate, there are several rinses containing topical anaesthetics for pain, and/or steroids for inflammation (Box 8.3). Topical anesthetics and their compounds can be used in conjunction with NSAIDs or synthetic opioids, with escalation to stronger oral opioids as necessary. Systemic analgesics/opioids might be necessary when the topical anaesthetic activity is short (5–15 min), a stinging sensation occurs, or when the altered taste or numbing sensation is not well tolerated.

Box 8.3 Topical anaesthetics for the management of mucositis pain.

1. Maalox® or kaolin/pectin combination and elixir of Benadryl® in a 1 : 1 mixture.
2. 2% viscous lidocaine or a lidocaine/Benadryl or lydocaine/Maalox combination.
3. Benadryl/Kaopectate 50 : 50.
4. Benzydamine (Difflam), if available.[a]
5. Dyclonine.
6. 'Magic' mouthwash (contents may have steroid, antifungal, antihistamine and/or topical anaesthetic depending on individual hospital pharmacy).

[a]Benzydamine is the only topical anaesthetic for which there is scientific evidence for efficacy from prospective trials (not available in the USA).

(b) *Xerostomia* (the subjective complaint of a dry mouth) and salivary hypofunction are common sequelae from RT, which can be palliated by the use of saliva substitute or water. Alternatively, pilocarpine hydrochloride (5–7.5 mg, 3–4 times/day) or cevimeline 30 mg PO, (3 times/day) can help to increase salivation. Caution should be exercised when using these muscarinic agonists in patients with asthma, blood pressure and cardiac problems. Parotid gland tissue, if in the radiation field, will often recover from <3000 cGy but it can be permanently destroyed from >5000 cGy. Protective immunoglobulin A and the buffering and remineralizing capacity of saliva are lost, with a resultant lowering of salivary pH. A neutral sodium fluoride rinse, brush-on fluoride gel or high content fluoride toothpaste should be used every evening after careful tooth brushing and flossing. Patients need dietary counselling along with routine and careful follow-up until the dry mouth resolves, or indefinitely for patients who continue to have any degree of dry mouth or increased incidence of caries.

(c) *Osteoradionecrosis* (ORN), or exposure of alveolar bone, is most likely to occur in patients receiving >5000 cGy to the mandible, although the maxilla can also be involved. It is caused by permanent damage to bone cells and their blood supply. The patient remains at indefinite risk of ORN from a removable dental prosthesis or any trauma to compromised mucosa, following oral surgery, or from oral infection. Hyperbaric oxygen (HBO) is widely felt to promote healing but the value of HBO as a preventive measure prior to extraction(s) in an irradiated patient has come under question.

(d) *Taste loss* is a common problem when the tongue and mid face are in the RT portals and is exacerbated by salivary hypofunction. It is usually transient except with high doses of RT. The greatest resolution occurs within 3 months of treatment but dysgeusia can persist for up to 1 year post-RT. Tongue hygiene and dietary considerations are important.

(e) *Infections*. Bacterial infection results from a variety of changes during radiotherapy: a presumed shift in the oral flora; loss of the protective activity of salivary antimicrobial proteins; systemic immunosuppression; and poor nutrition that includes an increase in refined carbohydrates.

Fungal infections are common during and following RT. Clotrimazole troches 4–5/day at the onset of infection and for the duration of RT will likely eliminate fungal infection or reduce its severity until the time that the mouth environment returns to its near pre-RT state. Sips of water may be necessary to help dissolve the clotrimazole troches in the presence of xerostomia, but prolonged contact with the affected mucosa is the goal. Miconazole is an alternative. Avoid antifungal troches that utilize sucrose to mask the taste in dentate individuals. Fluconazole is an option for systemic therapy.

The timing of dental treatment is important for this patient population. Invasive dental procedures (e.g. extractions) are best done prior to RT, with at least 7 (ideally more) days for healing. This is a greater concern with mandibular as opposed to maxillary and impacted teeth. Teeth unlikely to become affected by caries or periodontitis at any point in the future can be maintained with aggressive preventive care. Teeth requiring extraction should be removed as atraumatically as possible, with careful alveoloplasty and primary closure of the mucosa, if possible. Preoperative HBO can be considered for patients who have received high-dose RT and who require mandibular extractions but its efficacy is unproven. Some authorities recommend avoiding new removable prostheses for 6–24 months after RT, but the literature suggests that the regional vascularity does not improve and that it might continue to deteriorate with time.

C. Chemotherapy

1. Overview

Chemotherapy is the mainstay of treatment for a wide variety of cancers. Some chemotherapy protocols are of major concern with regard to oral sequellae and dental procedures because they have either a direct or indirect effect on the oral cavity, particularly the oral mucosa and its ability to heal and maintain homeostasis. Mucositis, mucosal infection and bacteraemia from breakdown of the mucosal surface during myelosuppression are common problems.

2. Assessment of the patient to be treated with chemotherapy

- Medical diagnosis: the nature, location and extent of the malignancy determine both the chemotherapy protocol and the overall prognosis.

- General status: nutrition, current blood counts overall (e.g. white blood cells and platelets), debilitation, ability to tolerate dental treatment.
- Blood counts: exercise caution if the patient has:
  - a total white blood cell count <2000, and more importantly, absolute polymorphonuclear leukocytes (PMN or polys) <500.
  - platelets <40 000 if invasive procedures are planned. However, prolonged mucosal/gingival bleeding from routine oral hygiene care is unlikely with a platelet count >25 000.
- Timing of chemotherapy: if chemotherapy occurred within the previous month, the oral mucosa and bone marrow might be significantly compromised.
- Risk of infection and/or bleeding from dental treatment: the appropriate dental treatment depends on the nature of the dental problem and the patient's medical status. Sequelae from no treatment must also be considered. For uncomplicated healing to occur following an invasive procedure, platelet counts should be maintained above 2000. The absolute neutrophil count should be maintained at greater than 1000 for 7–10 days. Patients might have a coagulopathy from their disease (e.g. leukaemia and poor platelet function) in addition to myelosuppression from cancer treatment.

3. *Oral complications from chemotherapy*

(a) Prevention of oral complications: if there is sufficient time before the patient becomes myelosuppressed, there are several preventive issues that should be addressed (Box 8.4). The timing is important with regard to other oral care, such as brushing/flossing, topical anaesthetics and antifungals, so as not to interfere with the benefit of each. For example, mouth care should be done first. Topical anaesthetics and antifungals should not be followed by another oral medication/rinses until sufficient time for their efficacy has abated.

Box 8.4 Considerations for the patient receiving cancer chemotherapy.

- Patients should have a thorough oral examination, including a full-mouth series of radiographs.
- Extraction of hopeless periodontally or cariously involved teeth.
- Thorough oral prophylaxis (cleaning) and oral hygiene instruction. Patients should be educated as to the relationship between odontogenic disease and problems during and following chemotherapy.
- Oral antifungal prophylaxis (miconazole or fluconazole) may be appropriate when the white count or absolute neutrophil count is significantly depressed, especially with prolonged periods of neutropaenia.
- Fluoride: neutral sodium fluoride rinses or fluoride gel, if the patient can tolerate it, will help to prevent and arrest incipient caries.

(b) Osteonecrosis of the jaws: exposure of the alveolar bone as a result of radiotherapy was a common occurrence 30 years ago, but a combination of major changes in the way these tumours are treated and the emphasis on prevention of oral complications has resulted in a significant decrease in incidence. Nevertheless, patients who have had tumoricidal doses of radiotherapy to the jaws are at lifetime risk for osteonecrosis. In recent times, there are increasing numbers of reports of osteonecrosis from the bisphosphonate class of drugs. While it is clear that there is a far greater risk from intravenous bisphosphonates, it is not clear to what extent the oral preparations present a risk. The major goal in both cases of osteonecrosis is prevention, since treatment of these lesions is currently lacking. The reader is referred to the evolving literature on this topic of osteonecrosis.

(c) Infection: periodontal and dental abscess formation can occur independent of the patient's medical status and treatment. Such infections must be managed quickly and definitively. Clearly, antibiotics are less effective in the presence of mylosuppression and consultation with the patient's medical oncologist may be appropriate to select an antibiotic that will cover what may be an altered oral flora. During severe neutropaenia (absolute neutrophil count < 500 microliter), broad-spectrum parenteral antibiotics may be necessary to cover for Gram-negative and anaerobic bacteria in addition to the usual Gram-positive oral flora. Elective dental treatment should wait until absolute neutrophil count rises to >1000 and platelets to >50 000.

(d) Bleeding: this usually occurs from the gingival crevice in the presence of a platelet count <20 000. If several minutes of moderate pressure from a saline dampened sponge fails to stop the bleeding, a topical thrombin-soaked sponge can be applied to the area and held in place for several minutes. Remove the sponge gently so as not to disturb the new clot. There is some concern with the use of topical thrombin because of sensitivity, and this should be discussed with the patient's physician. Avoid any gingival manipulation (e.g. chewing or brushing) within 48–72 hours of oral bleeding or until a significant increase in the platelet count.

(e) Mucosal pain from mucositis: there is little scientific evidence-base for the use of the many topical anaesthetics and mouth care products. Begin with one of several topical anaesthetics and switch to another if ineffective (Box 8.3). Change to systemic opioids if topical anaesthetics are inadequate or there are widespread lesions. Localized areas of painful mucosa can often be managed with topical Benzocaine in orabase or combined with other anaesthetic or anti-inflammatory preparations.

(f) Nutrition: weight loss can be a short to medium term side effect of a sore mouth or throat, nausea/vomiting, poor appetite or diarrhoea. Consultation with a dietitian may be indicated to find foods that are well tolerated and maintain adequate nutrition. For a sore, dry or ulcerated mouth, try frequent rinses with a bland solution (e.g. baking soda and water) to keep the mucosa moist and clean. In addition, a soft and/or liquid diet that might include ice cream and watermelon. Avoid tart or acidic foods (e.g. citrus juices and fruits, seasoning and spices), alcohol, cigarettes and hot or very cold foods. Sugarless candy or mints may stimulate saliva production, although sharp edges can injure the oral mucosa.

IV. Cardiovascular disorders

A. Overview

Patients can look well but have a major compromising cardiovascular condition that needs to be considered prior to stressful or invasive dental procedures. Once a medical history is taken, specific questions may need to be posed to the patient's primary care physician or cardiologist for details. What follows are common cardiac conditions of concern to dental practitioners.

Box 8.5 American Heart Association (2007) – Cardiac conditions associated with the highest risk of adverse outcome from endocarditis for which prophylaxis with dental procedures is reasonable.

- Prosthetic cardiac valve or prosthetic material used for cardiac valve repair.
- Previous infective endocarditis.
- Congenital heart disease (CHD):
  - Unrepaired cyanotic congenital heart disease, including those with palliative shunts and conduits.
  - Completely repaired CHD with prosthetic material or device either by surgery or catheter intervention during the first six months after the procedure.[a]
  - Repaired CHD with residual defects at the site or adjacent to the site of a prosthetic patch or prosthetic device (which inhibit endothelialization).
  - Except for the conditions listed above, antibiotic prophylaxis is no longer recommended for any other form of CHD.
- Cardiac transplantation recipients who develop cardiac valvulopathy.

[a]Prophylaxis is reasonable because endothelialization of prosthetic material occurs within 6 months after the procedure.

Box 8.6 American Heart Association (2007) – Dental procedures for which endocarditis prophylaxis is reasonable for patients in Box 8.5.

All dental procedures that involve manipulation of gingival tissue or the periapical region of teeth or perforation of the oral mucosa[a]

[a]The following procedures and events do not need prophylaxis: routine anaesthetic injections through non-infected tissue, taking dental radiographs, placement of removable prosthodontic or orthodontic appliances, adjustment of orthodontic appliances, placement of orthodontic brackets, shedding of deciduous teeth and bleeding from trauma to the lips or oral mucosa.

1. Infective endocarditis (IE) is an infection of the myocardium of the heart by pathogens that often originate from the oral cavity. The reader is urged to read the full 2007 American Heart Association (AHA) document for details on the issue of the dental management of the patient at risk for IE. The four higher risk conditions recommended for prophylaxis are (Box 8.5, 8.6 and Table 8.1):

(a) Artificial heart valves, either (1) porcine-derived, which have a shorter duration of efficacy but do not require anticoagulation, or (2) mechanical valves which commonly require life-long anticoagulation therapy with warfarin. Patients taking warfarin are monitored by routine INR blood tests. On rare occasions, they may need to have their warfarin dose reduced for highly invasive or extensive oral surgical procedures, but for the vast majority of outpatient dental procedures, to include extraction of erupted teeth, there is little or no indication for interfering with warfarin dosage. The risk associated with lowering the INR below the therapeutic range (e.g. stroke, thrombosis) invariably outweighs the risk of prolonged bleeding from a dental procedure.

(b) Previous endocarditis. These patients will have a history of hospitalization for the initial management of IE.

Table 8.1 American Heart Association (2007) – Regimens for a dental procedure

Situation	Agent	Regimen – single dose 30–60 minutes before procedure	
		Adults	Children
Oral	Amoxicillin	2 g	50 mg/kg
Unable to take oral medication	Ampicillin **OR**	2 g i.m. or i.v.[a]	50 mg/kg i.m. or i.v.
	Cefazolin or ceftriaxone	1 g i.m. or i.v.	50 mg/kg i.m. or i.v.
Allergic to penicillins or ampicillin – oral	Cephalexin[b,c] **OR**	2 g	50 mg/kg
	Clindamycin **OR**	600 mg	20 mg/kg
	Azithromycin or clarithromycin	500 mg	15 mg/kg
Allergic to penicillins or ampicillin and unable to take oral medication	Cefazolin or ceftriaxone[c] **OR**	1 g i.m. or i.v.	50 mg/kg i.m. or i.v.
	Clindamycin phosphate	600 mg i.m. or i.v.	20 mg/kg i.m. or i.v.

[a]i.m. – intramuscular; i.v. – intravenous.
[b]or other first or second generation oral cephalosporin in equivalent adult or pediatric dosage.
[c]Cephalosporins should not be used in an individual with a history of anaphylaxis, angioedema or urticaria with penicillins or ampicillin.

(c) Heart transplantation: the major concerns are immunosuppression and current cardiac status. Patients will be on specific immunosuppressives, likely with some degree of altered immune response to bacteria. IE prophylaxis is an issue for those transplant patients with valve damage.

(d) Congenital heart disease (CHD): successful surgical corrections for cardiac defects in children in the past 3–4 decades have resulted in increasing numbers of older patients with patches and conduits that might indicate the need for antibiotic prophylaxis. The 2007 AHA guidelines provide specifics as to which CHD patients are at higher risk.

B. Risk assessment for bacteraemia from dental procedures

The oral cavity, and the periodontal pocket in particular, has a large and varied population of bacteria, and bacteraemia can result from any manipulation of the gingival tissues. However, there are only anecdotal data to suggest that invasive oral procedures are a more important cause of cardiac infections than the frequent, transient bacteraemia that arise from routine daily events such as tooth-brushing and chewing food. In addition, there are insufficient data to determine which dental procedures, if any, put patients at risk. For example, routine cleaning (scaling) of teeth may be more invasive than tooth extraction(s) with respect to causing bacteraemia. When taking the medical history from a patient, it is helpful to ask specific questions that cover critical issues in the identification of patients at risk for distant-site infection such as IE. These questions should elicit information about previous hospitalizations, surgery, medications and physician visits in recent years. Standard health questionnaires will often bring out significant positives in the history but they cannot be relied upon as the sole source of information.

2. Myocardial infarction (MI): the major concern is prevention of additional infarction and heart muscle damage. Consult the patient's physician concerning coronary vessel and myocardial involvement, arrhythmias, medication(s), the presence of other vascular disease and whether or not the patient has a pacemaker or defibrillator. There is longstanding dogma concerning patients who have had an MI within the past 6 months, but this is based on old data that MIs occur more frequently during general surgery and under general anaesthesia in the 6 months following an MI. Nevertheless, it is prudent and in the best interest of the patient to defer elective dental care for the conventional period of 6 months. These patients may be more likely to have an MI but there are medically necessary dental procedures, such as the definitive relief of pain (e.g. single tooth extraction), that may be necessary in this time period if pharmacological management (i.e. antibiotics and analgesics) either fails or is inappropriate. The outcome from avoidance of such dental procedures might be more likely to precipitate a cardiac event. Consultation with the patient's physician for additional medical history prior to stressful or invasive procedures is prudent since these patients may also be on Warfarin or aspirin therapy for anticoagulation. Multiple short appointments may be preferable if the patient has a relatively easy trip from home to the dental office. Be cautious with epinephrine as a vasoconstrictor in local anaesthetics and consider nitrous oxide for sedation. Postoperative pain control is essential. Finally, follow patients for gingival hyperplasia that can occur with calcium channel blockers.

3. Coronary artery bypass graft (CABG): the major concern is myocardial infarction. Consult the patient's physician or the medical record for coronary vessel and myocardial involvement, arrhythmias, medication(s), the presence of other vascular disease and whether or not the patient has an implanted pacemaker or defibrillator.

With regard to invasive dental procedures, some clinicians feel that the same time determinants apply as for patients with a history of MI; that is, if the patient is within 6 months of CABG surgery, discuss the need for dental treatment with the patients physician. However, cardiac circulation should be improved following CABG surgery and there is no documented need to wait longer than 6 weeks in order to provide elective oral health care. There is no evidence for grafted coronary vessels becoming infected from a dental procedure.

4. Angina: the major concern is to reduce the possibility of an anginal attack. Question the patient as to precipitating factors (e.g. exercise, climbing stairs, emotional stress), frequency, duration, timing, severity and response to medication. Stable, or exertional angina, occurs with physical activity. It is usually relieved by rest and the frequency or intensity should not have increased in the recent past. It is important to have the following information: date of the last attack; frequency of attacks; spontaneous occurrence; relieved by rest or medication; medications needed for relief; and physical restrictions – although this can be difficult to acertain in the elderly patient. Elective treatment is reasonable if the angina is stable and well controlled by 1–2 nitroglycerin tablets, and if the episodes are less frequent than one per week – otherwise the angina is considered unstable (labile). Crescendo (increasing frequency) angina patients are at high risk for MI. Therefore, for unstable or crescendo angina, consult the patient's physician before treatment.

Assess the vital signs at each appointment. The patient's nitroglycerin medication should be readily available during the procedure. If attacks are more than one per week, or if the patient is fearful and non-elective care is planned, consider nitroglycerin use at the start of the appointment. Consider short appointments and nitrous oxide or an oral sedative. Do not oversedate because of a risk of hypotension. For restorative treatment on elderly patients, particularly for teeth with existing restorations, pulpal discomfort is likely to be minimal.

5. Coronary stents: coronary stents have become a common treatment option for coronary artery disease (CAD) and over 800 000 people worldwide undergo nonsurgical coronary artery intervention procedures yearly. Stent technology is still evolving as an alternative to bypass grafting and medical management of CAD. The most significant issue for dental patients with stents, beyond the issues raised above for CAD, is that of anticoagulation. All stent patients are anticoagulanted with either aspirin or another anti-platelet drug, such as clopidogrel, or both, for at least 6–12 months following stent placement. Antiplatelet therapy should never be stopped by a dentist without discussion with the treating physician. Although the likelihood of prolonged bleeding is increased with two anticoagulants (e.g. aspirin and clopidogrel), there are few, if any, indications to alter such anticoagulation for a dental procedure.

6. Cardiac pacemaker: the risk of pacemaker infection due to a dental procedure is very low or non-existent. Use of certain electronic dental devices, including ultrasonic scalers, electric pulp testers and electrosurgery units should be avoided because of possible interference with pacemaker function. Cell phones compete with some monitoring devices.

7. Congestive heart failure (CHF): it is important to acquire information on the degree of CHF. The patient will have variable levels of compensation and might be on multiple medications and dietary measures to control and balance cardiac function. If well compensated, patients can undergo elective dental treatment. If not, treatment should wait until the patient is stable. Signs of poor compensation and high risk for stressful dental procedures include:

- Paroxysmal nocturnal dyspnea: patient awakens at night short of breath as a result of pulmonary congestion.
- Orthopnea: patients who require two or more pillows to prevent pulmonary congestion during sleep.
- Shortness of breath or dyspnea on exertion: find out how many steps or flights of stairs the patient can climb without having to stop and rest.
- Pedal oedema: this results from right heart failure. Question the patient about swollen ankles and examine for a depression left after pressing a swollen ankle with a finger (pitting oedema).

Dental management considerations for patients with CHF include:

- Patients with orthopnoea may not tolerate the supine position in the dental chair and will need to be treated in the upright position. Since orthostatic hypotension can result from some cardiac medications, raise them to a sitting position in several stages over several minutes. Ask them to sit with their feet on floor for 2 minutes before standing upright.
- Patients might have urinary urgency during morning appointments in response to a diuretic. Ask if they would like to use the bathroom before the procedure.

8. Heart transplantation: in some situations it is preferable to accomplish all invasive, bacteraemic dental procedures before the heart transplantation, for example, when patients are relatively stable from an overall medical standpoint. However, a severely compromised patient in cardiac failure is likely at greater risk from elective dental treatment before transplantation, in spite of the concern for post-transplant immunosuppression.

9. Arrhythmias: there is a wide range of cardiac arrhythmias and varying degrees of concern for dental practice. Consult with the patient's physician if unsure about the nature of the arrhythmia and the current management. The patient might be anticoagulated for atrial fibrillation and have an increased risk for bleeding. Arrhythmias following MI are usually managed with medication. Epinephrine should be avoided and patients should be monitored carefully during

Table 8.2 Classification and management of blood pressure for adults

Classification of blood pressure for adults			
Blood pressure classification	**SBP**		**DBP**
Normal	<120 mm Hg	and	<90 mm Hg
Prehypertension	120–139 mm Hg	or	80–89 mm Hg
Stage 1 hypertension	140–159 mm Hg	or	90–99 mm Hg
Stage 2 hypertension	≥150 mm Hg	or	≥100 mm Hg

SBP = Systolic blood pressure;
DBP = Diastolic blood pressure.

dental procedures. Should the patient report syncope or unexplained loss of consciousness, consider deferring elective procedures and refer the patient for evaluation with their primary physician.

10. Hypertension: hypertension is defined as a resting blood pressure in excess of 140 mmHg systolic and/or 90 mmHg diastolic, and it is found in up to 20% of adults on random screening (Table 8.2). The major concern is precipitating a hypertensive crisis, stroke or MI, and it increases the risk of renal disease. Patients often show poor compliance with blood pressure medications and diet, and need reinforcement concerning the importance of medications in preventing vascular problems. Side effects of blood pressure medications include orthostatic hypotension, synergistic activity with narcotics, and potassium depletion. Beta-blockers will decrease the response to medications (e.g. epinephrine) used to treat anaphylaxis. Epinephrine use with these patients is controversial. However, the benefit from prolonged and more profound anaesthesia (and haemostasis) is thought to outweigh the risk of systemic effects. Do not use concentrations greater than 1 : 100 000 and use care to aspirate to avoid intravascular injection. Poorly controlled or uncontrolled patients should not be treated until their hypertension is under control. Elective treatment should be avoided if the blood pressure is significantly above the patient's baseline or if >180 mmHg systolic or >100 mmHg diastolic. Patients in pain might have some lowering of their pressures after local anaesthesia. Hypertension often leads to increased blood loss during surgery. Monitor the blood pressure before, during and after treatment. Patients should also be monitored for medication-related xerostomia and gingival overgrowth.

C. Other cardiac considerations

Cardiac drug interactions: caution should be used with respiratory depressants such as opioids, barbiturates and other sedatives which can worsen the cardiovascular status. Nitrous oxide/oxygen relative analgesia can be used safely in cardiac patients, but the oxygen content must not drop below 25%. Use of local anaesthetics with vasoconstrictors is controversial. The benefits of vasoconstrictors (e.g. more profound and longer anaesthetic effect) probably outweigh the risks in most cases. However, restricted outflow track defects (e.g. aortic stenosis, hypertrophic cardiomyopathy), some cardiac arrythmias, unstable angina, recent MI and uncontrolled CHF are exceptions. Avoid concentrations of epinephrine >1 : 100 000 and restrict the total volume of epinephrine at one appointment. The traditional limit of two dental syringe carpules has little if any basis in science and it is more important to deliver the injection slowly (after aspiration), monitor for elevated BP and heart rate and wait at least two minutes between injections.

V. Cerebral vascular disease

A. Overview

Cerebrovascular accident (CVA): a CVA, or stroke, presents as paralysis or weakness, often involving the facial muscles. The patient might have headache, nausea and vomiting and numbness or paralysis of one side of the body. Confusion and aphasia are also common.

A CVA can be caused by three events: (1) A thrombus of a small or large vessel (e.g. carotid), usually in people with hypertension and diabetes. This event comes on more slowly than an embolus. A transient ischaemic attack (TIA) might be a warning of an impending CVA; (2) an embolus, which usually originates from the heart or neck (e.g. the carotid bifurcation), or atrial fibrillation. The deficit is sudden and improves only slowly; and (3) a haemorrhage, which is usually spontaneous, or secondary to hypertension or an aneurysm, occasionally from a coagulopathy. The onset of symptoms is sudden.

B. Dental management considerations

Patients with CVA might be on an anticoagulant (e.g. warfarin, aspirin or clopidogrel) and this is a concern for hypertensive patients. An INR test, in the case of warfarin, is desirable to evaluate risk of bleeding from invasive dental procedures and to ensure that the patient is in the desired range of anticoagulation. One of the primary concerns for patients with stroke is their ability to maintain proper oral hygiene due to some combination of incoordination, weakness or cognitive problems. In such cases, care givers can have a measurable impact on the prevention of oral disease.

VI. Drug abuse and addiction

A. Overview

Drug abuse and addiction, beyond alcohol and tobacco products, is an uncommon finding in the geriatric population. However, alcohol abuse is common, depending on the definition used, and it must be reognized by oral health practitioners.

B. Alcoholism

This is a significant problem with older adults and it can be difficult to ascertain during medical history taking since they may live in a more isolated environment, unobserved by family, and not drive cars. Therefore, the behavioural changes (e.g. dementia) and legal problems (e.g. drunk driving charges) are less likely. The prevalence of psychiatric disorders such as depression is a factor in many cases. Misuse of drugs prescribed for medical conditions is also common. It has been called the 'invisible epidemic'. Although moderate use of alcohol is reported to be of benefit in the elderly for its cardiac protective effects, there are potential adverse effects for those patients who also take certain medications [e.g. patients with liver damage who take both warfarin and acetaminophen (paracetamol)] (see liver disease). Older people may not break down alcohol as effectively and may be less tolerant to the same volume of alcohol as a younger individual. Other problems include the consumption of non-nutritional calories, impaired cognitive function, risk of falls and insomnia.

C. Significant elements in the history and physical findings

A history of delirium tremens or gastrointestinal bleeding is important. Obtaining a social history of alcohol use is imperative, with more than two drinks per day or more than 7 drinks per week (women) and 14 drinks per week (men) indicating a high likelihood of alcohol abuse and dependence. Unfortunately, up to half of patients do not accurately report their alcohol intake. Presence of unexplained hypertension, depression, insomnia, tremors, confusion or spider angiomata can indicate occult alcohol abuse.

D. Dental management considerations

Dental findings may include an increased rate of caries and periodontal disease, either from neglect or changes in salivary fluid. Oral hygiene should be monitored carefully. Generally, morning appointments are best. Patients who are uncooperative or incoherent should not be treated because of the risk of injury, decreased gag reflex and problems of informed consent. Given the possibility of alcoholic liver disease from prolonged, heavy use of alcohol and the potential for bleeding, consider acquiring a PT/INR and platelet count to screen for the potential for bleeding from invasive dental procedures. Management considerations also include the possibility of an increased risk of oral cancer, especially in the presence of tobacco use. Finally, avoid the use of respiratory inhibitors such as opioids and medications that are metabolized in the liver [e.g. acetaminophen (paracetamol)], especially in the presence of liver failure.

VII. Endocrine disorders

A. Diabetes mellitus

1. Overview: diabetes mellitus is a group of metabolic disorders caused by defects in insulin secretion or tissue sensitivity, with a resultant hyperglycemia. Almost 20 per cent of adults over 65 years of age have diabetes, therefore dentists will be treating a larger number of these patients as our population ages. Patients presenting with persistent hyperglycemia may be unaware of their condition, resulting in a delayed diagnosis and greater chance for end-organ disease.

Diabetes classification:

- Type 1 (formerly insulin-dependent or juvenile onset) diabetes, constituting 5–10% of diabetes. Patients produce little or no insulin and there is a greater tendency to ketoacidosis.
- Type 2 (formerly non-insulin-dependent or adult onset) diabetes constituting 90–95% of diabetes. The insulin receptors display diminished sensitivity to insulin.

2. Significant elements in history: age of onset, antidiabetic medications (glycemic control), compliance with therapy and secondary complications. Symptoms include: excessive thirst, nocturia, malaise, decreased appetite leading to nausea, vomiting, hyperpnea and coma (diabetic acidosis). Make a note of the patient's diet, insulin dosage, route, frequency and timing of injection. The type of insulin should also be noted. Some patients might use an insulin pump to deliver steady doses of insulin. Record any hospital admissions for an uncontrolled state (e.g. insulin reactions, diabetic coma). Also note problems with infection, since hospital admission might be indicated for type 1 patients with severe oral infection.

3. Hyperglycemia has a long onset, and although it can result in diabetic coma it is far less likely to result in a dental office crisis. Signs include a flushed face, dry skin, dry mouth, nausea, vomiting, weakness, dehydration, Kussmaul (very deep and rapid) respirations, elevated pulse, decreased blood pressure and lethargy. Hyperglycemia can occur as a result of an infection (most common), weight gain, hyperthyroidism, steroids, fever, dehydration or non-compliance with medical care. It can lead to impaired granulocyte phagocytosis and chemotaxis. Hyperglycemia can progress to ketoacidosis and coma over several hours or days in patients with type 1 diabetes. Treatment for hyperglycemia includes early recognition and basic life support, if indicated. A sugar solution by mouth if awake or i.v. glucose if unable to give

by mouth should distinguish these symptoms from insulin shock from hypoglycemia. Medical assistance must be obtained immediately.

4. Hypoglycemia, or insulin shock, is the most common diabetic complication that occurs in the dental office. It can result in a loss of consciousness, which can occur rapidly if the blood glucose falls to <50 mg/100 cc. Common causes of hypoglycemia are omission or delay of meals, excessive exercise prior to meals, overdose of insulin or oral hypoglycemic agents and stress. Hypoglycemia usually appears first as decreased cerebral function, mental confusion, headache, dizziness, changes in mood, weakness, hunger, nausea, increased epinephrine activity (sweating, tachycardia, piloerection, increased anxiety) as an endogenous reaction to raised blood glucose. The patient can appear intoxicated and might progress to unconsciousness, convulsions and coma. Treatment for hypoglycemia includes early recognition of the condition, oral or parenteral simple carbohydrates, basic life support if necessary and medical assistance.

5. Dental management considerations: the major concerns in dental management are preventing hypoglycemia and the possibility of a poor response to dental and periodontal infections in poorly controlled diabetics. Although it is commonly felt that all diabetics have an increased risk of oral infection and impaired wound healing, this is not necessarily the case except for insulin-dependent and poorly controlled diabetics.

For well controlled diabetics, morning appointments are best, as blood sugar levels are generally higher at this time. Appointments should not be scheduled soon after insulin use, given the increased risk for hypoglycemia. Ensure that the patient has received his/her normal insulin dose if able to eat after the procedure, otherwise the insulin dose may need to be reduced. Also ensure that the patient has eaten a normal breakfast, supplemented with orange or other sugar-containing juice and have glucose available during dental treatment. Antibiotic prophylaxis is rarely indicated for surgical procedures since there are no scientific data to support this practice. Although there is *in vivo* evidence to suggest an increased risk of infection from decreased neutrophil function this does not seem to be evident clinically. However, diabetics do not tolerate infection well and their medical management can be complicated by even asymptomatic oral infection (e.g. generalized periodontitis). Resume normal insulin and oral intake immediately after the procedure.

For poorly controlled diabetics, consult the patient's physician and consider hospitalization for extensive invasive restorative or surgical procedures. Avoid stressful procedures and anticipate slower healing. The insulin requirement might be affected by poor tolerance to oral infection or generalized periodontal disease, and the insulin dose might need to be adjusted before and after treatment. It is proposed that there is a direct link between chronic, low grade periodontal disease and glycemic control. Furthermore, it has been suggested that active treatment of periodontal disease in a poorly controlled diabetic can improve glycemic control.

Salivary gland dysfunction, xerostomia and dehydration are common findings in diabetics. This predisposes patients to dental diseases, impaired retention of full removable prostheses, as well as the need for careful dental management. In addition, these changes to the oral mucosa, and likely changes in bacterial ecology, predispose diabetics to mucosal problems such as lichen planus, fungal infections and burning mouth syndrome.

In addition to other end-organ disease (e.g. retinopathy, neuropathy) be aware that type 1 diabetics have a more advanced state of cardiovascular disease at a younger age than non-diabetics. Diabetes is the major reason for kidney disease under the age of 25 and the main cause for dialysis at any age. The common comorbidities of hypertension, obesity, lipid disorders and smoking are important because of their role in the development of cardiovascular disease.

B. Thyroid gland disorders

1. Hyperthyroidism: thyroid disorders affect up to 5% of women in the USA, most commonly a result of unregulated production of thyroid hormones. Worldwide, iodine deficiency is the most common thyroid disorder. In Great Britain, the incidence is about 25–30 cases per 10 000 women. Thyroid hormones, thyroxine (T_4) and triiodothyromine (T_3) influence multiple metabolic processes, tissue growth and energy metabolism. Over or underproduction of thyroid hormones can result in serious medical complications if not managed properly. Many cases of hyperthyroidism are subclinical, but they often progress to overt disease. The majority of patients have Graves' disease. Thyroid storm (thyrotoxic crisis) can be precipitated by stress, trauma or acute infection if the patient is not well controlled on medication. Look for evidence of thyrotoxicosis – fever, nervousness, restlessness, altered mental status, sweating, tachycardia, heat intolerance, weight loss, nausea and vomiting, hypertension and exophthalmos. Weight loss and decreasing appetite may be more common with aging.

2. Hypothyroidism: caused by a congenital defect, hypothalamus or a pituitary defect, Hashimoto's thyroiditis, surgery or radiogenic (e.g. radioactive iodine therapy). The result is a decrease in production of hormone and therefore gland function. The risk from inadequate management is

poor response to stress, infection and trauma resulting in hypothyroid coma. Signs include hypotension, bradycardia, arrhythmias, decreased temperature, dry skin and weight gain. Use caution with sedatives and opioids.

3. Dental management considerations: important elements in the history include the cause of the impairment; thyroid hormone levels; current therapy; and symptoms. For hyperthyroidism, patients may have anorexia and wasting, and cardiac conditions such as atrial fibrillation and congestive heart failure. If possible, use pharmacological management (i.e. antibiotics/analgesics) for acute oral infections until the thyroid is under control. The accelerated bone turnover with excessive thyroid hormone may result in osteoporosis and a radiographic appearance of bone loss. Although the neutrophil count may be decreased, this likely has little impact on oral infection. Treatment should be postponed if the patient is untreated or poorly controlled or presents with symptoms suggestive of thyroid disease (e.g. tachycardia, hypertension, sweating). Use caution with stressful procedures. Prevention of infection is important to avoid a crisis. Caution must be used with the use of epinephrine and other pressor amine (e.g. gingival retraction cords) in local anaesthetic solutions, especially in patients who are poorly controlled. Well managed hyperthyroidism patients generally need no adjustment in their dental management. For hypothyroidism, the clinician must be aware of the susceptibility to cardiovascular disease. Avoid stressful situations and avoid the use of sedatives and narcotics in patients with poorly controlled hypothyroidism. Well controlled patients have no contraindications to dental care.

C. Adrenal disorders

1. Hyperadrenocorticism (Cushing's syndrome): this is hypersecretion of glucocorticoid as a result of various diseases affecting the hypothalamus, anterior pituitary or the adrenal gland. Features include hypertension; muscle weakness; 'moon facies'; truncal obesity; hirsutism; diabetes; osteoporosis; and coagulopathy. The result can be poor wound healing, easy bruising and increased risk of infection.

2. Hypoadrenocorticism (Addison's disease): this is hyposecretion of the glucocorticoid cortisol as a result of autoimmune destruction of the adrenal cortex, exogenous steroid therapy, therapeutic bilateral adrenalectomy or damage to the pituitary gland. Features include hyperpigmentation of the skin, buccal and labial mucosa and gingivae, weakness, fatigue, malaise, mental confusion, weight loss, fever, orthostatic hypotension, syncope and depressed vasoconstrictor response. Patients with a poor response to stress could precipitate cardiovascular collapse. Additional symptoms include nausea and vomiting, thirst, polyuria, hyperkalemia, arrhythmia, cardiac arrest.

3. Dental management considerations: older patients would most likely be diagnosed and under treatment if their hyper- or hypoadrenocorticism was severe enough to be a consideration for dental procedures. The concern for hypoadrenocorticism is the possibility, albeit remote, that the patient would have an adrenal crisis during a stressful procedure. This is a true medical emergency that can result in cardiovascular collapse, due in part to hypovolemia. For office-based procedures, the patient can be instructed to take their usual dose of corticosteroids on the morning of the procedure. If more stressful procedures are planned, consult with the treating physician regarding the use of stress-dose steroids.

4. Considerations for patients taking steroids: there are two primary clinical issues. First, patients with adrenal insufficiency or who are taking steroids for any reason may be at higher risk of infection. Second, the issue of prophylactic steroids prior to dental procedures is controversial. The major consideration is suppression of adrenal capacity to respond to stressful situations. The risk of an adrenal crisis occurring during dental treatment is overstated and it is a truly rare event. Nevertheless, patients who have been, or are currently, on systemic steroids are potentially at risk for adrenal (Addisonian) crisis during or following a stressful event such as a dental procedure or general anaesthetic.

Topical and other non-parenteral sources of steroids can suppress adrenal function with prolonged use and/or high dosage. Also, the likelihood of clinically significant adrenal suppression varies with the individual and no reliable formula exists to help the clinician. Single dose steroid supplementation is often given because it is easy, inexpensive and essentially non-threatening to the patient in comparison to the potentially disasterous outcome of an adrenal crisis. Increasing the patients' steroid dose for surgical procedures is rarely necessary but it is difficult to predict who might have an adrenal crisis under stress, and the risk to the patient from increasing the steroid dose is minimal to non-existent. Consult the patient's physician to determine the reason for, and duration of, steroid therapy and the need for increasing the steroid dose prior to and following dental procedures.

The general goal for supplementation is to have 80–100 mg hydrocortisone available systemically for procedures that are stressful from either a surgical or psychological standpoint. The normal daily output of hydrocortisone is 20 mg. Patients taking low doses of prednisone (e.g. 5 mg) for short time periods (e.g. less than 2 weeks) do not likely need a supplemental dose. For patients on larger doses or for longer periods, consider either doubling the patient's daily dose the morning of surgery up to the physiological output of the adrenal glands. Hospital patients can be given 100–200 mg of intramuscular or intravenous hydrocortisone 30 min prior to the planned procedure. For highly stressful procedures in patients at high risk, consider prednisone 60 mg or hydrocortisone 100 mg on the day of surgery, tapered rapidly over the next 3 days back to the patient's usual replacement dose. Patients on high doses (>40 mg/day) of prednisone would not normally require a supplemental dose, except perhaps for major surgery and/or general anaesthesia. Consideration might be given to steroid supplementation 12 h after the procedure to cover patients still in pain. Patients who have had a prolonged or significant dental infection might benefit most from supplemental corticosteroids, particularly if a long and/or stressful procedure is anticipated. Patients off long-term high-dose steroids for over 6 months can have the drug instituted the day prior to treatment, at the discretion of the physician. Keep in mind that a major precipitating factor in an adrenal crisis is hypovolaemia. Therefore, ensure that the patient is well hydrated prior to the procedure. Sedation may be considered to minimize stress.

VIII. Liver disease

A. Overview

The number of deaths due to liver disease increases greatly after the age of 45 years due in part to age-related loss of liver volume and impaired liver cell function and regeneration. A consequence of aging, therefore, is an increase in liver diseases as well as delayed and less efficient drug metabolism. A significant contributor to liver impairment is alcohol abuse. Other disorders include:

1 Hepatitis A, also known as infectious hepatitis, which is spread primarily via a fecal–oral route. The incubation time is 2–6 weeks. Some people display lifetime immunity. There is no known carrier state and hepatitis is rarely, if ever, fatal or parenterally transmitted.
2 Hepatitis B, also known as serum hepatitis, is transmitted primarily by parenteral inoculation, but it can also be spread by saliva, nasopharyngeal washings, semen, menstrual fluid, vaginal secretions, razors or toothbrushes. Over half of dialysis patients are chronic carriers and have a persisting concentration of hepatitis B surface antigen. The incubation period is 2–6 months. Five per cent of people infected develop chronic active hepatitis, 5–10% are carriers for 1–6 months, and 2% are carriers for life. Factors that increase the risk of exposure include drug abuse, long-term residential or institutional care and transfusion of blood and blood products. Almost all hepatitis A and over 85% of hepatitis B patients resolve completely. Cases are often mild or subclinical with only increased transaminase levels. Hepatitis B surface antigen is found in acute or chronic cases of hepatitis B and also in healthy carriers. Hepatitis B surface antigen concentration in patients with acute hepatitis B is usually transient. If it persists more than 4 months then a chronic disease state is possible. Carriers might be without a history of hepatitis and might have normal liver function tests.
3 Hepatitis C, also known as transfusion-associated hepatitis, accounts for the majority of non-A and non-B hepatitis. In addition to being transfusion-associated, there is a high prevalence among injecting drug-users. It can be transmitted by 0.0001cc plasma. The infection rate is 1 in 27 parenteral exposures. Sexual partners and household contacts are at risk of infection. The incubation period is from 6–9 weeks to 6 months. There is an icteric period with anorexia, nausea and right upper quadrant pain for 6–8 weeks. Eighty per cent are chronic carriers and most improve in 2–3 years. However, 20% develop cirrhosis and there is an increased incidence of hepatocellular carcinoma.
4 Hepatitis D (delta) has an epidemiology, transmission and concern in dental practice that are the same as for HBV and HCV. HBV vaccine also protects against HDV.

B. Dental management considerations

Of primary importance for dentistry is the liver's ability to metabolize drugs, and the implications that age and disease have on liver function and the reduced capacity for normal haemostasis. The following are general recommendations for the management of the patient with liver disease:

- Acquire a thorough medical history, to include current hepatic function and complications from cirrhosis (ascites, hypertension, coagulopathy).
- Avoid elective treatment on active hepatitis patients.
- Evaluate liver damage prior to prescribing certain medications [e.g. diazepam, acetaminophen (paracetamol)] because of poor drug metabolism. This also applies to some local anaesthetics, analgesics, sedatives and antibiotics. Liver-dependent factors involved in haemostasis should be checked prior to surgery; the PT/INR test is the most valuable.

C. Post-liver transplant considerations

- Immunosuppression: there is the potential for an increased risk for infection even though T-cells are targeted. Bacteraemia that might provoke sepsis should be avoided, particularly in the 6 months following the transplant when immunosuppressive agents are given in higher doses.
- Adrenal suppression secondary to the use of prednisone.
- There is no scientific evidence to suggest the use of prophylactic antibiotics in the setting of liver disease.

IX. Renal disorders

A. Overview

Renal disease is increasingly common and age increases the likelihood of renal failure. Chronic renal failure (CRF) has a wide spectrum of degree of compromise, and it is important to have an understanding of the patients' current renal status to avoid complications with invasive dental treatment and medications. In addition, the degree of chronic renal disease (CRD) and the presence of comorbid conditions must be determined. The incidence of CRF is growing due to the increase in diabetes – the single greatest cause of chronic renal disease in the USA. The loss of renal function results in a variety of problems for dental patients: that of elimination of drugs, uraemia and cardiovascular complications such as hypertension, CHF and ischaemic heart disease.

B. Dental management considerations

Renal haemodialysis requires that patients have an access (shunt) to the circulation. It is important that blood pressure not be measured in the arm with a shunt. Dental practitioners should be familiar with the dosing of antibiotics and antifungal agents in the patient with renal failure. The initial dose of the antifungal or antibiotic drug should be the same as for a patient with normal renal function to achieve a therapeutic blood level. The maintenance dose should then be reduced such that the blood concentration not continue to increase prior to the next dialysis appointment, at which time all of the drug will likely be eliminated. For example, potassium-containing penicillins are acceptable for short-term use (several days) but not long-term, due to high potassium levels in the absence of dialysis. Erythromycin is an alternative. Aminoglycosides, tetracyclines and cephalosporins should be avoided due to nephrotoxicity. Published guidelines should be consulted concerning drug dosage adjustment for invasive procedures.

It is desirable to treat dialysis patients closer to the time of finishing a dialysis appointment than in the hours before dialysis because of the problem of increasing uraemia and consequent impaired platelet function. Heparin is used during dialysis but there is little concern of bleeding from dental procedures given the short half life of heparin. Patients are usually tired after dialysis and might not tolerate dental appointments at that time. The morning after dialysis is probably the best alternative. Many patients are chronically anticoagulated due to increased risk of thromboembolic disease. PT/INR values should be obtained prior to surgical procedures for patients taking warfarin, but the desired INR target range is invariably low enough to permit routine dental procedures without adjustment of the warfarin dose. Although invasive procedures can usually be done safely with INR levels as high at 3.5–4.0, these patients often have more than one coagulopathy, which greatly increases the likelihood of prolonged bleeding following a dental procedure. There is a higher incidence of hepatitis B and C and anaemia in these patients. Antibiotic prophylaxis for dialysis patients undergoing dental procedures is greatly overemphasized and there are no data to suggest that it is of any benefit in the prevention of infection of dialysis shunts.

C. Renal transplant patients

Renal transplant patients are on life-long immunosuppressive drug(s). The issues of the need for antibiotic and/or steroid prophylaxis for dental procedures are unresolved, but likely of little or no benefit. Watch for gingival overgrowth if the patient is taking cyclosporine. Oral disease and infection should be treated aggressively to avoid the possiblity of an acute exacerbation of a chronic dental disease and complicating the medical management of immunosuppression.

X. Neurological and neuromuscular disorders

A. Alzheimer's disease

See Chapter 9 for details on Alzheimer's disease (AD) and Chapter 26 for details on dental management considerations.

B. Parkinson's disease

See Chapter 9 for details on Parkinson's disease and Chapter 26 for details on dental management considerations.

C. Dementia

See Chapter 9 for details on all common forms of dementia and Chapter 26 for details on dental management considerations.

D. Seizures and epilepsy

1. Overview

Seizures are one of the most common neurological disorders. The prevalence of seizures is highest among children, but the incidence of first-time seizures increases significantly after age 50 years. Epilepsy is characterized by recurrent, unprovoked seizures and they affect 0.4% of the population. There is a need to distinguish between epilepsy and reflex anoxic seizures, vasovagal syncope, breath-holding attacks, migraine, cardiac arrhythmias, Munchausen's syndrome and 'pseudo' seizures. Epilepsy is caused by brain damage from CVA or brain tumours, acute alcohol intoxication or they are idiopathic. Other causes of seizures include trauma, fever, diabetes, alcoholism and hyponatremia/kalaemia. There is a genetic predisposition.

2. Important medical history elements

The practitioner should enquire about the type of seizures the patient has experienced and how well they are controlled; the frequency and duration of the seizures; what triggers it; and the nature of the attacks. Consult the patient's physician for additional medical history on the patient's seizure status.

3. Dental management considerations

- If the patient is well controlled on medication, there are no contraindications to routine dental care.
- The dental staff must be aware of the potential for seizures, which are usually self-limiting. The level of seizure control can be determined at each dental visit by asking the patient when they had their last seizure and how many they have had in the preceeding weeks and months.
- The condition is active if seizures are reported within the preceding 2 years.
- Seizures that are prolonged in duration are considered status epilepticus, which is a medical emergency.
- All anaesthetic agents are cerebral irritants.
- Preventive care is vital because of numerous side effects of anti-seizure medications: xerostomia, gingival hypertrophy, dental neglect, caries (can be due to sugar-based liquid oral medicines, and the potential for dental trauma.
- Phenytoin will cause gingival hyperplasia in approximately 50% of patients. Scrupulous oral hygiene is necessary to help control or prevent gingival enlargement.
- Be aware of the side effects of seizure control drugs, such as oral ulceration with ethosuximide, benzodiazepines (e.g. clonazepam) and midazolam/flumazenil. Other common problems with anti-seizure drugs are sedation, pharmacokinetic interactions and, in the longer term, weight gain and seizures despite combination therapy.
- Fixed prosthetics may be safer for a patient with seizures due to concerns of dislodgement of dentures or partials during a seizure.

E. Degenerative neuromuscular disorders

1. Multiple sclerosis

There are 250 000–350 000 patients in the USA with multiple sclerosis. Eighty per cent of patients have the relapsing-remitting variant, which frequently escapes diagnosis for many years due to the remitting and various nature of presenting symptoms. The typical patient presents in the second and third decade of life and the disease has a 2 : 1 female predominance. As with any progressive neurological disorder, the main concern is for sensory, motor or coordination deficits that would interfere with normal oral function.

2. Dental management considerations

- The swallowing reflex can be affected and oral clearance is poor, so suction of secretions is important during dental treatment.
- General anaesthesia is contraindicated due to the potential for a prolonged hospitalization.
- Reduce the dosage of local anaesthesia since there is poor tolerance.
- Flaccid soft tissues, an open-mouth posture and muscle weakness suggest that oral hygiene may be unsatisfactory.

F. Motor neuron disease

This is a progressive neuromuscular condition seen primarily in older people. Its origin is unknown and it involves degenerative changes in anterior horn cells, cranial nerve nuclei and the pyramidal pathway. It is characterized by bulbar or pseudobulbar palsy – lower cranial nerve involvement, weakness of head and neck muscles, eating and swallowing difficulties. Dental considerations are the same as for other conditions where airway impairment is profound, for example, myasthenia gravis and muscular dystrophy.

XI. Pulmonary diseases

A. Asthma

1. Overview

This is an uncommon disorder in the elderly but the dental practitioner should be aware of the signs and symptoms of an asthmatic attack, especially if dental materials are the precipitants. Asthma is a syndrome of episodic and reversible acute or subacute narrowing of the airways, or bronchospasm. There is constriction of smooth muscle with oedema of the bronchial mucosa and formation of tenacious mucous, predisposing to infection. Stress is an important precipitator of attacks in dentistry but others include cold air, pollutants, respiratory infection, exercise, aspirin and medical non-compliance. Several dental materials have been reported to trigger attacks, including toothpaste, sealants, tooth enamel dust and methyl methacrylate.

Intrinsic asthma includes half of all asthmatics and it usually develops in adulthood. Attacks are usually precipitated by non-allergic factors such as infection, air pollutants, smoke, cold air, exercise, stress, emotional upset or physical exertion.

Significant elements in the history include the age at which attacks began, the frequency and severity of attacks and hospitalizations and/or frequency of emergency room visits. The use of steroids suggests severe asthma. If steroids are used, be alert for the possibility of adrenocortical insufficiency and oral candidiasis. Theophylline or aminophylline, erythromycin and clindamycin can increase the theophylline level and result in theophylline toxicity. Importantly, approximately 5% of asthma patients have aspirin sensitivity.

2. Dental management considerations

The primary emphasis for dental management is the prevention of an asthmatic attack in the dental office. The history should include the frequency of attacks, what triggers them, and the frequency of visits to the emergency room. As a general rule, elective dental care should be reserved for patients who are well-controlled.

Prevention of attacks involves avoiding dental treatment during respiratory infections and avoiding aspirin and NSAID-containing drugs, epinephrine (controversial) and antihistamines. Confirm that the patient has taken his/her most recent dose of anti-asthma medication. Ask the patient to bring medications to each appointment. Keep the appointments short and eliminate stress as much as possible. Sedation may minimize risk of attacks. Nitrous oxide may be helpful but caution should be used to prevent airway irritation, which may also be caused by instruments, enamel dust, water mist and other factors during dental care delivery.

Some studies suggest that asthma predisposes to an increased caries incidence due to the salivary drying effect of B_2 agonists. Given the reported loss of salivary function, candidal infections are more likely to occur, especially oropharyngeal candidiasis in chronic users of steroid inhalers.

B. Chronic obstructive pulmonary disease

1. Overview

Chronic obstructive pulmonary disease (COPD) is a major cause of death in the elderly and it occurs as a result of several pulmonary diseases, most commonly emphysema (usually from smoking), chronic bronchitis and asthma. These patients will typically have dyspnea, cough or wheezing. Important elements in the history include: triggering agents/events; duration of the disease; presence of asthma with COPD; use of bronchodilators and beta adrenergics; or chronic use of oral or inhaled steroids. The pathophysiology involves bronchospasm with increased resistance to airflow and destruction of alveolar units with a decrease in elastic recoil, bronchial fibrosis, air trapping and alveolar distention. There are excessive secretions in the tracheobronchial tree and mucosal swelling. COPD is usually the result of cigarette smoking.

2. Management considerations

Although it is uncommon for patients with COPD to be on chronic oral steroids, it is important to elicit that history. Accordingly, the clinician must be aware of the possibility for adrenocortical insufficiency and the potential need for steroid supplementation for stressful procedures and antibiotics for an active oral infection. If patients are on theophylline or aminophylline, use of erythromycin should be avoided due to the possiblity of an increased theophylline level and possible toxicity. Avoid sedatives, tranquilizers, hypnotics and opioids. Avoid high-flow oxygen because it can remove respiratory 'drive'. Watch for xerostomia-related problems such as increased caries incidence, gingivitis and candidiasis from a steroid inhaler. Anxiety control is important before and during dental appointments. While nitrous oxide may be indicated for patients with mild to moderate COPD, it should be avoided in patients with severe COPD since their drive to breathe is based on hypoxia. If there is concern of uncontrolled COPD or undiagnosed sleep apnea with hyypoxia or hypercarbia (elevated CO_2 levels) dental treatment should be deferred until the patient is evaluated and stabilized. Avoid the use of nonsteroidal anti-inflammatory drugs (e.g. aspirin), respiratory depressants, narcotics and sedatives.

C. Pulmonary tuberculosis

Pulmonary tuberculosis (TB) is one of the least transmissible respiratory diseases. However, given the emergence of multidrug-resistant (MDR) forms, appropriate masks must be worn as a preventive measure. Workplace modifications and use of HEPA filter respirators decrease the risk of occupational transmission. Patients should be referred to a physician for a chest film, cultures and purified protein derivative (PPD) if unsure of status. Avoid elective treatment in patients with active disease or positive sputum or those who are still coughing. Most patients have negative sputum cultures after 3–4 weeks of therapy (streptomycin, isoniazid, rifampin, ethambutol, etc.) and are non-infective. MDR TB strains have evolved due to patient non-compliance with anti-TB drug therapy. MDR TB is more prevalent in the HIV-infected population.

XII. Rheumatological diseases, osteoarthritis, osteoporosis and prosthetic joints

A. Rheumatoid arthritis

1. Overview

Rheumatoid arthritis (RA) affects over 2.5 million people in the USA and 40 million around the globe. Peak incidence is the third through fifth decade of life and the disease has a 3 : 1 female predominance. RA is a chronic and progressive inflammatory disorder that leads to joint destruction if not treated with disease-modifying anti-rheumatic drugs (DMARDS). Joint disease crtitical to recognize in the dental patient include the TMJ and upper cervical spine. TMJ involvement can limit access during dental procedures. Inflammatory and degenerative changes in the upper cervical spine, specifically C1 and C2, can lead to cervical cord impingement if the neck is hyperextended. RA is initially treated with glucocorticoids, followed by DMARD therapy such as hydroxycholoroquine, methotrexate or tumour-necrosis factor alpha (TNF-α) inhibitors. Assessing the DMARD therapy in a patient with RA is critical, especially in the face of an active infection.

2. Oral manifestations of rheumatoid arthritis

These are primarily related to medications the patient may be taking. For example, gingival overgrowth can result from cyclosporine and TMJ symptoms may arise from loss of the bone on the head of the condyle. Some patients will have secondary Sjögrens syndrome and chronic xerostomia, and all the attendant side affects associated with dry mouth.

3. Dental management considerations

Significant elements of the history include the use of salicylates or other anti-inflammatory agents: record the drug name, dosage and duration of use and a history of prosthetic joint surgery. Aspirin or other non-steroidal anti-inflammatory agents alter platelet function, but prolonged oral bleeding from a dental procedure is exceedingly unlikely in the absence of other coagulopathies.

Severe RA is a relative contraindication to hyperextension of the neck, and with ankylosing spondylitis the neck vertebrae may be fused, with resultant rigidity. Patients can have problems with oral hygiene secondary to impaired dexterity; they might also have difficulty rising from the dental chair without assistance. A patient in a wheelchair should be transferred to the dental chair whenever possible, for both the patient's and the clinician's well-being.

If the patient has a history of steroid use it might be prudent to increase the daily dosage for stressful procedures. Discuss this with patient's physician in regard to the degree of adrenocortical suppression. Patients with RA who have had joints replaced may be indicated for antibiotic prophylaxis (see prosthetic joints below).

Presence of active infection in a patient with RA should prompt a discussion with the patient's treating physician regarding interruption of their DMARD therapy, especially the use of TNF-α inhibitors.

B. Osteoarthritis

Advanced age, obesity and female gender are the strongest risk factors for the development of osteoarthritis (OA). It is a degenerative disease primarily affecting the weight-bearing joints of the lower extremities and is estimated to affect 80% of patients over the age of 55 and 95% of patients over the age of 65. Treatment often involves exercise, physical therapy, acetaminophen (paracetamol) and NSAIDS. Complications of degenerative osteoarthritis will rarely complicate dental treatment, including the use of NSAIDS (except aspirin) as they rarely predispose to significant bleeding.

C. Osteoporosis

1. Overview

Osteoporosis is a common diagnosis in the elderly, with 24% of women over the age of 65 meeting WHO criteria for the diagnosis. It results in 1.5 million fractures per year in the USA, at an annual direct cost of $18 billion. Standard treatment for osteoporosis includes weight-bearing exercise, calcium, vitamin D, bisphosphonates and selective oestrogen receptor antagonists. The use of oestrogen replacement therapy has declined rapidly for this indication with the finding that hormone replacement therapy increases the rate of breast cancer and cardiovascular events, particularly stroke.

2. Dental management considerations

Many patients are taking biphosphonate medications to slow the process of bone loss. Patients taking a parental drug are at greater risk of osteonecrosis and they should be followed closely for oral disease. Invasive procedures should be done with caution. It is not clear yet the extent to which oral bisposphonates increase the risk for exposed alveolar bone.

D. Prosthetic joints

1. Overview

It has been estimated that over 600 000 joint prostheses are placed each year in the USA. There has been a longstanding concern about the prevention of bacterial seeding of a prosthetic joint from the oral flora during dental treatment. Although the risk from dental procedures is extremely low, poorly documented case reports of joint infection from the oral cavity continue to appear in the literature. The issue of antibiotic prophylaxis to prevent distant site infections in general from invasive dental procedures is highly controversial due to lack of scientific evidence of efficacy. It has been proposed that for most, if not all, of these clinical situations the risk of anaphylaxis from an antibiotic likely outweighs the risk of distant infection from oral bacteraemia. The 2003 guidelines from the American Academy of Orthopaedic Surgeons (AAOS) and the American Dental Association (ADA) have been replaced by controversial guidelines from the AAOS in 2009. A two-year joint collaboration between the ADA and American Association of Orthopaedic Surgeons was published in 2012. These guidelines failed to resolve the controversy surrounding these issues of who needs antibiotic prophylaxis and for which procedures, as well as other considerations. The ADA Center for Evidence-based Dentistry and Council on Scientific Affairs re-reviewed the literature and published a Statement in January 2015 that should help to guide dentists on this issue.

2. Significant elements in the history

Date of surgery; surgeon's name and contact information; the location of the replaced joint; current or past use of steroids; and any history of arthritis, diabetes, chemotherapy and immune deficiency. Dental evaluation and management of the patient with a prosthetic joint infection should include a thorough oral exam, full mouth series of radiographs and treatment to rule out or eliminate sources of possible haematogenous route of bacteraemia from the oral cavity.

3. Dental management considerations

- Aggressive treatment of an overt dental infection with antibiotics.
- Patient should contact their orthopaedic surgeon if they experience pain in a prosthetic joint that was previously pain free.
- The recommendations in 2003 from a joint panel of the American Academy of Orthopedic Surgeons, American Dental Association and specialists in infectious diseases recommended antibiotics prior to all invasive dental procedures for 2 years after replacement of a prosthetic joint. They further state that, after 2 years, antibiotic coverage should be employed only in patients who are immunocompromised or immunosuppressed (e.g. RA), insulin-dependent (Type 1) diabetics, malnourished, haemophiliac, have HIV infection, malignancy or a history of previous joint infection.

Further reading

The elderly patient

Meurman, J.H. & Hamalainen, P. (2006) Oral health and morbidity–implications of oral infections on the elderly. *Gerodontology*, **23**(1), 3–16.

The medical history

Lockhart, P.B. (2013) (ed) *Oral Medicine and Medically Complex Patients*, 6th edn, Wiley-Blackwell, Ames, IA.

Common medical problems in the elderly with consequences for oral health care delivery

I. Allergy

II. Bleeding disorders

Brennan, M.T., Shariff, G., Kent, M.L., Fox, P.C. & Lockhart, P.B. (2002) Relationship between bleeding time test and postextraction bleeding in a healthy control population. *Oral Surgery, Oral Medicine, Oral Pathology, Oral Radiology and Endodontology*, **94**(4), 439–443.

Grines, C.L., Bonow, R.O., Casey, D.E., Jr.,, Gardner, T.J., Lockhart, P.B., Moliterno, D.J. *et al.* (2007) Prevention of premature discontinuation of dual antiplatelet therapy in patients with coronary artery stents: a science advisory from the American Heart Association, American College of Cardiology, Society for Cardiovascular Angiography and Interventions, American College of Surgeons, and American Dental Association, with representation from the American College of Physicians. *Journal of the American Dental Association*, **138**(5),652–655.

Lockhart, P.B., Gibson, J., Pond, S.H. & Leitch, J. (2003) Dental management considerations for the patient with an acquired coagulopathy. Part 1: Coagulopathies from systemic disease. *British Dental Journal*, **195**(8), 439–445.

Lockhart, P.B., Gibson, J., Pond, S.H. & Leitch, J. (2003) Dental management considerations for the patient with an acquired coagulopathy. Part 2: Coagulopathies from drugs. *British Dental Journal*, **195**(9), 495–501.

III. Cancer

Rubenstein, E.B., Peterson, D.E., Schubert, M., Keefe, D., McGuire, D., Epstein, J. *et al.* (2004) Clinical practice guidelines for the prevention and treatment of cancer therapy-induced oral and gastrointestinal mucositis. *Cancer*, **100**(S9), 2026–2046.

Sonis, S.T., Elting, L.S., Keefe, D., Peterson, D.E., Schubert, M., Hauer-Jensen, M. *et al.* (2004) Perspectives on cancer therapy-induced mucosal injury: pathogenesis, measurement, epidemiology, and consequences for patients. *Cancer*, **100**(S9), 1995–2025.

IV. Cardiovascular disorders

Bavitz, J.B. (2006) Dental management of patients with hypertension. *Dental Clinics of North America*, **50**(4), 547–562.

Brennan, M.T., Shariff, G., Kent, M.L., Fox, P.C. & Lockhart, P.B. (2002) Relationship between bleeding time test and postextraction bleeding in a healthy control population. *Oral Surgery, Oral Medicine, Oral Pathology, Oral Radiology and Endodontology*, **94**(4), 439–443.

Chobanian, A.V., Bakris, G.L., Black, H.R., Cushman, W.C., Green, L.A., Izzo, J.L., Jr., *et al.* (2003) The seventh report of the joint national committee on prevention, detection, evaluation, and treatment of high blood pressure: the JNC 7 report. *JAMA*, **289**(19), 2560–2572.

Grines, C.L., Bonow, R.O., Casey, D.E., Jr.,, Gardner, T.J., Lockhart, P.B., Moliterno, D.J. *et al.* (2007) Prevention of premature discontinuation of dual antiplatelet therapy in patients with coronary artery stents: a science advisory from the American Heart Association, American College of Cardiology, Society for Cardiovascular Angiography and Interventions, American College of Surgeons, and American Dental Association, with representation from the American College of Physicians. *Journal of the American Dental Association*, **138**(5), 652–655.

Lockhart, P.B., Gibson, J., Pond, S.H. & Leitch, J. (2003) Dental management considerations for the patient with an acquired coagulopathy. Part 2: Coagulopathies from drugs. *British Dental Journal*, **195**(9), 495–501.

Lockhart, P.B., Littmann, L. & Glick, M. (2007) Diseases of the cardiovascular system. In: M.S. Greenberg, M. Glick & J.A. Ship (eds) *Burket's Oral Medicine: Diagnosis and Treatment*. BC Decker Inc.

Lockhart, P.B., Loven, B., Brennan & M.T., Fox, P.C. (2007) The evidence base for the efficacy of antibiotic prophylaxis in dental practice. *Journal of the American Dental Association*, **138**(4), 458–474.

Roberts, H.W. & Mitnitsky, E.F. (2001) Cardiac risk stratification for postmyocardial infarction dental patients. *Oral Surgery, Oral Medicine, Oral Pathology, Oral Radiology and Endodontology*, **91**(6), 676–681.

Rose, L.F., Mealey, B., Minsk, L. & Cohen, D.W. (2002) Oral care for patients with cardiovascular disease and stroke. *Journal of the American Dental Association*, **133**(Suppl.), 37S–44S.

Wilson, W., Taubert, K.A., Gewitz, M., Lockhart, P.B., Baddour, L.M., Levison, M. *et al.* (2007) Prevention of Infective Endocarditis. Guidelines from the American Heart Association. A Guideline from the American Heart Association Rheumatic Fever, Endocarditis, and Kawasaki Disease Committee, Council on Cardiovascular Disease in the Young, and the Council on Clinical Cardiology, Council on Cardiovascular Surgery and Anesthesia, and the Quality of Care and Outcomes Research Interdisciplinary Working Group. *Circulation*, **116**, 1736–1754.

V. Cerebral vascular disease

VI. Drug abuse and addiction

Friedlander, A.H. & Norman, D.C. (2006) Geriatric alcoholism: pathophysiology and dental implications. *Journal of the American Dental Association*, **137**(3), 330–338.

Oral-Facial Emergencies. Diagnosis and Management, 1st edn, JBK Publishing, Portland, OR, 1994.

Saitz, R. (2005) Clinical practice. Unhealthy alcohol use. *New England Journal of Medicine*, **352**(6), 596–607.

Sorocco, K.H. & Ferrell, S.W. (2006) Alcohol use among older adults. *Journal of General Psychology*, **133**(4), 453–67.

VII. Endocrine disorders

Little, J.W. (2006) Thyroid disorders. Part I: hyperthyroidism. *Oral Surgery, Oral Medicine, Oral Pathology, Oral Radiology and Endodontology*, **101**(3), 276–284.

McKenna, S.J. (2006) Dental management of patients with diabetes. *Dental Clinics of North America*, **50**(4), 591–606.

Pinto, A. & Glick, M. (2002) Management of patients with thyroid disease: oral health considerations. *Journal of the American Dental Association*, **133**(7), 849–858.

VIII. Liver disease

Firriolo, F.J. (2006) Dental management of patients with end-stage liver disease. *Dental Clinics of North America*, **50**(4), 563–590.

Lockhart, P.B., Gibson, J., Pond, S.H. & Leitch, J. (2003) Dental management considerations for the patient with an acquired coagulopathy. Part 1: Coagulopathies from systemic disease. *British Dental Journal*, **195**(8), 439–445.

Schmucker, D.L. (2005) Age-related changes in liver structure and function: Implications for disease? *Experimental Gerontology*, **40**(8–9), 650–659.

IX. Renal disorders

Kerr, A.R. (2001) Update on renal disease for the dental practitioner. *Oral Surgery, Oral Medicine, Oral Pathology, Oral Radiology and Endodontology*, **92**(1), 9–16.

X. Neurological and neuromuscular disorders

Bryan, R.B. & Sullivan, S.M. (2006) Management of dental patients with seizure disorders. *Dental Clinics of North America*, **50**(4), 607–623.

Hong, C.H., Allred, R., Napenas, J.J., Brennan, M.T., Baddour, L.M. & Lockhart, P.B. (2010) Antibiotic prophylaxis for dental procedures to prevent indwelling venous catheter-related infections. *American Journal of Medicine*, **123**(12), 1128–1133.

Noseworthy, J.H., Lucchinetti, C., Rodriguez, M. & Weinshenker, B.G. (2000) Multiple sclerosis. *New England Journal of Medicine*, **343**(13), 938–952.

XI. Pulmonary diseases

Hupp, W.S. (2006) Dental management of patients with obstructive pulmonary diseases. *Dental Clinics of North America*, **50**(4), 513–527.

Steinbacher, D.M. & Glick, M. (2001) The dental patient with asthma. An update and oral health considerations. *Journal of the American Dental Association*, **132**(9), 1229–1239.

XII. Rheumatological diseases, osteoarthritis, osteoporosis and prosthetic joints

American Dental Association, American Academy of Orthopaedic Surgeons. (2003) Antibiotic prophylaxis for dental patients with total joint replacements Advisory Statement. *Journal of the American Dental Association*, **134**(7), 895–899.

Baddour, L.M., Epstein, A.E., Erickson, C.C., Knight, B.P., Levison, M.E., Lockhart, P.B. *et al.* (2010) Update on cardiovascular implantable electronic device infections and their management: a scientific statement from the American Heart Association. *Circulation*, **121**(3), 458–477.

Khosla, S., Burr, D., Cauley, J., Dempster, D.W., Ebeling, P.R., Felsenberg, D. *et al.* (2007) Bisphosphonate-associated psteonecrosis of the jaw: report of a task force of the American Society for Bone and Mineral Research. *Journal of Bone and Mineral Research*, **22**(10), 1479–1491.

Lockhart, P.B., Brennan, M.T., Fox, P.C., Norton, H.J., Jernigan, D.B., Strausbaugh, L.J. *et al.* (2002) Decision-making on the use of antimicrobial prophylaxis for dental procedures: A survey of infectious disease consultants and review. *Clinical Infectious Diseases*, **34**(12), 1621–1626.

Lockhart, P.B., Loven, B., Brennan, M.T. & Fox, P.C. (2007) The evidence base for the efficacy of antibiotic prophylaxis in dental practice. *Journal of the American Dental Association*, **138**(4), 458–474.

Lockhart, P.B., Wray, D., Peterson, D.E., Greenberg, M.S. (2007) Fourth world workshop on oral medicine. *Oral Surgery, Oral Medicine, Oral Pathology, Oral Radiology and Endodontology*, **103**(3 Suppl. 1).

O'Dell, J.R. (2004) Therapeutic strategies for rheumatoid arthritis *New England Journal of Medicine*, **350**(25), 2591–2602.

Rethman, M.P., Watters, W., Abt, E., Anderson, P.A., Carroll, K.C., Evans, R.P. *et al.* (2013) The American Academy of Orthopaedic Surgeons and the American Dental Association Clinical Practice Guideline on The Prevention of Orthopaedic Implant Infection in Patients Undergoing Dental Procedures. *Journal of Bone and Joint Surgery. American Volume*, **95**(8), 745–747.

Rosen, C.J. (2005) Clinical practice. Postmenopausal osteoporosis. *New England Journal of Medicine*, **353**(6), 595–603.

Treister, N. & Glick, M. (1999) Rheumatoid arthritis: a review and suggested dental care considerations. *Journal of the American Dental Association*, **130**(5), 689–698.

Woo, S.B., Hellstein, J.W. & Kalmar, J.R. (2006) Narrative [corrected] review: bisphosphonates and osteonecrosis of the jaws. *Annals of Internal Medicine*, **144**(10), 753–761.

CHAPTER 9

Psychiatric disorders in old age – implications for the dental practitioner

Angela R. Kamer*[1], Mony J. de Leon[2] and Martin J Sadowski*[3]
[1]Department of Periodontology and Implant Dentistry, NYU College of Dentistry, New York, USA
[2]Center for Brain Health, Department of Psychiatry, NYU School of Medicine, New York, USA
[3]Departments of Neurology, Psychiatry, Biochemistry and Molecular Pharmacology, NYU School of Medicine, New York, USA

Introduction

The proportion of elderly in the population is growing at a fast rate. By the year 2050 it is projected that the number of people older than 65 will reach almost 87 million with almost 25% being older than 85 years. Parallel to this increase, it is expected that the number of elderly with psychiatric conditions will increase as well. Caring for these people's general health, including oral health, is an important and challenging task. Oral diseases constitute significant problems in this population and the health care provider is challenged to address them effectively. Oral health characteristics in aging have changed during the past few years. In the United States, the percentage of total edentulism decreased in the past decade but is still present in almost 25% of adults 65 years and older. During the same period, the tooth retention increased and there was a decline in decayed, missing and filled permanent teeth and in the prevalence of moderate to severe periodontitis (Vital and Health Statistics, 2007). While these numbers are encouraging in general terms, the distribution of oral disease is not uniform. Continuing major health issues remain in the interactions between old age and psychiatric and oral conditions. This chapter will describe the most prevalent psychiatric conditions found in elderly populations and current treatment approaches. It will also describe age-related oral conditions and their implications for the oral health care provider.

* Address correspondence regarding neurological and psychiatric disease to Dr Martin J. Sadowski and for dental health issues to Dr Angela R. Kamer.

Psychiatric and neurological disorders in the elderly

1. Affective disorders

Depression

Depression is characterized by persistent symptoms of depressed mood, lack of motivation, energy, drive and/or markedly diminished interest or pleasure in activities. Depending on the severity of symptoms, two forms of depressive disorder are distinguished: major depressive disorder and dysthymia (non-major depressive). The incidence of depression as well as suicide significantly increases after the age of 65. Risk factors for increased frequency of depressive disorders in older patients include: a history of mood disorder earlier in life, co-existence of personality disorder traits, as well as social and personal changes ongoing in the lives of elderly subjects. Most typical examples include the death of a spouse, changes associated with retirement, lesser engagement in social and professional activities. There is significant comorbidity of depression and complex medical illness and/or dementia. Major depression has been found in 20–25% of older patients with medical illness. Among older patients presenting with major depressive disorder almost 90% were found to have at least one medical illness. Studies on comorbidity of depression and dementia have shown the presence of depression in up to 50% of patients with Alzheimer's disease (AD), whereas vascular dementia was associated with major depression in 20% and with dysthymia in another 20% of cases.

Symptoms of the depressive disorder include persistent symptoms of depressed mood for more than 48 h, lack of

Textbook of Geriatric Dentistry, Third Edition. Edited by Poul Holm-Pedersen, Angus W. G. Walls and Jonathan A. Ship.

motivation, energy and drive, tearfulness and/or markedly diminished interest or pleasure in activities. Frequently, depression is linked to fear, increased anxiety and feelings of hopelessness. Sleep disturbances, including nightmares or decreased amounts of sleep at night (or both), early awakening and difficulties in falling back to sleep, are frequent. Sexual drive is usually diminished, although this feature has to be critically assessed in the aged since the libido declines with age. Depression is also associated with limited attention and motivation; therefore, capacity of cognitive performance and memory in particular are diminished. Occurrence of depressive symptoms in the elderly almost always has a strong impact on cognitive performance. In subjects free of dementing illness depression may mimic dementia, whereas in subjects with mild cognitive impairment (MCI) or early dementia, co-existence of depression may worsen patient performance, mimicking later stages of the disease. Issues related to depression that the dental practitioner may come across include the tendency of a depressed patient, and in particular a patient with coexisting depression and dementing illness, to neglect oral hygiene and be inattentive to the requirements of dental treatment.

Treatment of depression in older individuals must take into consideration the complexity of medical care including medical comorbidities, a frequently extensive daily medication schedule, an age-associated decrease in renal and liver drug clearance and a high risk of drug-induced encephalopathy. Due to their relatively benign adverse-effect profile, selective serotonin reuptake inhibitors (SSRIs) are used as the first line of treatment. The most commonly used SSRIs include citalopram (Celexa), escitalopram (Lexapro), fluoxetine (Prozac), paroxetine (Paxil) and sertraline (Zoloft). They are usually administered once a day and have few possible side effects, which makes this class of drugs a primary choice in the aged. Adverse effects common for all SSRIs include gastrointestinal symptoms: abdominal cramps, diarrhea, constipation, nausea and rare vomiting. In addition, fluoxetine may cause insomnia and paroxetine may cause mild anticholinergic effects. Other frequently used medications include buproprion (Wellbutrin), mitrazapine (Remeron) and venlafaxine (Effexor). Tricyclic antidepressants are used sparingly because of their numerous adverse effects: anticholinergic symptoms, orthostatic hypotension, sedative effects and a slowing effect on the cardiac conduction system. A pretreatment EKG is required to establish absence of atrio-ventricular conduction defects in patients considered for tricyclic antidepressant therapy. Therefore, use of this class of drugs is mainly reserved for patients whose symptoms had been resistant to other forms of therapy. When used in elderly patients, desipramine (Norpramin) and nortryptyline (Aventyl, Pamelor) are preferred due to their low propensity to cause anticholinergic, orthostatic and sedative side effects. In cases that are resistant to pharmacological treatment or life threatening (e.g. refusal to eat and take oral medications) electroconvulsive therapy may constitute the treatment of choice. The risk of electroconvulsive therapy is very low but, as for each type of depression treatment, it must be weighed against the consequences of depression and risk of a patient's suicide. Psychotherapy can be used in the form of adjunct therapy, especially targeting non-demented patients and patients with cognitive impairment and early stages of dementia. It can be particularly useful in cases where depression has a strong association with age-related changes in life situation and family dynamics (family therapy).

Bipolar disorders in the elderly

The majority of cases of bipolar disorder begin before the age of 50 and manic episodes during the course of life-long bipolar disorder tend to decrease in frequency and intensity with age. The clinical picture of a manic episode in the elderly differs significantly from that seen in younger individuals. While euphoria and elation are less common, confusion, paranoia, irritability, dysphoria and distractibility nearly resembling dementia or delirium are seen more often. Treatment includes prevention of mood changes by chronic treatment with one of the mood stabilizing agents: valproic acid (Depakene, Depakote), carbamazepine (Tegretol), or lithium carbonate (Eskalith, Lithotabs, Lithonate). All three drugs require monitoring of blood level, liver function and electrolytes. Because of adverse effects on memory, cognitive performance, tremor and ataxia, lithium is used sparingly in the elderly population. As emphasized above, occurrence of a new onset bipolar disorder after the age of 65 is rare. Therefore, when assessing an elderly patient without a prior history of bipolar illness who presents with manic symptoms one is required to search for an underlying pathological process: CNS infection, stroke, tumour or neurodegenerative disease (e.g. frontotemporal dementia). General medical illness, including occult infection (e.g. abscess) and adverse effects from medications have to be ruled out as well.

2. Anxiety disorders

Anxiety disorders are characterized by unjustifiably excessive and maladaptive emotional response. Although in general anxiety disorders are becoming less common with age, their prevalence in 20% of elderly subjects makes them one of the most common issues encounterd in geriatric psychiatry. Morbid anxiety can manifest itself with cognitive, behavioural and physiological symptoms, and can range from excessive worrying about minor matters to panic attacks. Cognitive symptoms associated with anxiety may include nervousness, apprehension, racing thoughts, fearfulness, irritability and distractibility. Behavioural symptoms include repetitive motor acts, phobias, pressured speech and startle response. In more severe cases, one or more physiological symptoms like tachycardia, palpitations, chest pain, abdominal cramps, diarrhea, heaviness of the limbs, hyperventilation or parasthesias are present. Forms of anxiety disorders diagnosed in older patients are similar to those observed in younger subjects and examples include panic disorder, social phobia, simple phobia (agoraphobia, claustrophobia), generalized anxiety disorder, obsessive compulsive disorder and post-traumatic stress disorder. The last entity is especially prevalent among military veterans. Occurrence of anxiety in the elderly may also be associated with cognitive loss and thus it is frequently seen during mild cognitive impairment and early stages of dementia, especially in patients who remain professionally active.

Treatment of anxiety disorders in the elderly is complex and includes both pharmacological and psychological approaches. If the occurrence of anxiety is associated with cognitive impairment, withdrawal of a patient from anxiety-provoking activities appears to be very effective. Retirement from a job to eliminate daily stress and humiliation serves well as an example of such action. Pharmacological treatment includes use of different groups of medications to ameliorate anxiety symptoms and restore psychological comfort. Different pharmacological strategies have been developed to target various forms of phobia. Groups of medications used to treat anxiety disorders include SSRIs, benzodiazepines, antihistamines, buspirone, β-blockers and monoamine oxidase inhibitors. Although benzodiazepines are very effective in ameliorating symptoms of anxiety they have to be used with caution in the elderly as these drugs can particularly affect short-term memory, even causing amnestic syndrome, cognitive impairment and confusion. By affecting liver enzymes, benzodiazepines may also affect half-life of other medications. Adverse effects of benzodiazepine therapy are usually reversible.

3. Late-life delusional and paranoid psychoses

The prevalence of delusions (false beliefs not shared by others) and paranoias (a complex system of delusions that direct the patient to act) is markedly increased among elderly patients and very frequently occurs in subjects without premorbid history of psychopathology. They frequently arise on the bases of organic pathology including AD, other neurodegenerative disorders, stroke or vascular dementia. It has been estimated that about half of all patients with AD will experience psychotic symptoms at some time in the disease course. It is not unusual that an episode of psychosis or paranoid symptoms may precede onset of neurodegenerative dementing illness, even by several years. It has to be emphasized however that incidence of schizophrenia decreases with advancing age and diagnosis of new onset of thought disorder becomes extremely rare after the age of 65. In patients, with a life-long history of schizophrenia, the frequency of psychotic episodes tends to decrease with age (burned-out schizophrenia), negative symptoms prevail and these patients appear to have increased risk for developing dementia.

Paranoid and delusional symptoms in the elderly have diverse causes. They result from impaired judgment and abstract thinking, loss of control of social rules and poor orientation and memory that are associated with progressive neurodegenerative disease like AD or are a result of stroke. Sensory deprivation, which accompanies the aging process, is a significant contributory factor. The prevalence of lens cataracts is up to 50% in the 75–85 years age group and 70% have glaucoma. Significant numbers of elderly patients develop macular degeneration, microvascular retinopathy and other ocular pathologies contributing to visual disability. Furthermore, one third of the aged have some degree of auditory disability. These sensory changes are frequently either an initiation factor in developing delusions of hallucinations or factors that magnify ongoing psychopathological processes.

Common examples of delusions among elderly patients, especially in those with dementia, are delusions of suspicion (e.g. spouse infidelity), jealousy, persecution (e.g. being watched or poisoned), guilt or theft. In addition, beliefs that long-time deceased family members are still alive and beliefs that close family members are replaced by impostors (Capgrass symptoms) are frequent for old-age psychiatry. Very typical for young-onset schizophrenia, delusions of thought broadcasting, mind control or reference are infrequent among the elderly. Often delusions rise to the level of paranoia directing elderly patients to act in an aberrant way, making the patients even verbally or physically abusive The effect of delusions and paranoia on a patient's life may vary from disruption of family life (e.g. a patient barricading himself or eloping in search of long-gone relatives) to life-threatening situations (e.g. delusion of spouse infidelity leading to physical altercation, even including use of a firearm).

Infrequent isolated delusions, which are not associated with agitation, can be addressed by providing counselling to a caregiver who, when confronted with delusions, should stay calm and try to persuade a patient. In a situation when delusions become more frequent, rise to the level of paranoia and are associated with aberrant and disruptive behaviour, medical treatment should be considered. Atypical antipsychotic medications are effective drugs of choice although they should be used with caution in lower doses and with careful titration. Their use in the elderly population has been associated with an increased rate of sudden death or stroke, although the pathomechanism responsible for this relationship remains obscure. This led the FDA to add a 'black box' warning label. Therefore, it is a standard of good practice to have a documented discussion with the patient and/or family about the risk and benefits of antipsychotic treatment. The most commonly used antipsychotics include quetiapine (Seroquel), aripiprazole (Abilify), ziprasidone (Geodon), olanzapine (Zyprexa) and risperidone (Risperdal). Use of aripiprazole and olanzapine are associated with elevation of blood sugar, hence these drugs cannot be used in patients with concomitant diabetes. Due to its strong blocking effect on D2 dopaminergic receptor, prolonged use of Risperidone may be associated with occurrence of symptoms of Parkinsonism.

Typical, older antipsychotic agents also carry an increased risk of death in the aged and their adverse effects are more potent than those of atypical agents: anticholinergic symptoms, orthostatic hypotension, and strong preponderance for eliciting extrapyramidal symptoms. Therefore typical antipsychotic agents (e.g. haloperidol) are used sparingly and mainly in a hospital setting for a limited period.

4. Confusion and delirium

Confusion and delirium are extremely frequent among patients with dementia and they are not unusual among non-demented elderly subjects. They are frequently associated with underlying medical illness. Thus, confusion or delirium can be the first manifestation of pulmonary or urinary tract infection, abscess, dehydration, acute renal failure or be an adverse effect of medications. Confusion and delirium can also be caused by a process directly affecting the brain, like intracranial hemorrhage, meningitis, CNS vasculitis or encephalitis. Symptoms include disorientation and an altered level of responsiveness. Patients may become either withdrawn or, to the contrary, agitated. If agitation occurs, it is not usually associated with delusions which allows differentiation of delirium from paranoia. Cognitive symptoms may be associated with worsening of gait and occurrence of mild Parkinsonism. In the case of intracranial processes, focal symptoms including extremity weakness and/or cranial nerve lesions are frequent. A change in mental status is considered a medical emergency and requires prompt medical handling in a hospital emergency room. Basic workup includes non-contrast head CT to rule out a bleed and abscess, complete blood count, chemistry and liver function tests to rule out metabolic causes, chest X-ray and urine analysis to rule out pulmonary or urinary tract infection. Spinal tap and brain MRI should be performed if an intracranial process is suspected. In a case where systemic infection is suspected, blood cultures and a trans-esophageal cardiac echogram to rule out encocarditis should be obtained. Treatment should target underlying medical illness. Agitation should be cautiously treated with antipsychotic medications, avoiding escalation of doses.

Elderly patients are also prone to develop post-surgical delirium, especially when subjected to general anaesthesia. As a rule of thumb, an epidural block or local anaesthesia should be used rather than general anaesthesia. This principle is also relevant to cases of oral surgery. Increased sensitivity of elderly patients to narcotics prescribed for post-procedure pain is another reason for post-surgical confusion and delirium. Opiod induced confusion is always reversible, but it can be prevented by prescribing smaller doses than is done for younger patients. Involvement of caregivers in supervision of opiod administration is always helpful in preventing delirium.

5. Dementia

Dementia is a neurological disorder characterized by the loss of mental capacities, such as memory, reasoning and thinking, severe enough to interfere with daily activities. Alzheimer's disease (AD) is the most frequent cause of dementia accounting for approximately 60–70% of all cases. Other types of dementia include vascular, Lewy body and frontotemporal dementia.

Alzheimer's disease

Alzheimer's disease is a heterogeneous disorder with both familial and sporadic forms. The prevalence of dementia is below 1% in individuals aged 60–64 years but increases exponentially with age. The most significant risk factor for AD is aging. Genetic background also appears to be important since the extent of heritability for the sporadic disease is almost 80% and the presence of an *APOE* ε4 allele increases the risk of the disease by three times in heterozygotes and by 15 times in homozygotes. Other potential risk factors proposed include a decreased reserve capacity of the brain, low educational and occupational attainment, low mental ability in early life, reduced mental and physical activity during late life and head injury. Hypercholesterolaemia, hypertension, atherosclerosis, coronary heart disease, smoking, obesity, diabetes, peripheral infections and inflammations are currently being investigated. Since these factors are also important in vascular diseases, they may independently relate to AD or they may induce cerebrovascular pathology, which adds to the clinically silent AD disease pathology. Several dietary intake such as homocysteine-related vitamins (vitamin B_{12}

and folate), antioxidants (vitamin C and E), unsaturated fatty acids, moderate alcohol intake, especially wine, have been proposed to reduce the risk of AD but data so far are not conclusive enough to provide dietary recommendations.

AD is characterized by the presence of its characteristic lesions, the senile or neuritic plaques and neurofibrillary tangles in the medial temporal lobe structures and cortical areas of the brain, together with a degeneration of the neurons and synapses. Senile plaques are deposits of high-grade fibrillar beta amyloid filaments surrounded by dystrophic neuritis, reactive astrocytes and activated glial cells. The neurofibrillary tangles are bundles of filaments in the neuron cytoplasm and their main component is the hyperphosphorylated tau protein. The neuronal loss predominates in the hippocampus, entorhinal and temporoparietal cortex. Several hypotheses have been put forward to explain the initiation and the pathogenic process in AD. One such hypothesis is the amyloid cascade hypothesis according to which an imbalance between the production and clearance of amyloid-β (Aβ) in the brain is the initiating event, ultimately leading to neuronal degeneration and dementia. The Aβ is produced by neurons, astrocytes and glial cells from amyloid precursor protein (APP). APP is cleaved sequentially by β and γ secretases resulting in the production of Aβ peptides. Soluble Aβ may undergo a conformational change to high β-sheet content, rendering it prone to aggregate into soluble oligomers and larger insoluble fibrils in plaques. In this process, the fibrillogenic Aβ42 isoform peptide triggers the misfolding of other Aβ species. Initially, only Aβ deposited in plaques was assumed to be neurotoxic, but findings suggest that soluble Aβ oligomers might be the culprits, inhibiting hippocampal long-term potentiation, disrupting synaptic plasticity, inducing an inflammatory and oxidative stress and impairing neuronal and synaptic function. Tangles are composed of abnormally hyperphosphorylated tau protein. Tau is a normal axonal protein that binds to microtubules promoting microtubule assembly and stability. Tau hyperphosphorylation leads to sequestration of normal tau and other microtubule-associated proteins, which causes disassembly of microtubules and thus impaired axonal transport, compromising neuronal and synaptic function. Tau also becomes prone to aggregation into insoluble fibrils in tangles, further compromising neuronal function. Tau pathology starts early in the disease process in neurons in the transentorhinal region, spreads to the hippocampus and amygdala, and later to the neocortical association areas. Whether tau hyperphosphorylation and tangle formation are a cause or consequence of Alzheimer's disease is unknown.

Another prevalent hypothesis attempting to explain AD pathogenesis is the inflammatory hypothesis. The central theme of the 'inflammatory hypothesis' is the presence of an inflammatory process in the brain that is self-perpetuating and contributes to synapses dysfunction and neurodegeneration. It is not known what initiates and maintains brain inflammation in AD. However, it is suggested that it may be induced by the Aβ found in senile plaques, hyperphosphorylated tau protein (P-Tau) of neurofibrillary tangles or components of the degenerated neurons by activating the astrocytes and glial cells to produce proinflammatory cytokines such as TNF-α, Il-1β, Il-6 and inflammatory sensitive proteins such as CRP. The role of these molecules is twofold: (1) to maintain a vicious cycle by stimulating the glial cells and (2) to activate pathways leading to neurodegeneration. An associated hypothesis is that peripheral inflammatory processes may contribute to the progression of AD. Other hypotheses proposed included abnormalities in proteins regulating the cell cycle, oxidative stress and mitochondrial dysfunction with disruption in neuronal energy metabolism. Although each of these mechanisms could contribute to disease pathogenesis, to what extent they drive the neurodegenerative process is uncertain.

Alzheimer's disease is a slowly progressive disorder, with insidious onset and progressive impairment of episodic memory; instrumental signs include aphasia, apraxia and agnosia together with general cognitive symptoms, such as impaired judgment, decision-making and orientation. Neurodegeneration is estimated to start 20–30 years before the clinical onset of AD. During this preclinical phase plaque, and later the tangle load, increases and it is possible that at a certain threshold the first symptoms appear. The initial clinical phase is often called mild cognitive impairment (MCI), which is defined on the basis of subjective reports of memory loss that are verified by close personal informants and by objective measures adjusted for age and education. MCI is an etiologically heterogeneous entity because many patients with MCI have prodromal AD, whereas others have a benign form of MCI as part of the normal aging process and some have other disorders such as vascular dementia. The memory-predominant subtype amnestic MCI has been suggested to constitute a transitional stage between normal aging and AD but data show that many patients with amnestic MCI have the early neuropathological changes of AD and thus, in reality, represent early AD. In MCI, the conversion rate to AD with clinical dementia is 10–15% per year.

The clinical diagnosis of AD is commonly done using the criteria of the National Institute of Neurological and Communicative Diseases and Stroke and the Alzheimer's Disease and Related Disorders Association (NINCDS–ADRDA). According to these criteria the presence of a clinical diagnosis of possible or probable AD is done based on the presence of a dementia syndrome confirmed by neuropsychological testing. These neuropsychological tests specify eight cognitive domains that may be impaired in AD. These are memory, language, perceptual skills, attention, constructive abilities, orientation, problem solving and functional abilities. The medical history, clinical, neurological and psychiatric examination are used in the diagnostic work-up. Neuropsychological testing can help to obtain objective signs of memory disturbances particularly in early cases. Laboratory studies, such as thyroid-function tests and serum vitamin B_{12}, are used to rule out secondary causes of dementia and coexisting disorders that are common in elderly people. Similarly, neuroimaging, CT and MRI tests exclude alternative causes of dementia, such as brain tumour, subdural haematoma and cerebrovascular disease. According to the NINCDS–ADRDA criteria, AD cannot be diagnosed until the patient has Alzheimer's dementia, meaning cognitive signs severe enough to exceed an arbitrary threshold of interference with social or occupational activities. These criteria for probable AD largely depend on the exclusion of other dementias and therefore result in a sensitivity of around 80% and specificity of 70% in research centres and probably substantially lower figures in primary care settings and in patients with mild AD. A definite diagnosis of AD requires neuropathology diagnosis. Although this is regarded as the gold standard, as few as a third of patients with definite AD have pure Alzheimer pathology. Approximately 20–40% of non-demented individuals have enough plaques and tangles to warrant a neuropathological diagnosis of AD, around 50% of patients with neuropathological disease have significant concomitant cerebrovascular pathology and there is also a large overlap in pathology between AD and Lewy-body dementia (LBD).

To date, the treatment for AD is only symptomatic. Such groups of drugs are acetylcholinesterase inhibitors and N-methyl-D-aspartate (NMDA) receptor antagonists. Acetylcholinesterase inhibitors inhibit the acetylcholinesterase, the enzyme that degrades acetylcholine in the synaptic cleft, thus enhancing the cholinergic neurotransmission. N-Methyl-D-aspartate (NMDA) receptor antagonists interfere with the sustained activation of NMDA receptors thus facilitating the neuronal function. The acetylcholinesterase inhibitors donepezil, rivastigmine, and galantamine are approved for clinical use in AD. Donepezil and galantamine are selective acetylcholinesterase inhibitors, whereas rivastigmine inhibits acetylcholinesterase and buturylcholinesterase with similar affinity and galantamine also allosterically modulates presynaptic nicotinic receptors. Both donepezil and galantamine are metabolized in the liver by the cytochrome P450 enzymes and thus can interact with drugs that inhibit these enzymes, such as fluoxetine and paroxetine. Rivastigmine has a non-hepatic metabolism, making interactions rare. A non-competitive NMDA-receptor antagonist is memantine. Considering the mechanism of action for the acetylcholinesterase inhibitors and NMDA receptors antagonists they are not expected to change the natural course of AD, but only to temporarily mitigate some of the symptoms. Acetylcholinesterase inhibitors can be effective up to 2–5 years and are indicated in mild to moderate AD while memantine may be effective in moderate to severe disease for shorter periods. Additionally, combination therapy with donepezil and memantine may show positive effects on symptoms relative to donepezil alone in moderate to severe disease. In addition to cognititive symptoms often AD patients receive treatment for their behavioural signs. Aggression, psychomotor agitation and psychosis (hallucinations and delusions) are very common in patients with AD, especially in the late stages of the disease. Atypical antipsychotic drugs produce fewer extrapyramidal side effects (e.g. Parkinsonism and tardive dyskinesia) than conventional neuroleptics and are thus preferred for the management of psychosis or agitation. Several short-term trials show efficacy of risperidone and olanzapine in reducing the rate of aggression, agitation and psychosis. Alternative treatments include anticonvulsants, such as divalproate and carbamazepine, and short-acting benzodiazepines, such as lorazepam and oxazepam. Additionally, the cholinergic deficits can contribute to the development of behavioural symptoms, and treatment with acetylcholinesterase inhibitors also shows improvements in behavioural symptoms.

Vascular dementia

After AD, cerebrovascular disorders are the second cause of cognitive deficit in the aged. In autopsy series of dementia, various forms of vascular pathology, alone or in association with AD, are found in 40% of cases. Development of vascular cognitive impairment may be related to several processes separated by their distinct pathological mechanism and the type of cognitive deficit they produce.

1 Multi-infarct dementia resulting from repeated large vessel strokes.
2 Intracranial haemorrhage(s).
3 Leukoariosis – chronic ischaemic white matter disease.
4 Lacunar infarctions.

Multi-infarct (or large vessel dementia) is associated with atrial fibrillation, cardiomyopathy, endocarditis, inborn cardiac defects (e.g. patent foramen ovale) and atherosclerosis of large and medium size arteries (e.g. carotid stenosis). Intracranial haemorrhage can be sequel of untreated hypertension or an aneurysm. Repeated lobar haemorrhages are associated with deposition of vascular amyloid, which weakens arterial wall. Both recurrent large vessel ischaemic strokes and lobar haemorrhages produce step-wise cognitive deterioration, with the type and severity of symptomatology associated with the size and localization of the brain insult. The pattern of cognitive deficit associated with multi-infarct dementia (and in most cases with repeated lobar haemorrhages as well) is consistent with 'cortical dementia'. Its cardinal features are domain specific deficits (e.g. aphasia, apraxia, agnosia, acalculia) and normal cognitive speed. Unless a lesion is placed in fronto-orbital areas, hippocampus or mamillary bodies the memory is preserved. A significant level of cognitive deficit may also be observed after a single, but massive and/or strategically placed, vascular event (apoplectic dementia). A caveat with making diagnosis of dementia in such patients is to demonstrate deficit in more than one area of cognition, hence patients with aphasia are not automatically diagnosed with vascular dementia.

Leukoariosis (previously referred to as Binswanger disease) manifests on brain MRI as multiple or confluent areas of increased white matter signal on T2 or fluid-attenuation inversion recovery images (FLAIR). These areas correspond to ischaemic demyelination and gliosis which are associated with lipohyalinosis, a degenerative obturative process affecting small arterial vessel walls supplying the subcortical white matter, thalamus and basal ganglia. Uncontrolled blood sugar level in the course of diabetes, smoking, uncontrolled hypertension and hypercholesterolaemia are direct risk factors (given in order of decreasing importance) for developing lipohyalinosis. Rapid occlusion of a distal vessel that is the only vessel supplying a particular area gives rise to lacunar infarction. Therefore, leukoariosis and lacunar infarctions share pathological mechanism and risk factors and frequently coexist with each other. Leukoariosis, with or without coexisting lacunar infarctions, is also referred to as small-vessel dementia. It is responsible for 50% of all cases of vascular dementia and 16% of cases co-exist with multi-infarct large-vessel dementia. Unlike large vessel (multi-infarct) dementia, leukoariosis causes slowly progressing cognitive deficit with subcortical patterns. This pattern is characterized by impaired information processing, slowing of cognitive speed and deficit in information retrieval. Subcortical dementia is also frequently associated with psychiatric symptoms (labile mood, apathy, depression) and neurological signs (dysarthria, spasticity and gait disorders). Cortical functions like language or calculation are typically preserved.

In rare cases, leukoariosis is genetically determined. Cerebral autosomal dominant arteriopathy with subcortical infarcts and leukoencephalopathy (CADASIL) is an autosomal dominant disease caused by the notch3 gene mutation (chromosome 19q13) which manifests by extensive degeneration of walls in small arteries and multiple lacunar strokes, resulting in dementia by the sixth decade. When reviewing MRI results one has to be aware that detection of leukoaraiosis is not automatically equal to diagnosis of vascular dementia. Radiological observations always have to be correlated with clinical picture and presence of risk factors for small vessel disease. Some studies have indicated that a threshold volume of white matter damage (10 cm^2) has to be reached before cognitive deficit becomes apparent. Some degree of white matter changes can be detected in 27% of cognitively normal subjects. Its incidence increases with age and positively correlates with presence of vascular risk factors. Furthermore, a similar leukoaraiosis picture of white matter damage can be seen with multiple sclerosis, Lyme disease, vasculitis, mitochondrial disease or in a group of inherited diseases associated with abnormal formation or accelerated breakdown of myelin (leukodystrophies). Therefore, one has to assure that diagnosis of small-vessel dementia is continent with the clinical picture and cannot be made in the absence of vascular risk factors.

Unlike AD and other neurodegenerative disorders, progression of cognitive deficit associated with vascular disorders can be arrested. Addressing vascular risk factors and prevention of stroke recurrence are key management principles. This management includes tight control of blood pressure, lipid levels, blood sugar (in case of diabetes) and cessation of smoking. Prevention of further strokes and/or progression of leukoaraiosis includes daily administration of anti-platelet agents: aspirin, combination of aspirin and dypiridamole (available as two separate drugs or marketed in a combined formulation as Aggrenox) or Plavix. Anticoagulation with coumodin is reserved only for cardioembolic sources of stroke (e.g. atrial fibrillation) or for conditions associated with hypercoagulable state (e.g. antiphospholipid syndrome in the course of systemic lupus erythromatosus). Cardiac defects and high-grade carotid artery stenosis should be addressed surgically. Since the continuity of antiplatelet or anticoagulation therapy is critical for stroke prevention, dental practitioners should avoid stopping these medications for planned dental procedures or at least limit to the minimum the time patients are off the medications.

Modest clinic benefit in slowing down the rate of cognitive decline associated with vascular disorders was demonstrated for cholinesterase inhibitors. In patients with vascular dementia, these drugs should be used in the same doses as they are used for Alzheimer's patients.

Since 30% of patients who survived a stroke develop partial or generalized seizures, use of anti-epileptic agents in patients with vascular dementia is common. Examples of the most commonly used anticonvulsants include levetiracetam (Keppra), phenytoin (Dilantin), valproic acid (Depakote). Due to limited number of adverse effects, lack of interaction with other medications and no effect on liver metabolism, levetiracetam is gaining popularity as a medication of choice in the geriatric population for seizure disorders that are related to stroke or neurodegenerative diseases. All three listed agents can be administered in both an oral and an intravenous form. This flexibility is particularly crucial for patients undergoing a surgery under general anaesthesia or extensive dental surgery when access by mouth can be interrupted. In such instances, missing the schedule can be avoided by intravenous administration of the equivalent dose.

Depressed mood and major depression, which are frequently associated with cerebrovascular diseases, should be treated with SSRIs. SSRIs (especially sertraline) have been also found to be useful in treating emotional incontinence and labile mood, which are frequently associated with small-vessel dementia.

Other dementias

Frontotemporal dementias Frontotemporal dementias are a group of neurodegenerative diseases with heterogeneous neuropathological picture, which share common predilections for involvement of the frontal and temporal lobes. They have peak incidence between the ages of 40 and 60 years, hence two decades before the peak of onset of sporadic AD, and unlike AD, the incidence of frontotemporal dementias does not increase with advancing age. New onset of frontotemporal dementia after the age of 75 years is rare. Males and females are affected equally. Base on autopsy series, frontotemporal dementias make up 10% of the neurodegenerative dementias and the most common pathological variants include Pick's disease, familial cases associated with tau protein mutation, cases with ubiquitine positive neuronal inclusions and cases with ubiquitine and protein TDP-43 positive neuronal inclusions. The clinical picture of frontotemporal dementias is characterized by gradually progressive cognitive deficit, always associated with marked personality and behavioural changes, which are evident early in the course of the disease. Cognitive deficit affects primarily executive functions and language, whereas memory is relatively spared, especially in the early phase of the disease. A variant of frontotemporal dementia dominated by gradual and progressive loss of language function is called primary progressive aphasia. Behavioural and personality symptoms associated with frontotemporal dementias include difficulty modulating behaviour to the social demands or situation, lack of inhibition resulting in outbursts of frustration or lack of social tact, limited insight or lack of personal concern for his/her own actions. This lack of inhibition and self-restraint leads to pathological behaviour, examples of which may include excessive spending, gambling, excessive use of vulgar language or inappropriate sexual behaviour. Diagnosis of frontotemporal dementia is made based on the pattern of clinical symptoms and can be supported by FDG-PET imaging showing decreased metabolism in frontal and temporal lobes as well as cerebrospinal fluid (CSF) analysis demonstrating elevated level of tau and phospho-tau levels with normal level of Aβ, unlike in AD. Frontotemporal dementias have a progressive course with an average duration of eight years. Management is limited to addressing behavioural and psychiatric symptoms using SSRIs or atypical antipsychotics.

Dementia with Lewy bodies and dementia associated with Parkinsonism Dementia with Lewy bodies is characterized by coexistence of gradually progressive cognitive deficit and extrapyramidal symptoms. It is caused by intraneuronal deposition of α-synuclein, which form Lewy bodies. Formation of Levy bodies is a major cause of neuronal loss in the substantia nigra in Parkinson's disease. In the Lewy body dementia, similar lesions are found widespread in the association cortex and in the basal ganglia. Their detection on autopsy series is associated with 20% of all late-onset dementias. Very frequently they co-exist in combination with Alzheimer's pathology. Clinical symptoms of dementia with Lewy bodies can be organized in three categories: (1) gradually progressive cognitive deficit characterized by apraxia, confusion, memory loss and loss of visuospatial skills; (2) extrapyramidal symptoms including stooped posture, bradykinesia, muscle rigidity and tremor; and (3) psychiatric symptoms – visual hallucinations, delusions and depression. Extrapyramidal symptoms in the course of dementia with Lewy bodies may range from atypical to typical Parkinson's disease. Diagnosis is made based on the clinical picture and can be supported by demonstrating characteristics for this entity occipital lobe hypometabolism by FDG-PET or SPECT. Differential diagnosis of dementia with Lewy bodies must include other dementing syndromes which coexist with movement disorders. From 30 to 40% of patients with Parkinson's disease exhibit frank dementia and in most cases dementia is caused by AD. Unlike in dementia with Lewy bodies, where cognitive and extrapyramidal symptoms coexist from the beginning of the disease, in Parkinson's dementia the onset of cognitive deficit follows onset of movement disorder by several years. Another neurodegenerative disorder which may closely mimic dementia with Lewy bodies is progressive supranuclear palsy. Progressive supranuclear palsy is also characterized by coexistence of dementia and extrapyramidal symptoms but, early in the course of the disease, occurrence of progressive gaze palsy and dysfunction of cranial nerves 9 and 10 allows a differential diagnosis to be made.

Treatment of Lewy body dementia include use of rivastigmine (Exelon), which in clinical trial was found to be effective in ameliorating both cognitive deficit and behavioural symptoms – particularly hallucination and mental status fluctuation. Both typical and atypical neuroleptics should be avoided as their use is likely to exacerbate extrapyramidal and cognitive symptoms and may be even associated with autonomic dysfunction, leading to rapid, inexorable clinical decline or even death. No published clinical data exist on benefits of dopaminergic therapy for extrapyramidal symptoms of dementia with Lewy body. Sinemet is used on a case-by-case basis with low starting dose and careful titration.

Normal-pressure hydrocephalus Normal pressure hydrocephalus is characterized by a triad of gait disorder, cognitive deficit and urinary incontinence. It is one of the most common dementias. Gait dysfunction is characterized by slowed, magnetic gait and stooped posture. Cognitive deficit features decreased speed of cognitive processing, apraxia, visuospatial and memory dysfunction. Urinary incontinence is characterized by loss of bathroom reflex. Patients are unable to consciously overcome the urge to urinate when their bladder is full and frequently are indifferent to wetting themselves. Pathology of normal pressure hydrocephalus is associated with abnormal kinetics of the cerebrospinal fluid that leads to gradually progressing hydrocephalus. Symptoms of normal pressure hydrocephalus can be ameliorated by performing a ventriculoperitoneal shunting procedure, where a catheter tip is placed in the lateral ventricle and the CSF is drained through an adjustable valvular device placed under the skin outside the skull and then through a subcutaneous drain to the peritoneal cavity. A favourable response to the shunting procedure can be assessed preoperatively based on improvement of gait and cognitive performance after a diagnostic removal of 30 cc of CSF through lumbar puncture. This evidence can be further strengthened by demonstrating abnormal CSF kinetics using radioisotope cisternography. Because of significant comorbidity between normal-pressure hydrocephalus and AD, further deterioration of cognitive symptoms, despite improvement in gait performance in some subjects is observed.

Creutzfeldt–Jakob disease Creutzfeldt–Jakob disease is a rapidly progressing dementia. It occurs with one case per year per one million people, has peak incidence in the seventh decade and affects both genders equally. The pathological mechanism of Creutzfeldt–Jakob disease is associated with conformational transformation of PrP^{C} protein into a toxic, infectious and self-perpetuating conformer PrP^{Sc}. Initial symptomatology includes cognitive deficit, frequently associated with depression and/or anxiety, which rapidly progresses to dementia. Other neurological symptoms like ataxia and myoclonus are frequent. The average clinical course from the first symptoms to death is seven to nine months. Diagnosis is made based on a constellation of clinical symptoms, increased level of tau and 14-3-3 proteins in the CSF, demonstrating periodic sharp waves on an EEG, and a characteristic MRI picture which includes an increased signal on T2 weighted images in the brain cortex (cortical ribbon sign), basal ganglia (hockey stick and puck sign) and in the thalamus (pulvinar sign). Confirmation of clinical diagnosis can be obtained by brain biopsy or autopsy. No treatment, other than supportive medical management, is currently available for Creutzfeldt–Jakob disease.

A unique feature of Creutzfeldt–Jakob disease is its transmissibility, associated with resistance of PrP^{Sc} to withstand standard sterilization procedures. The disease can be transmitted from one patient to another (termed iatrogenic Creutzfeldt–Jakob disease) or from cattle affected by bovine spongiform encephalopathy to humans (termed the variant of Creutzfeldt–Jakob disease). In the case of variant Creutzfeldt–Jakob disease, transmission occurs through the alimentary tract and PrP^{Sc} replicates within the lymphatic organs for months to years prior to secondary involvement of the brain. This creates a phenomenon of disease carriers, who are infectious, but remain clinically asymptomatic. There are estimates that several thousands of asymptomatic carriers may live in Europe. Transmission of Creutzfeldt–Jakob disease from a person to another person may occur through surgical instruments, organ transplantation (e.g. corneal and dural transplants) and, in the case of variant Creutzfeldt–Jakob disease, through blood transfusion. Since the infectious PrP^{Sc} is widely spread in the lymphatic system of asymptomatic carriers, there is a potential risk of disease transmission through instruments used during dental procedures and occupational risks for dental practitioners. This risk is however considered to be very low, and thus far no evidence of transmission linked to a dental procedure has been provided.

Dementia associated with ethanol abuse Nearly 20% of older alcoholics show some level of dementia. Diagnosis of alcoholic dementia requires documented prolonged history of ethanol abuse, lack of organic lesions identified by MRI and other potential causes of dementia. Alcoholic dementia can not be determined in patients actively abusing alcohol. Persistent cognitive deficit has to be confirmed after at least two months of abstinence. The pattern of cognitive deficit that is typical for alcoholic dementia is characterized by deficit in executive functions, decreased cognitive speed and memory deficit. Other neurological symptoms like tremor, cerebellar ataxia and peripheral neuropathy can be present. The clinical picture of alcoholic dementia can be dominated by a distinct amnestic disorder (Korsakoff syndrome) where a patient presents with primary memory deficit associated with extensive confabulations produced in order to fill memory gaps. Lack of Korsakoff syndrome does not rule out alcoholic dementia. Management of this condition is focused on substance abuse treatment, counselling and on the treatment of associated psychiatric symptoms, which most frequently include anxiety and/or depression.

Dementias secondary to diverse physiological disturbances
Symptoms of reversible or irreversible cognitive dysfunction may occur secondary to over 50 etiologies other than described above. Examples include infectious diseases (AIDS, Lyme disease, syphilis), autoimmune disorders (systemic lupus erythematosus), multiple sclerosis, vitamin deficiencies (B_{12}, niacin), hormonal dysfunction (hypothyroidism, parathyroid dysfunction) or heavy metal poisoning. In most of these diseases, cognitive deficit is preceded and/or coexisting with systemic symptoms and focal neurological signs. They are diagnosed based on neuroimaging findings, CSF examination, laboratory workup and neuropsychological testing.

Oral health in patients with psychiatric disorders

Several studies evaluated the presence of oral diseases in elderly patients with psychiatric disorders. However, many of them suffered from significant limitations including lack of diagnosis criteria for psychiatric disorders and oral lesions, inclusion of heterogeneous populations, lack of appropriate controls and lack of appropriate presentation of data and their analysis. Nevertheless, they point to the existence of significant oral health disparities between the elderly with psychiatric disorders and subjects without these conditions. These findings are not surprising since these patients have a combination of several risk factors for oral diseases such as the psychiatric disorder itself, associated comorbidities, medications and use of other drugs. Therefore, the treatment protocols should implement preventive and treatment measures based on knowledge of the specific psychiatric and oral conditions, as well as the risk factors for these conditions.

1. Oral health in patients with affective disorders

Elderly patients with affective disorders are thought to have significantly more oral diseases than patients without affective disorders (Box 9.1). The prevalence of edentulism is difficult to evaluate from the existing literature. However, it is thought to be high. As the patients loose their teeth and replace them by dentures they may have difficulty in adapting physically and psychologically, with their new condition resulting in high disappointment rates. For example, it was found that, for each unit increase on the 15-point depression scale, the probability of denture dissatisfaction in subjects with depressive symptoms increased by 24%, suggesting that the severity of depression impacts treatment satisfaction. The dentures worn by these patients are often unrelined and uncared for, thus predisposing the individuals to higher rates of alveolar ridge resorptions and mucosal conditions.

Box 9.1 Oral conditions that may present in patients with affective disorders.

- Xerostomia
- Increased caries
- Increased gingival inflammation
- Dentures: uncared and unrelined
- Dissatisfaction with dentures
- Burning mouth syndrome
- Taste changes
- Mucosal changes
- Bruxism
- Temporomandibular disorders

The prevalence of tooth decay may also be increased in patients with affective disorders, although not all of the studies concurred. Patients taking antidepressant medication though have consistently shown higher caries rates and these rates were dependent on the number of medications taken. They also may have rampant caries. The relationship between depression and periodontitis is also uncertain. Some studies have failed to find a relationship between depression and periodontitis while other studies suggested that perhaps the coping mechanisms may be more important than the disease itself. However, a recent study showed that women with depression had more gingival inflammation, deeper periodontal pockets and higher levels of Il-6 in the gingival crevicular fluid, suggesting that depression may be associated with periodontal disease. Other oral conditions that may be associated with depression or the medications taken include burning mouth syndrome, taste changes, mucosal changes, bruxism and temporomandibular disorders.

2. Oral health in patients with psychotic disorders

The prevalence of oral disease in patients with psychotic disorders is thought to be significantly higher than in the general population (Box 9.2). Edentulism was reported to be as high as 66% and many of these patients may not wear their dentures. High prevalence of caries and periodontal diseases is also noticed. Up to 55% of psychiatric patients may have untreated caries and more than 80% may have periodontal diseases. Soft tissue lesions such as angular cheilitis, gingival hyperplasia, and factitious lesions may also be present. Poor oral health is not surprising considering the medical characteristics of this population. The nature of their disorder contributes to the neglect of oral health issues and hygiene practices. In addition the anti-psychotic medication and drug abuse by these patients may augment their apathy and disinterest in oral health. The side effects of antipsychotic drugs such as hyposalivation and oro-facial movement disorders add even more risk for oral diseases.

Box 9.2 Oral conditions that may present in patients with psychotic disorders.

- Xerostomia
- Increased caries
- Increased periodontal disease
- Increased plaque accumulation
- Increased denture prevalence
- Not wearing dentures in severe cases
- Extrapyramidal symptoms

3. Oral health in patients with dementia

The prevalence of oral diseases in patients with dementia is thought to be increased (Box 9.3). The frequency of edentulism in subjects with dementia or AD is difficult to evaluate from the existing studies although tooth loss is thought to be higher. However, when patients with dementia are edentulous, they are less likely to wear their dentures. Possible explanations for their behaviour are the lack of denture stability and difficulty in adjusting if new dentures are made. Their dentures are also older and less clean. These findings are significant since ill-fitted dentures may affect a patient's dietary quality, nutrient intake and quality of life.

Box 9.3 Oral conditions that may present in patients with dementia.

- Increased tooth loss
- Increased caries
- Increased gingival inflammation
- Increased plaque accumulation
- Older, unfitted and uncleaned dentures
- Dentures less likely to be worn
- Difficulty adjusting to new dentures
- Soft tissue lesions
- Xerostomia

Subjects with dementia have been reported to have a higher prevalence and incidence of both coronal and root caries, although not all studies concur. Although bacteria play an important ethiopathological role, many biological and social factors predispose an individual to dental caries. Xerostomia (dry mouth), systemic diseases and medication are important biological factors. Patients with dementia may have decreased salivary output. They may also have more systemic conditions and take more medications. Among social factors, oral hygiene delivery and functional ability as well as fewer visits to the dentist are important risk factors for dental caries in patients with dementia.

The prevalence of chronic periodontitis in dementia patients is unknown. Two studies reported that the presence of periodontitis in AD subjects was not significantly different from normal controls while another study reported it to be 100%. Due to methodological limitations these studies may not accurately estimate the presence of the disease. Considering the high prevalence of chronic periodontal disease in the elderly and the presence of other risk factors for periodontal disease in dementia patients, it is imperative to perform more studies evaluating the prevalence and the characteristics of these diseases in dementia patients.

The existence of soft tissue pathology in dementia patients was reported only in a limited number of studies. For example, one study reported that AD patients had more frequent denture stomititis and angular cheilitis compared to non-demented controls while another study did not report any difference. These conditions may cause significant pain and suffering among demented elders and therefore it is important that more studies be performed.

Oral hygiene and salivary dysfunctions are significant risk factors for oral diseases including caries, periodontal diseases and soft tissue lesions. Studies have consistently shown that patients with dementia have poorer oral hygiene compared to controls and this oral hygiene worsens with the severity of cognitive dysfunction. These results are not surprising since dementia progression is associated with further deterioration of mental faculties and motor skills. Difficulties with denture and teeth cleaning are increasing and the dementia patients often need a caregiver help. However, caregivers may encounter significant difficulties in providing care for dementia patients. Patients with dementia may refuse oral hygiene, may refuse to open their mouths and they are unable to spit or rinse and may show aggressiveness. When the oral hygiene is performed by caregivers, they are more likely to use a gauze and non-fluoridated mouthwashes, contributing further to poor oral hygiene and health. In addition, systemic diseases, medication and possible salivary dysfunction may also contribute to oral hygiene deterioration.

Risk factors/indicators for oral diseases in patients with psychiatric conditions

A list of possible risk factors/indicators is presented in Box 9.4. These risk factors/indicators may be related to the characteristics of the psychiatric disorder itself, its pathogenic mechanisms, the consequences of their treatment, associated comorbidities and their treatment or social factors. Patients with affective, psychotic and dementia disorders have altered mood, decreased lack of interest, forgetfulness and difficulties with self-care functions which impair their oral hygiene and visits to the dentist. These impairments obviously depend on the specific psychiatric condition and its severity. For example, subjects with a high number of depressive symptoms and dementia brushed their teeth and visited their dentist less frequently. Depressive disorders may also constitute a risk for oral diseases as these patients are likely to have high carbohydrate intake thus predisposing them to carious lesions. Patients with dementia, particularly AD, may have salivary gland dysfunction resulting in hyposalivation and its effects on oral diseases. In addition, patients with affective, psychotic disorders and dementia are often treated with medication with anticholinergic effects leading to hyposalivation and xerostomia (see Table 9.1). The presence of comorbidities and their treatment may also have similar effects. The lack of saliva with its buffering and immunological properties predisposes these patients to increased microbial colonization with subsequent caries, mucosal lesions, discomfort in wearing dentures and possible periodontal diseases. Another predisposing factor for oral diseases may be the existence of addictive behaviours. Some patients with affective and psychotic disorders are smokers and others may be abusing other types of drugs such as cocaine, which further increases their risk for oral diseases. And still other risks for oral diseases are the availability of a knowledgeable caregiver and access to appropriate dental care.

Box 9.4 Risk factors for poor oral health in elderly patients with psychiatric conditions.

- Specific diagnosis
- Severity and duration of the condition
- Severity of mental and functional impairment
- Drug treatment for the psychiatric condition
- Associated comorbidities
- Drug treatment for their comorbidities (antihypertensive)
- Addictive behaviour
- Caregivers' help and knowledge
- Visits to dentists (patient's knowledge, psychological and physical impairments, caregiver knowledge and burden, existence of dental insurance, convenience)

Dental management of patients with psychiatric disorders

Dental management of patients with psychiatric disorders is challenging and depends on the specific psychiatric diagnosis, its severity, associated comorbidities and the array of medication that the patient is taking. It also depends on the nature of the oral conditions and their severity, the existence of risk factors for the oral conditions and the goal that the dentist is aiming for.

The initial phase of the interaction between the dentist and the patient with psychiatric disorders is highly significant. This is the stage when the dentist should establish a comprehensive oral health plan. The aim of the dental treatment should not only be to eliminate pain and attend to the patient's chief complaint but also to obtain optimum oral health (Box 9.5). The dentist should become familiar with the patients' oral status and patients' risk of oral diseases, educate the patients as well as their families in oral health issues and organize regular check-ups. The importance of this treatment phase is tremendous as it establishes the basis for maintaining a good oral health in the future.

Box 9.5 Goals of the treatment for oral diseases in psychiatric patients.

- To treat the existing oral disease
- To prevent oral disease from occurring
- To prevent oral disease from progression
- To restore oral function, including aesthetics
- To prevent potential systemic effects
- To organize regular dental visits
- To develop a relationship with the patient

Table 9.1 Possible oral health effects of commonly used drugs for affective disorders

Disorder	Class of drug	Examples	Oral effects
Depressive disorders	*Selective serotonin reuptake inhibitors*	Citalopram (Celexa) Escitalopram (Lexapro)	Xerostomia Extrapiramidal symptoms
		Fluoxetine (Prozac)	Xerostomia Extrapiramidal symptoms Erythema multiforme Taste alteration
		Paroxetine (Paxil)	Xerostomia
		Sertraline (Zoloft)	Xerostomia Taste alteration
	Antidepressants, others	Buproprion (Wellbutrin)	Xerostomia Erythema multiforme Stevens–Johnson syndrome
		Mitrazapine (Remeron)	Xerostomia
		Venlafaxine (Effexor)	Xerostomia Taste alteration
	Tricyclic antidepressants	Desipramine (Norpramin)	Xerostomia
		Nortryptyline (Aventyl, Pamelor)	Xerostomia Taste alteration
Bipolar disorder		Valproic acid (Depakene, Depakote)	Erythema multiforme Stevens–Johnson syndrome Toxic epidermal necrolysis Hepatotoxicity Bleeding
		Carbamazepine (Tegretol)	Erythema multiforme Stevens–Johnson syndrome Toxic epidermal necrolysis Taste alteration
		Lithium carbonate (Eskalith, Lithotabs, Lithonate)	Xerostomia Taste alteration
Anxiety disorders	*Selective serotonin reuptake inhibitors*	Citalopram (Celexa) Escitalopram (Lexapro) Fluoxetine (Prozac) Paroxetine (Paxil) Sertraline (Zoloft)	See above
	Benzodiazepines *Antihistamines*		Dry mucous membanes
	Buspirone		Xerostomia Extrapyramidal symptoms
Late-life delusional and paranoid psychoses	Atypical antipsychotics	Quetiapine (Seroquel)	Xerostomia
		Aripiprazole (Abilify)	Xerostomia Extrapiramidal symptoms
		Ziprasidone (Geodon)	Xerostomia Extrapiramidal symptoms
		Olanzapine (Zyprexa)	Xerostomia Extrapiramidal symptoms (severe) Taste alteration
		Risperidone (Risperdal)	Xerostomia Salivation Extrapiramidal symptoms (severe) Tardive dyskinesia Taste alteration Parkinsonism
	Typical antipsychotics	Haloperidol (Haldol)	Extrapiramidal symptoms Tardive dyskinesia Xerostomia Parkinsonism
Confusion and delirium	Typical antipsychotics Atypical antipsychotics		See above
Vascular dementia	*Anti-platelets*	Aspirin	Taste alteration
		Clopidogrel (Plavix)	Erythema multiforme Stevens-Johnson syndrome Toxic epidermal necrolysis
		Aspirin and dypiridamole (Aggrenox)	Taste alteration
	Anticoagulants	Coumadin	Bleeding
	Cholinesterase inhibitors		
	N-methyl-D-aspartate (NMDA) receptor antagonists	Mementine (Namenda)	Stevens-Johnson syndrome
Seizure disorders	*Anticonvulsants*	Levetiracetam (Keppra)	
		Phenytoin (Dilantin)	Gingival enlargement Stevens–Johnson syndrome Toxic epidermal necrolysis Taste alteration
		Valproic acid (Depakote)	Pancreatitis Liver dysfunction Bleeding
	Selective serotonin reuptake inhibitors	Sertraline (Zoloft)	See above

(Continued)

Table 9.1 (*Continued*)

Disorder	Class of drug	Examples	Oral effects
Other dementia	*Atypical antipsychotics*	Quetiapine (Seroquel) Aripiprazole (Abilify) Ziprasidone (Geodon) Olanzapine (Zyprexa) Risperidone (Risperdal)	See above
	Selective serotonin reuptake inhibitors	Citalopram (Celexa) Escitalopram (Lexapro) Fluoxetine (Prozac) Paroxetine (Paxil) Sertraline (Zoloft) Rivastigmine (Exelon)	See above
Alzheimer's dementia	*Acetylcholinesterase inhibitors*	Donepezil Rivastigmine Galantamine	See above
	N-methyl-D-aspartate (NMDA) receptor antagonists	Memantine	
	Atypical antipsychotic		
	Anticonvulsants	Divalproate	
	Benzodiazepines	Lorazepam Oxazepam	

In the early stages of the psychiatric disease the patients are cooperative and capable of understanding their role in oral health. The dentist will be able to develop a relationship with the patient that will be crucial for maintaining the oral health at later stages of the psychiatric disease. At this stage, the patient is able to understand and follow instructions, be an active part of reducing the risks of oral diseases and treatment planning and undergo dental treatment. The patient will be able to form good oral habits and hopefully maintain them. The dental treatment should include all phases of prevention. Primary prevention aimed at preventing oral disease from occurring will identify and reduce modifiable risk factors. Comprehensive risk assessment for future oral disease should be performed. Based on the risk factors identified, individualized oral hygiene practices, fluoride applications, diet changes, smoking cessation and regular dental check-ups should be done. Secondary prevention aimed at preventing oral diseases from progressing will identify oral diseases in their early stages, implement preventive measures aimed at decreasing the risk of future lesion development and progression and treat them. And finally, tertiary prevention aimed at restoring oral function will identify patients' oral defects and disabilities and devise treatment protocols based on patients' needs, expectations, financial possibilities and treatment predictability, duration and feasibility. Although these preventive phases are defined independently they are interconnected.

Since bacteria in the dental plaque are associated with caries, periodontal diseases and soft tissue lesions, decreasing dental plaque accumulation is a very efficient method of prevention. Several steps can be taken to interfere with plaque accumulation. These are good oral hygiene practices, use of antimicrobials, and diet control. Brushing and flossing are very effective in reducing cariogenic and periodontopathic bacteria and preventing gingival inflammation. According to the American Dental Association, brushing and flossing twice a day is sufficient to control plaque. Although manual brushing is very effective, ultrasonic or mechanical brushes may be helpful if the manual dexterity is reduced or the removal of plaque is performed by caregivers.

Antimicrobial agents may be used as mouth rinses, gels or varnishes. Among antimicrobials, chlorhexidine digluconate is a very effective antiplaque agent. Chlorhexidine digluconate is a bis-biguanide whose effectiveness is due to its bacteriostatic/bactericidal effects and substantivity (the ability of an agent to bind to the tissues and then be released). Studies have consistently shown that oral rinses with 0.12% chlorhexidine solution reduced oral bacteria and inflammation. Periodontopatic bacteria may be reduced by 40–60% and cariogenic bacteria by 40%. However, chlorhexidine works best when it is preceded by mechanical plaque removal. Compounds containing essential oils such as Listerine are less effective, resulting in plaque reduction of 20–30%. Solutions of hydrogen peroxide up to 3% are often used by nurses but clinical data to support their efficacy and safety are lacking. However, most mouth rinses contain alcohol (up to 26.9%) and therefore caution should be exercised, particularly in patients with xerostomia, alcohol intolerance or medication interactive with alcohol. Chlorhexidine contains 11.6% alcohol and in Europe nonalcoholic formulations of chlorhexidine mouth rinses exist with effects comparable with the alcoholic ones. Gels or varnishes containing antimicrobials may be applied by the dentist, although their effect may be questionable.

Caries prevention and treatment protocols should follow the consensus principles of caries management by risk assessment (CAMBRA). These protocols are based on combining the assessment of risk factors for caries and a treatment that affects caries as a disease, is minimally invasive and predictable. Patients with psychiatric conditions are at high risk for caries development. Therefore, the protocols should include modification of the oral flora, patient education, use of calcium supplementation, remineralization of non-cavitated lesions of the enamel, dentine and cementum and minimal operative intervention. Although no clinical trials exist testing these principles in psychiatric patients, they are sound. Modifications of these principles may be required in individual cases.

Periodontal disease treatment should also start with periodontal risk assessment providing the dentist with an index for the risk of developing future periodontal disease and progression of the existing disease. In the early stages of the psychiatric condition, the treatment of periodontal disease should be comprehensive and tailored to that specific patient taking into account periodontal risk factors, severity of the periodontal condition, the possible deterioration of the psychiatric condition and the oral rehabilitation component. Treatment of other oral conditions may follow similar protocols.

The rehabilitation phase should be well planned and may include fixed, removable and implant-supported prostheses. Studies have shown that one of the major challenges facing the dentist is treating psychiatric patients when they are fully edentulous. Full edentulism is defined as loss of all teeth and is considered a disability by WHO. As soon as the teeth are lost or extracted the residual alveolar bone starts to resorb. The resorption continues for the life of the individual, is progressive and irreversible. The mandible resorption is four times more severe than that of the maxilla, contributing to the difficulty of mandibular rehabilitation and maintaining the bone base for a full mandibular denture. Psychiatric patients have difficulties wearing dentures. For example patients with dementia may not wear their dentures due to poor fit and difficulty in adjusting to them if they are relined or remade. The construction of overdentures supported by implants will delay the mandibular resorption in addition to increasing the stability and retention of the dentures. To date, overdentures over implants for mandibular rehabilitation constitute the standard of care. Randomized control studies testing their efficacy in patients with psychiatric disorders are lacking. However, until new data are produced, overdentures over implants should be used. Given the increased stability of the dentures, patients with psychiatric conditions may wear their dentures more often. The patients may also adjust easier if the dentures are relined or redone. Overall, this treatment may significantly improve a patient's quality of life.

At later stages of the psychiatric disorder, when the patient may have a higher degree of impairment, the dentist should continue to implement primary and secondary preventive measures. At this stage, treatment protocols and rehabilitation procedures should consider the patient's needs and the patient's ability to withstand dental treatment.

Further reading

Affective, psychotic disorders and dementia

Alexopoulos, G.S. (1991) Heterogeneity and Comorbidity in Dementia - Depression Syndromes. *International Journal of Geriatric Psychiatry*, **6**, 125–127.

Alexopoulos, G.S., Meyers. B.S., Young. R.C., Kakuma, T., Silbersweig, D. & Charlson, M. (1997) Clinically defined vascular depression. *American Journal of Psychiatry*, **154**, 562–565.

Conwell, Y., Nelson, J.C., Kim, K. & Mazure, C.M. (1989) Elderly Patients Admitted to the Psychiatric Unit of A General-Hospital. *Journal of the American Geriatrics Society*, **37**, 35–41.

Erkinjuntti, T., Kurz, A., Gauthier, S., Bullock, R., Lilienfeld, S. & Damaraju, C.V. (2002) Efficacy of galantamine in probable vascular dementia and Alzheimer's disease combined with cerebrovascular disease: a randomised trial. *Lancet*, **359**, 1283–1290.

Himmelfarb, S. & Murrell, S.A. (1984) The Prevalence and Correlates of Anxiety Symptoms in Older Adults. *Journal of Psychology*, **116**, 159–167.

Kalaria, R.N., Viitanen, M., Kalimo, H., Dichgans, M. & Tabira, T. (2004) The pathogenesis of CADASIL: an update. *Journal of Neurological Science*, **226**, 35–39.

Orgogozo, J.M., Rigaud, A.S., Stoffler, A., Mobius, H.J. & Forette, F. (2002) Efficacy and safety of memantine in patients with mild to moderate vascular dementia - A randomized, placebo-controlled trial (MMM 300). *Stroke*, **33**, 1834–1839.

Peden, A.H., Head, M.W., Ritchie, D.L., Bell, J.E. & Ironside, J.W. (2004) Preclinical vCJD after blood transfusion in a PRNP codon 129 heterozygous patient. *Lancet*, **364**, 527–529.

Porter, S.R. (2003) Prion disease - Possible implications for oral health care. *Journal of the American Dental Association*, **134**, 1486–1491.

Rodin, G. & Voshart, K. (1986) Depression in the Medically Ill - An Overview. *American Journal of Psychiatry*, **143**, 696–705.

Schneeweiss, S., Setoguchi, S., Brookhart, A., Dormuth, C. & Wang, P.S. (2007) Risk of death associated with the use of conventional versus atypical antipsychotic drugs among elderly patients. *Canadian Medical Association Journal*, **176**, 627–632.

Schneider, L.S., Tariot, P.N., Dagerman, K.S., Davis, S.M., Hsiao, J.K., Ismail, M.S. *et al.* (2006) Effectiveness of atypical antipsychotic drugs in patients with Alzheimer's disease. *New England Journal of Medicine*, **355**, 1525–1538.

Alzheimer's disease

Blennow, K., de Leon, M.J. & Zetterberg, H. (2006) Alzheimer's disease. *Lancet*, **368**(9533), 387–403.

McKhann, G.M., Knopman, D.S., Chertkow, H., Hyman, B.T., Jack, C.R., Jr. Kawas, C.H. *et al.* (2011) The diagnosis of dementia due to Alzheimer's disease: recommendations from the National Institute on Aging-Alzheimer's Association workgroups on diagnostic guidelines for Alzheimer's disease. *Alzheimer's & Dementia*, 7(3), 263–269.

Randall, C., Mosconi, L., de Leon, M. & Glodzik, L. (2013) Cerebrospinal fluid biomarkers of Alzheimer's disease in healthy elderly. *Frontiers in Bioscience*, **18**, 1150–1173.

Selkoe, D.J. (2003) Aging, amyloid, and Alzheimer's disease: a perspective in honor of Carl Cotman. *Neurochemical Research*, **28**(11), 1705–1713.

Oral health in psychiatric patients

Boehm, T.K. & Scannapieco, F.A. (2007) The epidemiology, consequences and management of periodontal disease in older adults. Journal of the American Dental Association, **138**(Suppl), 26S–33S.

Chalmers, J.M. & Ettinger, R.L. (2008) Public health issues in geriatric dentistry in the United States. *Dental Clinics of North America*, **52**(2), 423–446.

Chalmers, J.M., Carter, K.D. & Spencer, A.J. (2005) Caries incidence and increments in Adelaide nursing home residents. *Special Care in Dentistry*, **25**(2), 96–105.

Ellefsen, B., Holm-Pedersen, P., Morse, D.E., Schroll, M., Andersen, B.B. & Waldemar, G. (2008) Caries prevalence in older persons with and without dementia. *Journal of the American Geriatric Society*, **56**(1), 59–67.

Ekstrand, K., Martignon, S. & Holm-Pedersen, P. (2008) Development and evaluation of two root caries controlling programmes for home-based frail people older than 75 years. *Gerodontology*, **25**(2), 67–75.

Friedlander, A.H. & Marder, S.R. (2002) The psychopathology, medical management and dental implications of schizophrenia. *Journal of the American Dental Association*, **133**(5), 603–610; quiz 624-5.

Friedlander, A.H., Friedlander, I.K., Gallas, M. & Velasco, E. (2003) Late-life depression: its oral health significance. *International Dental Journal*, **53**(1), 41–50.

Friedlander, A.H., Norman, D.C., Mahler, M.E., Norman, K.M. & Yagiela, J.A. (2006) Alzheimer's disease: psychopathology, medical management and dental implications. *Journal of the American Dental Association*, **137**(9), 1240–1251.

Ghezzi, E.M. & Ship, J.A. (2000) Dementia and oral health. *Oral Surgery, Oral Medicine, Oral Pathology, Oral Radiology and Endodontology*, **89**(1), 2–5.

Ship, J.A., DeCarli, C., Friedland, R.P. & Baum, B.J. (1990) Diminished submandibular salivary flow in dementia of the Alzheimer type. *Journal of Gerontology*, **45**(2), M61–66.

Slots, J. (2002) Selection of antimicrobial agents in periodontal therapy. *Journal of Periodontal Research*, **37**(5), 389–398.

Turner, M., Jahangiri, L. & Ship, J.A. (2008) Hyposalivation, xerostomia and the complete denture: a systematic review. *Journal of the American Dental Association*, **139**(2), 146–150.

Whyman, R.A., Treasure, E.T., Brown, R.H. & MacFadyen, E.E. (1995) The oral health of long-term residents of a hospital for the intellectually handicapped and psychiatrically ill. *New Zealand Dental Journal*, **91**(404), 49–56.

Young, D.A., Featherstone, J.D., Roth, J.R., Anderson, M., Autio-Gold, J., Christensen, G.J., *et al.* (2007) Caries management by risk assessment: implementation guidelines. *Journal of the California Dental Association*, **35**(11), 799–805.

CHAPTER 10

Disability in old age – the relationship with oral health

Kirsten Avlund†
University of Copenhagen, Denmark

Like people in other age groups, older adults have very different thoughts about what it takes to have a good life. But on the whole one wish is common for all older adults: to have a good functional ability in everyday life, so that one can manage for as long as possible without help.

The prevalence of chronic diseases rises with age, and in old people it is common to have several diseases and symptoms at the same time. A combination of potential diseases, medical treatment and physiological/biological age-changes may cause problems with activities and opportunities for self-realization in daily life. These problems may be of great importance for the individual's feeling of self-worth and independence at the same time as disability may be decisive for change of dwelling or allocation of help. Accordingly, the main purpose of most health care intervention in older adults is to improve or sustain functional ability for as long as possible. This is the case with regard to medical treatment and rehabilitation, but also with regard to preventive work among community-dwelling older people.

Three terms are commonly used to identify vulnerable older adults: frailty, comorbidity and disability. *Frailty* is a physiological state of increased vulnerability to stressors that results from decreased physiological reserves, and even dysregulation, of multiple physiological systems. *Comorbidity* is defined as the concurrent presence of two or more medically diagnosed diseases in different organ systems in the same individual, with the diagnosis of each contributing disease based on established, widely recognized criteria. *Disability* is defined as difficulty or dependency in carrying out activities essential to independent living, including essential roles, tasks needed for living independently in a home and desired activities important to one's quality of life. Although early stages of these processes may be clinically silent, the syndrome may become detectable by looking at clinical, functional, behavioural and biological markers.

The disablement process

In 1994 Verbrugge and Jette introduced a theoretical model for the consequences of disease and aging to be used in epidemiological, gerontological and clinical research: 'The Disablement Process'. The model is a further development of WHO's 'International Classification of Impairments, Disabilities and Handicaps (ICIDH)', and describes 1) how chronic and acute conditions affect functioning in specific body systems, basic physical and mental actions and activities of daily life, and 2) the personal and environmental factors that speed or slow disablement. In recent years this conceptual model has been increasingly used in American and European gerontological research.

The main pathway to disability

According to the model, **pathology** refers to biochemical and physiological abnormalities that are detected and medically labelled as disease, injury or congenital/developmental conditions (e.g. osteoarthrosis and diabetes mellitus). Detection of pathology often relies on the evaluation of more manifest signs and symptoms. Defined this way pathology may be caused by a disease and/or by physiological and biological age-related declines in the individual.

† Author is deceased.

Textbook of Geriatric Dentistry, Third Edition. Edited by Poul Holm-Pedersen, Angus W. G. Walls and Jonathan A. Ship.

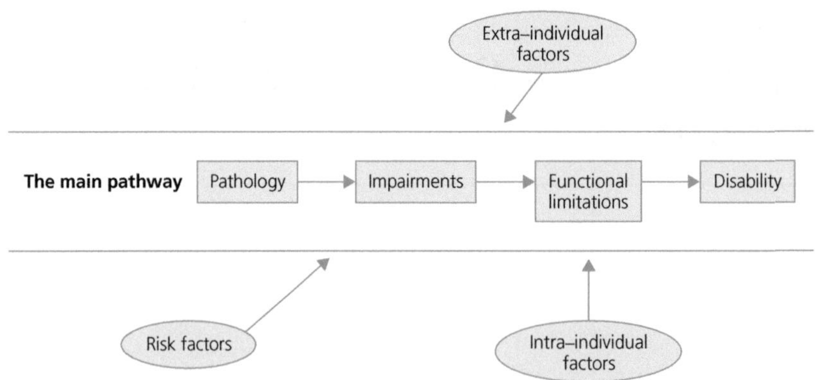

Figure 10.1 The Disablement Process.

Impairments are dysfunctions and significant structural abnormalities in specific body systems. Medical procedures to evaluate impairments include clinical examination, laboratory tests, and patients' medical history and symptom reports. Impairments reflect the consequences and degree of pathology (e.g. decrease of articular cartilage caused by osteoarthrosis of the hip).

Functional limitations are restrictions in performing basic physical and mental *actions* used in daily life by one's age–sex group. These are generic actions which direct the general abilities of body and mind to do purposeful 'work'. Fundamental physical actions include overall mobility and discrete motions and strengths. Basic mental actions include central cognitive and emotional functions. In short, such physical and mental actions constitute the basic interface between a person and the physical and social milieux in which she or he does daily activities.

Disability is experiencing difficulty doing *activities* in any domain of life (the domains typical for one's age–sex group) due to health or physical problems. According to Verbrugge and Jette the words 'action' and 'activity' are simple devices to distinguish the concepts of functional limitations and disability. They help convey the generic (situation-free) features of one and the social (situational) features of the other. Functional limitations refer to individual capability without reference to situational requirements. Disability is a social process – the pattern of behaviour arising from the loss or reduction of ability to perform expected or specified social role activities of extended duration because of a chronic disease or impairment. Disability thus refers to the expression of a functional limitation in a social context. Examples are that a frozen shoulder (pathology) causes problems with the dexterity of the shoulder (functional limitation), which again makes it difficult to pick apples (disability). Also osteoarthritis in the hip (pathology) will cause problems with general mobility of the hip joint (functional limitation), which may result in difficulty sitting at the floor and playing with the grandchildren. A decline in general mobility (functional limitation) may also make it difficult, e.g. to dance, to run to catch the train, to go to art exhibitions with many stairs or to take part in tours arranged by an organization for nature development.

Several factors contribute to shaping the dimensions and severity of disability. The individual's perception of the situation, e.g. by comparison to age-peers, and reactions to disability may be important factors in determining how the situation will turn out. The perception of the situation by others and their reactions and expectations may also play a role. Finally, the characteristics of the environment and the degree to which it is free from, or encumbered with, physical and sociocultural barriers may be important. The disablement process explicitly includes factors that affect the pace and direction of disablement. These factors can be external, e.g. the physical environment or the social relations and internal, e.g. health behaviour.

Over time, the disablement process can prompt some global outcomes and feedback effects. (1) Disability is a predictor of important outcomes such as hospitalization, institutionalization and death. It also has a powerful effect on happiness and life satisfaction. (2) A given disablement process can lead to a vicious circle and sometimes even cause new pathologies and associated consequences. Within a disablement process these feedback loops are often seen in frail people, e.g. a woman with painful arthritis may no longer be able to walk with her dog (disability); this eventually reduces her aerobic capacity and muscle strength (impairments), further reducing mobility and social activities (functional limitations and disability).

It may be argued that the model by Verbrugge and Jette is too rough, as it is based on the notion of one disease causing one impairment causing one functional limitation causing one kind of disability. Multiple co-occurring diseases and

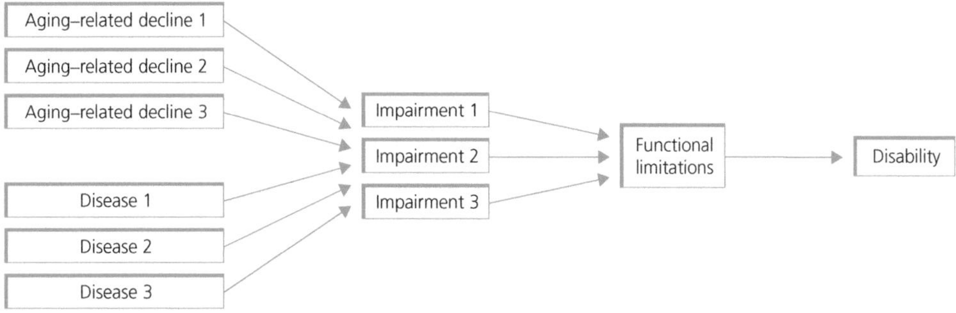

Figure 10.2 An expanded model of the Disablement Process.

impairments are common and each has a synergistic effect that is difficult to unravel. Thus, it might be appropriate to expand the model of the disablement process, as shown in Figure 10.2.

Risk factors for disability

There are a large number of longitudinal studies, which have examined risk factors for functional decline at the individual level. The majority of these studies have had a focus on factors in the main pathway of the disablement process.

It is thus well documented that a number of chronic diseases are observed more frequently in disabled older adults than in those who are nondisabled. However, not all diseases cause disability and some diseases cause more disability than others. Diseases with large effects on functional ability include stroke and other neurological diseases, heart diseases, cancer, respiratory diseases, high body mass index, diabetes, depression, dementia and musculoskeletal diseases. Although different medical conditions impose functional problems that are specific to each disease, musculoskeletal disease is the chronic disease which affects most dimensions of functional ability, including functional limitations and disability: *mobility, lower body limitations, upper body limitations, Physical Activities of Daily Living* and *Instrumental Activities of Daily Living.*

It has also been reported that the presence of more than one chronic disease in an individual – or co-morbidity – is related to the presence of disability and to that person's future risk of disability. For example, the number of chronic diseases in a disability-free group age 65 and older at baseline is directly associated with risk of losing mobility over 4 years. Also, after 4 years the risk of becoming disabled is 4-fold higher for a person with four chronic diseases than for a person with no chronic diseases. In some instances, a disease may not be sufficient to cause substantial disability in itself, but it may increase risk of subsequent functional decline when a new condition develops. A Danish study has found a step-wise increase in disability with increasing number of chronic conditions.

In addition, several types of impairments have been shown to be related to disability, e.g. hearing impairment, visual impairment, poor balance, weak muscle strength, loss of muscle mass, motor impairment, pulmonary impairment, and cognitive problems. A Finnish study showed that the burden of co-impairments on disability, e.g. having both poor balance and poor muscle strength seemed to be greater than the sum of the single impairments involved.

It is also well-established that social and behavioural risk factors play a large role in the disablement process. This has been shown for socio-economic position, social relations, smoking, nutrition and alcohol. However, physical activity is probably the factor which is most important for promoting health into the latest years of life. Exercise is relevant to primary, secondary and tertiary prevention; older adults at all levels of health and function can improve or maintain their exercise tolerance and strength through targeted exercise programmes. Lack of exercise is strongly associated with disability onset while, conversely, regular exercise appears protective in maintaining function. Longitudinal studies of aging have shown strong associations between health behaviour and the incidence of disability with substantial postponement of the onset of disability. An American study documented postponement of disability by 7.75 years in those people who exercised, had normal body mass indices and did not smoke compared to those who did not exercise, were obese and smoked. The cumulative lifetime disability of those with low risks was one fourth of that in those with high risks.

Measures of disability

Most current studies of **disability** among older people focus on the ability to carry out the activities of daily living (ADL), which involve daily activities in the home, at work and in leisure time. Most measures comprise two phenomena: PADL (Physical Activities of Daily Living) and IADL (Instrumental Activities of Daily Living). PADL include basic daily tasks that need to be performed by all people regardless of gender, culture, housing conditions, housing environment and leisure time interests. They include bathing, dressing, using the toilet, eating. IADL comprise more complex, outgoing activities that are essential for living an independent life in society. Work is the best example of an IADL activity but after retirement daily tasks become more relevant for living a meaningful life. The activities most often used in measures of IADL are use of the telephone and public transportation, shopping, cooking, housework and administration of medicine and personal finances.

During the last 40 years, hundreds of measures of physical, mental and social function have been developed, e.g. Barthel Index and Katz ADL Index. Both these scales are based on items on basic mobility-activities and Physical Activities of Daily Living. The Barthel Index is a well established assessment scale that is widespread in use among frail older adults. It is easy and quick to administer, acceptable to the individual and has been proven to be reliable and valid. It is fairly sensitive to describe change and especially useful to describe disability in disabled older people. The Katz Index of ADL is also widely used but is very insensitive to changes and can almost only be used for the categorization of patients.

Neither of these two measures is usable to describe variation and change in functional ability over time in the general population of older adults. During the last 20 years a new measure of functional ability has been developed that describes fatigue and need of help in daily mobility and Physical Activities of Daily Living: the Avlund Scales. The items used in these new scales have shown to be relevant and meaningful to all older adults, not only to disabled older people. The method meets the demands for reliability and validity and, using this method, it has been found that people with decreased functional ability have more chronic diseases, worse muscle- and lung function, poorer balance, more deterioration in cognitive performance and are more often depressive. In addition, it is indicated that people with these *early signs* of disability in everyday life have more problems using their social resources.

The scales have been developed and used in the Aging Studies in Glostrup, Denmark, with baseline study at age 70 in 1984 and with follow-ups with 5 year intervals at age 75, 80, 85 and 90. Examples of Avlund Scales are the Mob-T Scale and the Mob-H Scale. The Mob-T Scale (Mobility–Tiredness) describes whether the participants are able to perform their mobility activities without fatigue and is formed by answers to questions about the following six activities: transfer, walking indoors, going outdoors, walking outdoors in nice weather, walking outdoors in poor weather, and climbing stairs. The Mob-T Scale describes whether the participants perform the activities with or without fatigue afterwards and counts the number of items performed without fatigue. High scale values describe better function. The Mob-H Scale (Mobility–Help) is formed by answers to questions about the same activities as in the Mob-T Scale. It describes whether the participants perform the activities with or without help and counts the number of items performed without help.

Functional ability in an older population

Results from the Glostrup Aging Studies in Denmark show that the proportion of men and women who felt fatigued (The Mob-T Scale) and were in need of help in their daily activities (The Mob-H Scale) increased with age (Figure 10.3). About half of the study population felt fatigued when they were 70 years old compared to more than 75% of the 85-year-olds. Only 3/4% of the 70-year-old men/women needed help compared to 40/60% of the 85-year-olds. No gender differences were seen at age 70, but as the population grew older, significantly more women felt fatigued in their daily activities compared to the men.

Figures 10.4(a) and 10.4(b) show the individual changes in self-reported fatigue in daily activities and in need for help at mobility in the different follow-up periods. In all three follow-up periods a large proportion of old people had sustained fatigue. Up until the age of 80 a rather large proportion reported sustained no fatigue in the follow-up periods, and some people also recovered from a period with fatigue. However, the proportion of people with sustained no fatigue from age 80 to 85 was small and very few recovered from fatigue in that age group, while a substantial proportion declined. More women than men had sustained fatigue in all follow-up periods.

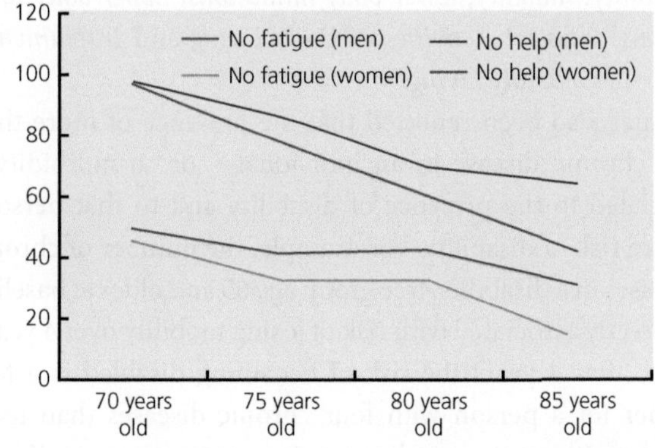

Figure 10.3 Proportion of 70, 75-, 80- and 85-year-old men and women with good functional ability. Reproduced from Avlund, 2004.

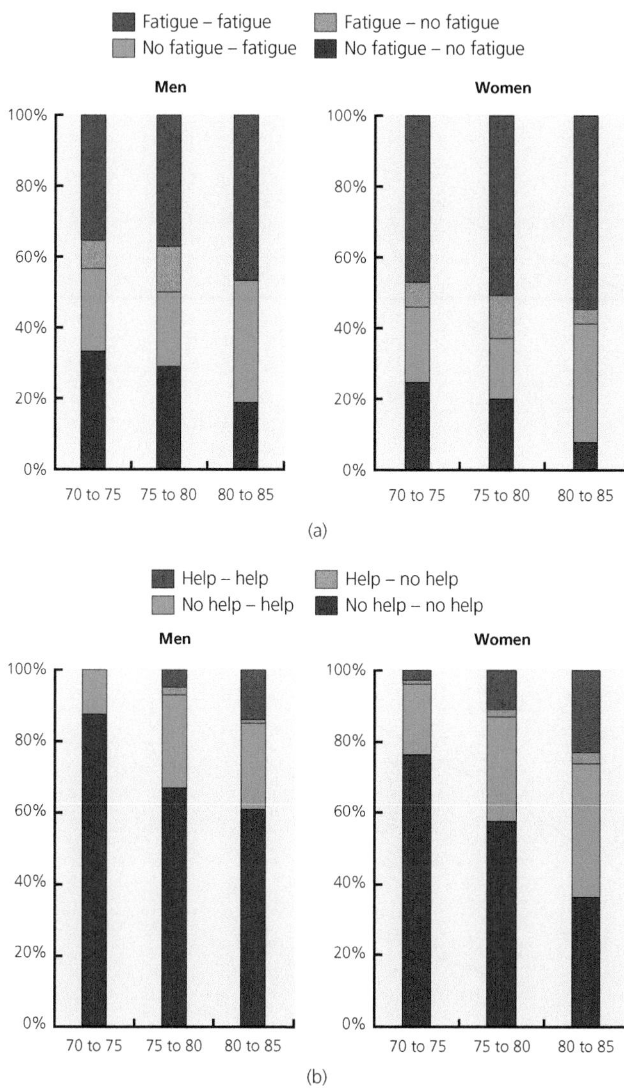

Figure 10.4 a) Changes in fatigue in daily activities (Mob-T) among men and women from age 70 to 75, 75 to 80 and 80 to 85. b) Changes in need of help in daily activities (Mob-H) among men and women from age 70 to 75, 75 to 80 and 80 to 85. Reproduced from Avlund, 2004.

From age 70 to 75 a large proportion had sustained no need of help and a rather small proportion became in need of help. Although this pattern changes over time it is still a rather large proportion of both men and women who had sustained no need of help from age 80 to 85, even though the proportion who became in need of help is substantial (See chapter by Olshansky). In all follow-up periods the women were worse off: they had more sustained need of help and more functional decline than the men. The results underline that older people are not homogeneous. Although some people deteriorate in their functional ability with age there are still a rather large proportion with sustained good functional ability at age 75 and 80 – and even some who improve over time. It is thus not everybody who deteriorates in their functional abilities with age. Therefore it should be taken seriously when a person has a decrease in their functional ability.

The finding of both improvement and deterioration over time is in agreement with several other studies. The results indicate that functional ability is not a stable construct; functional ability may not only deteriorate with age, but also improve. It may thus be possible to postpone both fatigue in daily activities and need of help. More improvement was seen with regard to fatigue than with regard to need of help. This indicates that it is easier to recover from fatigue than from need of help and supports the results by American studies that it is easier to recover from loss of function if the impairment is not severe.

Along this line, it is central to be able to identify people who are at risk of disability but who are not yet disabled. Especially in the large group of well-functioning older people it may be useful to identify individuals at high risk of functional decline before it actually occurs by characterizing an early functional state that is associated with later disability. Results from the Glostrup Aging Studies in Denmark have shown that fatigue in daily activities may be such an early sign of later disability.

Figures 10.5(a) and 10.5(b) describe fatigue in mobility (measured by the Mob-T Scale) as a predictor of onset of need of help. It can be seen that people who feel fatigued when they perform their daily mobility-activities in general have more need of help 5 years later. Among those who do not feel fatigued at age 70, 3% of the men and 6% of the women are in need of help 5 years later. Among those who feel fatigued when they perform all or nearly all activities at age 70, 25% of the men and 34% of the women need help 5 years later. The effects of fatigue can further be seen in relation to onset of need of help 10 and 15 years later. Additional analyses demonstrate that fatigue in daily activities among 70-year-olds is independently related to development of need of help after 5, 10 and 15 years, when adjusted for comorbidity and aerobic capacity. In addition, older people who feel fatigued at age 75 and 80 are also at larger risk of onset of need of help. This has been found both when onset of disability has been measured by self-reported questionnaires and by physical tests. In addition, fatigue in daily activities has been found to be related to use of home help, hospitalization and mortality.

Selection due to mortality

A special problem with regard to the measurement of functional change in old populations is the selection due to loss

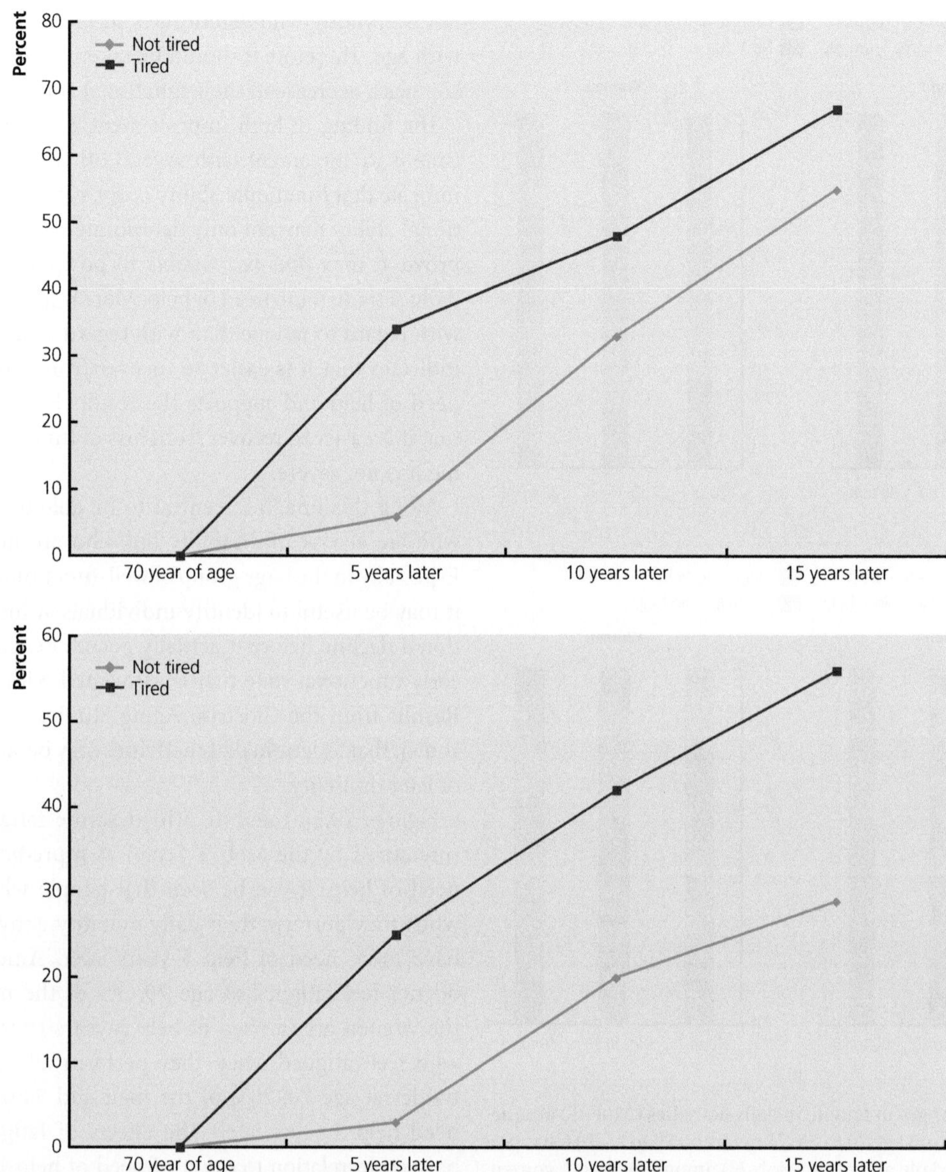

Figure 10.5 a) Proportion of fatigued and not fatigued 70-year-old women with functional decline during the next 15 years. b) Proportion of fatigued and not fatigued 70-year-old men with functional decline during the next 15 years.

at follow-up because of death or non-participation for other reasons. This may be especially problematic in very old study populations because of the high mortality rates among these groups. If people who die during follow-up periods are excluded from a study of functional decline there is a risk of missing important information both about different trajectories in function in old age and about the effect of different determinants on functional ability. There is also a risk of selection, however, because those with poorest functional ability at baseline are more likely to have died at follow-up.

Gender differences in the disablement process

An interesting finding about changes in functional ability is that women had both higher prevalence and higher incidence of disability than men, but that the men had higher risks of dying. This is in agreement with other studies, which found that women had consistently higher rates of prevalent and incident disability compared to men. These gender differences may have several explanations. It is possible that gender differences in the diseases underlying the

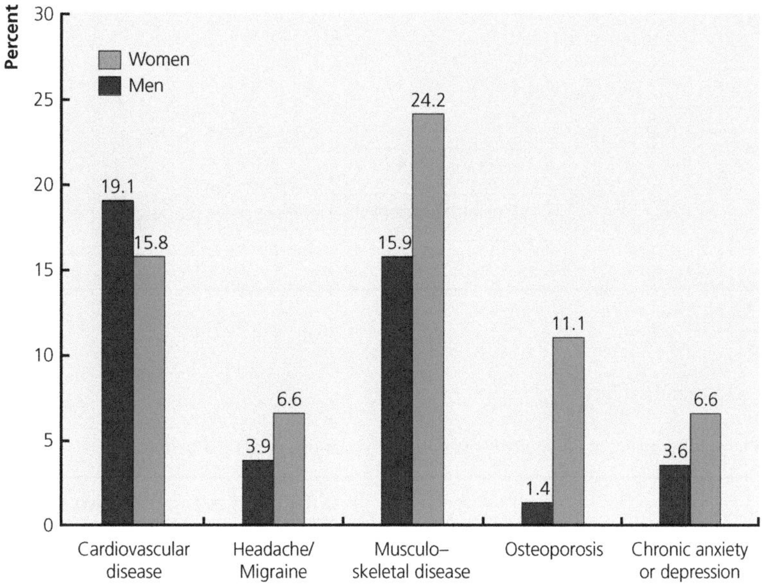

Figure 10.6 Percentage of 65+ year-old men and women with different diseases. Data from the Danish Health Interview Survey, 2005.

disablement process play a role in explaining this paradox. It is known that, compared to men, women have higher rates of disabling, non-fatal chronic disease. This is particularly true for musculoskeletal diseases, such as arthritis and osteoporosis. Other chronic conditions that disproportionately affect women include depression, varicose veins, migraine, cataracts and dementia. See Figure 10.6 which shows the proportion of men and women 65 years and older with some of these diseases, based on a representative Danish sample. Each of these conditions may contribute to disability in old age. It has also been demonstrated that women with peripheral arterial disease had a higher prevalence of leg pain on exertion and rest, poorer functioning and greater walking impairment from leg symptoms than men with the same disease. Contrary to this, men have higher rates of common fatal diseases, such as heart disease and cancer, and thus are more likely to die from these diseases before disabling chronic conditions progress to disability in old age.

Another explanation may be that men have a shorter duration of disability because they die from the conditions that cause their disability, such as heart disease and stroke. In addition, the number of chronic conditions also predicts incident mobility disability, suggesting a dose-like effect for these conditions on future occurrence of disability. Recent American evidence has demonstrated that in addition to having higher rates of the most common disabling conditions women also have higher co-morbidity – that is more co-occurring chronic conditions – another factor that may contribute to higher rates of disability in women. A Danish study showed a step-wise increase in prevalence of disability with an increasing number of chronic diseases.

Constitutional factors related to body composition may also predispose more women than men to becoming disabled. The higher risk of osteoporotic fracture in women compared to men is related to lower peak bone mass in women and accelerated bone loss beginning at menopause. Women have poorer pulmonary function and lower aerobic capacity than men and the age-related declines are larger for women compared to men. Women also have more loss of muscle mass and higher percentages of body fat than men. This relative difference in body composition may be a major contributor to the comparatively greater disability in older women. For example, a number of studies have suggested that muscle strength plays an important protective role in preventing disability. Lower initial muscle strength in women, compounded by further strength losses that occur with aging may place older women at greater risk of mobility problems in old age and help explain gender differences in disability. Many common tasks that are critical for independence, such as walking and climbing stairs, require the same amount of strength across gender. Certain tasks, including walking and rising from a chair, require threshold levels of strength and aerobic capacity and women are typically closer to these threshold levels than men.

The main pathway to oral disability

Over time, the general disablement process can prompt secondary conditions and dysfunctions. For example, a woman

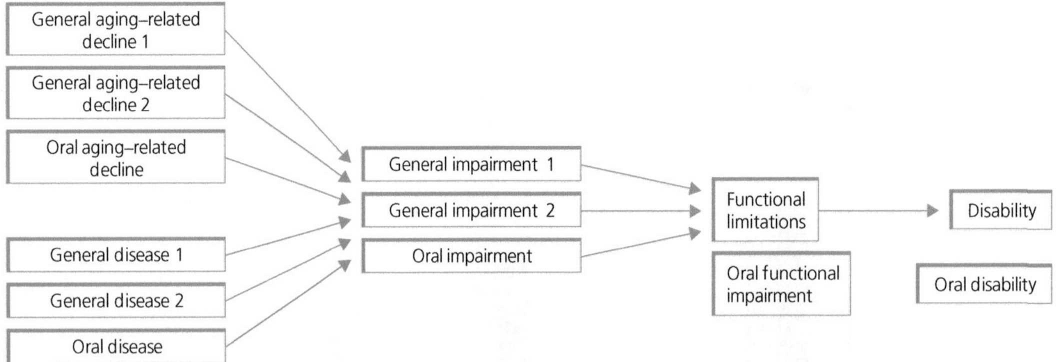

Figure 10.7 The main pathway to oral disability.

Table 10.1 Mobility in relation to number of teeth, difficulty chewing and regular use of dentist/denturist

		0–4 teeth		Difficulty chewing		No regular use of dentist/denturist	
Age 75	**(Total *n*)**	**%**	***p***	**%**	***p***	**%**	***p***
Mobility-related fatigue							
Fatigue	(263)	57%		52%		62%	
No fatigue	(147)	43%	0.009	44%	0.109	51%	0.026
Need of help in mobility							
Need help	(59)	63%		59%		73%	
No help	(351)	50%	0.080	48%	0.103	56%	0.014
Age 80							
Moblity-related fatigue							
Fatigue	(188)	53%		54%		56%	
No fatigue	(138)	43%	0.062	43%	0.068	41%	0.008
Need of help in mobility							
Need help	(99)	58%		55%		60%	
No help	(226)	45%	0.039	40%	0.016	46%	0.022
75 to 80							
Mobility-related fatigue							
No fatigue–no fatigue	(138)	43%		43%		41%	
Fatigue–no fatigue							
No fatigue–fatigue	(66)	50%		53%		55%	
Fatigue–fatigue	(122)	55%	0.143	54%	0.186	57%	0.029
Need of help in mobility							
No help–no help Help–no help	(226)	45%		45%		46%	
No help–help	(80)	55%		60%		56%	
Help–help	(19)	68%	0.068	58%	0.055	74%	0.028

Note: *p* describes *p*-values from chi-square tests of differences between mobility function and the oral health variables. Percentages have been rounded.

with painful arthritis may restrict her recreational walking disability; this eventually reduces her cardiopulmonary function and induces muscle weakness, further reducing mobility and social activity. The general disablement process may thus also have consequences for oral health.

The disablement process can also be looked at from an oral health point of view. Locker has proposed a model with a general pathway from disease via oral impairments (such as edentulism) and oral functional limitations (such as difficulty in chewing) through to disability (such as inability to consume a range of foods) and impacts on social roles (for example avoiding going out with others) (see Figure 10.7). It seems plausible that oral impairments, oral functional limitations and general functional limitations (e.g. mobility problems) are signs of disablement, that they are interrelated and that prevention should be aimed in all directions if the intention is to promote a good life in old age. Thus, oral health care should be seen in this broader perspective.

Cross-sectional results from the Glostrup Aging Studies (Table 10.1) show that 75- and 80-year-old people who felt fatigued (measured by the Mob-T Scale) had fewer teeth and tended to have more chewing difficulties than people who did not feel fatigued. Further, longitudinal analyses showed that people with onset of fatigue or sustained fatigue from age 75 to 80 tended to have fewer teeth and more chewing difficulties than others. It is of interest that this early sign of general disability is also related to poor oral health.

Table 10.1 also shows that 75- and 80-year-olds who were in need of help in mobility (measured by the Mob-H Scale) and people with onset of need of help from age 75 to 80 had fewer teeth and more chewing difficulties than people without these characteristics.

These findings support a few cross-sectional population studies that have shown that non-institutionalized older adults with physical disability have more dental impairments compared to nondisabled older adults. A Swedish study on three 70-year-old cohorts born at 5 year intervals ($n = 1380$) found that impaired ADL-function was related to dental state, measured by the Eichner index, based on existing natural tooth contacts between maxilla and mandible in the bilateral premolar and molar regions.

Another study of community-dwelling older adults aged 70 and older living within the six New England States ($n = 1156$) showed that older people with physical disability were at significantly increased risk of edentulism and active caries, using the National Institute of Dental Research (NIDR) diagnostic criteria for dental examinations as basic operational definition for coronal and root caries, but at no increased risk of periodontal disease compared with their physically able counterparts. Physical activities that require considerable upper extremity and fine motor skills, such as eating, bathing and toileting, were most strongly related to the prevalence of current decay regardless of respondents' age, gender, education, living arrangement, oral hygiene and dental care use. The study also showed that those older people with decreased mobility in areas such as bed transfers, walking and getting outside were more likely to have lost all of their natural teeth regardless of their age, gender, education and living arrangements.

In a Swedish study of 159 very old community-dwelling older people in Kungsholmen, Stockholm, it was shown that older adults with a decrease in functional ability during the preceding years had more root caries than others. Figure 10.8 shows the proportions with and without root caries. Among those with a good functional ability about half have caries, while nearly 80% of those with decreased functional ability have caries. Further, the study showed that people who were not able to perform IADL had more coronal caries.

Similar results have been found in studies of nursing home residents. In a Swedish study among 192 nursing home residents significant correlations were found between functional ability and ability to chew. The same patterns were found in a study of long-term care residents in Portland, Oregon. Here strong associations were found between four dexterity tests and plaque score, as defined by the Turesky modification of the Quigley–Hein plaque index. Similar results have been found in studies of nursing home residents in e.g. Canada, Spain and Belgium.

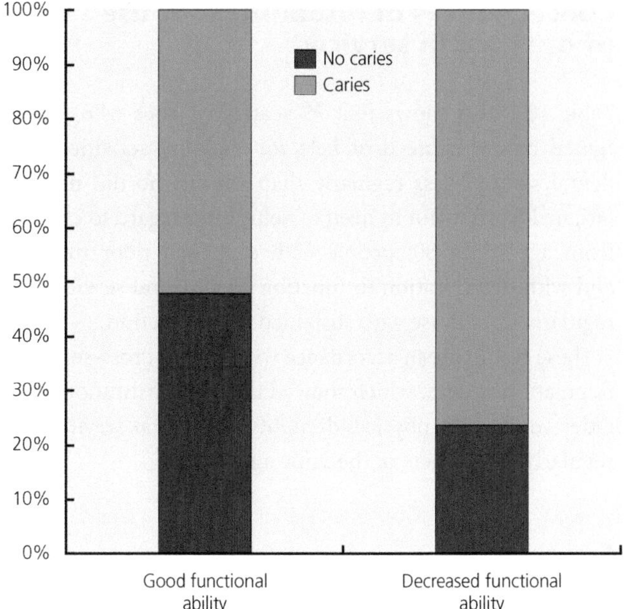

Figure 10.8 Percentage of men and women with and without caries in relation to their functional abilities. Reproduced from Avlund *et al.*, 2004.

One potential explanation for these patterns of associations is that physical limitations may make it more difficult for older people to take proper care of their teeth, thus contributing to the higher prevalence of current decay. It is thus obvious that tooth brushing and flossing become difficult to perform adequately with a decreased manual dexterity. In addition, loss of functional abilities may reduce self-esteem and individuals may lower the priority given to oral hygiene and regular dental care. Some older adults may feel that tooth loss is an inevitable part of growing old. Finally, it seems quite feasible that mobility disability may limit an older person's access to dental care. Lack of proper dental care for caries and/or periodontal disease might eventually lead to loss of natural teeth, with replacement by complete or partial dentures. This interpretation is supported further by a supplemental multiple regression analysis in some of the described studies, which showed that disability was no longer predictive of edentulism when controlling for recency of last dental visit. Among institutionalized older adults poor mobility reduces a resident's ability to access dental care outside the nursing home, and accessing care within the institutional setting is difficult because most dentists are not interested in providing services and/or feel inadequately trained.

Consequences of disabilities for use of oral health services

Table 10.1 also shows that 75-year-old Danes who felt fatigued or are in need of help for mobility-activities used dental services less regularly than those who did not feel fatigued or were not in need of help. With regard to changes from age 75 to 80, people with sustained poor function and with deterioration in function used dental services less regularly than those with sustained good function.

These results are in accordance with several cross-sectional population studies, which showed that non-institutionalized older adults with physical disability use dental services less regularly than others of the same age.

Conclusions

Older adults with early signs of disability and with actual disability are at larger risk of having oral health problems. This has several implications.

First, it should be recognized that prevention of disability in older adults will eventually also cause better oral health in the old people. This may be the case with regard to specific prevention of various diseases and with regard to health promotion, e.g. promotion of physical exercise and to stop smoking. Here, the effect may be indirect via functional ability, i.e. treatment of a disease or increased physical exercise may improve the functional ability of older adults, thus making it easier to take proper care of the teeth. But the effect may also be direct, i.e. treatment of a specific disease such as diabetes or stopping smoking may have a direct beneficial effect on oral health.

Second, it is important to be aware that older people who feel fatigued when they perform their daily activities are at larger risk of disability and of oral health problems. This should be recognized in the multidimensional interventions which take place in several communities, e.g. in Denmark, where all 75+ year-olds living at home in the municipalities are offered annual preventive home visits. Here the preventive home visitors should be aware of oral health problems as one possible consequence of feelings of fatigue.

Third, problems with fine motor activities caused by dexterity problems may make it difficult to take care of the teeth and periodontium. This may be relieved by an enlargened hand grip or an electric toothbrush, but if the person is severely disabled he/she may need daily help with tooth brushing and interproximal flossing. For institutionalized older adults one way may be to assist nursing staff through educational initiatives, which should encourage them to offer daily mouth care as an integral component of their personal hygiene care for all disabled older people in residential and home care. This care includes daily tooth brushing, quarterly or semiannual preventive assessments and service education for daily caregivers (nurses and aides), so that they learn the essential skills to provide daily mouth care for frail older adults.

Finally older people with personal care disability, for example, may require more frequent dental visits to compensate for their physical disability. Frail and functionally dependent older people living in long-term care facilities or at home, have special difficulties in accessing dental care because the problems of attending a dental clinic often appear insurmountable. The accessibility of the dental office is important too, especially for functionally disabled older patients (see chapter by Ettinger).

Further reading

Avlund, K. (1997) Methodological challenges in measurements of functional ability in gerontological research. A review. *Aging Clinical and Experimental Research*, **9**, 164–174.

Avlund, K. (2004) Disability in old age. Longitudinal population-based studies of the disablement process. *Danish Medical Bulletin*, **51**, 315–349.

Avlund, K. (2010) Fatigue in older adults: An early indicator of the aging process. *Aging Clinical and Experimental Research*, **22**, 100–115.

Avlund, K., Holm-Pedersen, P. & Schroll, M. (2001) Functional ability and oral health among older people: A longitudinal study from age 75 to 80. *Journal of the American Geriatric Society*, **49**, 954–962.

Avlund, K., Damsgaard, M.T., Sakari-Rantala, R., Laukkanen, P. & Schroll, M. (2002) Tiredness in daily activities among non-disabled old people as determinant of onset of disability. *Journal of Clinical Epidemiology*, **55**, 965–973.

Avlund, K., Holm-Pedersen, P., Morse, D.E., Viitanen, M. & Winblad, B. (2004) Tooth loss and caries prevalence in very old Swedish people: the relationship to cognitive function and functional ability. *Gerodontology*, **21**, 17–26.

Avlund, K., Rantanen, T. & Schroll, M. (2006) Tiredness and subsequent disability in older adults. *The role of walking limitations. Journal of Gerontology: Medical Sciences*, **61A**, 1201–1205.

De Visschere, L.M., Grooten, L., Theuniers, G. & Vanobbergen, J.N. (2006) Oral hygiene of elderly people in long-term care institutions – a cross-sectional study. *Gerodontology*, **23**, 195–204.

Dolan, T.A., Peek, C.W., Stuck, A. E. & Beck, J.C. (1998) Functional health and dental service use among older adults. *Journal of Gerontology: Medical Sciences*, **53A**, M413–M418.

Felder, R., James, K., Brown, C., Lemon, S. & Reveal, M. (1994) Dexterity testing as a predictor of oral care ability. *Journal of the American Geriatric Society*, **42**, 1081–1086.

Fried, L.P., Ferrucci, L., Darer, J., Williamson, J.D. & Anderson, G. (2004) Untangling the concepts of disability, frailty, and comorbidity: Implications for improved targeting and care. *Journal of Gerontology: Medical Sciences*, **59**, M255–M263.

Gift, H. C. & Newman, J. F. (1993) How older adults use oral health care services: Results of a national health interview survey. *Journal of the American Dental Association*, **124**, 89–93.

Guralnik, J.M. & Ferrucci, L. (2003) Assessing the building blocks of function. Utilizing measures of functional limitations. *American Journal Preventive Medicine*, **25**, 112–121.

Hawkins, R.J. (1999) Functional status and untreated dental caries among nursing home residents aged 65 and over. *Special Care in Dentistry*, **19**, 158–163.

Holm-Pedersen, P., Vigild, M., Nitschke, I. & Berkey, D.B. (2005) Dental care for aging populations in Denmark, Sweden, Norway, United Kingdom, and Germany. *Journal of Dental Education*, **69**, 987–997.

Jette, A.M., Feldman, H.A. & Douglass, C. (1993) Oral disease and physical disability in community-dwelling older persons. *Journal of the American Geriatric Society*, **41**, 1102–1108.

Locker, D. (1988) Measuring oral health: A conceptual framework. *Community Dental Health*, **5**, 3–18.

Lundgren, M., Emilson, C.-G., Österberg, T., Steen, G., Birhead, D. & Steen, B. (1997) Dental caries and related factors in 88- and 92-year-olds. Cross-sectional and longitudinal comparisons. *Acta Odontologica Scandinavica*, **55**, 282–291.

Macintyre, S., Hunt, K. & Sweeting, H. (1996) Gender differences in health: Are things really as simple as they seem? *Social Science & Medicine*, **42**, 617–624.

Mänty, M., de Leon, C.F., Rantanen, T., Era, P., Pedersen, A.N., Ekmann, A. *et al.* (2012) Mobility-related fatigue, walking speed and muscle strength in older people. *Journal of Gerontology: Medical Science*, **67**, 523–529.

Newman, A.B. & Brach, J.S. (2001) Gender gap in longevity and disability in older persons. *Epidemiologic Reviews*, **23**, 343–350.

Stuck, A.E., Walthert, J.M., Nikolaus, T., Büla, C.J., Hohmann, C. & Beck, J.C. (1999) Risk factors for functional status decline in community-living elderly people: a systematic literature review. *Social Science & Medicine*, **48**, 445–469.

Verbrugge, L.M. & Jette, A.M. (1994) The disablement process. *Social Science & Medicine*, **38**, 1–14.

Vita, A.J., Terry, R.B., Hubert, H.B. & Fries, J.F. (1998) Aging, health risks, and cumulative disability. *New England Journal of Medicine*, **338**, 1036–1041.

Österberg, T., Lundgren, M., Emilson, C.-G. & Sundh, V. (1998) Utilization of dental services in relation to socioeconomic and health factors in the middle-aged and elderly Swedish population. *Acta Odontologica Scandinavica*, **56**, 41–47.

CHAPTER 11

Nutrition and oral health for the older person

Angus W. G. Walls
University of Edinburgh, Edinburgh, UK

Introduction

Nutrition and health are inextricably linked together. Inadequate nutrient intake or absorption will result in overt or sub-clinical deficiency states which may have a significant effect on health outcomes for older people. There is significant evidence of malnourishment amongst older individuals, particularly those who are admitted to hospital, with a reported prevalence of between 20 and 70% in a range of clinical studies. This pattern is similar in free-living populations as well as those who are admitted to hospital for health care.

Nutritional and dietary requirements change with increasing age as a consequence of alterations in body composition or physiology that impact on nutritional status or nutrition, which are summarized in Table 11.1. The need for change however is not well communicated to older people in general and specifically to the frail and housebound.

Additionally there are a number of social and functional changes that impact on the availability of foods and their consumption. These include difficulties in shopping for food because of challenges with mobility, the physical ability to carry weights and vision. There are also social changes that impact on older people who can become increasingly isolated as partners and friends die. Eating and the enjoyment of eating and cooking are in part a social construct and as the social environment changes the enthusiasm for food preparation and eating diminishes.

The enjoyment of foods is also intimately tied up with the special senses of taste and smell, there are age-associated changes in these that again impact on the pleasure associated with eating foods among older people. These changes are reviewed later in this chapter and are worse in people who have oral dryness.

Table 11.1 Alterations in body composition or physiological function that affect macro- and micronutrient intake/requirements

Dietary intake	Physiological change	Effect
Energy	Altered body composition with reduced muscle bulk and relative increases in fat and connective tissue. Reduced levels of physical activity particularly with chronic disease.	Reduced energy requirements but no change in requirements for micronutrients so need for a changed, more nutrient dense diet.
Vitamin D	Altered effectiveness of skin synthesis of vitamin D along with a tendency for reduced exposure to sunlight with increasing age.	Need for micronutrient supplementation at the level of 10–15 μg/day
Vitamin B_{12}	Alterations in gastric pH, particularly with atrophic gastritis, leading to reduced absorption of B_{12}.	Need for micronutrient supplementation at the level of 15–25 μg/day

Whatever the cause, a failure to eat and malnourishment result in increased severity of disease outcomes and prolonged hospital stays for a significant number of older people; simple nutritional supplementation in this population can have a significant benefit in terms of health outcomes (Figure 11.1). One factor that also needs to be considered among the old who are ill is that they have a reduced ability to readapt their energy balance after a period of low or high intake. So an individual who has been acutely ill, and as a result may have had limited dietary intake, has a reduced ability to return to a normal dietary pattern with increasing age.

Furthermore, there are many systemic disease processes that may be related to oral disease in older people for which

Textbook of Geriatric Dentistry, Third Edition. Edited by Poul Holm-Pedersen, Angus W. G. Walls and Jonathan A. Ship.

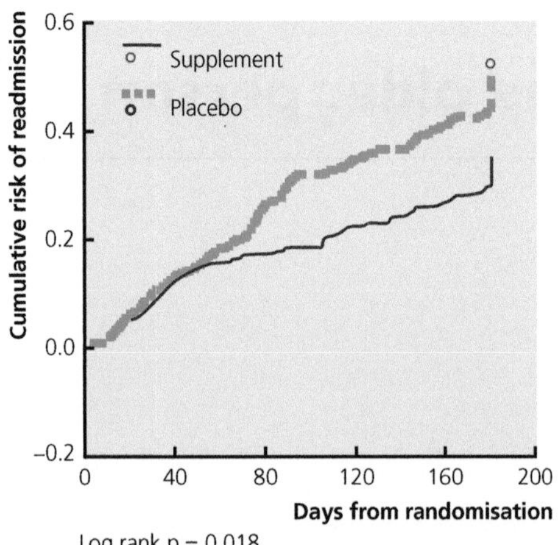

Figure 11.1 Reduced risk of hospital readmission among older people taking nutrient supplements compared with controls. *Source:* Gariballa *et al.*, 2006. Reproduced with permission of Elsevier.

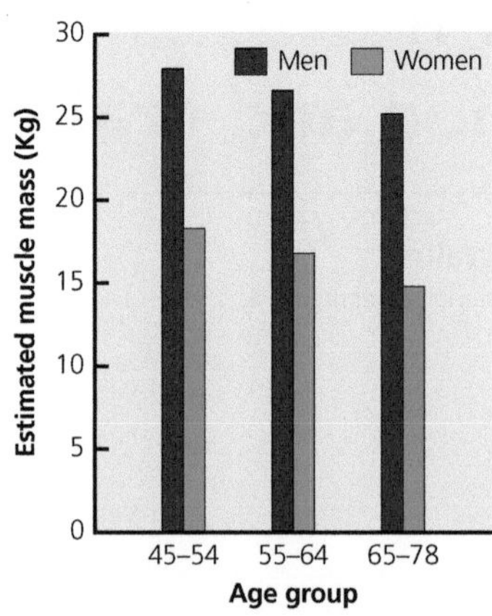

Figure 11.2 Reducing muscle mass (estimated from urinary creatinine excretion) with increasing age among men and women. Reproduced from Frontera *et al.*, 1991.

nutrition, either contemporary or historic, plays a key part in their aetiology, including metabolic syndrome and diabetes as well as cardiovascular disease (CVD) and cancer.

Oral health and function are also inextricably linked to nutritional status. The mouth is the portal of entry for foods; limitation in oral functional status is one of the variables that are associated with altered dietary habits and choice. Such alterations in oral functional status are more likely to occur in older people as most oral disease and tooth loss are irreversible processes. Furthermore, our enjoyment of foods (and hence our enthusiasm for eating) is achieved as a consequence of oral function, breaking up and releasing tastants from the food which are then available in solution in saliva for the oral taste buds or in gaseous form for smell receptors in the nasopharynx. Finally the texture of food is critical to our willingness to eat. If some textures are difficult to chew or cause discomfort in the oral environment then people will not choose to select those foods.

The purpose of this chapter is to review these issues in some depth and to clarify not only the role of nutrition in oral health but also the role of oral health in helping to sustain an adequate nutritional intake and the role of the dental team in helping our patients to achieve that.

Nutritional requirements with age

Energy requirements

There is a progressive alteration of body composition with age, with a reduction in skeletal muscle and a relative increase in adipose and connective tissue. At its worst, muscle wasting (sarcopenia) results in a significant reduction in problems with simple muscle activity and things like posture contributing to falls and instability in older age. Even at a 'normal' rate of reduction there will be progressive loss of muscle power, and the amount of energy required for basal metabolic activity is reduced as a consequence (Figure 11.2). The benefits of resistance exercise in terms of maintaining muscle bulk are however retained among older people; those who undertake regular resistance exercise reduce or prevent loss of muscle bulk.

Added to the impact of sarcopenia on muscle activity there is a general tendency for people to become progressively less active as they get older. This occurs among the vast majority of people in one form or another so, for example, while a 70-year-old trained athlete will likely do more exercise than the average person and will retain more muscle bulk as a consequence, they will still be doing less than they did when they were 30 years younger. This tendency is exacerbated in people who suffer chronic disease that impairs their ability to take exercise, for example those with rheumatoid arthritis or people who are obese.

The outcome of this reduction in muscle bulk and reduced physical activity is a reduction in the need for energy on a daily basis. Older people need to eat less than younger ones to avoid weight gain. This is reflected in the recommendations for daily energy intake provided by government (Table 11.2). Whilst the patterns for alterations in recommended energy intake are consistent between these various organizations/governments, there are variations in absolute values. The difference of about 1 MJ/day between UK/WHO and US recommendations over an adult lifetime (say from 20–65 years of age) is 16 452 MJ. It is estimated that fat mass in living people has an energy value of 29 MJ/kg, thus the difference between these recommendations equates to 566 kg of fat mass!

Table 11.2 Reference values for energy intake for males and females in MJ/day (kcal = MJ x 240)

Age	Male				Female			
	UK / WHO	USA	EU		UK / WHO	USA	EU	
			Low[a]	High[b]			Low[a]	High[b]
15–18	11.51	12.5	11.8		8.83	9.2	8.9	
19–50	10.6	12.1	11.3	12.0	8.1	9.2	8.4	9.0
51–59	10.6	9.6	11.3	12.0	8.0	9.2	8.4	9.0
60–64	9.93	9.6	8.5	9.2	7.99	9.2	7.2	7.8
65–74	9.71	9.6	8.5	9.2	7.96	9.2	7.2	7.8
75+	8.77	9.6	7.5	8.5	7.61	9.2	6.7	7.6

[a]No physical activity, desirable body weight.
[b]Recommended physical activity, desirable body weight.
Data from UK as Estimated Average Requirement (EAR), from USA as Average Energy Allowance (AEA).

Protein intake

Proteins are required for a variety of purposes, including maintenance of skeletal muscle as well as a source of energy. There is considerable debate in the literature whether there should be different protein intakes for older people compared with younger. This reflects a combination of the reduced skeletal muscle mass in older people suggesting that protein intake should be less. However, nitrogen balance studies suggest that older populations require at least as much protein as younger people. A recent European Foods Standards Agency report has concluded that there should be no difference in the Average Requirement of Population Reference Intake levels for protein for all adults. They did note though that the reduced energy requirements in older people would suggest that sedentary older adults should have a higher protein to energy ratio in their diets because of their lower need for energy.

Micronutrient intakes

There is no reduction currently in the recommendations for daily intake (Reference Nutrient Intake or RNI) for micronutrients in this population, current recommendations are the same for all adults over the age of 20. As a consequence, older people need to change their dietary habits if they are to sustain micronutrient intake with a reduced energy intake. They need to consume a more nutrient dense diet (one that contains more micronutrients per unit of energy). Such diets will need to be relatively higher in fruits, vegetables and whole-grain content with an appropriate amount of fat. Protein and carbohydrates are a more sensible form for the bulk of energy intake rather than fat as they are less nutrient-dense and also induce a greater sense of satiety than fats.

There is evidence from cross-sectional epidemiological studies of older people that there are some micronutrients where there are intakes significantly below the LRNI (Lowest Reference Nutrient Intake). More worryingly the evidence shows that low micronutrient status (based on haematological assessment) is considerably more prevalent than dietary intakes might suggest and this is a particular problem among people living in long-stay care. Tables 11.3 and 11.4 show data from the UK National Diet and Nutrition Survey for people aged 65 and over. These outcomes though are found varyingly in other similar studies internationally in Europe, Australia and the USA.

Table 11.3 Proportion of older people (65 and above) with micronutrient intakes from food below the Lower Reference Nutrient Intake (LRNI)(%)

	Free living		Long-stay care	
	Men	Women	Men	Women
Iron[a]	1	6	5	6
Vitamin C[a]	2	2	1	0
Folate[a]	1	6	4	5
Vitamin B_{12}	> 0.5	1	nil	nil
Thiamin	> 0.5	> 0.5	> 0.5	> 0.5
Riboflavin[a]	5	10	3	3
Vitamin D	97% below RNI		99% below RNI	
Magnesium[a]	21	23	39	22
Potassium[a]	17	39	28	42
Zinc	8	5	13	4

[a]Proportion increases with age.
Reproduced from Finch *et al.*, 1998.

It is unclear why micronutrient levels are lower than would be suggested by intake data; there are two possible explanations:

- In the long-stay care sample within the National Diet and Nutrition Survey, intake was based on foods given to the residents rather than consumed so plate wastage (food left on the plate at the end of the meal) was not taken into account.
- There may be changes in physiological function that impact on an individual's ability to absorb or synthesize micro nutrients.

Table 11.4 Proportion of older people (65 and above) with low haematological micronutrient status (%)

	Free living		Long-stay care	
	Men	Women	Men	Women
Iron (Hb)[a]	11	9	52	39
Vitamin C[a]	14	13	44	38
Folate	15	15	39	39
Vitamin B_{12}	6	6	9	9
Thiamin	8	9	11	15
Riboflavin	41	41	41	32
Vitamin D[a]	6	10	38	37

[a]Proportion increases with age.
Reproduced from Finch *et al.*, 1998.

Changes in physiological function

There are two sources of vitamin D in humans: dietary intake and skin synthesis. Skin synthesis is dependent on an individual having adequate skin exposure to the sun at times of year when the sun is sufficiently intense to trigger the synthetic process. Solar intensity is a potential problem in temperate climates where the sun is only sufficiently intense for a limited period of the year. For example vitamin D levels are lower in adults in Aberdeen in northern Scotland compared with those in Surrey in southern England. This synthetic activity is reduced with increasing age and older people are less likely to be out of doors in direct sunlight than younger individuals. It is obviously also impaired in ethnic groups where religious or other customs require the coverage of significant amounts of skin.

As a consequence there are now common recommendations for older people to increase their consumption of vitamin D orally to offset a combination of reduced skin exposure to sun to allow for vitamin D synthesis in the skin and reduced efficiency of vitamin D synthesis in the skin with increasing age. The level recommended by the UK Department of Health currently is 10 µg/day over the age of 65. This can only reasonably be achieved by consuming vitamin D supplements rather than through dietary change.

There may be alterations in absorption of some nutrients as a consequence of changes in the gut, for example acidity of the stomach is essential for absorption of some of the B complex vitamins, particularly B_{12}. Gastric pH rises with increasing age, most likely as a consequence of the high prevalence of atrophic gastritis in the over 65s.

The role of nutrition in the aetiology of major systemic disease that may be of relevance to oral health

Obesity

There is an international 'epidemic' of obesity in the developed world. The aetiology of obesity is complex, but fundamentally obesity represents an excess of energy intake compared with consumption. With the excess being stored as fat. Visceral or abdominal fat is thought to be more harmful than other patterns of fat storage

It is now widely recognized that adipose tissue is not just a simple storage organ for excess fat but is also a very active tissue, involved in maintenance of both triglyceride and free fatty acid levels. It has a role in influencing resistance to the effects of insulin and hence in glucose tolerance and has an active hormonal role in terms of both regulation of satiety through leptins and resistin as well as a pro-inflammatory effect with secretion of adipokines, TNFα and IL6. Finally it is a source of Plasminogen Activator Inhibitor 1 which reduces the rate of clot lysis.

Obesity generally and central obesity in particular are critical risk variables for hypertension, CVD and stroke, type 2 diabetes mellitus as well as gout and arthritis.

There are a number of genetic conditions that predispose to obesity but they are a very small part of the picture. During the period of most change in obesity rates there has been a marked alteration in dietary patterns that includes a significant increase in portion sizes of foods consumed, a change from diets rich in low energy-density carbohydrate-rich foods (typically potatoes or other starchy foods, vegetables, grains and wholemeal bread) to those with increased proportions of high energy-density high fat content foods such as meat and dairy products and a generalized reduction in the amount of physical activity undertaken by people. There are also links to obesity with reductions in sleep and increases in stress.

The regulation of food intake is dependent to an extent on a feeling of fullness or satiety during eating. This is regulated by the foods we eat and is greater per unit energy consumed for high carbohydrate foods and lower for fatty foods with their associated high energy-density.

Evidence would suggest that weight loss can only be reliably achieved with a combination of modest (and sustainable) increases in physical activity and reductions in caloric intake, particularly reductions in fat intake. Current thinking is that the contribution of alcohol, carbohydrate and protein in the diet to obesity is that they are metabolized first as sources of energy and fat consumed at the same time is stored, rather than their being converted to fat per se.

The significance of obesity to oral health is threefold. Diabetes and CVD are more prevalent in obese people and both are associated with the circulating markers of oral inflammation from mucosal inflammatory disease, either periodontitis or denture-associated stomatitis. There is evidence of a separate and independent increased risk for and severity of periodontal disease in obese people, probably linked to the pro-inflammatory actions of adipose tissue. Finally in practical terms the delivery of oral health care to the morbidly obese can require highly specific and costly dental equipment. The recommended weight limits for many modern dental chairs are relatively modest (around 140 kg or 300 lb which is relatively low in relation to obese patients).

Diabetes mellitus

Type 1

This is a result of autoimmune destruction of the β cells in the islets of Langerhans in the pancreas. As a consequence the individual's ability to produce insulin is impaired but their cellular response to insulin remains within normal limits. This disease most commonly manifests itself before the age of 40 and it is managed with a combination of injected insulin and diet.

Type 2

This is a result of either a reduction in insulin production from the pancreas or an increasing resistance to the effects of insulin on cellular metabolism. Insulin resistance increases with increasing age for reasons that are unknown at present. Insulin resistance is also a feature of metabolic syndrome that is believed to be a pre-diabetic state, and is enhanced in people who are obese, particularly those with central abdominal obesity. Type 2 diabetes mellitus (T2DM) is by far the more common form of this disease that occurs predominantly in people over the age of 40 although, with increases in adolescent and young adult obesity, type 2 diabetes is now also seen in younger people.

The prevalence of diabetes increases with age and varies considerably between countries and within ethnic groups. The population estimates for prevalence of T2DM in the 3rd US National Health and Nutrition and Examination Survey (NHANES III) was around 20% for 60–74-year-olds.

Obesity is by far the most significant risk variable for T2DM and its aetiology has already been discussed. The severity of insulin resistance in T2DM is affected by the inflammatory state of the body; any source of circulating inflammatory markers will reduce the body's ability to manage glucose in patients with T2DM. In addition both forms of diabetes mellitus are risk factors for progression of periodontal disease. Thus periodontitis is worst in people with diabetes mellitus and the management of patients with periodontal disease who have T2DM will result in an improvement in their ability to manage circulating glucose levels with reductions in their glycated haemoglobin ($HbA1_c$) levels. The benefit in terms of glycaemic control appears to be comparable to that achieved with normal oral hypoglycaemic agents.

Cancer

The major risk variables for oral cancer are alcohol and tobacco consumption, particularly those forms of tobacco that are held in contact with the oral mucosa for long periods of time like chewing tobacco in the USA or quid used in the Indian subcontinent with combinations of tobacco, betel and areca nut in association with slaked lime.

Table 11.5 Recommendations for dietary intake to minimize risk of cardiovascular disease

	WHO/FAO
Total fat	15–30%
Saturated fatty acids (SFA)	<10%
Cis-polyunsaturated fatty acids (PFA)	6–10%
Of which n-6 (PUFA)	5–8%
n-3 (PUFA)	1–2%
Cis-monounsaturated fatty acid	Remainder[a]
Trans-fatty acids (TFA)	<1%
Dietary cholesterol	<300 mg/day
Total carbohydrate	55–75%
of which free sugars	<10%
Dietary fibre (NSP)	From foods
Protein	10–15%
Salt	<5 g/day
Fruits and vegetables	>400 g/day

[a] *Cis*-monounsaturated fatty acid = total fat − (TFA + PFA + SFA).

There is some limited evidence of the benefit of fruits and vegetables intake, particularly in people who smoke/use tobacco products or drink alcohol to excess. There is also limited evidence for the benefits of dietary change in areas of the world where diets were historically low in antioxidant vitamins (increase in β-carotene, selenium and vitamin E in Chinese populations appears to be protective against oesophageal cancer in a population with previously low intakes of these nutrients).

Cardiovascular disease

Obesity, especially central obesity associated with raised waist circumference or waist : hip ratio once again is a key, nutritionally linked, risk variable for atherosclerotic vascular disease alongside dietary fat intake as an important component of CVD risk.

Disease risk is elevated in people with higher intakes of saturated and *trans*-unsaturated fats, while n-3 and n-6 polyunsaturated fats appear to have a protective effect. There are internationally recognized guidelines for the intake of macronutrients to help prevent CVD (Table 11.5). Saturated and *trans*-unsaturated fat intake results in an increase in plasma cholesterol and relatively high levels of high-density lipoprotein (HDL).

There is evidence of benefit from a variety of antioxidants in the diet, notably from vitamins C and E and β-carotene in addition to a wide range of plant flavonoids from berries, some vegetables and fruits. The latter may explain the low levels of CVD seen in France where there are relatively high levels of cholesterol in the population, but much lower levels of disease than seen in other European countries with a similar cholesterol profile. There is little evidence however to support any single element dietary supplement as being protective against CVD. However diets that are high in fruits and vegetables intake show some cardioprotective benefits, likely as a consequence of a wide mix of antioxidant activity. The features of a cardioprotective diet are:

- low levels of saturated and *trans*-unsaturated fats;
- high levels of fruits and vegetables intake along with cereals and wholegrains (care is required around cooking fruits and vegetables to prevent loss of vitamins and minerals);
- protein intake from fish, vegetables, seeds and nuts;
- if meat is part of the diet then it should be lean and in small quantities;
- balanced energy intake to minimize obesity.

These are in contrast with the dietary pattern commonly encountered among edentulous people with higher levels of fat intake and reduced intake of fruits and vegetables compared with people with some teeth. Interventions in edentulous subjects can affect change in fat intakes in a 'healthy' direction (see later).

Nutrition and oral health

Oral mucosa

Age-related alterations to the oral mucosa are covered in Chapter 12. That change does occur is accepted; however, the effect of that change on the relationship between oral mucosal integrity and nutritional deficiencies is unclear. Oral mucosa has a very rapid rate of turnover like most of the mucosal lining of the gastrointestinal tract. As a consequence, micronutrient deficiencies that affect mucosal turnover and integrity will result in oral mucosal lesions at an early stage.

Iron, vitamin B_{12} and folate

These micronutrients are critical for mucosal integrity; deficiency states will result in alterations to the mucosa of both the tongue and the oral vestibule. The clinical picture associated with these deficiency states is described in detail elsewhere (Chapter 18). The papillae of the tongue tend to flatten and the mucosal covering reduces in thickness and in keratinization resulting in a smooth surface that is red in appearance rather than the dusky pink of normal lingual mucosa.

Vestibular ulceration is more common with deficiency states, particularly minor apthae, as are red lesions (erythroplasias) of the oral mucosa. An erythroplasia needs to be investigated with care and urgency as they are regarded as premalignant lesions.

Iron deficiency is also associated with burning mouth syndrome and angular cheilitis (see Chapter 18), as well as stomatitis associated with the area beneath the plate of a denture. Candidal infections are commonly associated with both denture-induced stomatitis and angular cheilitis. In addition the angle lesions can be infected with Staphylococci.

Most of these conditions respond to simple micronutrient supplements; however where bacteria or fungi are also involved then appropriate antimicrobial therapy is also essential (see Chapter 12)

Alcohol

The relationship between oral health and alcohol consumption is complex due to the many and varied components in alcoholic beverages.

Oral cancer. There is an increase in both oral premalignant lesions (estimated as a 22% increased risk per drink per day) and in overt malignancy in individuals who consume alcohol. The evidence for premalignant lesions does not show any variation between spirits and beer or pattern of consumption but there is evidence of higher rates of overt malignant disease associated with drinking spirits. Furthermore, it has been suggested that polyphenols (present in wines rather than beers and spirits) in some forms of alcoholic beverage may moderate the effects of alcohol intake on risk for malignant disease.

Smoking

Smoking and alcohol consumption have a synergistic effect in terms of the development of oral premalignant lesions with higher relative risk of individuals who both smoke and drink developing lesions compared with the cumulative effect of drinking or smoking. The relative risk for individuals who both smoke and drink alcohol is approximately threefold that of people who only drink alcohol.

Chewing tobacco and other forms of chewed quid (notably betel and areca nut) are also associated with increased risk of oral cancer. The estimated relative risk of developing oral cancer in individuals who chew areca nut alone is 58.4 (95% CI 7.6–447.6); this is markedly higher than that for smoking alone, for example, at 6.63 (95% CI, 4.48–9.81). Chewing betel and areca quids is endemic in the Indian subcontinent and increasing among Indian ex-patriots elsewhere in the world. This combination of tobacco leaf and slaked lime which is mixed with the nut pulp is particularly harmful, resulting initially in a characteristic sub-mucous fibrosis and subsequently in overt squamous carcinoma.

There are some other nutritional links to oral malignancy; premalignant lesions (particularly erythroplasias) are associated with iron deficiency and high levels of alcohol intake, and there are specific problems associated with tobacco use (either when smoked or in smokeless forms).

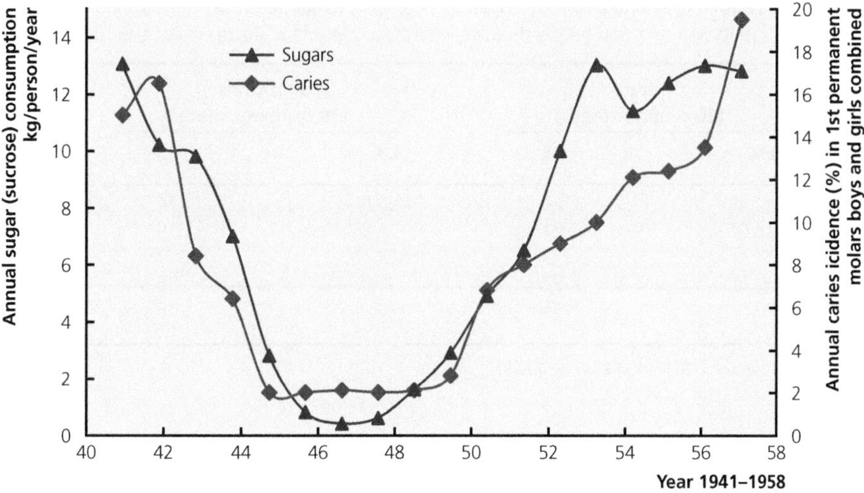

Figure 11.3 The relationship between sugar (sucrose) consumption and dental caries in Japanese children between 1941 and 1958.

Dental caries

Sugars

Dental caries occurs as a consequence of interactions between bacteria on the surface of teeth and within demineralized enamel and dentine and fermentable carbohydrates in food. The bacterial biofilm begins to form on the surface of a tooth immediately after it has been cleaned, but the biofilm (dental plaque) does not reach acidogenic *maturity* until it is about 4 days old. Mature dental plaque has a characteristic microbial flora and is capable of metabolizing some carbohydrates to produce acids. The microbiology of dental plaque is complex and is discussed elsewhere, but our understanding of this process is expanding continuously as molecular biology techniques permit the identification of bacterial species within plaque which currently cannot be cultured by conventional means.

Sugars are an inescapable component of all diets and yet they are also causatively linked with tooth decay. There is consistent evidence linking caries to sugars intake in younger people, including national epidemiological studies (Figure 11.3). However, there are fewer data linking decay in older adults to sugars consumption. Those data that are available suggest that root caries is linked to high sugars intakes (Table 11.6) and to the use of sugar (sucrose) as a sweetener in tea or coffee, particularly in men. One particular area of concern is the high level of untreated dental caries in institutionalized populations (see Chapter 25). This is the result of a relatively cariogenic diet with a high frequency of sugars intake daily to try to maintain energy consumption at adequate levels in frail older people and poor access to dental care and preventive services.

Table 11.6 Variables and their odds ratios (OR) for primary root caries risk from the UK National Diet and Nutrition Survey programme

Variable	OR
Cleans teeth less than once daily	3.4
Severe plaque deposits in combination with RPD	2.5
Any teeth with 9 mm + loss of attachment	2.2
Sugars rich foods – 9 or more intakes daily	2.1
Number of vulnerable roots	1.5[a]
Number of exposed but sound roots	0.7[a]
Number of teeth with restored but sound crowns	0.9[a]

[a] These odds ratios were per tooth (or root); to compute the odds ratio per person this figure would be raised to the power of the number of teeth/roots present in this condition. So for a person with 10 vulnerable but sound roots the OR would be 0.7^{10} or 0.028. Odds ratios below 1 are indicative of a variable which infers reduced risk in this model.
Reproduced from Steele *et al.*, 2001.

Is frequency or quantity of sugars intake important?

Sugars that are taken into the oral environment can be metabolized by plaque bacteria to produce acids. The acid in turn results in a reduction in pH on the surface of the tooth causing demineralization and potentially caries. The oral environment is very effective at remineralizing tooth structure providing that salivary function is maintained. However, it takes time for the oral and plaque pH to rise above the demineralization threshold for tooth tissue, particularly dentine and it takes time for the remineralization to occur. Hence there is a maximum number of de- and re-mineralization cycles that the natural defence mechanisms of the mouth can cope with. If the total number of episodes of demineralization exceed this maximum the outcome will favour overall demineralization of tooth tissue, which can manifest itself as either caries or erosive pattern tooth wear. Within

Table 11.7 Dietary intake of specific nutrients among adults aged over 65 according to dental status. The UK data are from the National Diet and Nutrition Survey for people aged 65 years and over and the US data are from the US Veterans' Association Longitudinal Dental Survey

	Intact (20 or more teeth)		Compromised (19 or fewer teeth)		Edentulous (No teeth)	
	UK	US	UK	US	UK	US
Protein (63 g/day)	72.3	80	66.6	74	60.1	68
NSP (25 g/day)	16.2[a]	21[a]	12.9[a]	19[a]	11.0[a]	16[a]
Calcium (800 mg/day)	883	773[a]	812	677[a]	722[a]	689[a]
Niacin (15 mg/day)	33.8	32	31.0	28	27.0	34
Vitamin C (60 mg/day)	82	156	73	146	60	127

[a]These values are below the recommended daily intake values (RNI).
Reproduced from Krall *et al.*, 1998; Sheiham *et al.*, 2001.

limits, the absolute quantity of sugars that are consumed at any one time are irrelevant to this relationship. There is no evidence on what frequency of sugars intakes might be regarded as safe for preventing caries in older populations. The 'rule of thumb' for young people is four sugars containing intakes per day but the increased risks seen in older people, particularly those with dry mouth, may make even this level unacceptable. It is of note that the mean number of sugars intakes daily for the 'free-living' 65+ population in the UK was 5.1, rising to 7.9 for the 'institution' sample in the 65+ National Diet and Nutrition Survey. It was in this population that frequency of sugars intake was associated with root caries activity (Table 11.6). There are no data relating to coronal caries activity and sugars intake for older people.

Sugars in medicines

Sugars are used in prescribed products in two circumstances, either as energy supplements for the ill or as a preservative and sweetener in conventional drugs.

High energy food supplements in liquid or syrup form are used to maintain an adequate calorific intake in debilitated patients. They contain large quantities of sugars and are sipped over long periods of time. Furthermore, the syrupy nature of these preparations reduces the rate of oral clearance, particularly in individuals with impaired salivary flow.

Sugars that are used as preservatives in syrups and mixtures, and to hide the bitter flavour of drugs are also a problem for older people where the use of liquid medicines and those that are sucked again becomes common. The campaign for the replacement of sugars in medicines for children has been long and successful, but there has been no similar programme for older adults. Similarly, chewable preparations that have an intrinsically low pH (for example, vitamin C preparations) will add to the overall acid burden of the oral environment.

Which sugars are important?

Added sugars (non-milk extrinsic sugars or NMES) are the most harmful in terms of their ease of metabolism and ready availability when consumed; this applies particularly to sucrose but also to glucose, fructose and maltose. The natural fruit sugars, like fructose and those in milk (lactose), can also be metabolized by plaque bacteria to produce acids but are more difficult for the bacteria to metabolize and hence are less acidogenic. They are usually less readily available from foods in the oral environment and diets which include high frequency of intake of such sugars are unusual. Finely ground starch can also be metabolized to produce acids by oral bacteria but again at lower levels than seen with sucrose. There is also a significant starch/sucrose interaction where combinations of starches and sucrose, when taken together, are highly cariogenic; this combination occurs in starchy snack foods commonly used as between meals adjuncts to diet.

Refined sugars are used extensively as both sweetening agents and preservatives in foods, often being described as hidden sugars in this latter role as savoury food can often contain significant quantities of added sugar (examples would be tomato ketchup, tinned vegetables and baked beans).

Alcohol

Alcoholic drinks also contain sugars which can initiate decay and acids which also dissolve tooth tissue. This increased acid burden in the mouth associated with generalized neglect in individuals who become addicted to alcohol can result in very extensive carious lesions on multiple teeth.

Smoking

Smokers have a higher incidence of caries than past or non-smokers. The mechanism for this phenomenon is unclear; a salivary link is unlikely as they show greater levels of output than non-smokers. However, smokers are more likely to consume sugars-containing drinks and snacks than non-smokers; furthermore, their oral hygiene tends to be poorer. These effects influence both coronal and root surfaces of teeth.

Erosive or acid-mediated dissolution of tooth tissue

This term is usually used to describe loss of tooth structure from acid which is not a metabolic product from sugars by bacteria in dental plaque. The acids involved can be either extrinsic, usually from foods/drinks or intrinsic, as a result of Gastro Esophageal Reflux Disease. There is no epidemiological evidence linking loss of tooth structure in older adults and dietary acid; there is compelling evidence from national surveys of children's and adults' dental health from the UK of high levels of erosive pattern tooth tissue loss. Whilst acids soften tooth substance, physical removal of that softened surface is thought to occur through contact with foods or by tooth to tooth contact. The patterns of tooth wear in older people reflect a life-time's exposure of teeth to acids, oral functional contacts and often dental care, making the identification of specific causality in a cross-sectional study very difficult. The extent and severity of erosive pattern wear that is seen in younger people is of particular concern for the future. Such wear is irreversible and will pose a long-term management problem for the remainder of the lives of the individuals concerned.

Alcoholic drinks

Erosive pattern tooth wear is seen in professional wine tasters due to the acidity of many wines and the way in which they are atomized in the mouth during the tasting process. Individuals who suffer from alcoholism also present with wear from a combination of pH of the drink itself plus chronic regurgitation of gastric contents resulting from gastric mucosal irritation.

Periodontal disease

This is a chronic inflammatory process which is addressed in detail elsewhere in this book (see Chapter 17). As a disease process driven by inflammation, it is susceptible to those variables which influence the chronic inflammatory response. There is increasing evidence for the role of reactive oxygen species (ROS) in moderating the effects of inflammation and hence interest in the antioxidant activity in peripheral blood. The effect of ROS seems to extend beyond simple interactions with tissues as they are also thought to be implicated in the mechanisms for increased tissue destruction in both smoking and type II diabetes. There have been attempts to affect the severity of this disease with both local and systemic application of antioxidant supplements; however these have shown limited benefit as yet. There is some evidence for vitamin C depletion and replenishment having a moderating effect on gingival bleeding in periodontally healthy individuals.

Smoking

There are strong links between periodontal attachment loss and smoking (see Chapter 17). Smoking not only influences the development of and flora that comprise dental plaque but it also exerts direct effects on the tissues, modifying the blood flow through these tissues and influencing fibroblast function. It also affects the immune responses which are key to defence against any inflammatory disease.

These effects occur with both smoked and smokeless tobacco, but are reversible within disease pathogenesis so that treatment outcomes are improved in those who stop smoking compared with those who continue, although the effects of smoking impact on periodontal outcomes for up to 10 years after cessation.

Oral health and foods choice

Chewing efficiency, digestion and foods choice

Teeth serve a primary function in foods consumption: breaking down large pieces of food into smaller particles and mixing them with saliva to allow a bolus of food to be formed for swallowing. This comminution of food along with salivary enzyme activity, is an important component of the initiation of digestion of foods.

The process of breaking up food and converting it into a bolus to be swallowed is associated with the release of tastants from the food enhancing our enjoyment of the things we eat.

Impaired chewing function will affect all of these components. People with poorer masticatory function are less efficient at breaking food down to facilitate bolus formation. They tend to use fewer chewing strokes and 'accept' larger food particle sizes in the food bolus prior to swallowing. Whilst there are no documented problems associated with this, there could be an increased risk of choking in people who chew their food less effectively and who also have impaired swallowing, for example people with dysphagia post stroke.

Saliva is also critical to this process; changes in saliva in health and disease are reviewed in depth in Chapter 19. However, those individuals who have reduced salivary flow, through disease of the salivary glands, radiation damage or as a side effect of drugs, will experience increasing challenges in terms of chewing and swallowing (as the lubricant effect of saliva will be less) and of forming food particles into a bolus for swallowing as saliva is the *glue* which holds the bolus together.

The number and distribution of remaining natural teeth and/or the presence of complete or partial dentures are likely to influence the ease of chewing. There is a particular problem when trying to chew with conventionally retained dentures where the prostheses are controlled by the oral musculature and the forces of adhesion and cohesion between the salivary film between the denture base and the oral mucosa. Food particles will act as a profound destabilizing influence during chewing as forces are applied eccentrically to the dentures so stabilizing pressure is required from the tongue musculature. This is a difficult learned skill which is easily lost if dentures are left out of the mouth for any period of time (for example during periods of illness), furthermore it is a skill that is likely to be more difficult to learn with increasing age. The current trends in tooth loss would suggest that the age at which people are being rendered edentulous is progressively rising.

If edentulism is one of the key determinants of oral function it is worth noting that a proportion of older dentate people are edentate in one arch (predominantly the upper). There are few data on the prevalence of this pattern of oral health but proportions of 2.7% for the adult population in Switzerland and 23% over 65s in the UK have been reported. These individuals function in a similar manner to those who are edentulous. People who are edentulous in the lower jaw and function with denture against some natural teeth in the upper jaw report more problems with chewing and swallowing foods than any other combination.

Masticatory efficiency

Variables which influence the ability to break down foods by chewing are usually assessed by measuring the size of test foods that have been chewed for a specific number of chewing cycles or have been chewed until the study participants would feel the particles were small enough to swallow. The test food is then removed from the mouth and the particle size analysed using a graded sieving method or image analysis techniques.

This methodology has demonstrated reduced chewing efficiency with smaller numbers of teeth, with teeth and removable partial dentures (RPDs) compared with natural teeth, and with complete dentures compared with a natural dentition. The effect of age alone on chewing efficiency is negligible, although there is some reduction in oral motor function in older people, probably relating to altered muscle bulk.

Understandably, chewing efficiency is affected by the number and distribution of teeth; maximum biting force is reduced in people with advanced periodontal disease and increasing tooth mobility. The relationship between masticatory efficiency and biting force is unclear. This is particularly difficult to clarify in subjects who have periodontal disease with mobile teeth as they also tend to have fewer teeth. The relative impact of the effect of mobility of teeth compared with numbers of teeth has not been clarified.

Masticatory efficiency and digestion

In the 1950s Farrell demonstrated that our ability to digest food is not influenced by chewing with a modern diet. The quality of digestion was dependent on the food type but was independent of the extent by which the food had been chewed. These data were derived from studies involving young dentate volunteers so the relevance of this work in an older population is unclear. There are profound changes in the bowel with age, which include reductions in gastric motility and atrophy of the villi on the walls of the small bowel. These changes are likely to influence the ability of an older person to digest and absorb foods. Farrell's work has never been repeated. There has been very little further work in this area; there is some evidence of altered availability of sugars from food if foods are swallowed whole rather than having been chewed, and gastric emptying times are reduced when foods are chewed more thoroughly.

Masticatory efficiency and food choice

Digestion *per se* may not be influenced by the amount food is chewed; there is significant evidence that foods choice is affected by chewing ability. As masticatory efficiency is progressively impaired through tooth loss individuals report progressive increase in their perceived difficulty chewing foods. If a person finds a specific food difficult to chew then as a rule they choose to avoid that food rather than persevering with the challenge. There are specific groups of foods that are more difficult to chew, which include raw carrot, nuts, fibrous vegetables and some fruits, which are affected by this phenomenon. Additionally foods where there is a social challenge associated with consumption are also avoided. Thus, green leafy vegetables are a particular problem for denture wearers, the moist leaf can stick to the surface of the acrylic of the denture making the individual uncomfortable. In this circumstance the leaf has to be removed mechanically from the plastic either by taking the denture out of the mouth or by pushing against the leaf with a finger; obviously this is not socially acceptable, so again an avoidance strategy is taken. People become handicapped by their oral status; consequently they suffer impaired intakes of certain fruits and vegetables and the associated key nutrients. One specific area of concern is the markedly reduced area intake of non-starch polysaccharides (dietary fibre) when compared with national dietary reference values. It is common for intake to be less than 50% of that which would be regarded as necessary for good health.

There is also some evidence of dietary change towards a less healthy diet with increased intakes of saturated fats and cholesterol and an increasing proportion of foods energy derived from fats in older people with reducing numbers of teeth (Table 11.7).

Further detailed analysis of the dental, nutritional and biochemical data from three large studies, (the Veterans Administration Longitudinal Study on Ageing in Boston, the cross-sectional National Diet and Nutrition Survey for adults aged over 65 years in the UK and National Health and Nutrition Examination Series III survey in the USA) have demonstrated clear associations between oral health status, nutrient intake and biochemical markers of nutritional status. Summaries are given in Tables 11.3 and 11.4 for both nutrient intake and biochemical markers of nutritional status. These analyses have made allowance for the effects of age, gender, regional variation within a country and socio-economic group.

One of the coping strategies that people adopt when they can no longer chew some foods is to change the method they use for foods preparation. This occurs both during the transition to edentulousness but also recent evidence from the US Health Professional study has shown similar trends among people who had five or more teeth extracted over an 8-year period. Those who had had more teeth extracted were more likely to have stopped eating apples, pears and raw carrots and showed smaller reductions in intake of cholesterol, greater reductions in consumption of polyunsaturated fat and smaller increases in consumption of dietary fibre and whole fruit than those who had no teeth extracted during the time period.

Therefore there is an increased risk of foods being over-prepared (for example, removal of the skin from fruits and vegetables) or over-cooked to allow them to be chewed by a person with reduced chewing efficiency. A broad range of nutrients can be affected by these phenomena. Some of the change may be beneficial, for example carotene is more bioavailable from cooked compared with raw carrot, but others will be lost either as a consequence of denaturation of proteins during cooking or as they are contained within specific zones of a food (for example the vitamin C in potato is located very close to the skin, if this is removed the vitamin C goes with it). The damage predominantly affects micronutrients, some of which are important in terms of cellular defence and potentially combating the effects of aging (e.g. the antioxidant micronutrients vitamins C and E). Obviously any reduction in dietary fibre may impact more broadly in terms of cardiovascular disease and cancer prevention.

Prevention of dietary change

There have been a number of studies that have looked at oral health interventions in terms of chewing function and dietary change. Almost without exception an oral health intervention designed to improve chewing efficiency, whether it involves making removable dentures, bridgework or implant supported prostheses, showed similar outcomes – that the participants felt able to chew better but they did not then go on to make any change to their diet.

Change in dietary habit (or any social habit) is a complex process as part of which the individual has to be aware of the need for, and rationale associated with, any specific change. There is now some evidence that when an oral health intervention is paired with tailored dietary advice aimed at the 'stage of awareness of need to change' of the individual concerned, significant improvements in fruits and vegetables consumption can be achieved, although the long-term maintenance of the change has yet to be demonstrated.

Taste and smell

National estimates from the US Health Information Survey of 1984 showed that 1.4% of the population had disorders of smell and 0.6% had disorders of taste, with a strong age-related trend such that 40% of those with chemosensory problems were 65 or older. General health status, other sensory impairment, functional problems and a variety of other health-related characteristics were also associated with chemosensory difficulties.

Taste perception with age

Taste is perceived through the taste buds on the dorsum of the tongue, the soft palate, the pharynx, larynx epiglottis and in the upper third of the oesophagus. The quantity and distribution of taste cells do not appear to change in normal, healthy adults with increasing age.

Tastants must be dissolved in fluid, derived from saliva, to allow the specific taste to be perceived. Individuals cannot taste their own saliva as a product of habituation, but there are changes in the ionic composition of saliva and in the salivary mucins with age (see Chapter 19) that must result in progressive change in this background flavour. However, this change may go some way to explaining the variations in taste perception with increasing age.

Like all age changes, the manifestation of altered taste varies from individual to individual but the changes generally comprise both alteration in the ability to discriminate tastes (that they are present at all when compared with water) and in recognizing the five different taste qualities in a food compared with the young. There are five principal tastes: bitter, salty, sour, sweet and umami (umami is the taste of savoury which is perceived separately from salt and sour). Bitter, salt, sour and to an extent sweet are reduced by aging in healthy, unmedicated adults. It has also been shown that these effects are amplified in people who take multiple medications and in those who are chronically ill. It is interesting to speculate that this amplification may also be associated with changes in saliva and other oral secretions in individuals who are taking multiple drugs. The effect extends to all the principal tastes, with increase in detection thresholds of 11.6-fold for sodium salts, 7-fold for bitter, 5-fold for umami, 4.3-fold for acid and 2.7-fold for sweet.

People with complete dentures often complain of impaired taste which they attribute to full palatal coverage with the denture base. The rationale for this is less clear as there are few, if any, taste buds on the hard palate. Impaired taste is more likely to be associated with poorer release of tastants from foods which are not chewed well.

An obvious solution to altered taste is to explore the value of flavour enhancers on foods consumption. Flavour enhancement can take the form either of adding artificial flavours to *fortify* the food, or adding something that amplifies natural taste. The most common chemical in this latter group is monosodium glutamate. Some beneficial effects, either as an arrest in decline of food intake or of overt increases in energy intake and even increases in body weight, have been seen with this approach.

Perception of smell with age

Reductions in smell are generally more profound and more consistent than changes in taste. Nearly two thirds of all adults over the age of 80 show some level of disturbed sense of smell. Rates of change are higher in men, current smokers and those with stroke and epilepsy.

Olfactory thresholds are elevated for all odours by between 2- and 15-fold when younger populations are compared with the old. Central nervous system pathology will also impact on olfactory perception including facial trauma and both Alzheimer's and Parkinson's diseases. Indeed, reduced olfactory ability has been suggested as a marker for cognitive decline.

Smell and taste are inextricably linked to our enjoyment of food. The amount of *taste* that we smell is obvious when people have an upper respiratory tract infection and all food *tastes* bland. Reductions in chemosensory ability can result in altered foods choice and reduced energy intake, and there have been suggestions that individuals may also be at increased risk of food poisoning as they would not be able to detect rotten foods by their smell.

Texture

Foods texture plays an important and little recognized part in the ability to process the food in the mouth. This ability changes with increasing age, associated both with altered oral status and reduced muscle bulk limiting chewing strength. There are some attempts to compensate for this by older people by increasing the number of chewing strokes used to process a mouthful of food. Despite this, older subjects swallow the food bolus with larger particle sizes of foods than in younger cohorts. Alternate coping strategies are to avoid foods whose texture make them harder to chew and swallow. Foods that are avoided are those that require high forces or prolonged chewing to reduce them to a state suitable for swallowing, as well as those that adhere to dentures and/or teeth. Roininen and co-workers conclude that both elderly and young respondents found fruit and vegetables easy to eat if they were ready-to-eat, but those that were hard, fibrous, adhere to the teeth and require preparation were perceived as troublesome for all.

One final variable that also influences perceived texture in the oral environment is salivary function. Individuals with poorer salivary flow have more difficulty chewing and swallowing foods in general, as the lubricating and binding actions of the saliva are reduced. This will have its greatest effect with foods that are perceived more difficult to chew.

Summary

Older people have altered nutritional needs, requiring less energy with a more nutrient dense diet to maintain micronutrient intakes. This is characterized by a diet low in fats and added sugars and high in carbohydrates, wholegrains and fruits and vegetables. Oral health status may pose a barrier to achieving this dietary change in those who have few or no natural teeth.

Diet also plays an important role in disease risk for the oral environment, not only in terms of dental caries but also tooth wear, periodontal disease and oral cancer.

Further reading

Baqir, W. & Maguire, A. (2000) Consumption of prescribed and over-the-counter medicines with prolonged oral clearance used by the elderly in the Northern Region of England, with special regard to generic prescribing, dose form and sugars content. *Public Health*, **114**(5), 367–373.

Blot, W.J., Li, J.Y., Taylor, P.R., Guo, W., Dawsey, S., Wang, G.Q. *et al.* (1993) Nutrition intervention trials in Linxian, China: supplementation with specific vitamin/mineral combinations, cancer incidence, and disease-specific mortality in the general population. *Journal of the National Cancer Institute*, **85**(18), 1483–1492.

Bradbury, J., Thomason, J.M., Jepson, N.J., Walls, A.W., Allen, P.F. & Moynihan, P.J. (2006) Nutrition counseling increases fruit and vegetable intake in the edentulous. *Journal of Dental Research*, **85**(5), 463–468.

Chadwick, B. & Pendry, L. (2004) *Report 3 Non-carious dental conditions*. ONS, London.

Chaffee, B.W. & Weston, S.J. (2010) Association between chronic periodontal disease and obesity: a systematic review and meta-analysis. *Journal of Periodontology*, **81**(12), 1708–1724.

EFSA Panel on Dietetic Products, Nutrition and Allergies (NDA) (2012) Scientific Opinion on Dietary Reference Values for protein. *EFSA Journal*, **10**(2), 2557.

Farrell, J.H. (1956) The effect of mastication on the digestion of food. *British Dental Journal*, **100**, 149–155.

Finch, S., Doyle, W., Lowe, C., Bates, C.J., Prentice, A., Smithers, G. *et al.* (1998) *National Diet and Nutrition Survey: People Aged 65 Years and Over. Volume 1: Report of the Diet and Nutrition Survey London.*

Freedman, N.D., Park, Y., Subar, A.F., Hollenbeck, A.R., Leitzmann, M.F., Schatzkin, A. *et al.* (2008) Fruit and vegetable intake and head and neck cancer risk in a large United States prospective cohort study. *International Journal of Cancer,* **122**(10), 2330–2336.

Frontera, W.R., Hughes, V.A., Lutz, K.J. & Evans, W.J. (1991) A cross-sectional study of muscle strength and mass in 45- to 78-yr-old men and women. *Journal of Applied Physiology*, **71**(2), 644–650.

Gariballa, S., Forster, S., Walters, S. & Powers, H. (2006) A randomized, double-blind, placebo-controlled trial of nutritional supplementation during acute illness. *The American Journal of Medicine*, **119**(8), 693–699.

Hung, H.C., Willett, W., Ascherio, A., Rosner, B.A., Rimm, E. & Joshipura, K.J. (2003) Tooth loss and dietary intake. *Journal of the American Dental Association*, **134**(9), 1185–1192.

Kovacic, J.C., Castellano, J.M. & Fuster, V. (2012) Cardiovascular defense challenges at the basic, clinical, and population levels. *Annals of the New York Academy of Sciences*, **1254**, 1–6.

Krall, E., Hayes, C. & Garcia, R. (1998) How dentition status and masticatory function affect nutrient intake. *Journal of the American Dental Association*, **129**(September), 1261–1269.

Mathey, M.F., Siebelink, E., de Graaf, C. & Van Staveren, W.A. (2001) Flavor enhancement of food improves dietary intake and nutritional status of elderly nursing home residents. *The Journals of Gerontology Series A, Biological Sciences and Medical Sciences*, **56**(4), M200–M205.

Mavroeidi, A., O'Neill, F., Lee, P.A., Darling, A.L., Fraser, W.D. & Berry, J.L. *et al.* (2010) Seasonal 25-hydroxyvitamin D changes in British postmenopausal women at 57 degrees N and 51 degrees N: a longitudinal study. *The Journal of Steroid Biochemistry and Molecular Biology*, **121**(1–2), 459–461.

Roininen, K., Tuorila, H., Zandstra, E.H., de Graaf, C., Vehkalahti, K., Stubenitsky, K. & Mela, D.J. (2001) Differences in health and taste attitudes and reported behaviour among Finnish, Dutch and British consumers: a cross-national validation of the Health and Taste Attitude Scales (HTAS). *Appetite*, **37**(1), 33–45.

SACN (2012) Dietary Reference Values for Energy London.

Saman, D.M. (2012) A review of the epidemiology of oral and pharyngeal carcinoma: update. *Head & Neck Oncology*, **4**, 1.

Sheiham, A., Steele, J.G., Marcenes, W., Lowe, C., Finch, S., Bates, C.J. *et al.* (2001) The relationship among dental status, nutrient intake, and nutritional status in older people. *Journal of Dental Research*, **80**(2), 408–413.

Steele, J.G., Sheiham, A., Marcenes, W., Fay, N. & Walls, A.W. (2001) Clinical and behavioural risk indicators for root caries in older people. *Gerodontology*, **18**(2), 95–101.

Takahashi, K. (1961) Statistical study on caries incidence in the first molar in relation to the amount of sugar consumption. *Bulletin of Tokyo Dental College*, **2**, 44–57.

van der Putten, G.J., Vanobbergen, J., De Visschere, L., Schols, J. & de Baat, C. (2009) Association of some specific nutrient deficiencies with periodontal disease in elderly people: A systematic literature review. *Nutrition*, **25**(7–8), 717–722.

Vehkalahti, M.M. & Paunio, I.K. (1988) Occurrence of root caries in relation to dental health behavior. *Journal of Dental Research*, **67**(6), 911–914.

Welge-Lussen, A. (2009) Ageing, neurodegeneration, and olfactory and gustatory loss. *B-ENT*, **5**(Suppl 13), 129–132.

CHAPTER 12
Pharmacology and aging

Elisa M. Chávez and Peter L. Jacobsen
University of the Pacific, Arthur A. Dugoni School of Dentistry, San Francisco, CA,

Pharmacology and aging: introduction

In 2004 it was estimated that in developed countries, approximately 20% of the population was over age 60. By the year 2050 that percentage is expected to climb to 33%. The rise in the oldest old population, or those over 80 years old, will be even more dramatic, climbing from 86 million in 2005 to 394 million in 2050 worldwide. In the United States, people over 65 currently comprise 13% of the population but they consume approximately a third of all drugs prescribed. As the population ages, the number of patients with chronic diseases who take multiple medications (polypharmacy) increases. The presence of these diseases, and the drugs used to treat them, makes managing these patients in the dental office increasingly complex.

An adverse drug reaction (ADR) (See Table 12.1) may occur with the administration of even a single drug. Some drugs present an increased risk of an ADR in older individuals, even when there are no drug interactions reported.

There are seven different types of adverse drug reactions. Each has a wide range of severity. The adverse reaction may take the form of a localized oral change like mucositis or xerostomia or a life threatening event such as anaphylaxis secondary to drug allergy or excessive bleeding due to a drug–drug interaction. The risk of an ADR increases as the number of drugs the patient is taking increases. Forty per cent of older adults take an average of three medications. ADRs occurring in elders are often due to polypharmacy. The risk increases for those who are malnourished or have renal or hepatic diseases, diabetes, asthma or other systemic diseases. The risk of an adverse reaction rises from 6% with two drugs, to 50% with five, and 100% with eight or more medications.

Table 12.1 Types of adverse drug reactions

Allergic	Administration of the drug causes an undesirable immunological response, e.g. rash, anaphylaxis, which is often unpredictable.
Side effect	An undesirable effect occurs which is expected or predictable at therapeutic doses, e.g. nausea, dry mouth. Side effects are the most common adverse drug reactions.
Drug toxicity	A drug dose high enough to cause damage to a physiological system. Usually the dose is higher than recommended therapeutic levels. This occurs most commonly in children and frail elders.
Drug–drug interaction	The absorption, distribution, metabolism and/or excretion of one drug is altered by the administration of another drug e.g. erythromycin taken with digoxin increasing the digoxin level, or NSAIDs and methotrexate taken together resulting in renal failure. Such interactions are usually predictable.
Drug–physiology interaction	The presence of a drug at therapeutic levels adversely alters a physiological system. This ADR can overlap with a side effect e.g. administration of Clindamycin can result in colitis and diarrhoea. Such interactions are usually predictable.
Drug–laboratory test interaction	There is no effect on the physiological system being tested, but false positive or false negative test results e.g. amoxicillin can cause a false-positive urine glucose test. Such interactions are usually predictable.
Idiosyncratic	By definition these are unpredicted physiological or psychological responses occurring at therapeutic doses. These are unique to an individual.

Studies have shown prevalence rates of 10–35% for adverse drug reactions in community dwelling elders. Several studies examining community dwelling elders and institutionalized frail and hospitalized elders have shown that as the number of prescribed drugs increases, the occurrence of ADRs also increases.

Textbook of Geriatric Dentistry, Third Edition. Edited by Poul Holm-Pedersen, Angus W. G. Walls and Jonathan A. Ship.

Another reason ADRs occur in older adults is lack of compliance or inability to comply with a complicated drug regimen. This may result in either under or overuse of prescribed medications. Some patients are unwilling or incapable of following a prescribed drug regimen. But there are many other social, psychological, physical and economic reasons for poor compliance and mistakes in drug usage that may occur more often as people age, but not as a direct result of the aging process.

A thorough health history, increased care when prescribing certain drug classes and careful monitoring of the patient can prevent most of these adverse drug reactions, whether they are secondary to compliance issues or some other reason. There are six issues to consider when managing and prescribing for older patients taking medications:

- Medication as an indicator of medical conditions.
- Current medical conditions and medications as they impact dental care.
- Oral side effect of medications.
- Pharmacodynamics as it impacts dental management.
- Current medical conditions and medications as they impact dental prescribing.
- Non-compliance to medication use

Medication as an indicator of medical conditions

If a patient is taking a prescription medication, then a healthcare provider thinks the problem is sufficiently significant to necessitate pharmacological treatment. The dentist should ask the patient to list, or bring a list, of all the medications they currently take and should review, with them, the indication for the medication. This will allow the dentist the opportunity to clarify the health history and discover important information about the patient and any potential risks or management issues to be considered when treating the patient. In some cases the patient will not be able to communicate their health issues effectively, in which case their medication list may be the oral health clinician's only immediate resource for identifying medical problems sufficiently significant that they require pharmacological intervention. For example, a patient may not report that they have hypertension, but their medication list may include Furosemide, a diuretic. Both the hypertension and the diuretic can have implications on the provision of dental care as well as direct and indirect effects on the patient's oral health. (See Box 12.1)

Box 12.1 Steps for reviewing the existing medication list.

1 **Could any of these drugs be required during a medical emergency?**
e.g. Nitroglycerin – angina, inhalers – COPD exacerbation.

2 **Why is the patient taking these particular medications? Group by category to aid in assessing overall risk in patient care and management.**
e.g. Antihypertensive, anticoagulant, immunosuppressive, antidepressant etc.

3 **Do any drugs have the potential to contribute to a complication or even create an emergency situation?**
e.g. Warfarin – excessive bleeding, prednisone – adrenal insufficiency, insulin – hypoglycemia, bisphosphonates – osteonecrosis.

4 **Could any of these drugs compromise our desired treatment outcome?**
e.g. Vincristine – delayed healing, echinacea – potentiates inhibition of liver enzymes from erythromycin and ketoconazole.

5 **Do any of these drugs have potential oral side effects?**
e.g. Dilantin, nifedipine - gingival hyperplasia; chlorthiazide diuretics – lichenoid reactions; antihistamines – xerostomia.

The clinician should also inquire whether the patient uses over-the-counter (OTC) products/medications and whether they use any herbal products. This information provides insight into the patient's self-diagnosed problems, concerns and perceived risks. Furthermore, OTC medications/treatments can impact dental management (e.g. bleeding secondary to aspirin and garlic use) and must be recorded by all healthcare providers (see Table 12.2).

Current medical conditions and medications as they impact dental care

A patient's medical conditions and their medical management can have an impact on the provision of dental care. The patient's drugs should be categorized to identify immediate safety considerations. For example, does the patient require nitroglycerin for angina or an inhaler for dyspnea? If so, these drugs should be available during the dental appointment. Secondly, do any of the drugs on the list have the potential

Table 12.2 Natural products that may alter dental management

Compound	Possible relevant problem
Feverfew Garlic Ginger Ginko biloba Bilberry Dong quai	May increase bleeding.
St. John's Wort Echinacea St. John's Wort	These herbs inhibit liver enzymes so they may potentiate the liver enzyme (cytochrome P450) inhibiting the effect of erythromycin and ketoconazole.
Ephedra (Ma-Huang)	May increase blood pressure and heart rate due to anxiety or if epinephrine/vasoconstrictor used.
Bitter orange Kava-Kava	Hepatotoxicity, especially in those taking other medications metabolized in the liver, can alter the metabolism of other drugs metabolized by the liver.
Valerian	May potentiate the effects of sedative-hypnotics and anti-anxiety drugs

Table 12.3 Potential drug-related oral health/management complications

Drug groups	Example drugs	Management problems
Anticoagulants	Aspirin, warfarin[a]	Excessive bleeding
Immunosuppressants	Corticosteroids[a] Immunosuppressants for organ transplants[a]	Increase risk of bacterial and fungal infection, poor stress response
Chemotherapeutic agents	Vincristine	Delayed healing, mucositis, fungal infections
Sedative hypnotics,[a] narcotics, barbiturates	Acetaminophen with codeine, Valium, Demerol	Respiratory suppression, fall risk
Hypoglycemics	Insulin,[a] sulfonylureas	Hypoglycemia
Bisphosphonate bone stabilizers (esp. i.v. bisphosphonates)	Pamidronate (Aredia) Zoledronic acid (Zometa) Alendronate (Fosamax)	Delayed bone healing, bone necrosis

[a]Highly titrated drugs with a narrow margin of safety.

to complicate dental treatment? For example, has the patient taken their dose of insulin, but not eaten, placing them at risk of hypoglycemia? Third, could any of the medications compromise our treatment outcomes? For example is the healing time or risk of infection increased because the patient is on an immunosuppressant such as prednisone or a cancer chemotherapeutic agent or is there a risk of osteonecrosis because the patient is taking an oral bisphosphonate (e.g. Fosamax) for osteoporosis or an intravenous bisphosphonate (e.g. Zometa) for the treatment of bone pathology secondary to cancer. Special attention should be given to highly titrated drugs with a narrow margin of safety. These drugs run the greatest risk of an adverse drug event (See Table 12.3).

Oral side effect of medications

Many drugs have adverse intra-oral side effects. Drugs with the potential for these side effects should be identified. Certain classes of drugs are more likely to result in specific types of oral pathology so identifying drugs by class is also important (See Table 12.4). For example, ACE inhibitors and other drugs are associated with lichenoid reactions, diuretics and antidepressants often contribute to salivary hypofunction and xerostomia, calcium channel blockers and some anti-seizure and immunosuppressant drugs can cause gingival hyperplasia. Many medications result in altered taste sensations that, in severe cases, can result in nutritional deficiencies and malnutrition which can also lead to oral changes. Salivary hypofunction and xerostomia are frequently caused by medications and can cause a host of oral-pharyngeal side effects, such as increase in caries and an increased susceptibility to oral fungal infections. In the aged it can also result in easily traumatized mucosal tissues (see also Chapter 7 and Chapter 19). Dry mouth can reduce or alter the sensation of taste, as well as impair speech and swallowing function. The dentist should consider consulting with the patient's physician about changing one xerostomic medication to another with similar indications but fewer side effects. However, for patients on numerous medications that cause xerostomia, palliative therapy (e.g. salivary substitutes, lubricants) may be the only possible treatments. For dentate patients with polypharmacy-induced salivary hypofunction, caries prevention is critical.

Oral mucosal disorders develop from specific medications, such as gingival enlargement in patients taking Dilantin for seizure disorders, and are exacerbated by poor oral hygiene. Some medications, such as aspirin, may produce a chemical burn if they are misused and placed directly on the oral tissue. Interestingly, even adult teeth can become discoloured from tetracycline – specifically long term use of minocycline. These oral conditions may require treatment, palliation and/or preventive measures, which could include adding another medication to an already long list.

Oral healthcare providers may be the clinician to first document a patient's complaint of altered taste or smell (see Chapter 4 for more details). Taste and smell disturbances can be caused by a variety of physical and chemical factors. Chemosensory ability also decreases with age. This decrease is independent of environmental factors and should be taken into account when evaluating a patient for their concerns of chemosensory loss.

If a patient's complaint of chemosensory loss could be associated with a drug the dentist has prescribed, the most effective way of establishing the connection is to discontinue

Table 12.4 Oral side effects of drug classes and their possible uses

Oral side effect	Drug class	Example (Generic)	May be used to treat:
Xerostomia and salivary hypofunction	Antihistamine	Claritin (Loratadine)	Hay fever
	Antidepressant	Zoloft (Sertraline)	Obsessive compulsive disorder
	Antihypertensive Calcium channel blocker	Norvasc (Amlodipine)	Hypertension
	Diuretics	Lasix (Furosemide)	Hypertension
Fungal infection	Antibiotics	Tetracap (Tetracycline)	Periodontal disease
	Immunosuppressant	Cortan (Prednisone)	Rheumatoid arthritis
Mucositis	Anti-neoplastic	Adrucil (5-Fluorouracil)	Chemotherapeutic for breast cancer
Tooth discolouration	Antibiotics	Minocin (Minocycline)	Gastric ulcers caused by *Helicobacter pylori*
Dysgeusia	Oral hypoglycemics	Glucotrol (Glipizide)	Diabetes
	Anti-hypertensive Ace inhibitor	Vasotec (Enalapril)	Hypertension
Gingival enlargement	Anticonvulsant	Dilantin (Phenytoin)	Epilepsy
	Anti-hypertensive Calcium channel blocker	Procardia(Nifedipine)	Hypertension
	Immunosuppressant	Sandimmune (Cyclosporin)	Prevent organ transplant rejection
Stomatitis	Anti-hypertensive		
Lichenoid reactions	ACE inhibitor	Capoten (Captopril)	Hypertension
	Diuretics	Thiazide(HCTZ)	Hypertension
	Anti-inflammatory		
Mucosal burns		Ecotrin (Aspirin) if dissolved in the mouth	Osteoarthritis

the use of the drug. Drugs should only be discontinued by the healthcare provider who prescribed the drug. If the medication cannot be discontinued, then the lowest effective dose should be established. The impact of medication on taste and smell is commonly dose-related and utilizing the lowest effective dose may minimize or eliminate the drug-associated chemosensory disorder. If chemosensory loss is associated with a drug, discontinuing the drug should reverse the problem within a few days. Infrequently it may take up to a week. This assumes that there has been no permanent damage to the taste and smell sensory receptors and nerves. Permanent damage is uncommon. If the chemosensory loss does not improve and all other oral/dental causes have been ruled out, the patient can be referred to a specialized clinic for a thorough evaluation of their smell and taste function.

Pharmacodynamics as it impacts dental management

What impact does advanced age have upon the absorption, distribution, metabolism and elimination of the drugs a patient is taking and those that the provider plans to prescribe? In order to avoid drug toxicity, the prescriber must be aware of how the medication will be eliminated when selecting a drug or determining dosages. This is especially important if the patient has known renal or hepatic disease, since these are the most common routes of elimination. If they are available, some laboratory test values may serve as guidelines for prescribing drugs eliminated by the kidney or liver (see Table 12.5).

Older adults are at increased risk of experiencing the respiratory depressive effects of some medications such as benzodiazepines and opioids. They may be less able to compensate quickly for medications that alter cardiovascular function, such as epinephrine, and they may have an atypical adverse drug response such as altered mental status. It should be noted that few adverse drug events have been clearly attributed to the changes that occur in the processes of absorption, distribution and elimination as a result of normal aging. Risks associated with altered drug metabolism and elimination are almost always due to the presence of a known systemic disease affecting cardiac, kidney or liver function.

Some drugs present an increased risk of toxicity in older individuals, even without a drug interaction. In addition to screening for potential adverse drug interactions, knowledge of maximum doses of the drugs to be prescribed for a dental purpose is critical whether the individual is a child, healthy adult, an individual with renal failure or medically complex older adult. A decrease in dosage for aged individuals may

Table 12.5 Guidelines for compromised renal or hepatic function

Potential impairment	Examples of drugs for oral-facial disorders	Laboratory test	Laboratory value	Dosing recommendation
Renal	Amoxicillin Cephalosporin Penicillin	Glomelular Filtration Rate (GFR)	<10 mL/min 10–50 mL/min >50 mL/min	One dose q 24 hours One dose q 8–12 hours One dose q 8 hours
Hepatic	Acetaminophen Codeine Diazepam Erythromycin Ibuprofen Ketoconazole Lidocaine Lorazepam Prednisone	Liver Function Tests (LFTs): AST, ALT, (aka: liver transaminases)	>4 times normal values	Do not use drugs that are toxic to, or metabolized by, the liver

be recommended for some medications commonly used in dentistry (see Table 12.6). Due to normal physiological changes in elimination associated with aging and altered distribution as a result of decreased body mass, dosage of these drugs should be reduced by 50%, or to the lowest therapeutic dose for individuals under 100 pounds (45.45 kg) and patients over 85 years of age.

Current medical conditions and medications as they impact dental prescribing

The patient's current list of medications may alter the dentist's prescribing patterns for pharmaceuticals used in the practice of dentistry and oral medicine. The practitioner must be aware of drug characteristics that he/she prescribes. In addition to the short duration of use, the number of frequently prescribed medications is limited and their associated adverse drug reactions are well documented and are found readily in reference materials (see Boxes 12.3–12.5). Drug classes commonly used in general dentistry include analgesics, antibiotics, antifungals, antivirals, anesthetics, vasoconstrictors and sedatives. There are generally three to five commonly used medications in each class; however, most practitioners limit their prescribing pattern to one or two in each class. A limited list of these drugs and their potential drug interactions is found in Table 12.6. In addition to thorough knowledge of the drugs the dental provider will commonly use, it is important to ask a routine series of questions when assessing and prescribing medications for any patient, but especially an older patient who may have several risk factors for experiencing an ADR. A recommended sequence of prescriber considerations is listed in Box 12.2.

Box 12.2 Considerations for administering or prescribing medications for oral-facial disorders.

1. **Does this person have a specific drug allergy to a drug you intend to prescribe?**
   e.g. Taking penicillin has resulted in a skin rash.
2. **Is this drug contraindicated for use given any of this patient's medical conditions?**
   e.g. NSAIDs with history of gastrointestinal ulcers or liver disease.
3. **Is there a potential for an adverse drug interaction with the patient's existing medications?**
   e.g. Erythromycin reducing warfarin clearance by 30%.
4. **Where will the new drugs be metabolized and is there any indication that drug elimination will be a problem for this patient?**
   e.g. The elderly may have decreased ability to eliminate penicillin, cephalosporin, erythromycin.
5. **Could any of the new drugs contribute to an emergency situation?**
   e.g. Prednisone – risk of non-compliance and patient failing to take prescribed dose resulting in adrenal crisis.
6. **Is the dose prescribed in a safe range for the patient's weight and state of health (i.e. at or below the maximum safe dose)?**
   e.g. Acetaminophen prescribed should not exceed 4 g per day for adults, but hepatotoxicity has occurred with < 4 g in patients with cirrhosis.
7. **Have you carefully reviewed with the patient, or their caregiver, the indication for and appropriate use of the newly prescribed medication?**

Table 12.6 Adverse outcomes and interactions with common 'dental drugs' (Drugs listed may interact with more than the example drug listed)

Drug class	Common drugs used in dentistry	Interacts with a drug already prescribed (example)	Potential adverse outcome(s)
Analgesic Narcotic	Acetaminophen with codeine	Benzodiazepines	Respiratory depression
Non-narcotic	NSAIDs	Warfarin	Excessive bleeding
		ACE inhibitors	Decreased hypotensive action
	Acetaminophen	Lithium	Increased serum concentration
		Methotrexate	Renal failure
		NSAIDs	Nephrotoxicity
Antibiotic	Clindamycin[a]	[c]	Colitis and diarrhea
	Cephalosporin[a]	Warfarin	Excessive bleeding
	Erythromycin[b]	Digoxin	Increases digoxin level
	Penicillin	Probenecid	Increases PEN concentration
	Metronidazole	Warfarin	Excessive bleeding
Antifungal	Ketoconazole[b]	Glyburide	Increased hypoglycemic effect
	Nystatin	None known	None known
	Clotrimazole	None known	None known
	Fluconazole	Warfarin	Anticoagulant effect
Antiviral	Acyclovir	None known	None known
	Val acyclovir	None known	None known
Anti-inflammatory	Prednisone	NSAIDs, acetaminophen (paracetamol)	Hepatotoxicity
Anesthetic	Lidocaine	Beta-blocker, H2 blockers	Increased serum concentrations leading to toxicity
	Prilocaine	CNS depressants	Respiratory depression
	Articaine	CNS depressants	Respiratory depression
Vasoconstrictor	Epinephrine	MAO inhibitors, beta-blockers	Increased blood pressure
	Levonordephrine	Beta-blockers	
Sedatives	Diazepam[a]	CNS depressant	Respiratory depression, fall risk
	Lorazepam	CNS depressant	Respiratory depression, fall risk

[a]Increased risk of toxicity and adverse event in older adults – even without a drug interaction.
[b]Do not use these drugs in patients taking other drugs to avoid the risk of drug–drug interaction.
[c]There is not a known example of a drug that interacts with clindamycin to increase the risk of colitis, although it may interact with other drugs to produce a different adverse outcome or could be prescribed with other drugs that also have the potential to cause adverse gastrointestinal side effects.

After carefully reviewing the existing medications to assess the patient's systemic condition and considering the potential effects of the medication on oral health, the next consideration relates to drugs administered or prescribed for the patient, by the dentist. The first consideration is whether there are any absolute contraindications to the medication that will be prescribed, such as a drug allergy. Does the drug have the potential to exacerbate any of the patient's medical conditions (i.e. drug–physiology interaction), such as NSAIDs increasing the risk of gastrointestinal bleeding in a patient with gastric ulcers? Does the drug have the potential to interact with any of the over-the-counter, herbal supplements or medications reportedly taken by the patient such as erythromycin inhibiting liver enzymes and decreasing the metabolism of the anticoagulant Coumadin? Patients taking two or more drugs and those whose drug list includes, but is not limited to, anticonvulsants, barbiturates, antibiotics, digoxin, warfarin, amidarone or dexamethasone are at high risk of developing drug–drug interactions. Many of these drugs are highly titrated and a small change in their blood levels can have a large physiological impact.

Four drugs commonly used in dentistry inhibit cytochrome P450 enzymes: erythromycin, clarithromycin, metronidazole and ketoconazole. These enzymes are responsible for metabolizing many drugs. The inhibition of these enzymes by drugs prescribed by the oral health practitioner can significantly decrease the rate of drug metabolism and create a high potential for an ADR. Erythromycin and ketoconazole have the greatest potential to cause such inhibition. To avoid the risk of such drug–drug interactions, these medications should be used very carefully in patients taking other drugs.

Depending on the prescriber's level of concern, and the complexity of the patient's medication list, it may be useful to review reference books or websites to see if there are any contraindications or precautions to prescribing a particular drug to a patient with a coexisting medical condition, or with their currently prescribed medications. These references/resources may also help elucidate potential outcomes of ingesting a group of medications at one time. Some resources allow you to enter the drug or drugs in question and cross check for ADRs. Importantly, pharmacists can also be consulted to clarify seemingly ambiguous information.

Box 12.3 Useful internet-based websites relative to drugs and drug information.

Note: some of the referenced websites are commercial. The inclusion of such sites does not mean an endorsement of the product/company, but it does mean that the site provides a unique and informative resource, not available on other sites.

www.ada.org The American Dental Association website contains resources and connects to a variety of medically-related sites. Members can look through a long, well-researched list of useful websites related to drugs and health.

www.drugs.com A comprehensive and up-to-date prescription drug information site for consumers and professionals, with fast, easy searching of over 24 000 approved medications.

www.drweil.com Contains pages called 'Herbal Medicine Chest' and 'Home Health Remedies' which describe availability, dosages and warnings for a wide range of natural products. The site is available to the general public.

www.epocrates.com Offers freeware drug and infectious disease databases. Includes system requirements, tour of features and auto update information.

www.fda.gov/Drugs/default.htm The Center for Drug Evaluation and Research web page has information on all the drugs regulated by the FDA, which is all drugs.

www.hiv-druginteractions.org Provides HIV drug interactions as well as interactions with recreational/abuse drugs and with herbs.

www.hivinsite.ucsf.edu/ Provides comprehensive and up to date information on medications used in the treatment of HIV and AIDS.

www.lexi.com This site offers handheld software, downloadable updates, access to Lexi-Comp Online for member health professionals including Lexi-Interact and Lexi-Drugs for Dentistry, new drug information and special alerts and patient education.

www.medscape.com This is a searchable site with an extensive medical-based homepage that can be customized for your personal interests. It will send topics, such as pharmacology updates, to your computer, to allow you to keep current on areas of interest.

www.naturaldatabase.com Contains a drug interaction checker for natural products and an interactive component for health professionals. It also contains evaluations of natural products.

www.nlm.nih.gov Has a powerful search feature that looks at a large range of databases and searches out complete articles on specific topics.

www.pdr.net Registration is free, includes information on pharmaceuticals and herbals.

www.personalhealthzone.com/pg000059.html Prescription drug interactions and warnings relative to herbs and supplements.

www.purecaps.com Members and nonmembers can access the site for information on alternative medicinals that includes: botany, usage, active constituents and mechanisms of action, dosages, cautions and contraindications as well as depletions and interactions by drug name.

www.rxlist.com A comprehensive list of drug indications, contraindications, interactions, etc. It also has an extensive list of medical diseases and how they are managed. Some of the explanations of the diseases are presented in a short video interview format, which makes it an interesting educational resource.

www.seniorcarepharmacist.com Provides seniors with information about managing the medications they are taking and issues specific to elders and medications. The site also assists users in locating specialists in geriatric pharmacology in their area (this directed me to: ascp.com/find-senior-care-pharmacist).

Box 12.4 Author's choice of drug text references to keep in the office.

Texts may be found in medical bookstores or online. The resources below are personal preferences. There are other useful books/resources available. Given the rapid changes in drugs and medical management, utilize the most current edition(s) of the resource(s).

PDR Books (2015) *Physician's Desk Reference.*

PDR Books (2015) *Physician's Desk Reference for Non-prescription Drugs and Dietary Supplements.*

American Dental Association (2015) *ADA/PDR Dental Therapeutics Online.*

Wynn, R.L. & Meiller, T.F. (eds) (2014–15) *Lexicomp's Drug Information Handbook for Dentistry*, 20th edn.

Semla, T.P., Beizer, J.L. & Higbee, M.D. (eds) (2014–15) *Lexicomp's Geriatric Dosage Handbook*, 20th edn.

Jacobsen, P.L. (ed) (2014–15) *The Little Dental Drug Booklet*, 20th edn.

Jeske, A.H. (ed) (2013) *Mosby's Dental Drug Book*, 11th edn.

Therapeutic Research Faculty (2015) *Natural Medicines Comprehensive Database.*

US Pharmacopeial Convention (2014) *US Pharmacopeia, The Official Compendia of Standards.*

Boxes 12.3, 12.4 and 12.5 list a variety of resources and references for drug information. As is apparent on review of these tables, books, computer programs, online/internet resources and applications for phones and tablets are converging. A prudent clinician should build their own 'library' of useful, up-to-date, scientific information resources that can evolve as the technology evolves. Resources are available that regularly update pharmaceutical information.

Importantly, most medications prescribed for dental and oral-facial conditions are prescribed for only a short duration and many have a large margin of safety, which reduces the risk of adverse drug reactions. It may also be possible,

Box 12.5 Available computer and PDA drug information software.

Note: there are other online resources besides those listed.
Lexi-Comp On-Hand Databases: Lexi-Drugs for Dentistry, Lexi-Interact , Lexi-Dental Complete
Mobile Physician's Desk Reference
Natural Medicines Comprehensive Database

although seldom necessary, in consultation with the patient's physician, to temporarily change or suspend an interacting medication they have prescribed, for the duration of the dental prescription.

Most potential adverse drug effects, events and interactions can and should be anticipated so that they can be prevented. If, after all precautions have been taken, an unexpected adverse drug reaction appears to have occurred, either from a single prescription or a combination, a report can be made to the Federal Drug Administration: http://www.fda.gov/medwatch/report/hcp.htm

The oral health care provider ultimately assumes total responsibility for ADRs related to medications he/she has prescribed. The oral health care provider does not have the responsibility of identifying and eliminating risks for ADRs among medications prescribed by other providers. However, if an ADR is suspected or evident, it should be brought to the attention of the provider(s) who prescribed the drug(s).

Non-compliance to medication use

Oral health care providers must consider compliance when prescribing drugs. Though such a consideration sounds self-evident, lack of attention to compliance is a common reason drugs do not work as expected. The reasons patients are non-compliant with drug regimens are varied and may be as basic as misunderstanding directions to a complex psychosocial issue. Some patients cannot recall which medications to take or when to take them. Others cannot remember whether to take them with food, or on an empty stomach, or they do not understand the importance of taking them exactly as prescribed. This can be due to inadequate communication between providers and patients. Patients with mild to severe cognitive impairments or physical impairments are at risk for drug non-compliance. Other patients may develop a dependence on a medication and take more than prescribed. Some patients may not be able to afford the medication prescribed. Many of these reasons may not be readily evident to the provider. Recognizing those patients at risk for non-compliance, and finding ways to ensure they take their drugs as directed, can be difficult.

Solutions can be as simple as writing instructions down for the patient/caregiver in large lettering if they have difficulty with their vision, prescribing a liquid form of a medication if the patient has difficulty swallowing a tablet form or having the patient add the medication to their current drug calendar so they have a ready reminder to take it as directed. See Table 12.7 for suggestions to address potential causes of drug use errors. Some solutions may be more complex, such as enlisting family members or caregivers to help patients follow a regimen appropriately or even contacting adult protective services or a local Ombudsman, if there is evidence a medication is being withheld or used inappropriately by a caregiver.

Conclusion

Proper dental management and insuring desired treatment outcomes take knowledge and diligence. Decreasing the potential for adverse treatment outcomes in the aged is often complicated and includes an evaluation for the presence of chronic diseases or conditions, multiple drugs and possibly impaired communication, cognition and/or ability to comply with a complicated drug or treatment regimen. The medical conditions necessitating drugs and the medications themselves can impact the patient's oral health and the way in which oral health practitioners provide dental care. The complexity of these situations calls for attention to detail and necessitates a complete and careful review of the patient's health history and the prescription and non-prescription medications they are taking. The practitioner should have a sound knowledge of medically complex patients, the appropriate uses and limitations of prescribed drugs for oral-facial conditions, and the ability to utilize drug information resources to ensure their drug knowledge is complete and up-to-date.

Table 12.7 Medication non-compliance in the elderly and strategies for improving compliance

Barriers	Strategies for minimizing errors and improving compliance
Provider	
Poor communication	Clearly state the diagnosis and need for medication. Review and ask patient to repeat regimen and any special instructions. Print instructions for patient and/or caregiver to take home.
Negative attitude	Listen carefully to and address the patient's concerns and questions.
Patient	
Advanced age	Identify any physical and/or cognitive barriers to compliance.
Depression	Reinforce the need for the drug, if patient agrees, enlist family, friends to encourage compliance.
Cognitive impairment	Give written instructions, simplify regimen, involve caregivers or, if patient agrees, enlist family, friends to assist with compliance.
Attitudes	Follow up with patients who indicate they will not or have not followed regimen. Reinforce the need for the prescription and to take it as directed. Document non-compliance.
Medication	
High cost	Prescribe generics when possible.
Frequent dosing	Prescribe single or less frequent doses if possible.
Unpleasant side effects	Attempt to alleviate the side effect, consider changing the medication if necessary.
Abuse/dependence	Limit and monitor number of narcotics and sedative hypnotics prescribed.
Multiple medications	Utilize drug dispensers.
Systems	
Follow-up reminders	Call the patient to follow up, specifically asking about compliance with drug regimen.
Labelling	Request large labelling and/or individualized colour labels for family members.
Packaging	Consider easy-open lids.
Inadequate education	Encourage the patient to meet with the pharmacist when filling the prescription, especially if the patient takes multiple drugs.
Neglect and elder abuse	Report to adult protective services or Ombudsman.

Further reading

American Association of Oral and Maxillofacial Surgeons Position Paper (2014) Medication Related Osteonecrosis of the Jaw—2014 update, aaoms.org/docs/position_papers/mronj_position _paper?pdf?pdf=mronj-Position-Paper (accessed 1 February 2015).

Haas, D.A. (1999) Adverse drug interactions in dental practice: interactions associated with analgesics, Part III in a series. *Journal of the American Dental Association*, **130**(3), 397–407.

Halter, J.B., Ouslander, J.G., Tinetti, M.D., Studenski, S., High, K. & Asthana, S. (eds) *Hazzard's Principles of Geriatric Medicine and Gerontology*, 6th edn, McGraw-Hill Inc, USA.

Hersh, E.V. (1999) Adverse drug interactions in dental practice: interactions involving antibiotics, Part II of a series. *Journal of the American Dental Association*, **130**(2), 236–251.

Jacobsen, P.J. & Chavez, E.M. (2005) Clinical management of the dental patient taking multiple drugs. *The Journal of Contemporary Dental Practice* [Electronic Resource], **6**(4), 144–151.

Johnson, T.E., Boccia, A.D. and Strayer, M.S. (2001) Elder abuse and neglect: detection, reporting and intervention. *Special Care in Dentistry*, **21**(4), 141–146.

Lacy, C.F., Armstrong, L.L., Goldman, M.P. & Lance, L.L. (eds) (2012–2013) *Drug Information Handbook*, 21st edn, Lexicomp, Hudson, OH.

Little, J.W., Miller, C., Rhodus, N.L. & Falace, D.A. (eds) (2012) *Dental Management of the Medically Compromised Patient*, 8th edn, Mosby, St. Louis, MO.

Merck Manual of Health and Aging (2005) Merck and Co Inc., New York, Aoa.gov/AoA-programs/Special_Projects/Global_Aging /index.aspx (accessed 1 February 2015).

Merck Research Laboratories (2000) *Merck Manual of Geriatrics*, 3rd edn, Merck Research Laboratories, Whitehouse Station, NJ.

Moore, P.A. (1999) Adverse drug interactions in dental practice: interactions associated with local anesthetics, sedatives and anxiolytics, Part IV of a series. *Journal of the American Dental Association*, **130**(4), 541–554.

Moore, P.A. & Hersh, E.V. (eds) (2002) Dental Therapeutics Update, *Dental Clinics of North America*, **46**(4), xv–xviii.

Ruggiero, S., Gralow, J., Marx, R.E., Hoff, A.O., Schubert, M.M., Huyrn, J. *et al.* (2006) Practical guidelines for the prevention, diagnosis, and treatment of osteonecrosis of the jaw in patients with cancer. *Journal of Oncology Practice*, **2**(1), 7–14.

Rutkauskas, J.S. (ed) (1997) Clinical decision making in geriatric dentistry in *Dental Clinics of North America*, **41**(4).

Semla, T.P., Beizer, J.L. & Higbee, M.D. (eds) (2009) *Geriatric Dosage Book*, 15th edn, Lexicomp, Hudson, OH.

Laudenbach, J.M. (ed) (2010) *The Clinician's Guide to Oral Health in Geriatric Patients*, 3rd edn, American Academy of Oral Medicine, BC Decker Inc, Ontario.

Silverman, S., Jr, Eversole, L., Truelove, E., (ed) (2001) *Essentials of Oral Medicine*. BC Decker Inc, Hamilton, London.

Spielman, A.I. & Ship, J.A. Taste and smell. (2004) In: T.S. Miles, B. Nauntofte & P. Svensson (eds) *Clinical Oral Physiology*. pp. 53–70, 1st edn, Quintessence Publishing Co., Ltd, Copenhagen.

Yagiela, J.A. (1999) Adverse drug interactions in dental practice: interactions associated with vasoconstrictors, Part V of a series. *Journal of the American Dental Association*, **130**(5), 701–709.

CHAPTER 13

Preventive oral health care for elderly people

J. H. Meurman
University of Helsinki, Finland

The oral cavity is an ideal habitat for microorganisms. There are different surfaces in the mouth for microbial attachment, usually a frequent supply of energy and optimal temperature and moisture conditions. Today elderly people retain their own teeth in increasing numbers and they often have received restorative treatments not meeting the present day quality standards. This fosters accumulation of plaque. Dental prostheses further enhance the colonization of bacteria and yeasts in the mouth. On the other hand, salivary flow and defensive systems, which play an important role in controlling plaque-borne infections, may become impaired in the elderly, mainly due to drugs used daily for systemic diseases and due to the diseases themselves. Finally, decreased manual dexterity of the elderly poses difficulties in maintaining satisfactory oral hygiene. Dietary habits can change with increasing age with elderly people often favouring soft foodstuffs and carbohydrate rich food instead of vegetables and a fibre rich diet. Oral microorganisms readily ferment such carbohydrates for energy metabolism and subsequent growth. Microflora in the oral cavity are exceptionally dense and voluminous in dental plaque. 1 mg of plaque contains 10^{11} bacteria and over 700 bacterial species have been identified in the mouth [1].

In addition to dental plaque, oral mucosal surfaces are also colonized by other microorganisms. *Candida* sp., of which *C. albicans* predominates, are particularly important and may cause local and systemic infections [2]. In mucosal infections non-*albicans* strains such as *C. krusei* and *C. glabrata* are identified in increasing numbers among older people. These strains tend to be resistant to the commonly used antifungal drugs. In general, the increased global use of antimicrobial drugs results in selection pressure for resistant strains which may be a cause for concern in the oral environment.

From the oral cavity, microorganisms may gain access to blood circulation and spread all over the body. Odontogenic bacteraemia is a well-known entity and its role in the development and progression of systemic diseases has become a topic of great concern. The theories that oral microorganisms may play a role in the development of atherosclerosis are of particular concern [3]. Such bacteraemia is not a threat in healthy individuals because the body's defensive systems clear microorganisms from the circulating blood and prevent systemic harm. However, in patients with poor health or compromised defensive mechanisms bacteraemia can be dangerous. Poor oral health has been shown to increase mortality among the elderly [4]. Consequently, preventive oral health care cannot be overemphasized. The following sections describe evidence-based observations of oral health care among the elderly with some practical recommendations and visions for the future.

Prevention of plaque induced diseases

Plaque induced diseases mainly comprise dental caries and periodontal disease. The best strategy to prevent these diseases is the elimination of plaque, which in reality is not possible. However, successful control of plaque, by mechanical cleaning of the teeth, has been shown to reduce the frequency of both caries and periodontal disease. Chemical plaque control is another possibility but it is restricted to short-term strategies due to the potential side effects of the currently available agents. It should be emphasized that controlling dental plaque not only affects the dental diseases but also reduces potential systemic consequences by reducing the number of microorganisms of oral origin and their subsequent spread to other organs.

Textbook of Geriatric Dentistry, Third Edition. Edited by Poul Holm-Pedersen, Angus W. G. Walls and Jonathan A. Ship.

Mechanical cleaning

Daily mechanical cleaning of the teeth, dental prostheses and oral mucosa is the cornerstone of oral health care in the elderly. Poor oral hygiene has been shown to associate with bronchopneumonia; the mechanism is thought to be direct spread of oral microorganisms by aspiration to the lower parts of the respiratory tract. This association is particularly strong in individuals with periodontal disease [5]. In a study from Japan, elderly patients were randomly assigned to an oral care group and non-oral care group; nurses then cleaned the teeth of the intervention group after every meal and necessary dental treatment was given. During follow-up, pneumonias, duration of febrile illness and death from pneumonia were reduced significantly in the treatment group [6]. The putative mechanism for the effect of improved oral hygiene observed is reduction in the aspiration of bacteria of oral origin. Oral health care was beneficial both in the edentulous and in dentate subjects. However, there may be other factors involved in this outcome as good oral health care among the elderly has been associated with improvement in the sensitivity of their cough reflex [7].

Daily oral hygiene of residents in nursing homes is often ignored and they might not want or understand the need to ask for help. A satisfactory level of hygiene may also be difficult to maintain in home-dwelling older adults due to impaired manual dexterity. This in turn may lead to the accumulation of voluminous dental plaque (Figure 13.1). Powered toothbrushes with an oscillation–rotation action are more effective in reducing plaque and improving gingival health than manual toothbrushes. Elderly individuals accept powered toothbrushes the same way as younger ones [8].

Hence, regular twice daily mechanical cleaning should always be recommended. If an older person's motor functions are impaired, an electric toothbrush and other specially developed mechanical aids, such as tongue scrapers, can be recommended. Eating is also an important part of maintaining a healthy microflora in the oral cavity as parenteral feeding, for example through a naso-gastric tube, is associated with alterations in the oral microflora towards a more pathogenic one.

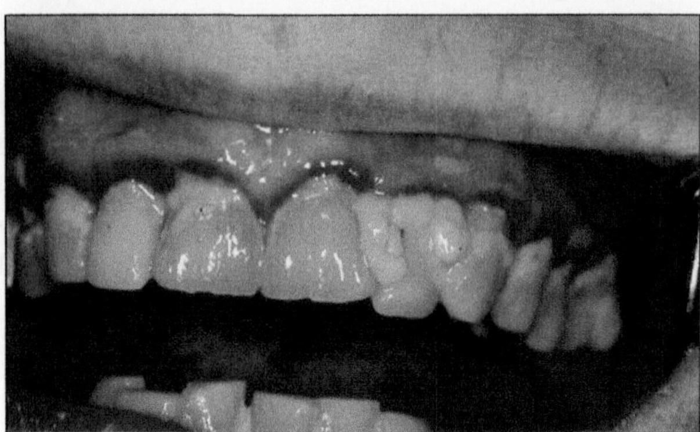

Figure 13.1 Neglected daily oral hygiene has led to voluminous dental plaque accumulation in an elderly lady with dementia.

Chemical plaque control

Combining frequent mechanical cleaning (tooth brushing and flossing) with antimicrobial agents such as chlorhexidine mouth rinse further decreases the number of bacteria in the mouth. Use of chlorhexidine has been shown to reduce the incidence of ventilator-associated pneumonia [9]. Chlorhexidine mouth rinse can also be used to control the number of *Candida* in patients with removable dentures. Chlorhexidine is indeed the gold standard in chemical plaque control. However, due to its unpleasant side effects of altered taste and staining of the teeth, continuous use of chlorhexidine is not advisable as a daily means of controlling oral hygiene unless the patient is at high risk of pneumonia or other systemic complications. A variety of other chemical agents have been investigated for controlling dental plaque in older people. These include daily use of a combination of amine fluoride and stannous fluoride mouth rinse, which also appears to have antifungal effect, povidone-iodine, cetyl pyridinium chloride, essential oils, zinc citrate, triclosan, tea tree oil and sanguinarine. Local delivery of antibiotics, such as tetracycline derivates, has also been investigated to facilitate dental plaque control but for obvious reasons this is not a strategy for long-term population base preventive programs. Box 13.1 presents some of the challenges of chemical plaque control among the elderly.

Box 13.1 Problems with chemical plaque control in the elderly.

- Compatibility with the oral environment and developing resistance of bacteria in long-term use.
- Strong and unpleasant taste of many commercial preparations.
- Impaired oro-motor function.
- High cost of preparations.
- Local side effects such as burning sensation of mouth mucosa.
- Staining of teeth and prostheses.

Fluorides

There is no doubt that fluorides are effective in the prevention of dental caries [10, 11]. However, use of fluorides in toothpaste or mouthwash for dental caries prevention has been mainly investigated in children and adolescents. In old age, root caries is usually the problem, and there is only limited evidence to show that fluorides may prevent or retard its progression. The few studies that have been performed in older adults suggest that fluoride toothpaste and, in the case of high caries risk individuals, the adjunctive use of other fluoride delivery systems, may be effective in preventing coronal and root caries [8]. The actual chemical nature of fluoride used in mouth rinse or toothpaste does not seem to play a key role in the efficacy of a product as long as the concentration of fluoride is optimal. However, it needs to be re-emphasized that there is only limited evidence of use of fluorides in caries prevention in the elderly. Further information about the role of fluorides in management of caries can be found in Chapter 15.

Prevention of dental erosion

Dental erosion is the dissolution of dental hard tissues in a chemical process that does not involve bacteria. All foodstuffs, drinks or regurgitated gastric juice with a pH value below the critical pH of dental enamel, pH 5.5, or dentine when this is exposed at pH 6.0 causes acid-mediated softening of the surface of the tooth. If the frequency of acidic assault exceeds the capacity of the oral environment for repair and remineralization erosive damage ensues. Hence, reduction in frequency of eating or drinking acid-containing products and treating any underlying gastrointestinal diseases is a life-long challenge in the prevention of irreversible lesions on the teeth. In patients with malignant disease an additional threat in this regard is cytotoxic drug treatment which can frequently cause vomiting. So far dental erosion has not been reported to be a specific problem in elderly generations but as the number of old people who have retained their own teeth increases it is expected that more erosion will be seen. It is often difficult to identify specific aspects of tooth wear in older people that may be associated with erosion alone against a background of a life-time's 'physiological' wear and tear to tooth tissue. The only effective prevention for erosion is eliminating the cause and/or treating any underlying systemic pathology.

Prevention of oral mucosal diseases

The prevalence of yeast infections increases with increasing age. Therefore, control of *Candida* is important in the elderly. Removable dental prostheses, in particular, increase oral *Candida* counts and care must be taken to mechanically clean them properly after every meal. If nothing else, rinsing the removable prostheses under running water is recommended. Cleaning the prostheses alone in edentulous patients, however, does not effectively decrease the number of microbes in the mouth. Mechanical cleaning of dentures will remove plaque from the surface of the plastic, but older resins become porous and the surface becomes colonised with *Candida* species. The only way to effectively clean such surfaces is by soaking the denture in an antimicrobial solution. One of the most effective is a 1% sodium hypochlorite solution with an overnight soak (1% hypochlorite is the concentration commonly used/recommended for sterilization of baby products). Cleaning oral mucosa with moistened cotton swabs may be needed for better oral hygiene, in particular among bedridden patients. However, care should be taken not to use acid-containing pre-moistened swabs frequently because of the risk of dental erosion of natural teeth [12]. Unfortunately such preparations have been used in many hospital wards.

Ill-fitting dental prostheses may cause mucosal lesions and in the worst cases may be associated with malignant transformation in the epithelium. Consequently, frequent check-ups are called for in patients with dental prostheses. Clinical experience has unfortunately shown that edentulous subjects often stop visiting dentists after they get total prostheses. The best way to prevent stomatitis caused by ill-fitting prostheses is to assure frequent dental examinations and appropriate hygiene advice.

Prevention of oral mucositis has mainly been investigated in connection with the side effects of radio- or chemotherapy used in the management of cancer. Various cytoprotecting agents and antimicrobial agents have been studied. However, no clear pattern has been identified regarding patient type, cancer treatment or type of antimicrobial agent used, and inconsistent assessment of oral mucositis has made comparison of outcomes difficult [13].

There are no evidence-based data on the prevention of other mucosal diseases such as lichen planus or vesico-bullous diseases. Similarly, the aetiology of oral leukoplakia and erythroplakia is not fully understood but because some of these mucosal conditions are thought to be premalignant, close and frequent follow-up examinations are recommended for patients presenting with these mucosal changes, with biopsy as required for suspicious areas. However, scientific evidence is weak in this area and treatment protocols are based on clinical experience alone.

There is every reason to believe that maintaining good systemic and oral health in general reduces the risk of exacerbation of mucosal diseases. It is evident that if the oral mucosal symptoms and signs are caused by underlying systemic disease (for example, such as rheumatic disease, diabetes or celiac disease) control of the disease in question is also of key importance to reduce the severity of oral mucosal lesions. For local symptomatic treatment, vegetable oil such as olive oil can be recommended. Some patients with mucosal diseases benefit from use of sour milk products and vitamin B-preparations have also been recommended. Box 13.2 outlines some of these recommendations. It should be reinforced that these recommendations do not meet the rigorous criteria of evidence-based care but are based on tradition and clinical experience. For prevention of repeated herpes episodes, however, specific drugs are available and should be prescribed in such patients. Mild herpetic cases can be controlled by topical anti-herpes preparations while severe cases call for administration of systemic drugs.

Box 13.2 Agents used for symptomatic treatment of mucosal diseases irrespective of their aetiology. The recommendations are not evidence based but rather derived from clinical practice.

- Olive oil
- Tea tree oil
- Other vegetable oil
- Vitamin B
- Sour milk products such as natural yoghurt

Prevention of xerostomia and burning mouth

Reduced salivary flow renders the patient susceptible to dental and oral mucosal problems and oral discomfort. There is sound evidence that dry mouth negatively affects quality of life. Medications such as diuretics, anti-hypertensive drugs, anticholinergics, anxiolytics and antipsychotics may significantly reduce salivary flow. This, in turn, reduces the salivary clearance effect in the mouth which may lead to plaque accumulation. Low salivary flow also affects buffering capacity with resultant increased risk of caries and erosion and reduces humoral defensive systems in the oral cavity which may lead to mucosal problems.

Xerostomia (subjective feeling of dry mouth) and hyposalivation (measured low salivary output) are very common problems among elderly subjects [14]. Reduced salivary flow increases the individual's risk of oral infections. This together with frailty may add to the detrimental effects of oral disease. Impaired saliva flow may simply be associated with dehydration; a sufficient daily intake of water is important for everyone. Elderly people often drink much less than the recommended intake of 1–1.5 L of water per day for a variety of reasons; poor sensory desire for thirst, a need for assistance in drinking and a fear of urinary incontinence often discourage people from drinking an adequate amount of fluid.

A variety of commercial preparations for dry mouth is also available. In isolated cases cholinergic drugs such as pilocarpine can be prescribed for older adults with reduced salivary flow. However, pharmacotherapy for reduced salivary flow has mainly been investigated in patients with cancer or Sjögren's syndrome and its use is of limited value in the elderly populations due to potential drug interactions. Box 13.3 summarizes some aspects of xerostomia prevention and a more detailed discussion can be found in Chapter 19.

Box 13.3 Prevention and treatment of reduced salivary flow and xerostomia (see also Chapter 19).

- Avoidance of drugs with anticholinergic effect.
- Avoidance of multiple concomitant medications.
- Control of hyposalivation-associated systemic diseases such as rheumatic diseases and diabetes.
- Strict control of radiotherapy affecting salivary glands.
- Drinking frequently and enough: 1–2 L/day
- Moisturization of mucosal membranes with vegetable oil or by use of commercial preparations.
- Administration of cholinergic drugs such as pilocarpine.

Burning mouth syndrome is described as burning or itching and/or painful sensation in oral mucosa (including the tongue, when it is called glossodynia) of patients where no medical or dental reason is to be found [15]. In other words, there are no clinical signs explaining the patient's complaint. The symptoms characteristically develop during the morning with full blown sensation later during the course of the day. The sensation can be extremely painful, leading to significant morbidity. The prevalence in populations is not known but being female and over 50 years of age seem to be risk factors for burning mouth. Because the reason for burning mouth is not known, there is no prevention. However, some peri- and postmenopausal women benefit from hormone replacement therapy although the scientific evidence is still weak. Burning mouth often goes hand-in-hand with xerostomia and reduced salivary flow appears to be a risk factor for it. Thus, the same preventive protocol as presented for dry mouth can also be recommended for burning mouth patients. These patients often benefit from the use of vegetable oil to lubricate their mouth mucosa (Box 13.2.). Oral discomfort of this type can also be associated with iron deficiency, when appropriate replacement therapy will be beneficial.

Prevention of oral cancer

Aetiology and pathogenic mechanisms of cancer are not fully understood. However, use of tobacco and alcohol are well-known risk factors of cancer in the mouth too, like in any other part of the body. Over 90% of patients with oral cancer use tobacco in some form. The risk of oral cancer associated with smoking is both dose and duration dependent while smoking cessation leads to a reduction in risk. Respectively, 75–80% of oral cancer patients frequently consume alcohol and alcohol is the principal risk factor in non-smokers. Risk increases linearly with amount of alcohol consumed over 4 units of alcohol per day (1 unit is 8 g of alcohol: about 250 mL of beer at 4% alcohol or 25 ml of spirits at 40%). The alcohol concentration also seems to increase the risk with people who consume spirits regularly being more at risk than wine or beer drinkers. Consequently, strategies for the prevention of oral cancer should be focused on these behavioural factors. Elderly patients who smoke should be advised to quit smoking and those who consume alcohol daily should be advised to restrict the intake of alcoholic beverages and, in particular, avoid straight liquor [16].

Oral squamous cell carcinoma is sixth in frequency in the global map of malignant diseases. The incidence rate varies widely throughout the world. In India it is the most common cancer, with an annual incidence rate in males of 27 per 100 000, accounting for over 50% of all cancers. Throughout the world, oral cancer occurs more frequently in men than in women, with the male to female ratio greater than 2 : 1. In the United States, oral squamous cell carcinoma is the tenth most common cancer among males, with an annual incidence rate of 11.5 per 100 000 person-years [17].

Recently, studies have shown that oral cancer might be affected by the level of oral hygiene. The pathogenesis behind these observations is the fact that several oral microbial species metabolize ethanol to acetaldehyde, the latter chemical being carcinogenic [18]. Thus, life-long good oral hygiene may reduce the risk of oral and upper gastrointestinal tract cancer. Box 13.4 summarizes means for putative prevention of oral cancer.

Box 13.4 Prevention of oral cancer.[a]

- Reduction in tobacco use (including smoking, chewed tobacco
products and quids).
- Reduced consumption of alcohol.
- Management of ill-fitting prostheses and poor restorations to reduce local trauma.
- Maintenance of good oral hygiene.
- Avoidance of papilloma-virus and HIV infections.
- Frequent follow-up of patients who have undergone treatment of any malignancy.

[a]Due to the complex aetiology of cancer, prevention of malignant disease may never totally succeed.

Prevention of bone loss

Alveolar bone that supports the teeth is lost if teeth are being lost. When teeth are lost, chewing is greatly hindered and speaking may become difficult too. The facial structures look different without the support teeth normally provide for the lips, cheeks, nose and chin. The loss of alveolar bone may make getting dentures that are stable and retentive much harder. Consequently, keeping a healthy natural dentition is the prerequisite in the prevention of jaw bone loss. Because periodontal disease and dental caries are the leading causes for loss of teeth, preventive strategies should be focused on preventing these conditions.

Systemic diseases such as osteoporosis, however, may greatly modify the clinical picture.

Osteoporosis was defined by WHO as bone mass that is two standard deviations or more below the young adult mean bone mass. The main consequence of osteoporosis is bone fracture. The majority of fractures are seen in older people, particularly postmenopausal women. By age 70, more than 25% of European women have sustained at least one osteoporotic fracture. The highest incidence of hip fracture has been found in Scandinavian women older than age 50 [19].

The association between osteoporosis and alveolar bone loss, however, is not clear. Most of the studies so far are confined to postmenopausal women and several other factors contributing to bone loss, such as hormone intake, sex, age, race, smoking and stress, need to be addressed when assessing the relationship between osteoporosis and alveolar bone loss. Nevertheless, periodontal disease inevitably leads to general horizontal alveolar bone loss and vertical bone pockets adjacent to the affected teeth. Consequently, effective plaque control should be emphasized for patients at risk. The management of osteoporosis is not without its oral consequences; bisphosphonates are drugs that inhibit osteoclastic activity and hence reduce bone loss. However they are also associated with bisphosphonate-associated osteonecrosis of the jaws; the aetiology and management of this condition and of patients taking these drugs are covered in Chapter 8.

In addition to idiopathic osteoporosis, there are several secondary reasons for systemic bone loss. These include long-term corticosteroid medication, renal diseases, gastrointestinal diseases such as coeliac disease, hepatic diseases, Parkinson's disease and chronic pulmonary diseases. Obviously, successful prevention of alveolar bone loss in these cases calls for control of the systemic disease in question. Box 13.5 summarizes the possibilities for the prevention of alveolar bone loss.

Box 13.5 Prevention of alveolar bone loss.

- Keeping the patient's natural dentition.
- Maintenance of 'key' teeth for over-dentures at the end stage of the dentition.
- Use of osseointegrated dental implants.
- Control of periodontal disease.
- Smoking cessation.
- Control of osteoporosis and other bone metabolism affecting systemic diseases.[a]
- Avoidance of long-term corticosteroid therapy.[a]
- Hormone replacement therapy in postmenopausal women.[a]

[a]Efficacy on alveolar bone loss specifically has not been verified; great care is required when providing dental care for subjects taking bisphosphonates to manage osteoporosis.

Prevention of temporomandibular dysfunction and myofascial pain

Elderly people rarely suffer from temporomandibular dysfunction (TMD) pain even though objective signs of joint dysfunction are prevalent in old age [20]. TMD and myofascial pain disorders, on the other hand, seem to fluctuate with a relatively good remission capacity and objective radiographic signs of joint pathology do not associate with subjective symptoms [21, 22]. The aetiology of TMD remains elusive, but it may be related to tension and neck symptoms in most cases where no joint pathology is seen [23]. However, temporomandibular joint osteoarthrosis may be a consequence of old age but even these patients seldom suffer from painful symptoms. Thus, prevention of these disorders is difficult if no distinct reason is to be found for the symptoms.

Planning preventive services

Elderly people are individuals like all people are. Subsequently, oral treatment and preventive services need to be planned and tailor-made on an individual basis. On this level, the manual dexterity and mental capacity of a patient largely dictates what kind of oral hygiene procedures, for example, can be recommended and implemented. In free living older people, daily oral hygiene and dietary recommendations, prescription of fluoride products and so on do not differ from those in a more youthful population. In dependent and/or institutionalized subjects, however, there may be problems in all areas of daily activities and maintaining oral hygiene at a satisfactory level often calls for outside help. Similarly, the planning of preventive oral health procedures and strategies is different on the population level than on the individual or special needs care level.

A quote from the WHO policy describes the situation: 'Public policies to support community awareness and acceptance of broad-based preventive behaviour to preserve oral health in old age are essential. Policies also must provide guidance on how to proceed when disabling disease occurs, provide for regular research and updating of information, and ensure access to cost-effective and high-quality services for all.' [24]. However, there are no systematic cost-effectiveness studies on the effect of certain preventive programmes on costs to the society and such studies would be unethical to conduct. There is enough evidence to show that maintaining good oral health does improve general health and affects the quality of life.

Barriers to prevention in older populations

Barriers to prevention can be discussed on the individual and population levels. Old age inevitably causes reduction in functional capacity which, however, is as highly individual as the aging process itself. Subsequently, maintaining daily oral hygiene may become difficult due to impaired manual dexterity, and choice of foodstuff and drinks may also become altered due to difficulties in chewing and swallowing. Dementia of various degrees modifies the understanding of the importance of maintaining satisfactory oral and dental health. Furthermore, strong tasting oral hygiene products such as toothpastes and mouth rinse preparations may not be accepted if mucosal membranes of the mouth have become thin and sensitive and saliva secretion is reduced. The latter is often due to multiple medications. On the other hand it has been shown that institutionalized elderly people readily accept oral hygiene products provided that frequent counselling is undertaken [25]. The latter is often restricted by lack of competent personnel and hospitalized patients are in special need in this regard. Further detail in this area is given in Chapters 25 and 26.

On a population level, elderly patients may not comply with daily oral hygiene and preventive care instructions as readily as younger generations. There is also a lack of tradition in societies regarding implementing oral health care and prevention strategies for the elderly. Cost is an additional aspect that must not be forgotten. In societies with a functioning public health service system, prevention and particularly prevention of oral and dental diseases are not of high priority in comparison with other health interventions such as controlling hypertension and obesity. WHO further points out that different oral health strategies may be needed for women and men due to biophysiological differences between sexes [26]. Box 13.6 summarizes problems in the prevention of oral diseases in the elderly population.

Box 13.6 Problems in the prevention of oral diseases of the elderly.

- Poor understanding of the importance of prevention.
- Impaired compliance of use of preventive strategies.
- Reduced manual dexterity in maintaining daily oral hygiene.
- Costs of oral hygiene products.
- Diet counselling difficult due to fixed habits and conceptions.

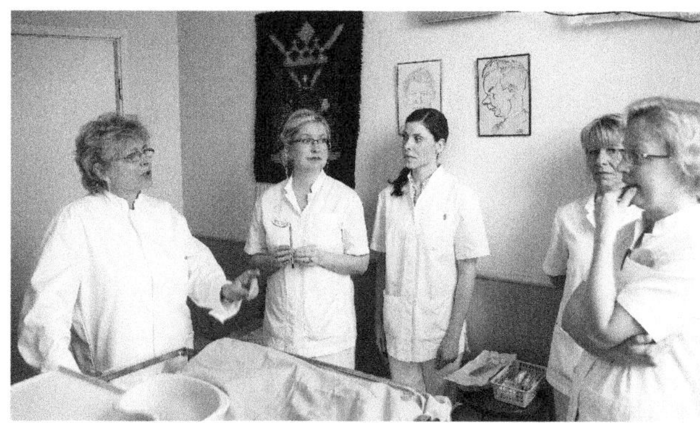

Figure 13.2 Dental hygienist visits a geriatric hospital ward and instructs the nurses and the patient on daily oral hygiene protocol of a patient.

Examples of prevention in practice

Preventive guidelines for home-living elderly patients are the same as for any adult patient, with dietary counselling towards healthy food habits and avoidance of fermentable carbohydrates, maintaining satisfactory oral hygiene and use of fluoride-containing toothpaste and mouthwash as the cornerstones for good oral health. However, older individuals with reduced manual dexterity, often together with a dry mouth, need special attention and enhanced preventive therapy. Community nurses and other formal and informal carers need to be educated about the need for and delivery of oral health maintenance because these personnel frequently visit the housebound elderly, unlike dental personnel. Emphasizing the benefit of drinking enough fluids daily needs to be repeated over and over again for individuals who are suffering from xerostomia. If dry mouth is caused by multiple medications, as is the common case, and this greatly disturbs the patient, then the patient's physician needs to be consulted as it may be possible to replace drugs with severe xerostomia as a side effect. Unfortunately, however, it is seldom possible to modify the medication on oral health grounds alone.

Institutionalized elderly call for special attention. These patients are of poor general condition, often bedridden and unable to take care of their daily oral hygiene. Providing advice and support for the carers within an institution through frequent visits by the oral health team to the institutions or nursing homes is necessary. Figure 13.2 shows how a dental hygienist instructs both the patient and hospital ward personnel in this regard. After some instruction and practise the hospital ward personnel can learn to help the patients by cleaning their teeth and dental prostheses (Figures 13.3 and 13.4). It has been shown that the best outcomes in terms of oral health and hygiene occur when nursing staff take responsibility for the delivery of oral hygiene in the ward [27].

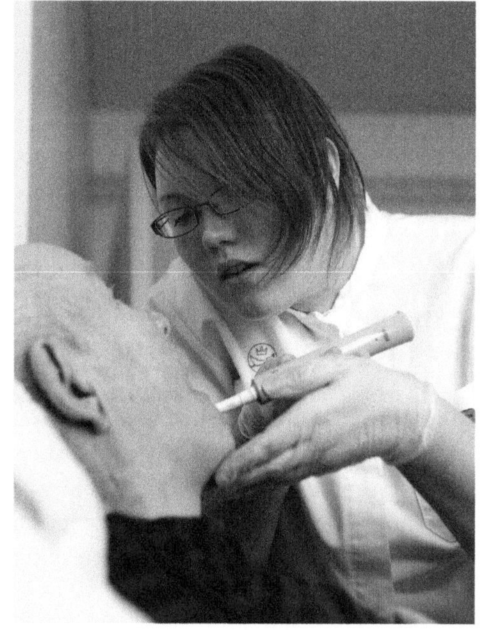

Figure 13.3 An electric toothbrush helps tremendously in daily cleaning of a patient's teeth. A nurse of the ward has been taught to clean a dependent patient's teeth.

Denture hygiene is another issue and is covered in some detail in Chapters 14 and 22. Personnel in nursing homes and geriatric hospital wards need to be given appropriate advice in this regard too. Removable prostheses must be cleaned daily and the use of antiseptic preparations is often recommended. However, the personnel must be advised that to prevent oral mucosal irritation after keeping the prostheses in antiseptic solutions they need to be thoroughly rinsed under running water before inserting them back to mouth.

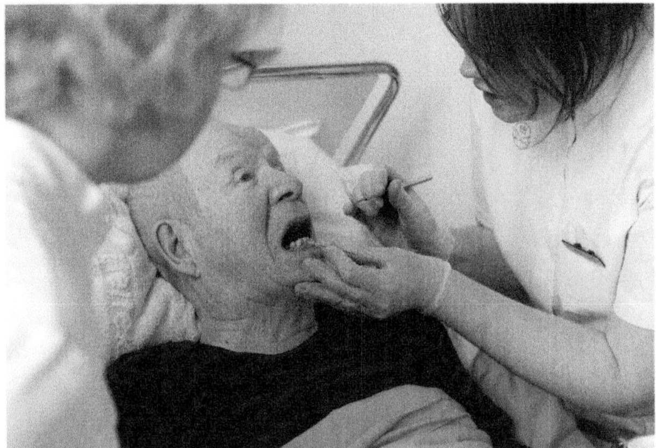

Figure 13.4 A nurse cleans the teeth of a bedridden patient in a geriatric hospital ward using an interdental brush after being advised by a dental hygienist.

In the future, protocols for improving oral health of the elderly may include use of novel methods such as administration of probiotics. These health-promoting bacteria given in daily used foodstuffs have been shown to reduce oral *Candida* counts in the elderly when compared with placebo [28].

Role of the oral health team in promoting healthier lifestyle

Dentists and other members of the oral health team have the privilege of regularly seeing most of their patients, year after year. However, due to the disabilities of old age, elderly patients may not be able to follow regular dental check-up schemes like younger individuals. Another obstacle for implementing life-long health counselling is the unfortunate fact that those people who are in highest objective need for prevention and control of diseases often are those who are most likely to neglect taking care of themselves and are not willing to quit detrimental habits such as smoking and excessive alcohol consumption. This polarization also holds true in the elderly. However, it should never be too late for preventive intervention even though one must be realistic and take the capacity of the patient carefully into account.

Smoking cessation can be encouraged using the same tools as in younger patients, namely pointing out the delay in wound healing among smokers and increased risk of periodontal disease and oral cancer and malignancy in general.

Dietary counselling also follows the same protocol as in any age group of patients. Diminished chewing capacity with eventual swallowing difficulties may lead to decreased intake of fibre-rich diet and shifting daily food habits towards carbohydrate-rich items of soft consistency. The patient should be advised about the detrimental consequences of such diets for general and oral and dental health, and the opportunities offered during the provision of dental care should be taken. Dietary interventions to improve fruits and vegetables intake in older people have been shown to be effective when associated with construction of new dentures for example.

Physical activity is inevitably reduced in old age. The oral health team has little to do in encouraging the patient to exercise more if motor functions are severely impaired. However, maintaining the daily practices of cleaning the teeth and mouth should be encouraged as long as possible. If the patient feels that help is needed, it should then be provided. In health promotion the role of good oral health in systemic health in general should be emphasized, thus motivating the elderly patients to take good care of themselves.

Consequences for geriatric preventive services

The time has come to also focus on preventive health care in the elderly with respect to oral diseases [26]. Changes in global demographics with subsequent global increases in the number of elderly who wish to maintain their own teeth for their lifetime calls for more action than hitherto. Good oral health in old age positively affects the quality of life and reduces the risk of dentogenic bacteraemia with its potentially severe consequences. Research evidence has shown that poor oral health is also associated with overall mortality. Hence, in this perspective funding used to deliver preventive oral health care of the elderly should have manifest effects both

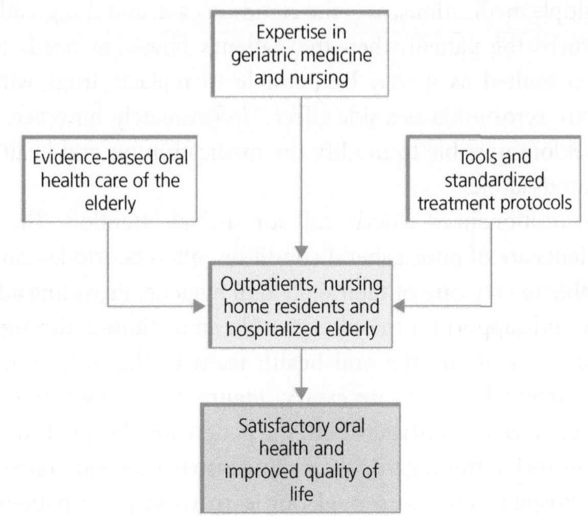

Figure 13.5 Theoretical model depicting the elements necessary for improved oral health of the elderly.

at the individual and the societal level. However, it should be borne in mind that the course of frailty is progressive with increase in co-morbidity and disability and thus all treatment plans including oral health protocols must be realistic [29]. Figure 13.5 summarizes the principal components of preventive philosophy in oral health care of the elderly.

References

1 Paster, B.J., Boches, S.K., Galvin, J.L., Ericson, R.E., Lau, C.N., Levanos, V.A. *et al.* (2001) Bacterial diversity in human subgingival plaque. *Journal of Bacteriology*, **183**, 3770–3783.
2 Ellepola, A.N. & Samaranayake, L.P. (2000) Oral candidal infections and antimycotics. *Critical Reviews in Oral Biology & Medicine*, **11**, 172–198.
3 Meurman, J.H., Sanz, M. & Janket, S.-J. (2004) Oral health, atherosclerosis and cardiovascular disease. *Critical Reviews in Oral Biology & Medicine*, **15**, 403–413.
4 Meurman, J.H. & Hamalainen, P. (2006) Oral health and morbidity--implications of oral infections on the elderly. *Gerodontology*, **23**, 3–16.
5 Scannapieco, F.A., Papandonatos, G.D. & Dunford, R.G. (1998) Associations between oral conditions and respiratory disease in a national sample survey population. *Annals of Periodontology*, **3**, 251–256.
6 Yoneyama, T., Yoshida, M., Ohrui, T., Mukaiyama, H., Okamoto, H., Hoshiba, K. *et al.* (2002) Oral care reduces pneumonia in older patients in nursing homes. *Journal of the American Geriatric Society*, **50**, 430–433.
7 Watando, A., Ebihara, S., Ebihara, T., Okazaki, T., Takahashi, H., Asada, M. *et al.* (2004) Daily oral care and cough reflex sensitivity in elderly nursing home patients. *Chest*, **126**, 1066–1070.
8 Davies, R.M. (2004) The rational use of oral care products in the elderly, *Clinical Oral Investigations*, **8**, 2–5.
9 Koeman, M., van der Ven, A.J., Hak, E., Joore, H.C., Kaasjager, K., de Smet, A.G. *et al.* (2006) Oral decontamination with chlorhexidine reduces incidence of ventilator-associated pneumonia. *American Journal of Respiratory and Critical Care Medicine*, **173**, 1348–1355.
10 Twetman, S., Axelsson, S., Dahlgren, H., Holm, A.K., Kallestal, C., Lagerlof, F. *et al.* (2003) Caries-preventive effect of fluoride toothpaste: a systematic review. *Acta Odontologica Scandinavica*, **61**, 347–355.
11 Twetman, S., Petersson, L.G., Axelsson, S., Dahlgren, H., Holm, A.K., Kallestal, C. *et al.* (2004) Caries-preventive effect of sodium fluoride mouthrinses: a systematic review of controlled clinical trials. *Acta Odontologica Scandinavica*, **62**, 223–230.
12 Meurman, J.H., Sorvari, R., Pelttari, A., Rytömaa, I., Franssila, S. & Kroon, L. (1996) Hospital mouth-cleaning aids may cause dental erosion. *Special Care in Dentistry*, **16**, 247–250.
13 Donnelly, J.P., Bellm, L.A., Epstein, J.B., Sonis, S.T. & Symonds, R.P. (2003) Antimicrobial therapy to prevent or treat oral mucositis. *Lancet Infectious Diseases*, **3**, 405–412.
14 Janket, S.-J., Jones, J., Sharron, R., Van Dyke, T.E., Garcia, R. & Meurman, J.H. (2007) Oral health outcomes and intake of xerogenic medications: The Veteran's Dental Study (Part II). *Oral Surgery, Oral Medicine, Oral Pathology, Oral Radiology and Endodontology*, **103**, 223–230.
15 Grushka, M., Ching, V. & Epstein, J. (2006) Burning mouth syndrome. *Advances in Oto-Rhino-Laryngology*, **63**, 278–287.
16 www.info.cancerresearchuk.org/cancerstats/types/oral/riskfactors
17 Warnakulasuriya, S. (2009) Global epidemiology of oral and oropharyngeal cancer. *Oral Oncology*, **45**, 309–316.
18 Salaspuro, M.P. (2003) Acetaldehyde, microbes, and cancer of the digestive tract. *Critical Reviews in Clinical Laboratory Sciences*, **40**, 183–208.
19 www.merckmedicus.com/pp/us/hcp/diseasemodules/osteoporosis/epidemiology.jsp
20 Schmitter, M., Rammelsberg, P. & Hassel, A. (2005) The prevalence of signs and symptoms of temporomandibular disorders in very old subjects. *Journal of Oral Rehabilitation*, **32**, 467–473.
21 Sato, H., Osterberg, T., Ahlqwist, M., Carlsson, G.E., Grondahl, H.G. and Rubinstein, B. (1996) Association between radiographic findings in the mandibular condyle and temporomandibular dysfunction in an elderly population. *Acta Odontologica Scandinavica*, **54**, 384–390.
22 Ohlmann, B., Rammelsberg, P., Henschel, V., Kress, B., Gabbert, O. & Schmitter, M. (2006) Prediction of TMJ arthralgia according to clinical diagnosis and MRI findings. *International Journal of Prosthodontics*, **19**, 333–338.
23 Curtis, A.W. (1980) Myofascial pain-dysfunction syndrome: the role of nonmasticatory muscles in 91 patients. *Otolaryngology – Head and Neck Surgery*, **88**, 361–367.
24 Barmes, D.E. (2001) Public policy on oral health and old age: a global view. *Journal of Public Health Dentistry*, **60**, 335–337.
25 Meurman, J.H., Kari, K., Aikas, A. & Kallio, P. (2001) One-year compliance and effects of amine and stannous fluoride on some salivary biochemical constituents and oral microbes in institutionalized elderly. *Special Care in Dentistry*, **21**, 31–36.
26 World Health Organization. (2006) *Oral health in aging societies. Integration of oral health and general health.* WHO Press, Geneva.
27 Peltola, P., Vehkalahti, M. & Simola, R. (2007) Effects of 11-month intervention on oral cleanliness among the longterm hospitalised elderly. *Gerodontology*, **24**, 14–21.
28 Hatakka, K., Ahola, A.J., Yli-Knuuttila, H., Richardson, M., Poussa, T., Meurman, J.H. *et al.* (2007) Probiotics reduce the prevalence of oral candida in the elderly--a randomized controlled trial. *Journal of Dental Research*, **86**, 125–130.
29 Stranberg, T.E. & Pitkälä, K.H. (2007) Frailty in elderly people. *Lancet*, **3690**, 1328–1329.

CHAPTER 14

Treatment planning for the geriatric patient

Frederick Hains and Judith Jones
Boston University Goldman School of Dental Medicine, Boston, MA, USA

Treatment planning is a 'complex process that should include a frank consideration of treatment alternatives that will provide maximum benefit to the patient' [1]. This definition of treatment planning as a process is a particularly important concept in caring for geriatric dental patients. A myriad of choices and consequences will present themselves and the decision as to the best approach must be made in concert with patients' wishes and consent. Moreover, geriatric dental patients are complex and must be evaluated physically, mentally, pharmacologically, functionally and socially (see Chapter 7 on clinical assessment). It is therefore essential to gather and process a wide range of patient-related information. Any decisions made may require input from a number of sources. Thus, treatment planning in the geriatric patient is ideally 'a social process that includes the dentist, the patient and sometimes other family members and insurers' [2].

The appropriateness of the care should also be considered in the treatment of geriatric patients. Appropriate care is care for which the benefits outweigh the risks by a wide margin [3]. Particularly among older, frail patients, pains should be taken not to underuse (not providing care that is appropriate), misuse (when otherwise appropriate care is provided in a way that leads to avoidable complications, e.g. prescribing antibiotics to which a patient is allergic) or overuse (providing care for which the risks outweigh the benefits) care.

While a geriatric patient may be older and more complex, his or her interests may be the same as those of patients from the general population. However, the interests of geriatric patients are often complicated by a variety of factors unique to the geriatric population. The purpose of this chapter is to consider how treatment planning for older, frail adults differs from the rest of the population, taking into account the medical, pharmacological, psychological, physical, functional, access to care and financial issues that are common among elders. Ethical issues in decision making will be discussed, along with approaches to different types of care. Finally, several patients are presented as examples of how decisions can be different in older patients.

Geriatric dental practice is different to providing care in traditional practice

Six issues that differentiate geriatric dentistry from the traditional practice of dentistry include the following [4].

1. The population is aged 65 years and over.
2. Eighty-six per cent of this population has at least one major chronic disorder, most commonly arthritis, osteoporosis, cardiovascular disease, cancer, neurological disorder, diabetes, mental illness and respiratory disease (see Chapter 7).
3. Polypharmacy - the geriatric patient typically consumes multiple prescriptions on a daily basis (see Chapter 12 on pharmacology).
4. Twenty per cent of this population suffers from cognitive dysfunction or depression. [5] (see Chapter 5 on psychology).
5. The geriatric population often suffers from physical disabilities which may impact on their ability to comply with instructions (see Chapter 10 on disability).
6. The combined effects of physical, psychological and mental disorders confound the dentist's ability to plan and execute dental treatment.

Who are the geriatric patients?

The clearest definition of the aging patient population is the population aged 65 years and over. This population is rapidly growing, diverse and complex. According to the US Department of Health and Human Services (DHHS), 36.3 million persons were over 65 years in 2004 [6]. The

Textbook of Geriatric Dentistry, Third Edition. Edited by Poul Holm-Pedersen, Angus W. G. Walls and Jonathan A. Ship.

DHHS projects that this number will increase by 39% by 2024. This population is living longer and healthier lives and is more prosperous than previous generations [6]. The aging population will have significant and profound effects on societies throughout the developed world. The year 2011 marked the entrance of the first individuals of the Baby Boomer Generation into the geriatric population, accelerating the trend. In some countries this graying population will outnumber the population of individuals less than 15 years of age [7].

Who are these geriatric patients who will be presenting to dental offices in larger numbers than before and how will they be treated? What will be their demands and expectations of the dental professionals? The 65+ year-old patient is not easily categorized; some older adult patients are healthy, active people with adequate finances while others are older than their years, in poor health and living on small, fixed incomes (see Chapter 7 on assessment). Therefore, it is important to better describe this population and then look at the process of making decisions as to how to best care for their dental health.

The primary dimensions that affect the dental treatment planning for the 65+ population are shown in Table 14.1. At any age the older adult patient might be unaffected in any of these categories or he or she may be profoundly affected in all categories. For many people, as they age there is a transition through this table and many of its categories will become concerns in the process of developing an appropriate plan of dental therapy. As one moves from well, community dwelling elders to functionally dependent, sick elders, the goals of care also change. Comfort, safety, dignity, prevention of new problems and maintenance of function in the existing dentition become more important than restoring the distolingual cusp on a second molar [8]. The concept of futility is also important. As patients near the end of life, the best treatment is sometimes no treatment, or treatment related to comfort only.

Atul Gawande presented a clear analogy, taken from the university researcher Leonid Grvrilov, of the course of events after 65 by comparing a human's life to a complex system such as a power plant [9]. Such a complex system is full of critical components that must function and survive for many years; it does so by depending on redundancy and backup systems.

This analogy describes human beings as failing randomly and gradually. Defects are replaced by backup systems that take over and operate until, eventually, there are too many defects, the backup systems fail and the plant must be closed. The condition cited would be best described as frailty in the human. The charge to the health care providers should be to provide 'enough function for active engagement in the world' [9] while supporting quality of life by mitigating the ravages of disease.

Applying this concept of progressive frailty to health care for frail elders, one sees a clear parallel with medicine. Some geriatricians use the phrase 'homeostenosis' to describe this process, whereby the body's normal homeostatic mechanisms are compromised by a combination of age-related and disease-related changes. Aging plus disease puts substantial stress on even the best maintained oral environment. Wear is inevitable, even in enamel, the hardest tissue in the human body [9]. The supporting structures of the dentition are subject to systemic and localized factors that contribute to a journey towards frailty. The advancement of age is at times associated with a decline in caloric intake and malnutrition; such declines focus the need to provide optimal oral function and maintain the mouth as an integral part of the whole body's health.

Disturbances in the oral environment are often the initial clues to systemic diseases in any patient; these disturbances are of particular importance in the aging dental patient.

Table 14.1 Dimensions critical to planning and delivery of dental care in the elderly (American Society of Anesthesiologists (ASA) [10])

Health concerns	Financial concerns	Mobility- ability to get around	Independence	Mental status	Dexterity
None ASA 1	None	Driving	Able to make independent decisions	Clear	No issue
Mild ASA 2	Concerned	Dependent on others	Requires assistance and input of partner or family	Forgetful, difficulty following oral and written instructions	Limited problems
Major ASA 3	Major consideration	House bound or bedridden Nursing home	Medical proxy	Confused and reliant on others for care	Significant problems to dependence on others
ASA 4	At risk of loss of life	Hospital Nursing home Hospice	Medical proxy	Unresponsive, unable to participate in decision making	Dependent on others

For example, a dehydrated patient will present with a dry tongue and mouth. A dentist evaluating an elderly dental patient taking multiple medications with this condition may be the first to recognize dehydration and its associated risks. Consultation with the patient's primary care physician concerning the intra-oral findings might prevent serious consequences to the patient's well-being. The dehydrated patient is at risk for dizziness and more prone to falling [9]. Annually, three hundred and fifty thousand Americans fall and break their hips [9]. The primary risk factors for falling and hip fracture are poor balance, taking more than four prescriptions and muscle weakness. Some of the major causes of dehydration include medications commonly prescribed to control blood pressure and depression. This is often further complicated by the fact that the elderly frequently do not consume adequate quantities of water. An illustration of this common phenomenon is a conversation with an octogenarian patient; when asked about what she drank daily, she answered 'one to two cups of coffee, some milk with my cereal and a cocktail in the evening'. To 'but what about water?', she replied, 'I don't like water, never drink it'. This is an example of when an observant dentist can initiate a dialogue of change that can have a profound impact on the well-being of an elderly patient.

Fundamentals of treatment planning for the older adults

The easiest patient to plan treatment for is one who has a good dental IQ, understands his or her options, is compliant, follows instructions, keeps his or her appointments and is an active, effective participant in his or her own care. Further, this patient is financially capable of allowing the selection of the best solutions to his or her problems and does not have physical, mental or medical issues that interfere with the execution and delivery of care. These patients are the easiest patients in a dental practice and, in general, receive the best care possible. The treatment plans of these patients can be ideal and one can focus on the delivery of optimal dentistry as required.

Challenge enters the treatment planning process as one moves right and down in Table 14.1. Taking each category in order, when treating a patient with a significant medical history, the difficulties are focused on how his or her medical health affects the ability to tolerate planned dental procedures and the delivery of planned care. What are the risks associated with the treatment at any level for this patient? American Society of Anesthesiologists (ASA) Risk Physical Status Classification [10] is an invaluable tool in classifying a patient's health and may serve as a guide to determine how well he or she will tolerate medical and dental procedures (see Table 14.2).

The hypertensive patient, for example, must be monitored for compliance with his or her medication regime and for his or her tolerance to the proposed procedure. This patient would be an ASA II or III patient depending on the control of the hypertension. The dental treatment plan would have to take into consideration the type and quantity of anaesthetic to use, the time of day to best schedule the patient, the length of the procedure and the level of stress, perceived or actual, that a particular dental procedure would cause (see Chapter 8 on medical issues). Hypertension is a chronic condition that affects over half of the US population 65 and older (see Chapter 7 on assessment). But it is only one of a list of chronic conditions that impact on the 65+ population. Increasingly, chronic disorders such as arthritis, diabetes, heart disease, hearing and vision impairment also affect the graying population either in isolation or more commonly in combination.

Each of these conditions by themselves can be significant enough to affect one's ability to participate in the activities of daily living [11]. Generally, combinations of these conditions are present in the geriatric population and challenge the patient and clinician alike. Common to this population and perhaps more problematic and insidious, are the pharmaceutical agents consumed by the geriatric patient (see Chapter 12 on pharmacology). Many of these medications contribute to a variety of dental conditions or exacerbate existing diseases. The most prevalent condition associated with pharmaceutical agents taken by the elderly is dry mouth (see Chapter 19 on saliva). More than 500 drugs in 42 drug categories can affect salivary flow [12]. Gingival enlargements, alterations in taste and tardive dyskinesia are other known side effects of commonly prescribed medications. Root caries, smooth surface and interproximal dental caries and oral bacterial and fungal infections are common consequences of drug-induced salivary gland dysfunction.

Ethical issues

How do we plan treatment for this ever growing complex population? What do we have by virtue of our training that will permit us to serve this aging population?

The ADA code of ethics includes five principles that direct us to provide care that is ethical and moral (Table 14.3). That code places importance on the autonomy of the individual. *Autonomy* requires that the patient be consulted before performing any treatment, informed of the risks inherent in the procedure, the consequences of not treating and treatment alternatives. The patient is then afforded the opportunity to accept or reject our proposals. Where the patient is not able to

Table 14.2 Dental care by ASA classification [10]

ASA classification	Definition	Expectations	Examples	Dental care alterations
ASA I	No systemic condition; a normal health individual that can undergo routine care.	Any routine dental care can be provided that the patient understands and for which they can give consent.	Healthy individuals with little to no dental anxiety.	No alterations to care.
ASA II	Mild to moderate systemic condition and/or a significant health risk factor	Medically stable person that may have a medical condition that is not incapacitating, nor limits activities BP 159/99	Well controlled non insulin-dependent diabetes, controlled epilepsy or patients with well controlled hyperthyroid or hypothyroid disorders or well controlled asthmatics. A patient that may be pregnant, or have a drug allergy or other active allergies. A patient with greater level of anxiety. Smokers.	Address the anxiety issues. Make sure the patient's medical condition is controlled.
ASA III	Severe systemic condition, not incapacitating but limits activity.	Stable angina pectoris. Status post myocardial infarction >6 months with no residual signs and symptoms. Status post cerebrovascular accident >6 months with no residual signs and symptoms. Well controlled insulin-dependent diabetes (IDDM). Congestive heart failure (CHF) with orthopnea and ankle oedema. Chronic obstructive pulmonary disease (COPD). Exercise induced asthma. Less well-controlled epilepsy. Hyperthyroid or hypothyroid disorders who are symptomatic. Adult blood pressure between 160 to 179 torr systolic and/or 100 to 109 torr diastolic	Patient with angina, congestive heart failure, hypertension.	Epinephrine use in L.A. is contraindicated. Use semi sitting position during treatment. Short appointments. Treat early in the morning. Best after a good night's sleep.
			Osteoarthritis, chronic respiratory disease, colostomy	Late morning so that they have had time to limber up, cleared their lungs and had an opportunity to use the toilet after breakfast.
			Diabetic patients, hypoglycemic	Midmorning appointments when insulin not at a peak.
			Angina, CV disease	Short morning appointments, nitroglycerine at hand. Adequate anaesthesia to reduce stress.
ASA IV	Severe systemic condition, incapacitating, limited activity	Debilitating systemic disease(s) that immobilizes them and is a constant threat to life. Usually, these patients have more than one distressing symptom or disabling signal that occur at rest or during normal activity.	Unstable angina pectoris (preinfarction angina). Myocardial infarction within the past 6 months. CVA within the past 6 months. Adult blood pressure greater than 200 torr and/or 115 torr. Severe CHF or COPD (requiring O_2 supplementation and/or confined to wheelchair). Uncontrolled epilepsy (with history of hospitalization). Uncontrolled insulin-dependent diabetes (with history of hospitalization).	Elective dental care should be postponed until the patient's medical condition has improved to at least an ASA III classification.
ASA V	Moribund, not expected to live.	Hospitalized or hospice patient in their final days.	Emergency care to improve the patient's comfort during this time if possible.	

Table 14.3 Professional code of ethics and conduct

Autonomy	Patient desires, patient's permission
Non maleficence	Do no harm
Beneficence	Do good
Justice	Treat patients fairly
Veracity	Be honest and truthful

participate in the decision making process due to mental or behavioural impairment, we are guided by the second principle of '*non-malificence*'. This principle of 'do no harm' is in effect with the mentally alert, but it especially must guide our decision making process when there is no one else available to participate in the decision process. *Substitutive judgment* is also a consideration here: 'What would the patient have wanted if he or she could have made the decision.' *Advance preferences* codify this judgment and have a place in practices where there are significant numbers of patients with dementia. For example, when you see an elderly patient with mild dementia who has a broken, abscessed tooth, you might ask: 'What is your approach to dental care in general? Do you prefer to wait until something bothers you or do you want all problems addressed at the earliest possible time?' The answer to this question documented and cosigned by the patient in the chart, will provide future guidance for both dentist and caregiver. The caregiver, significant other or proxy holder may also offer input, and the dental professional will be called upon for direction and advice. Generally the final treatment decision will be made in close consultation with the dentist and the caregiver or guardian. It is incumbent on any professional to be aware of the legal basis for any such proxy consent in their own country as it may be affected by national law or case law.

The third principle of *beneficence* or 'do good' comes into play especially when the treatment proposed is risky or outside our skill, knowledge and/or ability. Here we must appeal to a higher level principle such as *non-malificence.* We should be ready to refer when appropriate and in the patient's best interest. The fourth principle of *justice* is of particular importance in a population that is easily subjected to the prejudice of 'ageism'. The practitioner may think that the stereotypical geriatric patient can't hear, can't think for him or herself, can't remember and is depressed and unproductive [R. Dupree, 2005, *Geriatrics – 2005*, Personal communication from a lecture delivered at Tufts University Dental School, Boston, MA]. It is easy to dismiss such a patient but the fourth principle of *justice* reminds us to treat all patients the same without regard to age, race, creed, sexual preference or means. This principle becomes all the more important when considering the life expectancy of older people. Some older people are disinclined to accept treatment because they are 'too old'. But the life-expectancy of the average 65-year-old in 2004 in the US was 19 years and that of the average 75-year-old was 12 years [13, 14]. These figures are similar in the demography of many western nations. Because these average life expectancies continue to increase slowly, the ageist view that someone is too old for a certain treatment is losing traction, for good reason.

Finally, the fifth principle of *veracity* requires that we are truthful about the treatment we recommend. We need to be clear about risks and benefits. We need to convey a true sense of what a patient can expect from the proposed treatment. We must inform the patient in an honest, objective way the prognosis of the treatment and the consequence of non-treatment. Finally, we need to be truthful about our skills, knowledge and ability to perform the suggested treatment.

Use evidence to evaluate alternatives

The philosophy that treatment should be evidence-based, realistic and the minimum required for optimizing oral health, aesthetics and function should guide the dental provider. Treatment should be maintainable by our patients. These philosophies, along with our ethical principles, should be in our minds as we perform the hands-on steps that will lead to an appropriate plan of dental therapy.

Accurate data and diagnoses are key elements of effective treatment planning

Treatment planning begins with objective and accurate data gathering (see Chapter 7 on assessment): a thorough patient interview with particular attention to the patient's health status, anxiety level and need for special considerations (see Chapter 8 on medical issues). Many elderly patients will request that they remain upright in the chair and they may harbinger antiquated ideas of dentistry as performed without anaesthetics. It is important to assess their ability to function in life, to eat food and obtain an idea of the quantity and variety of foods consumed. The assessment must come from what is said by the patient as well as what is not articulated by the patient. The octogenarian cited earlier saw no problem with the consumption of liquids and it did not occur to her that the diuretic effects of coffee and alcohol were contributing to her dehydration that in turn was causing systemic and cognitive problems. Careful, probing questions provided the clues to a lifestyle that was deleterious to her overall health and longevity as an active, functional and autonomous person.

Careful recording and evaluation of the medications being taken and an assessment of what the patient thinks these medications do for him or her must be performed. At times a spouse or other member of the patient's support team will need to be contacted to further elucidate the rationale for the prescriptions and to get a sense of the patient's compliance.

The medical history is essential in determining the patient's well-being and level of risk. Inquiring as to the patient's last hospitalization, the reason for the admission and his or her last visit to a primary care physician give insight into the level of medical care required and his or her ability to access that care. Does the patient have a physician and is he or she able to access medical care? The name of the patient's physician is also important information to list and, when necessary, contact information should be obtained when a formal assessment of the patient's medical status is required.

A thorough assessment of a patient's past dental care would follow the medical assessments and gives insight to the level of dental care sought in the past. Does the patient seek regular dental care? Is the patient under the care of a dental specialist? Does the patient seek treatment on an as-needed or emergency basis?

Many edentulous and partially dentate patients will be episodic in their approach to continuing dental care. They will wait until the prosthesis no longer fits and/or is causing discomfort before seeking treatment [15]. Similarly, some patients that have undergone extensive prosthetic and or periodontal therapy in the past may not have been aware of the need for constant monitoring and recall appointments.

At some point in the patient interview the dentist needs to assess the patient's mental capacity, psychological status, financial means and functional capabilities.

The patient will often present with a specific complaint or series of issues which we would consider the 'chief complaint'. Careful listening to the description of the problem, problems or concerns must be performed so that a mental differential diagnosis can begin and the correct selection of diagnostic test(s) conducted to further clarify the cause of the concerns. The patient will frequently express certain wants and desires. Special attention should be paid to these communications as often they provide clues into other, unexpressed concerns. Here the astute dentist will begin to formulate an opinion on the patient's expectations. A patient's expectation without regard to age can be challenging and, at times, unachievable. Knowing this early in the care of the patient and having a frank discussion about reality will prevent patient disappointment and loss of confidence.

The extra-oral and intra-oral examination of the patient should detail the dental hard and soft tissue findings as well as the findings not dentally associated. For example, a mole, unhealed lesion, or pigmented area that might look suspicious and require a medical, surgical or dermatological consultation. Often these conditions are without symptoms and are disregarded by the patient (see Chapter 18, mucous membrane diseases).

During the intra-oral examinations observe and list all problems detected and carefully examine the salivary glands for the quality and quantity of secretions (see Chapter 19 on saliva). The parotid is responsible for predominately aqueous excretions whereas the submandibular and sublingual, as well as the some 450 to 750 smaller accessory glands produce more mucinous secretions [16]. The healthy individual produces saliva at a rate of approximately 1 mL per minute. The salivary fluid is buffered by bicarbonate at a pH of 6.8–7.0 [17]. If there is an alteration in the quantity and composition of saliva the host will suffer and manifest these changes. These changes may herald several disease states or maybe a side effect of pharmaceuticals [18]. The health and appearance of the tongue will give insight as to the patient's nutritional status, state of dehydration and evidence of intra-oral infections.

Changes in tongue colour can be a particularly strong clue to clinical decline in older patients with deficient amounts of niacin, riboflavin, pyridoxine, folic acid, vitamin B_{12} and biotin. Atrophy of filiform or fungiform papillae on the tongue occurs during iron or protein deficiency [19].

The most common misperception of the aging oral cavity centred on the issue of whether tooth loss was part of the normal aging process [20]. The reality is that the elderly are more likely to possess a larger complement of teeth than ever before. The current trend is for the Baby Boomer Generation to lose fewer teeth as they age. That means they will have more teeth that are at risk for dental caries and periodontal diseases throughout life and they will have higher expectations and will continue to seek cosmetic dental procedures [21]. This is particularly true since teeth undergo change as we age. They become more brittle. The enamel is less permeable and undergoes light reflective changes which make the teeth appear darker. Additionally, the dentine, which is yellow, increases in the teeth of the elderly making them less translucent and yellow in colour [22].

A study by the National Institute for Dental Research of Employed Adults and Seniors [21] indicated that examination of the teeth and supporting structures in older adults and seniors showed a high prevalence of moderate periodontal diseases (gingivitis, moderate pocket depths and recession) and a lower prevalence of severe pocket depths and recession. Coronal caries was also a significant problem for older adults and root caries was present in 57% of the senior population. Caries has historically been thought to be a progressive disease. The end result is destruction of the tooth unless the dentist intervenes. However, the 2001 NIH 'Diagnosis and Management of Dental Caries throughout Life' Consensus

Statement recognized a paradigm shift in the management of caries. The emphasis that came from the Consensus Statement was to be better at diagnosis of non-cavitated, incipient lesions and treatment for prevention and arresting such carious lesions [23].

Restorations repair teeth; they do not stop caries. They have a finite life and the tooth tissue around the restoration remains susceptible to disease. We need to detect caries earlier and in the non-cavitated stage. We then need to diagnose the disease process and identify risk factors such as diet and bacteria as well as the non-etiological risk factors such as socioeconomic status. Because of this, treatment planning must go beyond caries removal and address modification of factors to eliminate, arrest and reverse non-cavitated lesions and prevent future lesions. Similarly, we need to maintain the periodontium throughout old age through regular maintenance and reinforcement of good oral hygiene.

Prior to indirect restorations, impressions are required for careful occlusal analysis in addition to the patient examination and interview. This will allow the practitioner to carefully analyze the patient's condition and develop a plan of action based on needs and problem intervention, with special emphasis on the analysis of those teeth that have a particular importance to the patient's function and occlusion.

The plan

Dental education leads us to think first in terms of an ideal plan of therapy. Thus, we will typically approach the decision process from a technical point of view. The objective of an ideal treatment plan is the best dental prognosis without taking into consideration modifying factors [24]. When the elderly patient is involved, the modifying factors are generally significant and must be part of the planning process.

Treatment planning is most challenging when there is insufficient knowledge regarding the possible outcomes of the various treatment options. When an elder's situation is complex, and there is uncertainty as to the results of various options, it is difficult to identify one definitive answer. While we strive for the optimal prognosis and predictability, without clarity what options do we have?

To help obtain clarity keep in mind the following patient factors [25]:

1 Patient attitude and motivation. Does the patient see the need for treatment and does he or she want to undergo what is necessary to accomplish the results? Does the patient see a value in completing the treatment? Will the patient give consent? Is he or she able to give consent? Does the patient have the resources to pursue this care?
2 Patient health concerns. Are there health issues that will affect treatment decisions? A healthy person with the potential for longevity will necessarily be approached differently than one who is terminally ill.
3 How will our treatment affect the quality of the patient's life? Is the treatment likely to improve the patient's quality of life in a positive way or will the cost of the therapy in stress, discomfort and financial terms outweigh the potential benefit?
4 Can the patient maintain his or her oral health? Does the patient have the motor skills, visual acuity and cognitive ability to care for his or her mouth and the dental treatment planned?
5 What is the chance of an untoward result in the performance of the therapy? What is the possibility of an iatrogenic result in attempting the therapy, either in terms of the dental outcome or in terms of an adverse event in the patient's health or quality of life?
6 What is the prognosis of the proposed therapy? What will happen if no treatment is rendered? What is the worse case scenario?
7 What skills does the dentist have? What is his or her experience with this type of problem? Are the equipment and materials necessary to accomplish the proposed therapy available and part of the provider's knowledge base?

Then we must consider orally related factors [25]:

1 What is the problem?
2 Why did it occur?
3 How bad is the condition? What is the degree of dental and/or periodontal disease? If it is a tooth in question, how badly decayed is it? Is it restorable? Is it abscessed?
4 What is the overall oral health status? What is the ability to maintain oral hygiene?
5 What is the importance of the tooth to the patient's ability to function? What is the tooth's importance to the patient's occlusion?
6 What is the caries or other disease risk or experience for the patient? [25]

The next step will be to approach the therapeutic plan systematically. Once the patient's problems have been identified, diagnosed and a resolution selected, it is time to organize and implement.

Box 14.1 Phases of a treatment plan.

1 Diagnosis and emergency
2 Stabilization
3 Terminal
4 Recall and re-evaluation

The initial phase of the planning process has been discussed and it would be described as the data collection and diagnostic step in the treatment planning of a patient. Once problems have been identified, it is necessary to prioritize them.

The pressing conditions that need prompt attention will be addressed first. They can be considered an emergency when the patient is in pain or presents with an infection. These conditions require attention to the causative agent of the pain or infection, particularly when the infection is so severe as to cause delirium or cognitive changes. This must be delivered within the context of the patient-level factors cited above. The importance of the intervention at this point is to remove or ameliorate the condition that is causing pain or address the infection. This may be something that the dentist can do or may require referral to a site that can address the patient's emergency needs.

The second phase of a treatment plan would involve those procedures that will stabilize the patient's oral status. The objectives of this phase are to correct active disease entities so they do not progress, and complete initial therapies that have an influence on the definitive treatment proposed. At this time, it is also critical to evaluate the patient's control of environmental factors, ability and willingness to participate in their maintenance. Oral hygiene is evaluated; efforts are made to show the patient how it needs to improve to optimize oral health. Homecare efforts can be supplemented with dietary counselling and fluoride applications as appropriate.

Consider the need to alter the plan of treatment based on the outcome of the first two phases of treatment. Then prepare the patient for definitive treatment if that is part of the plan of treatment.

The third phase of a treatment plan is the terminal or rehabilitative phase.

The objective of this phase is to complete definitive treatment procedures that will restore the oral condition to optimal health and function. Recall that in the geriatric patient that definition includes the patient factors discussed previously.

Finally, there is a phase of the treatment plan that typically occurs at the completion of all treatment but should be in constant consideration throughout the execution of all phases of the plan of treatment. This fourth phase would be outcomes assessment or evaluation of the effectiveness of treatment and solutions to problems, recall and maintenance. The objective of this phase is to assess the success of therapy, evaluate the reasons for failure if they occur and reinforce proper patient maintenance. This re-evaluation phase needs to occur constantly to assure that the plan of therapy is on track and that it is effectively meeting the needs of the patient and correcting the identified problems.

High on the list of needed observations that are of very serious consideration to the elderly patient is the ability to anticipate and prevent problems [26].

Treatment

The dentate patient will present with needs that are common to all patients of all ages and they will have conditions that are specifically common to the elderly. When we deal with patients in general, and not just the elderly, we as dentists have certain mechanical approaches to the problems with which patients present.

When the patient is dentate the typical approach is to restore teeth back to form and function. If we are dealing with carious lesions our approach and material selected will be dictated by the surfaces involved, the depth of the caries. When possible, we will be placing an appropriate direct restorative material. If the damage either due to caries or loss of tooth structure is extensive, our choices may be an indirect restorative approach to achieve the goal of returning the tooth to form and function.

When the dentition is missing and replacement is sought we will consider removable prosthetics in the form of complete dentures or partial dentures. When there is adequate tooth support in the edentulous areas to allow the placement of fixed prosthodontics, tooth borne therapy should be a consideration. Finally, we should also consider implants when conditions permit as there is no evidence other than patient health issues and economic conditions to contraindicate the implementation of implant therapy in the treatment planning of the geriatric patient [27].

Endodontic therapy (see Chapter 16 on pulp diseases) and periodontal therapy (see Chapter 17 on periodontal diseases) do not change because of age and the therapy, when indicated, will proceed with outcomes that are similar to other population groups. However, endodontic therapy among elders is more likely to be complicated by pulpal sclerosis.

The geriatric population group does require us to consider the appropriateness of any of these therapies in the context of what is in the patient's best interest and what will be the benefit they will gain from accepting these therapies.

Looking carefully at each of the treatment options

Caries is a chronic infectious disease [28] that is common in the elderly. The causative agents are identified as *Streptococcus mutans* and to a lesser extent *Lactobacilli* [29]. The definition of caries is the destruction caused by progressive decalcification of the mineralized tissue as a result of acids produced by plaque bacteria from the surface towards the pulp. Classification is generally based on the surface the caries is found and the severity of the lesion is based on the activity and degree of damage caused by the process [30].

Many geriatric patients have gingival recession with exposure of additional root and interproximal surfaces. A generalized decline in the ability to maintain plaque free tooth surfaces and other patient-related factors leads to a particular susceptibility to root caries.

In 1989 Billings published an index for root surface lesions to assist in assigning treatment choices [31] (see Table 14.4).

The materials available to accomplish the restoration of the form and function of the damaged teeth are: dental amalgam, composite resin, glass ionomer and indirect restorations (crown and inlays/onlays). Because restorations have a finite life expectancy and there is an attendant risk of recurrent caries and new caries, we need to also include the prevention of new caries using other options such as fluoride (See Chapter 15 on caries).

Treatment options can be varied but generally are determined by the size and severity of the lesion (see Table 14.5) and the benefits restoring this tooth will have to the patient's overall condition. Incipient lesions may respond to homecare instruction and the use of fluoride. When the appearance of the surface suspected of being caries is hard, smooth and polished in appearance, treatment should be conservative. When this lesion is soft, the affected areas should be removed conservatively and restored with amalgam, composite or glass ionomer. The choices of the restorative material may be dictated by aesthetics and ability to obtain retention in or on the remaining tooth structure.

Glass ionomer, with its ability to be adherent to the tooth surface by chelation, is a popular material to use. It also has an advantage of containing fluoride which may decrease the recurrence of decay in the adjacent surfaces [32].

Composite resin allows a rapid and simple approach to treatment of many restorative needs in a single visit. It has an additional benefit in that repairs and additions can be made to these restorations by proper preparation and re-etching of the appropriate surfaces. Composite resin restorative materials rely on bonding to etched tooth surfaces (enamel and dentine). Enamel surfaces that are properly etched provide the best bond strengths. Dentine bond strengths are typically weaker. The dentine bond strength is dependent on the dentinal tubules and collagen. The dentinal tubules are where the micromechanical retention occurs. Teeth of the elderly have had more time to accumulate the effects of attrition, erosion and abrasion and sclerotic dentine making it more difficult to successfully bond to their teeth. The restorative dentist must therefore keep this in mind when treating the teeth of the elderly and maximize the potential bond strengths by careful adherence to the principles of bonding (isolation, maximization of quality collagen, moist demineralized dentine and maximum enamel surface areas). Various generations of bonding systems have evolved with the goals of simplifying the process and improving the bond strength to enamel and dentine.

Table 14.4 Index for root caries severity [31]

Grade	Surface texture	Surface defect	Pigmentation
Grade 1 Incipient	Soft, can penetrate with an explorer	No surface defect	Light tan to brown
Grade 2 Shallow	Soft, irregular, rough can be penetrated with an explorer	0.5 mm or less in depth	Tan to dark brown
Grade 3 Cavitation	Soft can penetrate with an explorer soft	Penetrating lesion cavitation present greater than 0.5 mm	Light brown to dark brown
Grade 4 Pulpal	Deeply penetrating	Defect that has pulpal involvement	Brown to dark brown

Table 14.5 Treatment considerations for root caries [31]

Grade	Treatment and materials	Advantages	Limitations	Adjunctive treatment
Incipient	Polish only with flexible discs, polishing points and prophylaxis paste	Noninvasive	Access, especially interproximal	Topical fluoride
Shallow	Recontour and smooth with abrasive points and fine diamonds then treat as in the Incipient Grade	Minimal invasive	Access, especially interproximal	Topical fluoride
Cavitated	Restore with glass-ionomer, possibly composite resin	Minimal preparation and fluoride release with glass ionomer	Access, especially interproximal and at margins of other restorative materials	Topical fluoride

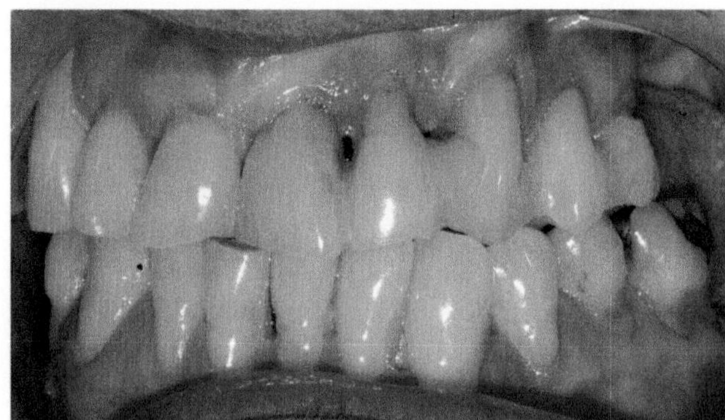

Figure 14.1 Splinting saves teeth.

Composite restorative material has the added benefit of being used to splint teeth. Periodontally involved teeth that are mobile can be stabilized and their longevity improved by a simple procedure of bonding teeth together with composite and a fibre material. Splinting can also be used as an inexpensive alternative to a fixed solution when a single tooth needs to be replaced. The extracted tooth or a replica can be splinted to the adjacent teeth and provide the patient with an inexpensive alternative to the restoration of the edentulous site with an indirect solution. Care needs to be taken with these direct approaches to ensure that the resultant architecture is cleansable by the patient.

Prosthodontic care

Frequently complete and partial removable dentures are necessary to restore function and facial support to the geriatric patient. When a patient lacks sufficient supportive occlusal units, a partial denture is indicated. This restorative therapy can provide occlusal support and return function to the patient. Having occlusal support protects the temporomandibular joint. It also improves function, allowing the ability to provide proper nutrition through better mastication of a variety of food substances. The tooth supported removable partial denture will have the added benefit of force distribution and protection of the remaining teeth from excessive occlusal forces on the unsupported dentition. The use of a partial denture will also provide needed stability to complete dentures. The distal extension partial denture is particularly useful in the improvement of the stability of a complete denture, improvement of mastication and support to the temporomandibular joint [33]. The treating dentist needs to recognize that this type of prosthesis must be maintained and relined as the supporting ridge undergoes atrophy and the partial becomes ill-fitting. Timely relining will ensure that it continues to fit well and that it does not burden the supporting dentition. The treating dentist should also recognize that this type of treatment is not required in a patient that does not manifest signs or symptoms of functional disturbances or a subjective demand for this type of treatment. The dentist must make the patient aware that removable therapy is ongoing and that monitoring, relining and replacement are parts of this therapy.

The design of all prosthetics should include a provision for failure. This will permit a provision for repair or correction of the existing prosthesis's with minimal expense and disruption of the patient's life.

Complete denture therapy usually falls under the following categories: the patient broke or lost his or her denture; the denture has become excessively worn and no longer functions or fits; the dentition is beyond hope and/or is insufficient to support any other reasonable solution. Aesthetics forces some patients to seek a new denture and this may be instigated by the patient or frequently a family member.

The completely edentulous geriatric patient often has atrophic supporting alveolar structures and changes in the vertical dimension of occlusion. Care must be exercised in the construction of the new denture. One must address the need to increase vertical dimensions carefully. Tooth placement must be guided by impression techniques that capture the 'neutral zone' [34]. The neutral zone (see Figure 14.2) is defined as 'the area in the mouth where, during function, the forces of the tongue pressing outwards are neutralized by the forces of the cheeks and lips pressing inwards' [34]. The 'neutral zone' philosophy is based upon the concept that for each individual patient there exists within the denture space a specific area where the function of the musculature will not unseat the denture and where forces generated by the tongue are neutralized by the forces generated by the lips and cheeks. The influence of tooth position and flange contour on denture stability is equal to or greater than that of any other factor.

Those dentists who ascribe to this philosophy of denture fabrication feel one should not be dogmatic and insist that teeth be placed over the crest of the ridge, or buccal or lingual to the ridge; rather teeth should be placed as dictated by the musculature, and this will vary for different patients.

Positioning artificial teeth in the neutral zone achieves two objectives. First, the teeth will not interfere with the normal muscle function and second, the forces exerted by the musculature against the dentures are more favourable for stability and retention [35].Where there is a highly atrophic ridge and a history of denture instability, a denture that is shaped by muscle function and that is in harmony with the surrounding oral structures will be more effective [35]. This technique is adaptable to partial dentures with extensive edentulous replacement areas and overdentures.

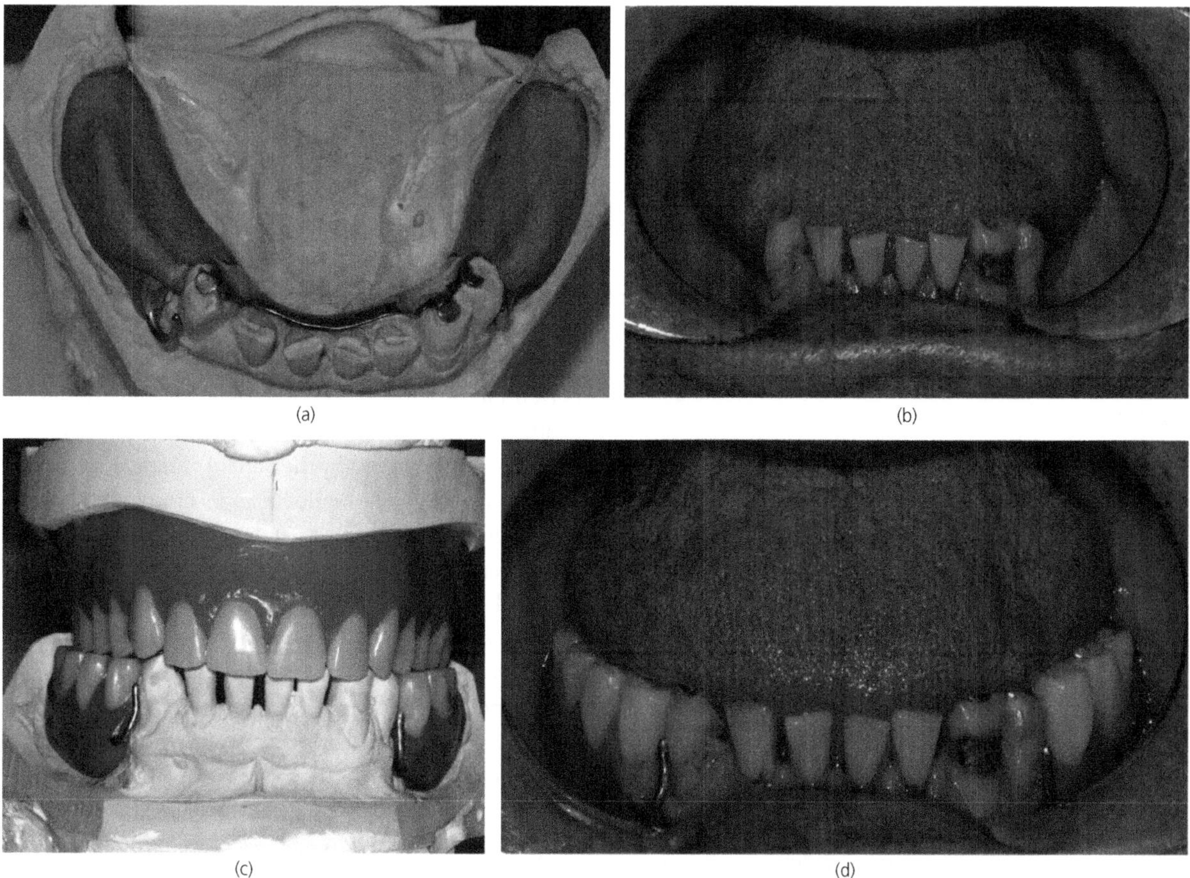

Figure 14.2 Positioning of teeth in the neutral zone. **a)** Midline of ridge and conventional place teeth are placed VS neutral zone directed. **b)** Tongue size and location will interfere with tooth positioned over the ridge. **c)** Result in a cross bite set-up. **d)** Harmony of the tongue and buccinator muscles with tooth location in the neutral zone.

Overlay dentures or removable partial dentures are options that should not be overlooked in patients with some remaining teeth. The retained roots provide support and stabilization to the removable prosthesis. The retained periodontal ligament provides proprioception giving the patient a better sense of discrimination than with a conventional denture. The alveolar bone is preserved by the existence of the retained roots and this will minimize future resorption of the alveolar ridge. The retained roots may be a site for retentive devices that will aid in the success of wearing the denture. A deterrent associated with this therapy is the added expense of the endodontic treatment that may be required and continuing preventive treatment required to preserve the retained root structure [33]. One of the most common reasons for failure of overdenture abutments is caries.

Fixed restorations may be required when the damage is extensive and the ability to return the tooth or teeth to form and function requires this level of treatment. Here the dentist must look at the necessity of the treatment and the ability of the patient to benefit from this therapy. Not all teeth are equally important in function and need to be restored or replaced. Third molars and second molars for example are expendable in a mouth that has a stable occlusion involving first molars and premolars [36]. There are a number of studies that point to 'sufficient adaptive capacity to maintain adequate oral function when at least four posterior occlusal units remain' [36, 37]. Contemporary adhesive approaches to prostheses retention add a further dimension to the prosthodontics dynamic (see Chapter 22).

Periodontal care

The fact that more geriatric patients are retaining their teeth and doing so for longer periods of their lives makes them at risk for periodontal disease. The diagnostic procedures and techniques for treatment do not change because the patient is elderly. It is well accepted that the response to periodontal therapy is similar to younger adult patients [38].

The concept that should be a guiding principle for treatment is the appropriateness of these therapies in the context of what is in the patient's best interest and what will be the benefit they will gain from accepting these therapies. Treatment should not be limited by the patient's age but by their medical condition, physical and functional capacity to accept treatment and financial resources.

Routine preventive care is very important in this population. By keeping a patient in an active prevention programme we limit the damage caused by untreated periodontal disease. The elderly patient will benefit from an aggressive preventive approach and may be able to avoid surgical intervention by recall appointments that are as frequent as every two months [39].

Implants

Dental implants have become a common first treatment choice when dentists consider options for tooth replacement. This therapy has the capacity to make significant contributions to a patient's health and well-being. The elderly dental patient is a potential beneficiary of this technology when it is not contraindicated by medical risk, patient resources or is without merit in the patient's treatment desires or needs.

The use of implants in combination with the restorative options in the treatment of the fully edentulous patient has made a significant improvement to the health, function and self esteem of those that choose this treatment option. It is generally considered the standard of care to offer an overdenture retained by two implants in the mandibular arch [40].

The restoration of the edentulous maxillary arch will also benefit from the incorporation of implants in the design but the maxilla is different to the mandible in the resorptive pattern, loading pattern, bone quality and volume. This makes rehabilitation of the maxillary arch comparatively more challenging. The standard of care for maxillary implant use in terms of the minimal number is still being debated and may be a variable that is driven by the patient's anatomy.

The patient's desires must be matched to the diagnostic realities. The patient's tooth display, inter arch space, quality and quantity of bone are factors that must be considered in the planning of the implant supported rehabilitation. The general options that can be offered to the patient address the support and retention of the restorations. The choices are removable and fixed and within the removable category there are sub categories of resilient and rigid. The cost and sophistication of the treatment accelerates as one progresses from the resilient to the fixed option.

Examples of geriatric patient treatment plans

Patient BJ is an 85-year-old Caucasian female who lives independently and has hypertension (180/95), osteoarthritis of the hands and hips, high cholesterol and has undergone a knee replacement. She is on a limited, fixed income and functions adequately with some strategic teeth and an upper partial denture. The lower arch has premolars that provide occlusal stops and support when the maxillary partial is in place. Homecare is a struggle for this patient and she is encouraged to return for prophylaxis and oral hygiene instruction on a quarterly basis. Unfortunately, she feels a semiannual visit is adequate. Her poor homecare and infrequent recall visits have led to recurrent decay on the root surfaces of the heavily restored maxillary incisor teeth. Her periodontal status is presently stable but there has been loss of attachment and boney support in localized areas. Gingival health is compromised by the patient's inadequate homecare. Her treatment plan should include monitoring BP, meds, and overall health status, and to continue to encourage the patient to seek more frequent care and to supplement her oral hygiene regime with a high fluoride containing dentifrice (Prevident 5000™ Colgate). Restoratively, the caries will be removed and the resulting cavity restored with glass ionomer (Ketac Molar™) (Figure 14.3). The existing restorations are considered stable and will not be replaced. Ideal therapy may have been to crown these teeth but the periodontal status of these teeth made them a poor risk and the patient's economics made this option impossible.

Patient OT is a 90-year-old Caucasian male who is still driving a car and is the primary care giver for a spouse with Alzheimer's disease. He takes 14 medications daily and suffers from a dry mouth that is exacerbated by his mouth breathing habit. The intra-oral exam found a dry mouth and smooth pale tongue, the hallmark of a poor diet. During the interview it was discovered that this patient did not have much of an appetite and had difficulty eating. His financial resources are severely limited and he is in need of extensive dental care. A treatment plan was developed for OT. At the time he presented he was wearing only an ill-fitting maxillary partial denture. His occlusion was not supported because he was missing posterior teeth in the mandibular right quadrant. He had some root surface caries and a chronic, generalized mild periodontitis with localized areas of moderate periodontitis, mild to moderate recession. During the treatment plan discussion with this patient, a maxillary denture was suggested and a lower partial denture recommended. The restorative needs were discussed and they were nominal. The patient expressed a strong desire to keep all remaining teeth and did not want to wear a maxillary denture. He understood and accepted the fact that tooth #26 had a poor long-term prognosis. Tooth #26 also had 4 mm of recession, class two buccal and distal furcation involvement and about 50% bone loss; this tooth was however stable.

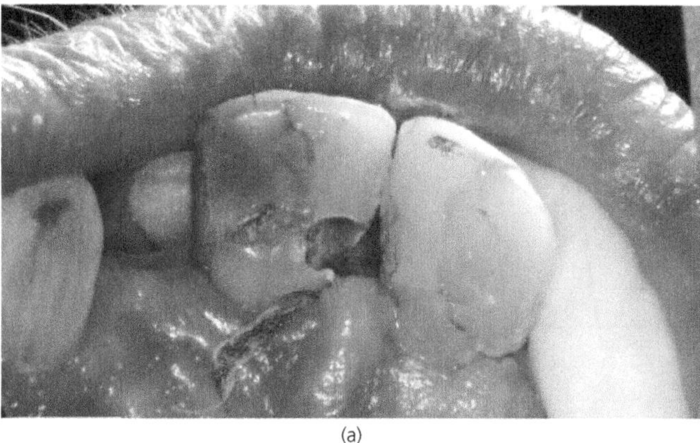

(a)

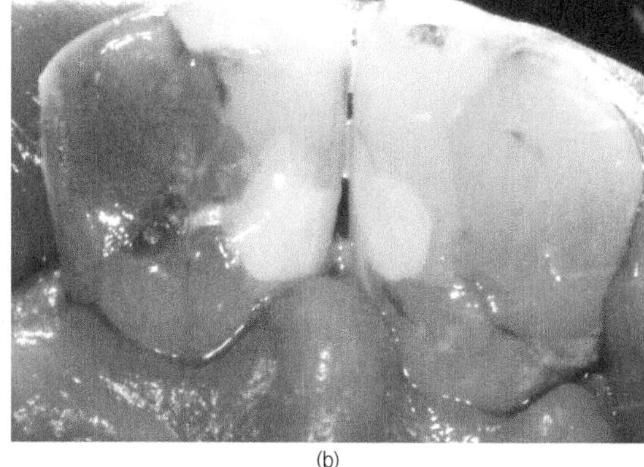

(b)

Figure 14.3 **a)** Carious lesion. **b)** Restored with glass ionomer (Ketac Molar™).

Transitional partial dentures were made for each arch and the four teeth that required simple treatment were restored. Tooth #26 was strategic to the retention of the partial denture but was a poor risk from a periodontal point of view; therefore, no aggressive therapy was planned for this tooth. A year after the treatment plan was completed, the patient developed symptoms in tooth #26. The diagnosis was irreversible pulpitis and endodontic therapy would be the appropriate treatment if the tooth was not a periodontal risk. The cost of this therapy was not affordable and the poor prognosis for this tooth made endodontic treatment inappropriate. In discussion with the patient, the poor/hopeless prognosis for this tooth was explained and extraction was discussed. Had we extracted this tooth, the ability to wear the denture would be compromised. The agreed upon alternative treatment was to extirpate the pulp and place a glass ionomer restoration (Ketac Molar™) with the agreement that if this treatment was unsuccessful this tooth would have to be extracted. The treatment was performed and the tooth continues to provide retention for the maxillary partial over two years later (Figure 14.4). He was encouraged to supplement his diet with liquid supplements.

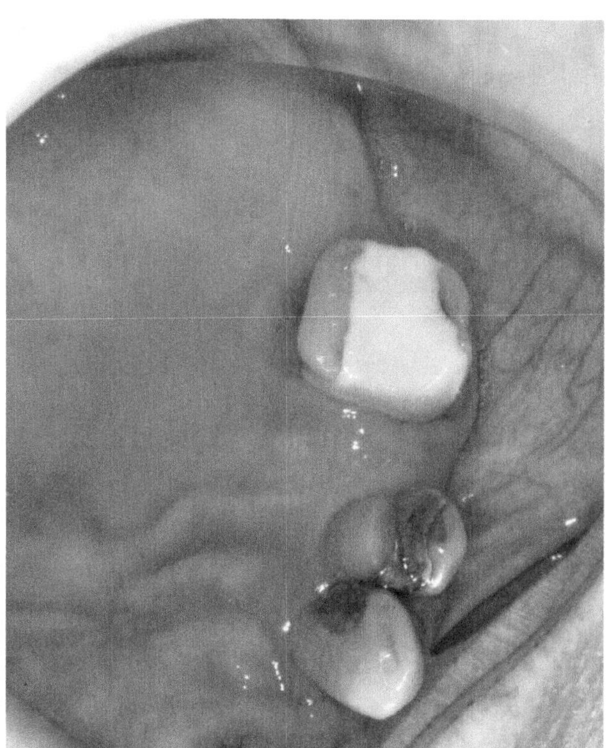

Figure 14.4 Glass ionomer (Ketac Molar™) provisional restoration 2 years post placement.

Patient CS is an 86-year-old Caucasian male with congestive obstructive pulmonary disease. He has been an active member of the dental practice for over 20 years. During that time he has undergone maxillary and mandibular reconstruction using fixed prosthodontics, i.e. crowns and bridges. Over time he has had endodontic failures and episodes of aggressive periodontal disease. His treatment post reconstruction has centred on prevention and maintenance. The 'shortened dental arch' [36] concept and splinting of teeth to add support to weak teeth has been responsible for this reconstruction being successful for more than 20 years (Figure 14.5). This patient demonstrates good plaque control and is very motivated. He uses a variety of dental cleaning devices and a high fluoride content dentifrice (1.1% NaF fluoride gel or paste). Recently, a mandibular anterior tooth had to be removed and this tooth was a terminal abutment of a three unit mandibular anterior bridge. Replacement of this prosthesis would involve a six unit replacement and that was deemed excessive, given his age and health. The alternative treatment was a partial denture. The placement of a partial denture was an option that would always be available and, knowing this, it was decided to attempt maintaining the existing bridge by splinting the extracted tooth/crown to the

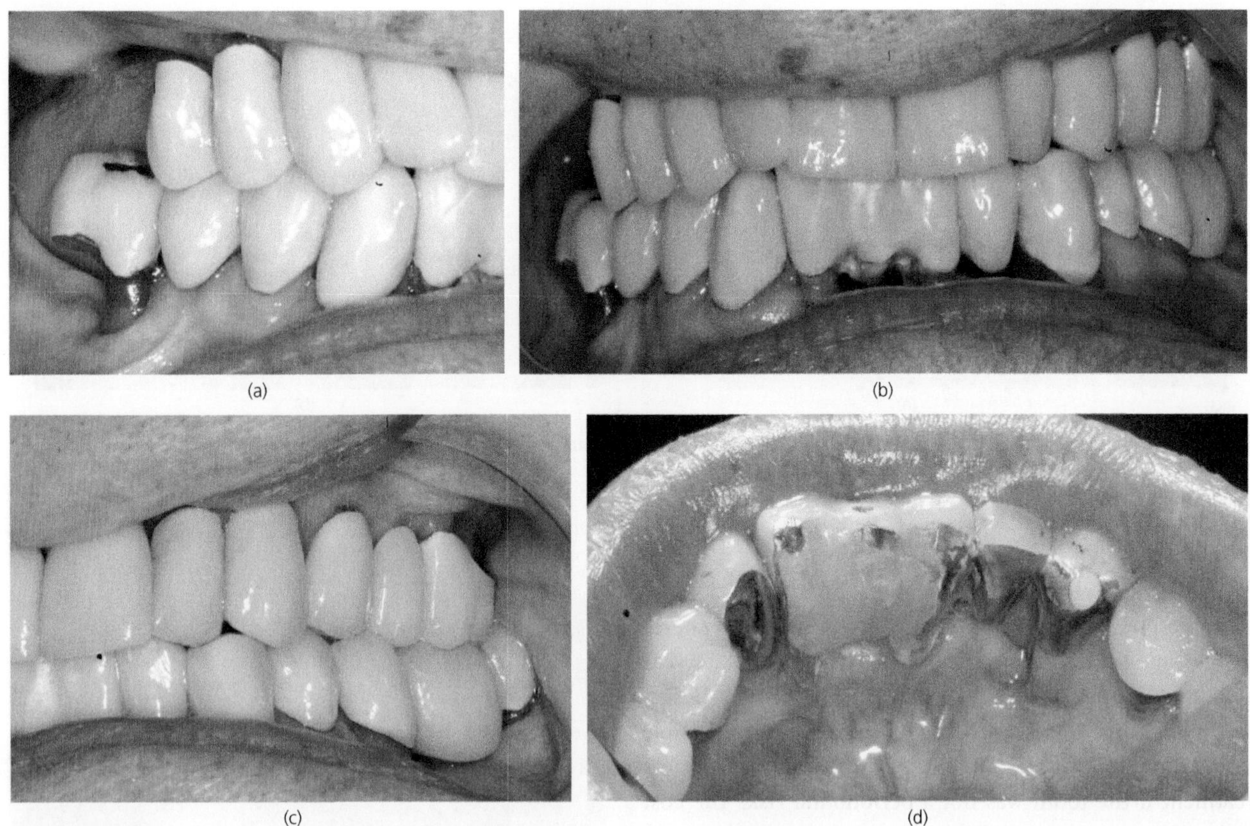

Figure 14.5 A 20-year-old reconstruction.

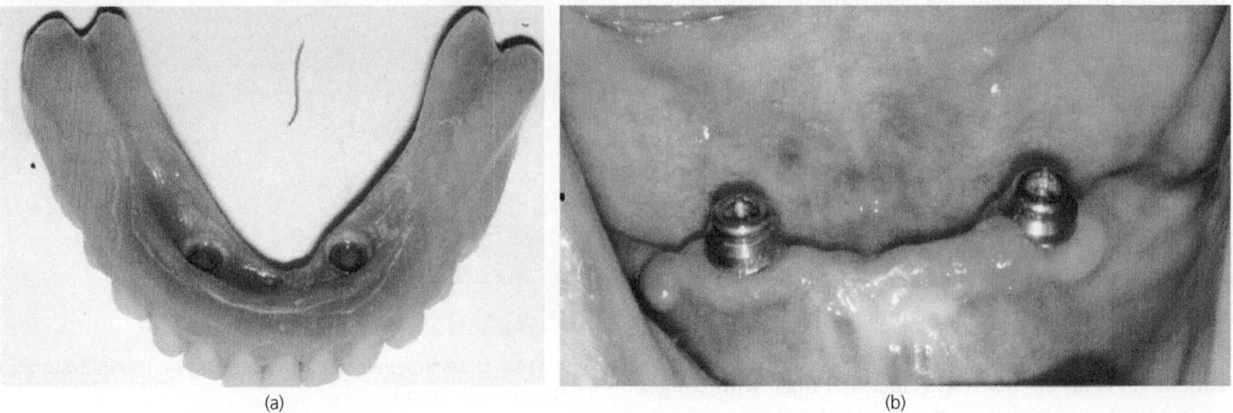

Figure 14.6 Implant-retained lower overdenture.

remaining intact fixed splint by using composite and resin fibre. This alternative therapy has been a successful solution for over two years and has kept this patient from having to wear a mandibular partial denture.

Patient CS is a 70-year-old Caucasian female who presented with the chief complaint of an inability to wear a mandibular partial denture and an ill-fitting complete maxillary denture. Both of these removable prostheses were ten or more years old and the patient had not been under the regular care of a dentist once these prostheses were inserted. During the exam it was found that the anterior teeth which supported a bilateral distal extension removable partial denture were periodontally hopeless, with over 90% bone loss and vertical mobility. They were uncomfortable to the patient and interfered with her ability to eat. The ill-fitting upper denture and lower partial had been responsible for accelerated ridge resorption and successful removable therapy was in question. The treatment plan was to initially extract all remaining teeth, and then fabricate a new set of complete maxillary and mandibular dentures and utilize the 'neutral zone' technique. In the discussion of treatment the option of implants was presented. The plan called for the fabrication of the dentures, and if added retention was desired, implants would be placed and the denture retrofitted to an overdenture with implant supported attachments (Locators™). Delivery of the conventional complete dentures went well, with the exception of the mandibular denture. Despite a technically excellent mandibular prosthesis, the patient was unable to wear it on her severely resorbed mandibular ridge without resorting to denture adhesive. The implant option was exercised and the mandibular denture converted to an implant-retained overdenture, with implants in the area of 33 and 43. The final result is pictured in Figure 14.6 and the patient has been a very successful denture wearer.

Conclusion

In conclusion, this chapter outlines a pragmatic approach to treatment planning that is based on a comprehensive dental, medical, psychological, social and functional assessment of the patient. The patient's desires and perceived needs must be considered, as well as the ethical issues involved in decision making, including the concepts of autonomy, beneficence, non-maleficence, justice and veracity. Appropriate care was defined as care where the benefits outweigh the risks by a wide margin. Critical attributes of geriatric practitioners are compassion, caring and a thoughtful deliberation on the best solution along with a discussion with the patient (or caregiver) of the risks and benefits of alternative forms of treatment. Finally, and the most critical issue in treatment planning and treatment of the geriatric patient, is the competence of the practitioner.

References

1 Hargreaves, K. (2007) *Endodontics Colleagues for Excellence; Treatment Planning: Comparing the Restored Endodontic Tooth and the Dental Implant*. American Association of Endodontics.

2 Grembowski, D., Milgrom, P. & Fiset, L. (1988) *Factors Influencing Dental Decision Making. Journal of Public Health Dentistry*, **48**(3), 159.

3 Committee on Health Care in America. Institute of Medicine. (2001) *Crossing the Quality Chasm: A New Health Care System for the 21st Century*. pp. 226–236, National Academy Press. Washington, DC.

4 Mohammad, A.R. & Preshaw, P.M. (2003) Current Status of Predoctoral Geriatric Education in U.S. Dental Schools. *Journal of Dental Education*, **67**, 509–514.

5 National Institute on Aging, National Institute of Health. (2007) *Growing Old in America: The Health and Retirement Study*. US Department of Health and Human Services, NIH No. 07-5757.

6 National Center for Health Statistics (2006) *Federal Interagency Forum on Aging Related Statistics*. National Center for Health Statistics, pp. 12–30, Hyattsville, MA.

7 Institute of Aging. *The Future is Aging*, p. 3, Canadian Institutes of Health Research, University of British Columbia, Vancouver, BC.

8 Jones, J.A. & Brown, E.J. (2000) Target Outcomes for Long Term Oral Health Care: a Delphi Approach. *Journal of Public Health Dentistry*, **60**(4), 330–334.

9 Gawande, A. (2007) The Annals of Medicine, The Way We Age Now. *The New Yorker*, (April 30).

10 Hwang, D., & Wang, H. (2006) Medical Contraindications to Implant Therapy: Part 1: Absolute Contraindications. *Implant Dentistry*, **15**(4), 353–360

11 Cigolle, C.T., Langa, K.M., Kabeto, M.U., Tian, Z. & Blaum, C.S. (2007) Geriatric Conditions and Disability: The Health and Retirement Study. *Annals of Internal Medicine*, **147**(8), 156–164.

12 Schwartz, M. (2000) The Oral Health of the Long-Term Patient: Clinical Care and Aging. *Annals of Long-Term Care*, **8**(12), 41–46.

13 Grove, R.D & Hetzel, A.M. (1968) *Vital Statistics in the United States, 1940-1960*. US Government Printing Office, Washington, DC.

14 Arias, E. (2004) *United States Life Tables, 2004*. Center for Disease Control and Prevention, National Center for Health Statistics, National Vital Statistics System, Hyattsville, MD.

15 Smith, J.M., & Sheiham, A. (1979) How Dental Conditions Handicap the Elderly. *Community Dentistry and Oral Epidemiology*, **7**, 305–310.

16 Sreebny, L.M. (2000) Saliva in Health and Disease: An Appraisal and Update. *International Dental Journal*, **5**(3), 140–161.

17 Mandel, I.D. (1989) The Role of Saliva in Maintaining Oral Homeostasis. *Journal of the American Dental Association*, **119**, 298–304.

18 Ghezzi, E.M., & Ship, J.A. (2000) Systemic Diseases and Their Treatments in the Elderly: Impact on Oral Health. *Journal of Public Health Dentistry*, **60**(4) 289–296.

19 Baker, H. (2007) Nutrition in the Elderly: Hypovitaminosis and Its Implications. *Geriatrics*, **62**(8), 22–26.

20 Baum, B.J., Caruso, A.J., Ship, J.A., & Wolff, A. (1991). Oral Physiology, In: A. Papas & H. Chauncey (eds), *Geriatric Dentistry Aging and Oral Health*, pp. 71–80, Mosby, St. Louis, MO.

21 National Institute of Dental Research. *Oral health of United States adults: The National Survey of Oral Health in U.S. Employed Adults and Seniors: 1985–1986*. NIH Publication 87-2868, National Institutes of Health, Bethesda, MD.

22 Levy, B.M. (1991) Disease-related Changes in Older Adults, In: A. Papas & H. Chauncey (eds), *Geriatric Dentistry Aging and Oral Health*. p. 87, Mosby, St. Louis, MO.

23 Fontana, M., & Zero, D. (2006) Assessing Patients' Caries Risk. *Journal of the American Dental Association*, **137**(9), 1231–1239.

24 Barsh, L.I. (1981) Dental Treatment Planning for the Adult Patient, *152-303*, WB Saunders Company, Philadelphia, PA.

25 Ettinger, R. L., & Berkey, D.B. (1991). Treatment Planning for the Older Patient. In: A. Papas & H. Chauncey (eds), *Geriatric*

Dentistry Aging and Oral Health, pp. 126–137; Mosby, St. Louis, MO.

26 Fishman, N. (1979) Overview of the Practitioner-Patient Relationship in Aged Persons. In: *Geriatric Dentistry*, Ch. 20, pp. 243–246, Lexington Books, Lexington, MA.

27 Stanford, C.M. (2007) Dental Implants a Role in Geriatric Dentistry for the General Practice? *Journal of the American Dental Association*, **138**(9), 34s–39s.

28 US Department of Health and Human Services. *Oral Health in America: A Report of the Surgeon General*. National Institutes of Health, National Institute of Dental and Craniofacial Research, HHS, Rockville, MD.

29 Hintao, J., Teanpaaisan, R., Chongsuvivatwong, V., Dahlen, G., & Rattarasarn, C. (2007) Root Surface and Coronal Caries in Adults with Type 2 Diabetes Mellitus. *Community Dentistry and Oral Epidemiology*, **35**(4), 302–309.

30 Banting, D.W. (1991) Management of Dental Caries in the Older Patient. In: A. Papas & H. Chauncey (eds), *Geriatric Dentistry Aging and Oral Health*, Ch. 9, pp. 141–164, Mosby Co., St. Louis, MO.

31 Billings, R.J. (1989) Restoration of Carious Lesions of the Root. *Gerontology*, **5**(1), 43.

32 Matis, B.A., Cochran, M., & Carlson, T. (1996) Longevity of Glass-ionomer Restorative Materials: Results of a 10-year Evaluation. *Quintessence International*, **27**(6), 373–382.

33 Budtz-Jorgensen, E. (1986). Prosthetic Considerations in Geriatric Dentistry, In: P. Holm-Pedersen & H. Löe, *Geriatric Dentistry: a Textbook of Oral Gerontology*. Ch. 24, pp. 321–351, Mosby Co., St. Louis, MO.

34 Beresin, V., & Schiesser, F. (2006) The Neutral Zone in Complete Dentures. *The Journal of Prosthetic Dentistry*, **95**(2), 93–100.

35 Gahan, M.J., & Walmsley, A.D. (2005). The Neutral Zone Impression Revisited. *British Dental Journal*, **198**(5), 269–272.

36 Kayser, A.F. (1981). Shortened Dental Arches and Oral Function. *Journal of Oral Rehabilitation*, **8**(5), 457.

37 Ramfjord S.P. & Ash M.M., (1976) *Periodontology and Periodontics*, WB Saunders Co., Philadelphia, PA.

38 Boehm, T. K., & Scannapieco, F.A. (2007). The Epidemiology, Consequences and Management of Periodontal Disease in Older Adults. *Journal of the American Dental Association*, **138**, 34s–39s.

39 Suzuki, J.B., Niessen, L.C. & Fedele, D.J. (1991). Periodontal Disease in the Older Adult. *Geriatric Dentistry Aging and Oral Health*, **11**, 189–201.

40 Das, K.P., Jahangiri, L. & Katz, R.V. (2012) The first-choice standard of care for an edentulous mandible; A Delphi method survey of academic prosthodontist in the United States. *Journal of the American Dental Association*, **143**(8), 881–889.

CHAPTER 15

Caries in the older person

Angus W. G. Walls[1] **and David Ricketts**[2]
University of Edinburgh, Edinburgh, UK; University of Dundee, Dundee, UK

Introduction

Tooth decay is one of the most common bacterial diseases in man. Evidence of tooth decay has been identified from skeletal remains that are thousands of years old, so this disease is not 'new' in the sense that it is something that has developed or become of more clinical significance in recent times. (Unlike, for example, erosive pattern tooth wear which seems to be undergoing a rapid increase at present.) However, it is also not a disease that would have had any significant influence in terms of evolution of teeth and the oral environment. Primitive man evolved over thousands of years with the simple diet of the hunter gatherer. This would be low in sugars intake, particularly readily fermentable carbohydrate, so caries was not a great cause of tooth loss. It becomes a recorded cause of damage to teeth with the development of civilizations where sugars formed an important component of diet, particularly added sugars. Thus there is evidence of caries from ancient Egypt and the other civilizations from that time to the present day.

The consequences of caries include loss of tooth structure, potential pain and ultimately loss of teeth, giving rise to impaired appearance and oral function (see Chapter 22). It is the management of this damage that forms the basis of much of the work that is undertaken by the practising dentist. Unfortunately the majority of the effort from the profession is directed at managing the physical damage to teeth (by placing restorations, or doing endodontics or extracting teeth in the worst case scenario), rather than trying to facilitate the prevention of this disease. This chapter will address both the aetiology, diagnosis and management of caries in the older adult, with a specific emphasis on trying to assist the practitioner in identifying those people who are at risk of developing this disease and hence facilitating effective, targeted prevention.

There are significant areas of overlap between the prevention of caries and the aetiology and management of xerostomia in older people. In an effort to minimize duplication this chapter will NOT address the aetiology and management of this condition but will include xerostomia as part of the risk assessment for caries. The reader is referred to Chapters 19 and 25 for detailed information about xerostomia.

Epidemiology

The traditional view of caries risk for older people identifies root caries as one of the principal challenges provided by the older person. However, contemporary epidemiological evidence would suggest that both coronal and root caries remain at high levels of prevalence in an older cohort (Figure 15.1). Indeed these data would suggest that coronal caries may have higher prevalence rates than root disease; however this assertion may be difficult to defend as all coronal surfaces are 'automatically' at risk from developing new disease whereas only those teeth where gingival recession has occurred have exposed root surfaces rendering the roots susceptible to caries. Hence, while the absolute prevalence of coronal disease is reported to be higher than root lesions, the number of teeth or surfaces at risk from disease may not be the same so the proportion of at risk surfaces that develop caries is likely to be different. Furthermore, much coronal caries occurs round existing restorations (so called recurrent carious lesions or more appropriately known as Caries Associated with Restorations and Sealants or CARS) while root caries tends to develop de novo on exposed tooth tissue.

There are a dearth of data which relate to caries risk or appropriate management strategies for coronal caries in the older population. There is an assumption that strategies

Textbook of Geriatric Dentistry, Third Edition. Edited by Poul Holm-Pedersen, Angus W. G. Walls and Jonathan A. Ship.

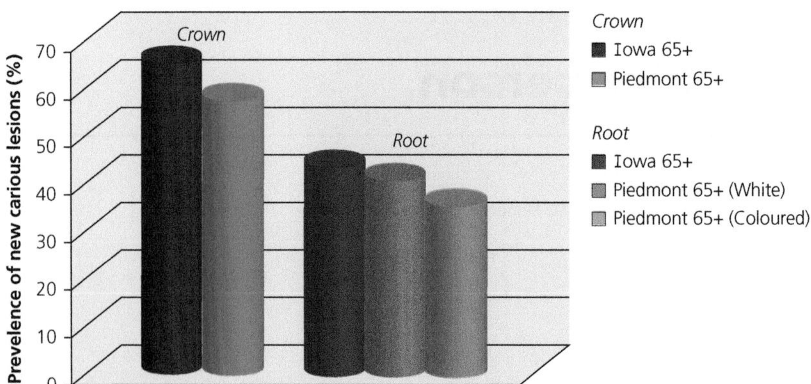

Figure 15.1 Caries prevalence in older population groups during longitudinal follow-up studies in Iowa and Piedmont. Significant levels of new carious lesions were seen over a 3-year follow-up period with coronal lesions being more common than root lesions.

that would be appropriate for coronal lesions in younger populations will also be relevant and effective for the older population. There are considerable data relating to root caries and those strategies that are directed at the tooth root will also likely prevent caries on the crown of the tooth, not least because it requires a lesser cariogenic challenge to develop caries on a dentine surface compared with an enamel surface.

Reporting caries in epidemiological studies

There are significant challenges associated with the reporting of caries in epidemiological studies of older people for three reasons:

Numbers of teeth

The number of teeth present is normally assumed to have been either 28 or 32 at baseline for most epidemiological programmes. In older population studies these numbers are more likely to be in the region of 15–20 at most and there is no way of determining accurately why missing teeth were extracted. Thus the M component of the standard epidemiological tool for describing caries, the DMF (Decayed, Missing, Filled) index, tends to be high and is of little value in determining disease activity. Teeth that were extracted for orthodontic purposes or because of periodontal disease may have been carious or have had restorations in them but there is simply no way of knowing. The M component can so dominate the DMF figure that changes in either D or F are difficult to detect.

Surfaces at risk

The crown of a tooth is generally fully exposed into the mouth in adults and hence any tooth which is present is likely to have a crown at risk of caries (the number of teeth used for overdenture abutments is very small on an epidemiological scale). The same cannot be said of roots. Gingival recession or periodontal disease has to occur before a root surface becomes exposed into the oral environment. Hence it is NOT safe to assume that all teeth have exposed roots and a simple report of the number of carious or restored roots may underestimate the level of disease activity. For example in a mouth with 20 teeth where there are 4 root lesions or restorations the prevalence of root caries could vary from as low as 20% (if all the teeth had exposed roots) to 100% (if only 4 had exposed roots). This problem has been recognised for some time and has been addressed with the relatively widespread use of the Root Caries Index (which is the proportion of exposed roots that have signs of active or treated disease).

Restorations

In younger people it is reasonable to assume that the surface of a tooth is restored because a dentist made a diagnosis of caries and prepared a cavity to assist with the management of the disease. This assumption is NOT valid for older people, particularly where prosthetic crowns are present and even (as far as surface scores are concerned) with large restorations. Teeth can and often are crowned because of tooth wear or fracture rather than decay and yet these surfaces are restored. Equally, teeth with large restorations often undergo fracture of weakened areas of the tooth structure requiring the replacement with even more extensive restorations. If data are reported as surface scores rather than at the tooth level (DMFS compared with DMFT) then this will result in an increase in the surface score which is not necessarily associated with caries. Finally, as far as the roots of teeth are concerned, dentists restore roots for two reasons: to manage decay and to manage cervical wear/sensitivity. Evidence from the UK suggests that about 55% of root restorations are placed because of sensitivity or wear with greater proportions in younger people. If restored surfaces are ignored

Table 15.1 Variables associated with caries risk from a population of older adults (data from the *UK National Diet and Nutrition Survey for People Aged 65 Years and Over*, oral health component)

	65–74	75–84	85+	Attenders	Non-attenders	Free living	Institution
Vulnerable roots	13.7	12.8	9.6	14.7	10.9	13.3	9.3
Filled but sound	1.9	1.8	1.5	2.6	0.6	1.9	0.8
Gross decay	0.3	0.4	0.6	0.1	0.8	0.3	0.7
New decay	0.8	0.8	1.3	0.6	1.2	0.8	1.7
Unsound restoration	0.2	0.1	0.2	0.2	0.1	0.2	0.3
RCI[a]	23%	24%	38%	24%	25%	24%	38%
RCI(c)[b]	16%	16%	29%	14%	22%	16%	33%
RCI(d)[c]	9%	10%	22%	6%	19%	10%	29%
Total	16.1	14.4	10.1	17.5	11.9	15.5	10.7

[a]RCI is the root caries index.
[b]RCI(c) is the root caries index corrected for the potential that 45% of the restorations seen in this population are there because of cervical wear or sensitivity rather than caries (after Walls *et al.* 2000).
[c]RCI(d) is the decay component of the root caries index alone
Note that decay is much more common in the older age group (85+), in those who do not attend the dentist regularly and in people living in long-stay care.

then caries prevalence will be underestimated and if they are included it will be overestimated (Table 15.1). It is likely that the pattern of provision of restorations on root surfaces will be specific within health care systems; currently there are no data available for the reasons for provision of restorations on root surfaces from any other countries.

Coronal caries

There are relatively few data about coronal caries risk in older people. It is likely that the majority of new coronal carious lesions in this age group will be lesions associated with restorations. There is considerable debate in the caries literature whether the term recurrent decay is a valid one as it implies continuation of a pre-existing problem rather than a new carious lesion developing around the periphery of a restoration. For the purposes of this chapter we will refer to all new carious lesions as that, whether or not they originate at a new hard tissue sight or at the interface between a restorative material and tooth structure.

Table 15.2 gives a summary of some of the studies that report coronal caries increment during a period of longitudinal follow-up among older individuals. As can be seen, there is wide variation in levels of caries activity and this picture is confused by both attrition bias in longitudinal studies and also that in the longer studies caries was also the most common reason for tooth extraction among the participants, so the overall caries increment will be an underestimate of caries activity as some will be masked by the loss of teeth. Whilst these studies report varied levels of caries activity, those that address caries activity among different age groups in the 'older' cohorts suggest that there is a relative reduction in coronal caries increment as the subjects age. The reason behind this phenomenon is unclear; there is no reason to think that caries risk per se decreases with age, however the numbers and distribution of teeth present in older people are different to the *young* even within the age cohorts investigated here. These changes are characterized by older people having fewer molar and premolar (bicuspid) teeth remaining as the numbers of teeth in their mouths fall. As a broad generalization, molar and premolar (bicuspid) teeth are more subject to coronal caries so it could simply be that the older cohorts investigated have had a different pattern of tooth retention rather than varying susceptibility to decay per se. Despite these variations, coronal caries is at least as common in older populations as root caries (Figure 15.1).

Root caries distribution within and between maxillary and mandibular arches has also been investigated. In the mandible, molar teeth are more commonly affected followed by premolar (bicuspid) teeth followed by anterior teeth. In the maxilla, risk is more evenly distributed. This may be due to the influence of the major salivary glands and the presence of the beneficial effects of saliva. It is unlikely to be due to ease of oral hygiene as the upper anterior teeth are most readily cleaned in the maxilla but most commonly affected by root caries.

There are very few studies that have looked specifically at risk variables for decay developing around existing restorations, particularly in older subjects. There is a broad acceptance that those generic variables which are associated with increased caries risk will affect both coronal and root surfaces of the teeth and around restorations on those surfaces (see below). There is also an ongoing debate whether specific restorations are more or less susceptible to the development of carious lesions at their periphery.

The value of fluoride within the restorative material seems to be limited when it comes to preventing new carious lesions around coronal restorations, and is only demonstrable in high-caries-risk populations.

Root caries

Root caries is often regarded as a specific problem in older people, in part because the exposure of root surface takes time to occur in the majority of people hence decay does not begin to develop for some time. That root dentine does develop caries is undisputed, and that the numbers of carious lesions present in older people on the surfaces of their teeth increases as they get older is also obvious. However there are few data that address the question whether or not there is a genuine age-associated increase in caries risk for older people on the root surface. A constant level of risk over 30 or 40 years would result in the overall numbers of restorations increasing with time (for example if the incidence of carious lesions was one surface every 10 years then there would be four carious/restored surfaces in a 40 year period). An increase in risk with age should be accompanied by an increasing rate of incidence of disease. There are relatively few studies that address this age associated risk, two of the studies in Table 15.2 do suggest that in a Scandinavian population there is an increase in caries in the older age groups. This is supported by Figure 15.2 which is a composite graph of root caries index against age for the UK using data from both the *1998 Adult Dental Health Survey* and the *UK National Diet and Nutrition Survey for People Aged 65 years and Over* where diagnostic criteria and training were identical and these data were collected within 18 months of each other. This seems to show constant risk of root caries up until the late 70s and then a sharp increase beyond that.

Any epidemiological data for root caries prevalence must be viewed in light of the concerns mentioned above about restored surfaces. This is particularly acute for the roots of teeth due to the use of restorations to manage both cervical wear defects and sensitivity. There are few data available which try to clarify when these conditions are more likely to be managed; those that are available would suggest that restorations

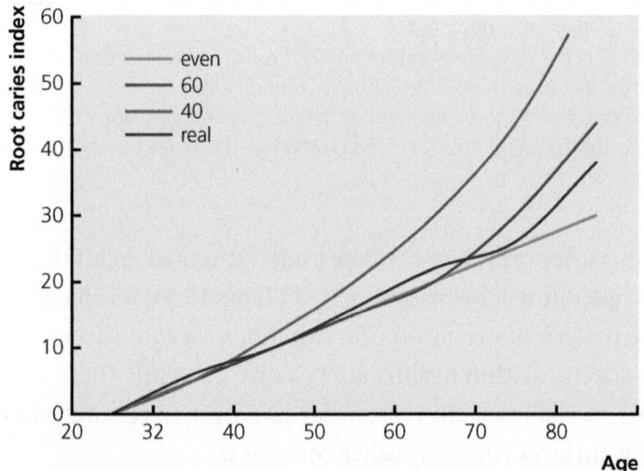

Figure 15.2 Root caries index profiles for three different levels of caries risk; constant risk is shown by the orange line, risk increasing at ages 40 and 60 are shown by the blue and red lines labelled 40 and 60. The real data plot (in purple) is a composite taken from data from the *UK Adult Dental Health Survey* for 1998 and the oral health component of the *UK National Diet and Nutrition Survey for People Aged 65 Years and Over*. The steep rise between the 70- and 80-year-old cohorts would suggest an age-associated change in risk.

Table 15.2 Coronal and root caries increments from a variety of longitudinal follow-up studies

Study	Age group	Follow-up	Coronal caries increment	Coronal/100 surfaces	Root caries increment	Root/100 surfaces
Lundgren *et al.*, 1997	88–92	4 years	1.3	4.5	3.6	17.5
Fure & Zickert, 1997	60	5 years	2.3		1.4	
	70	5 years	3.7		2.4	
	80	5 years	5.3		5.5	
Fure, 2003	55	10 years	6.0		5.3	
	65	10 years	3.8		8.1	
	75	10 years	1.9		14.3	
Hamassah *et al.*, 2005	65	9–11 years	18.3		1.27	
Hand *et al.*, 1988	'Elderly'	18 months	0.87[a]	1.4[a]	0.57[a]	2.6[a]
Drake *et al.*, 1997	65+ black	3 years	1.6	0.8[a]		
	65+ white		2.1	1.6[a]		
Lawrence *et al.*	65+ black	3 years			0.55	
	65+ white				0.8	
Chalmers *et al.*, 2005	82	1 year[b]	2.5		1.0	
Takano *et al.*, 2003	70	2 years			0.9	

[a]These are annualised data.

[b]These are data for nursing home residents.

are much more likely to be placed in young people to manage sensitivity and wear and in older people to manage caries. One further confounding variable is that many of the new lesions reported in some of the longitudinal follow-up studies seen in Table 15.2 were reported to occur around existing restorations rather than on previously unrestored surfaces. Some of those restorations are likely to have been placed originally to manage a worn or sensitive root surface rather than a carious lesion, but failure of the restoration with marginal breakdown makes an ideal environment for the development of a carious lesion on a surface that may not have undergone decay had it not previously been restored. Table 15.1 shows some of the effects of this sort of correction on root caries measurement and also the impact of age, habitual attendance patterns and being in long-term residential care on caries activity (caries is increased with older age groups, in people who don't habitually attend the dentist and in people living in long-term care).

Risk factors

Tissues exposed

Much of the focus on management and prevention of caries has focused historically on enamel and it is well documented that the pH for demineralization of enamel is of the order of 5.4.

However, when the root of the tooth becomes exposed in the mouth two other dental tissues can become involved in carious lesions, cementum and dentine. To all intent and purpose cementum is irrelevant in this context. It is a very thin layer of mineralized tissue that has a specialized function in maintaining the anchorage for the periodontal ligament providing tooth support. Once the periodontal ligament has been destroyed this tissue loses its vitality and one of the key objectives of periodontal therapy is removal of non-vital cementum from the surface of the root. Hence it is unlikely that there will be significant quantities of cementum involved in any carious lesion on a root. The bulk of the root comprises dentine, which has lower mineral content than enamel with a critical pH for demineralization of about 6. This has obvious implications for both the bacterial species that may be linked to root caries (in that bacteria which aren't capable of producing acids to reduce pH to 5.4 may be able to reduce it to between 6 and 5.4) and also the cycle of de- and remineralization associated with an acidic challenge. The Stephan curve will stay below pH 6 for longer than it will below 5.4 so for any given episode of acidic challenge the demineralization phase will be longer. Hence, the dynamic relationship between de- and remineralization is altered in relation to dentine compared with enamel (Figure 15.3).

Caries history

There is an association between root caries and previous caries experience, both coronal and root decay, and between the rate of development of new carious lesions around existing restorations with general caries activity. There are equivocal data for the relationship between past coronal caries experience (measured by the presence of restorations in teeth) and the likelihood of new root caries lesions. This is probably a reflection of variation in caries risk and also changes in dietary and other caries-related behaviours with age. Furthermore, the extent of restorations present in someone's mouth in old age may reflect past treatment practices by dentists rather than disease history, for example the use of the *prophylactic odontotomy* or cusp replacement when cusps are perceived to be weakened through decay.

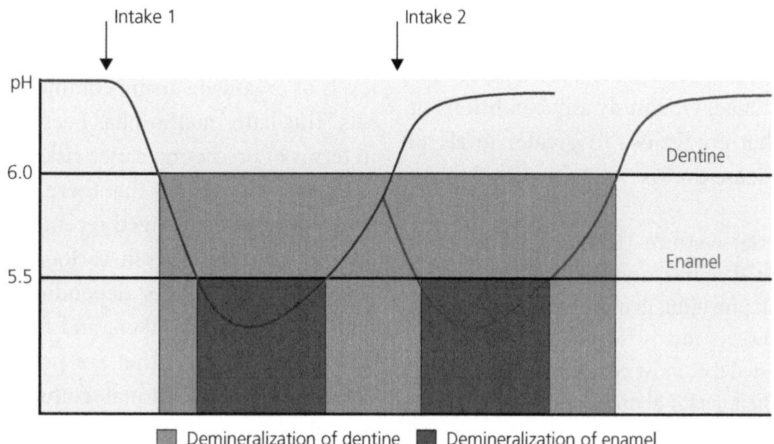

Figure 15.3 The impact of the pH of demineralization of dentine on the length of time that the tissue is exposed to demineralization for a *standard* episode of demineralization.

The association of risk for new root caries lesions with previous root caries experience is stronger than that for coronal decay, so that an individual who has a history of having had root caries in the past is more likely to develop a new root caries lesion than someone who has not. This association becomes stronger with increasing age of the individual. Again there is the potential for confounding here because a restoration on a root surface may not be there because of caries. Having said that, there is some evidence that the majority of restorations placed for older people on the roots of teeth are replacements of existing restorations and there are no data which correlate the reason why a restoration was first placed with the subsequent need for replacement. The estimated median longevity of tooth coloured restoration on root surfaces is of the order of 5–7 years, with some variation between composite resin and glass ionomer cement materials.

Periodontal disease

The relationship between periodontal disease and root caries is pivotal. Without attachment loss there would be no exposed root surfaces and hence root caries could not occur. Furthermore, caries is more likely to occur in patients with untreated periodontal disease compared with those who have been appropriately managed and can, and does, occur on root faces exposed in the mouth but which lie sub-gingivally within a periodontal pocket, making diagnosis and management more complex. People who are in the initial phase of periodontal therapy are also more susceptible to caries lesions developing than those whose treatment is complete. This appears to be associated with an increase in the numbers of *Streptococcus mutans* in the mouths of individuals in the initial phase of periodontal care, but is also likely to be linked to recent instrumentation of the root surface removing the hypermineralized layer which forms as a result of 'maturation' of the dentine surface with age.

Plaque and microflora

Plaque needs to be present on the surface of teeth before the carious lesion can be initiated. Obviously any conditions or clinical circumstances that predispose to greater levels of plaque retention will increase the risk of caries developing. These would include:

- **the presence of a partial denture (RPD).** There is good evidence to suggest that dentures need NOT be associated with increased caries risk providing denture and personal oral hygiene are optimal. However this is frequently not the case, indeed it has been suggested that most people who have partial dentures do so *because* their personal oral health care has been sub-optimal. Hence, without a significant change in personal health behaviour there will be an inevitable increased risk of disease. This increase in risk does not only affect the arch in which the denture is located. There are increases in plaque burden both in association with the denture itself and in the opposing dental arch if there isn't a denture there also.
- **impaired ability to perform personal oral hygiene.** Oral hygiene is a complex learned skill, which becomes more challenging as we age and the architecture an individual is trying to maintain plaque free becomes more complex. The challenges of appropriate personal oral health care become more acute in older people because of associated disease (for example someone with severe rheumatoid arthritis who has limited manual dexterity) or simply because of age changes to muscle which result in some muscle wasting (sarcopenia). Loss of muscle mass, particularly the fine motor fibres, makes fatigue during oral hygiene a clinical problem that needs to be addressed (see below).
- **alterations to the gingival architecture.** This is a particular problem with molar teeth and furcation involvement in attachment loss. Both the area within the furcation and the surfaces of the root that face towards each other can be particularly difficult to clean effectively. As an example, the surfaces of a lower molar's roots that face towards each other are, or tend to be, concave. This makes effective cleaning difficult necessitating the use of spiral brushes which can be a significant clinical challenge for older people because of physical limitations or simply because they have difficulty seeing what they are doing in a bathroom mirror.
- **altered visual acuity.** Many older people develop presbyopia as the lens of the eye hardens requiring spectacles for close vision. If someone has vari- or multifocal lenses in their spectacles then the close vision component is in the lower third of the lens frame making it difficult to see inside the mouth in a bathroom mirror.

The presence of a mature microbial plaque is a prerequisite for caries to occur. One of the debates associated with the higher pH for demineralization of dentine compared with that for enamel has been whether bacterial species that can ferment sugars to produce acids, but only result in a reduction of plaque pH that is above that for the demineralization of enamel, would have a significant role in the initiation or progression of root caries lesions.

The flora that is associated with caries is complex and can be assessed either by direct sampling or by screening for salivary levels of organisms using commercially available assessment kits. This latter method has been shown to have some value in terms of predicting caries risk

The traditional view that there is a characteristic *cariogenic flora* has been challenged recently with the recognition that culture of bacteria from carious lesions produces dramatically different results depending upon the pH at which the culture is undertaken, and furthermore that fewer than 50% of the bacteria that are present in the mouth can be detected by conventional culture techniques. A complex microbial flora is now being identified that is predominantly aciduric and includes *Lactobacilli*, *Actinomyces israelii* and *Strep mutans* from carious lesions, *Actinomyces gerencseriae* from sound root surfaces in patients with active lesions elsewhere in their mouths and *Streptococcus anginosus* and *Streptococcus oralis* in patients without root caries. There is no single grouping of bacteria that is pathognomonic of disease risk although salivary levels of both *Strep mutans* and *Lactobacilli* have been shown to be increased in caries active mouths. It is unclear which of these bacterial species are causative in terms of the carious lesion and which simply thrive better in an acidic environment.

There are some reports which also link *Candida* species to caries activity; again it is unclear what, if any, the role of *Candida* species is in the caries process although there are some suggestions that the collagenase that these yeast excrete may facilitate the spread of caries laterally through the dentine. They are also aciduric and may simply thrive better in this low pH environment.

Diet

Diet is just as important in relation to caries on dentine as it is for coronal caries. The frequency of sugars consumption remains important in the development of root caries. Between meals snacking, particularly in association with increased social activity in people who have retired, may be an important risk factor. The risk associated with increased frequency of sugars consumption extends to include the use of a sugar as a sweetener in tea and coffee, particularly in men. The overall quantity of sugars consumption is not as important as frequency, however there are few data covering this aspect of the aetiology of root decay. It should be remembered that highly refined/milled starches are also cariogenic. This can be influential in relation to between-meals snacking and advice to patients on choice of snack foods. It is however difficult to differentiate between the effects of quantity and frequency of sugars intake as the two are not surprisingly highly correlated and the effects of finely milled starch as this tends to be presented into the mouth in association with sugars, even in apparently savoury foods like bread.

Saliva

Salivary flow is an important risk factor in the development of caries in older adults.

Salivary flow is not influenced by age alone; the healthy fit older adult retains an adequate ability to produce saliva, despite the changes in glandular anatomy with reductions in numbers of acini and increased fatty infiltration.

The salivary reserve (the difference between the glands' maximum potential output and the quantity of saliva required for homoeostasis in normal function) is reduced as a consequence of the histological changes seen in older people. Consequently, any intrinsic challenge to salivary secretion is more likely to exert an effect on salivary output in an older population group compared with a younger age cohort.

It would appear that in healthy subjects unstimulated saliva has a greater influence on caries development than stimulated flow rate; furthermore subjects with high levels of phosphate, protein and amylase in their unstimulated saliva appear to be protected from the development of carious lesions.

A more extensive discussion of salivary change with age and caries risk can be found in Chapter 19.

Fluoride

Fluoridation of water supplies has long been established as an effective measure in prevention of coronal caries, with life-long reductions in caries activity. It has also been shown to be effective in reducing the amount of root decay for life-long residents in a fluoridate community.

Recently evidence has emerged showing a benefit for people who have lived in a non-fluoridated area as children, during their tooth development, and have then moved to an area with water fluoridation or where a fluoridation scheme has been introduced. These data suggest that 30-years residence in a fluoridated community results in reduced caries prevalence and 40-years residence in reductions both in the prevalence and the numbers of carious lesions in teeth. These findings add support to the current concept that the role of fluoride is more related to a long-term topical effect on both enamel and dentine surfaces than any benefit that might ensue from incorporation of fluoride into the mineral component of enamel or dentine during tooth development.

This topical effect is thought to be associated with the frequent episodes of de- and remineralization that characterize normal oral function. All acids cause some surface demineralization. Saliva is an extremely effective remineralizing solution; consequently any demineralized surfaces are rapidly remineralized in the presence of adequate salivary function. This remineralization process is more effective in the presence of fluoride and results in the incorporation of not only fluoride but also other trace elements into the surface of the enamel or dentine. This *mature* surface is, by the nature of the chemical processes involved, more resistant to further episodes of acidic attack.

There has only been one study comparing a conventional (1000 ppm or thereabouts) fluoridated with a non-fluoridated toothpaste in root caries prevention. This showed conclusively that caries was reduced in those using a conventional fluoridated paste.

Clinical appearance of root caries

Dental caries in the elderly can affect the enamel, coronal dentine beneath the enamel, cementum and root dentine.

The structure of each tissue, their relationship to one another, tooth morphology and anatomy will affect the appearance of any carious lesion that develops both clinically and histologically. Despite this the disease process itself remains fundamentally the same, a cariogenic biofilm producing acids and proteolytic enzymes from a suitable substrate causing demineralization and eventual breakdown of the tooth structure. The latter is not an inevitable consequence of the disease though, as caries is a dynamic process involving fluctuations of demineralization and remineralization depending on circumstance; the outcome of an early lesion being dependent on the dominant process. This is true for caries affecting any of the dental tissues.

The clinical appearance and histopathology of coronal caries in enamel and dentine have been well documented as a result of much research in children and young adults. Relatively little attention has been given to caries in relation to the exposed roots of the elderly.

Loss of gingival attachment and exposure of the root is an obvious prerequisite for root caries. Root caries can either be confined to the root, it can spread to undermine the enamel at the cement enamel junction or it can occur at the margins of restorations which finish on the root. It has even been suggested that 10–20% of root caries can occur in the gingival sulcus or periodontal pocket; however, others would claim that this is not possible and this is simply a lesion that developed supra-gingivally and became covered with gingival tissue that has become inflamed and swollen in a response to the plaque. Irrespective of this argument, root caries removal in preparation for a restoration often results in sub-gingival margins and problems with gingival bleeding.

Normally, demineralization initially occurs as a discrete lesion in plaque stagnation areas. These lesions can spread around the root face, merge and in extreme cases can completely encircle the root, making management extremely difficult. Whilst these lesions involve a large area of the root dentine they may not be particularly deep. This having been said, the depth of dentine from the surface of the root to the pulp is also small and pulpal complications can arise.

Root caries can be very variable in appearance from simply a minor colour change from sound dentine to dark discolouration. Lesions can be soft or leathery in consistency when gently probed and can have an apparent intact surface or demonstrate surface breakdown and cavitation. It is even possible for the appearance, texture and surface integrity to vary throughout a large lesion depending on localized microenvirons. These varying clinical presentations have been attributed to whether the lesions are active or inactive.

Lesion activity

From a single clinical examination a dentist would like to know whether a carious lesion is active or not and whether the lesion is likely to progress. With this in mind researchers have tried to characterize lesions accordingly and active lesions have been described as lighter in colour, soft and plaque covered, whereas inactive lesions are darker, firm/leathery to gentle probing and clean of plaque. Based upon the microbiology within the lesion and level of infection of the dentine as a 'gold standard' for lesion activity, colour has been found to be less of a predictor of lesion activity than texture, with proximity to the gingival margin in a plaque stagnation area a strong predictor of activity.

Predicting lesion activity from a single examination is difficult; at the extremes this may be easy, but most lesions fall in a haze between the two extremes and true lesion activity can only be confirmed over a period of time as to whether the lesion has progressed or not. For the clinician, caries activity and the likelihood of a lesion progressing is further aided by other risk factors that are taken into consideration either consciously or subconsciously and that can be built up over time. These factors are discussed elsewhere in this chapter.

Histopathology of root caries and pulp dentine complex reactions

The histopathology of root caries cannot be dealt with in isolation, as from the time the root surface becomes exposed and initial lesions occur pulp dentine complex reactions take place.

Caries affecting cementum

When cementum remains on the root surface, microradiographic examination of sections of extracted teeth with initial caries show that, in the majority of cases, there is a generalized demineralization of the cementum and underlying dentine. When dentine is involved, the cementum tends to have a higher mineral content than the demineralized dentine and has pronounced demarcation of incremental lines within the cementum. In areas where there is microcavitation within the cementum, demineralization radiates out from the base of the cavity towards the cement dentine junction. Undecalcified sections of such sites show clefts that pass through the thickness of the cementum and into dentine, which become filled with microorganisms. Such microcavitations and clefts could easily be created and exacerbated by probing. When dentine becomes exposed the surrounding cementum becomes undermined with microorganisms, but with minimum invasion of the dentine.

Initial and advanced root dentine caries

Often root caries begins on the roots that have undergone some degree of periodontal instrumentation and as such cementum is absent and the cariogenic biofilm lies directly on the root dentine. Cariogenic activity within this biofilm leads to demineralization of the dentine and ions which are dissolved are thought to diffuse outward towards the surface area of the lesion and reprecipitate there, forming a hypermineralized surface zone of approximately 10 μm depth. Demineralization of the dentine is then followed by breakdown of the intertubular collagen matrix by bacterial enzymes. Like lesions originating on cementum, cementum-free carious root dentine demonstrates cleft formation.

As the lesion becomes more advanced there is almost complete demineralization of the intratubular dentine and peritubular dentine, with early bacterial invasion of the dentinal tubules, their side branches and laterally into the intertubular dentine. This could explain the saucer shape of root caries in cross-section and lateral spread of the lesion. In addition to this, microradiographs of such lesions show a hypermineralized band at the pulpal front of the lesion as a consequence of the pulp dentine complex response leading to tubular sclerosis also resisting further spread of the lesion in a pulpal direction.

Arrested root caries

In arrested root caries, in addition to the prominent remineralized surface zone and mineralization at the advancing front of the lesion, irregular remineralization takes place within the intertubular dentine. Such reactions reduce the permeability of the dentine to exogenous and endogenous (pulpal) substrate for the bacteria within the lesion, leading to gradual arrest. Such arrest is obviously dependent on the severity of the lesion and the level of bacterial infection. However, even when cavitated but cleansable lesions are observed, arrest with remineralization at the base of the cavity can occur.

Caries diagnosis

Conventional visual and radiographic examination

Caries diagnosis is a complex process involving the initial identification or detection of the disease in the form of a carious lesion. A dentist then takes into consideration the severity of the lesion, any caries risk factors and the clinical features discussed in this chapter and then makes a decision as to whether the lesion is active or not; only then can a true diagnosis be reached. Once this information has been assimilated in the form of a diagnosis, a treatment plan can be formulated. It is important that caries is detected at a very early stage so that prevention can be targeted to individual patients and lesions. Where root caries is concerned this can be particularly difficult, despite the fact that periodontal attachment loss and gingival recession allow better visualization of the roots. Factors that complicate root caries detection are the presence of plaque and debris, varying descriptions of what constitutes root caries and the location of the lesion.

Presence of plaque

It is important that, before a definitive clinical examination is carried out, the teeth are cleaned. The carious process takes place in the bacterial biofilm on the surface of the tooth and the carious lesion beneath is the result of this process. Therefore, in order to see the early lesion the bacterial biofilm needs to be removed. Failure to remove the plaque and the acquired pellicle could lead to an underestimation of disease in the order of 20%, with an associated missed opportunity to identify disease early and institute prevention rather than relying later on operative intervention.

What constitutes root caries?

We have seen that the visual appearance of root caries is very variable, and investigators who have studied root caries have used differing descriptions as to the signs of the disease. Such criteria include contour, colour and cavitation and terms such as 'shallow and ill-defined', 'well established', 'discrete', 'well-defined', 'yellow–orange', 'tan' and 'light brown' have all been used to describe root caries. These terms are confusing and some diametrically opposed. As such, studies recording caries prevalence and incidence cannot be compared. Indeed, some of the great variation in the prevalence of root caries recorded in various studies may be due to differences in diagnostic thresholds and criteria used.

The difficulty in detecting root caries is also illustrated by the fact that examiners are not consistent within themselves or between examiners even when using a relatively simple four category visual tactile classification system. Kappa values for intra-examiner reproducibility range from 0.47 to 0.51 and for inter-examiner reproducibility range from 0.30 to 0.51. The most recent version of the ICDAS system has been modified to recognise and enable the recording of root-caries codes. However, this has not been used widely in clinical studies and there are no reliable data to date.

Location of the lesion

More than half root carious lesions occur on the proximal surfaces of teeth, which in posterior teeth, makes visual detection and assessment more difficult, especially when the lesion is adjacent to a restoration. Whilst there is a wealth of information on the diagnostic accuracy of a visual examination in relation to coronal caries, little has been published in relation to root caries. Bitewing radiographs can be taken to supplement a clinical examination of posterior teeth, however agreement between visual examination and bitewing radiographic examination for root caries has been estimated at 80%. Where disagreement occurs, this could be a result of false positive decisions from the radiograph where the appearance of root caries is difficult to distinguish from cervical burnout.

Caries detection tools

None of the criteria used to define root caries are objective, therefore if one detects an early lesion, makes a decision that it is active and institutes a preventive regime there is no clear way of determining whether the treatment has been successful in arresting the lesion, unless a careful and accurate description of the lesion is recorded with longitudinal monitoring of surface texture or sequential clinical photographs are taken. This is where diagnostic tools have the potential to aid a clinical examination in detecting early lesions and allowing objective monitoring with time.

Quantitative laser fluorescence

Quantitative laser fluorescence (QLF) is a technique best suited to coronal caries as sound enamel fluoresces when illuminated by laser light of specific wavelengths. Demineralized enamel results in a decrease in fluorescence compared to surrounding sound enamel and this percentage reduction can be quantified and is related to the amount of mineral lost. Whilst QLF has potential in the future for coronal caries detection and quantification, it has not been used in relation to root caries per se. Early experimentation with fluorescein-enhanced quantitative light-induced fluorescence to monitor de- and remineralization of *in vitro* root caries has been carried out. This has been shown to be possible due to the amount of fluorescein penetration being dependent on the level of demineralization. QLF therefore has limited potential in the elderly patient.

The DIAGNOdent (Kavo, Germany)

The DIAGNOdent and the more recently introduced DIAGNOdent pen are also laser fluorescence devices, but work on a slightly different principle to the QLF described previously. When red laser light is directed towards a carious lesion it fluoresces; the fluorescent light is then picked up by optical fibres, reflected laser light is filtered out and the amount of fluorescent light is quantified giving an objective reading. The fluorescence is thought to be due to bacterial by-products within the lesion, namely porphyrins. The DIAGNOdent has been used in many studies on coronal caries and in particular occlusal caries. For this purpose it has been shown to have an acceptable reproducibility and to have a high sensitivity value (correct identification of caries) compared to visual examination. However, plaque, calculus and staining also fluoresce with the DIAGNOdent and more false positive readings are given, resulting in lower specificity (correct identification of sound sites). This is a potential problem if the device is used to base operative intervention on. If it is solely used to detect and monitor lesions which are being managed preventively then it is a suitable, commercially available adjunct ONLY to a thorough clinical examination for coronal caries.

Relatively little work has been carried out with the DIAGNOdent on root caries. Those that have, have shown good reproducibility of readings and a moderate relationship between DIAGNOdent readings and depth of lesion and remaining thickness of sound dentine between the lesion and the pulp. It would therefore appear to have potential in monitoring root caries preventive treatment.

Electronic caries monitor

Much of the work on diagnostic tools has been driven by detection of coronal caries. The work with the electronic caries monitor (ECM) is no exception and it was originally devised to assist occlusal caries detection and monitoring. The basis of this technique is that sound enamel is an excellent electrical insulator. Pores that are created during the carious process fill with moisture and ions from saliva leading to an increased conductance of an electrical current. The ECM consists of a specially designed probe that exits centrally from a hollow tube connected to an air supply. As soon as the probe is placed in contact with the tooth a circuit is completed to a hand-held connector and air is blown around the probe tip breaking down any film of saliva over the tooth, so preventing conductance to soft tissues and a falsely high conductance reading. This is the most common way in which the ECM is used, giving site-specific readings. The ECM has also been used to give surface specific readings, by drying the tooth and then applying an electrical contact medium on the surface of the tooth in question and seating the probe tip in this medium. Conductance will then take place through the medium and to the deepest lesion on the surface.

Using the site-specific method to take readings, the ECM has been shown to accurately detect early occlusal caries, have an acceptable reproducibility and has been shown to give readings which strongly correlate with lesion depth and mineral content within the enamel lesion. As with the DIAGNOdent, false positive readings are a potential problem, especially in the young where newly erupted teeth with immature enamel give high conductance readings.

The ECM has also been used in the elderly to detect and assess root caries. In general, the conductance in sound dentine is much lower due to the porous nature of the tissue, but even in this lower range the ECM readings have been shown to be reproducible and to have a moderate relationship with lesion depth. It has been used clinically to monitor remineralization in a caries preventive program and has been able to differentiate between test and control groups.

The ECM operates on a low single frequency (23 Hz) alternating current, which measures the 'bulk resistance' of teeth. Work has however taken place to develop a new electrical impedance spectroscopy device that scans a range of frequencies, giving more information on impedance, capacitance and other parameters. This process has the potential to provide more detail on the physical structure of dental tissues and caries and may also prove to be useful in root caries detection and assessment in the future.

The diagnostic devices described here are the ones most likely to be available to the dentist now and in the near future. Other devices are available which could assist a clinical examination but either lack an objective reading (e.g. fibre optic transillumination) or are many years away from routine clinical use. It is important to emphasize that these devices should only assist a thorough clinical examination of clean, dry teeth with the aid of magnification and radiographs. They are in no way a substitute for a wet fingered dentist's assimilation of information on an individual patient basis to make a diagnosis and treatment plan.

Prevention of caries

Prevention remains the cornerstone for caries management in older as well as in young people. However, whilst prevention may have limited costs on an individual basis, if it is delivered to all the cost-benefit of the intervention is reduced. Eighty per cent of new root caries lesions are found in 20 per cent of the population (Figure 15.4). Accurate identification of these 20 per cent would allow effective targeting of preventive measures, making efficient use of preventive techniques both realistic and cost effective. Management of root caries from a non-operative point of view is also important as cavity preparation and restoration is extremely difficult, especially for those lesions that appear to circumnavigate the root.

Identification and reduction of risk

Bacteria

Cariogenic bacteria thrive in a mouth where there are poor standards of personal oral hygiene and increased frequency of food intakes containing fermentable carbohydrates. The cornerstone to prevention must be modifications to both diet and to personal oral health care.

The risk from bacteria can be derived using commercially available kits that attempt to assess the microbiological load or the potential acidogenicity of plaque. One approach uses a chair-side culture kit with whole saliva as the sample medium. The culture tray has selective media on one side for *Strep mutans* and for *Lactobacilli* on the other. The culture results can be read after 2 days and give a broad measure

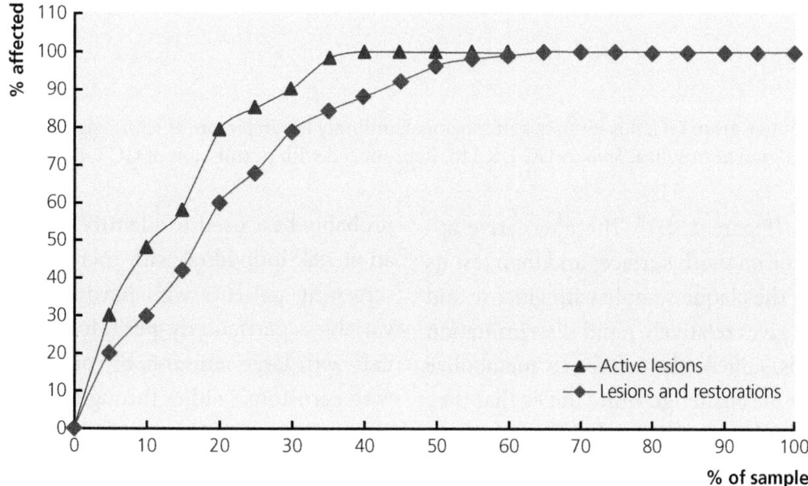

Figure 15.4 Pattern of root caries activity from a representative sample of older adults (*UK National Diet and Nutrition Survey for People aged 65 Years and Over*, oral health component): 20% of the population have 60% of all carious lesions and restorations on roots and 80% of all active lesions.

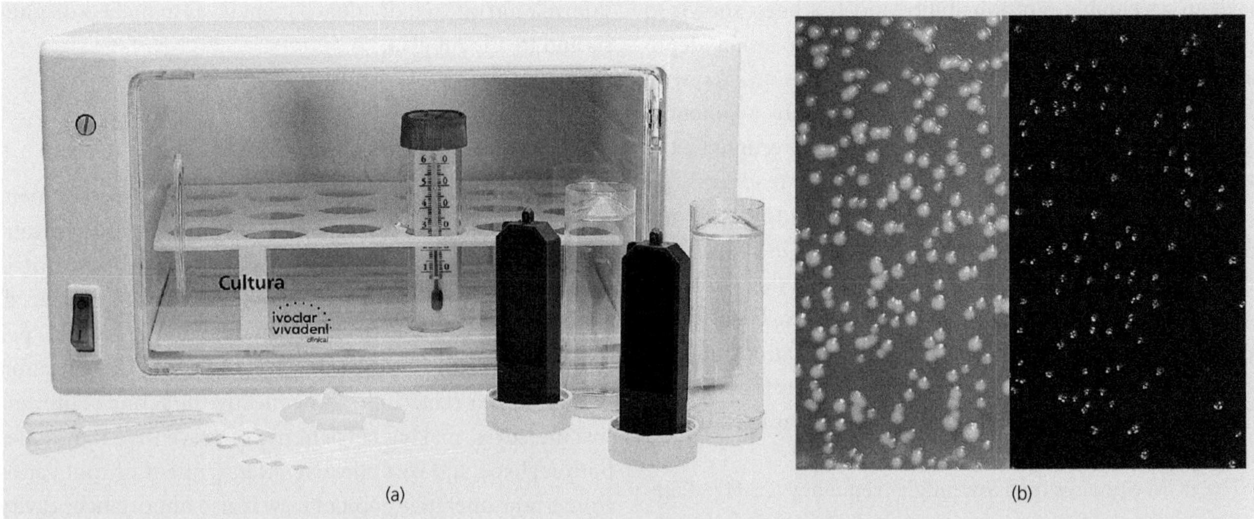

Figure 15.5 a) CRT from Ivoclar, the agar slides are double-sided with one side (green) for *Lactobacilli* and the other (blue) for *Strep mutans*. The slides are cultured in the small oven in a carbon dioxide-rich environment before reading. b) The image on the left is a positive culture for *Lactobacilli*, that on the right is a positive culture for *Strep mutans*. *Source:* Ivoclar Vivadent UK. Reproduced with permission of Ivoclar Vivadent UK.

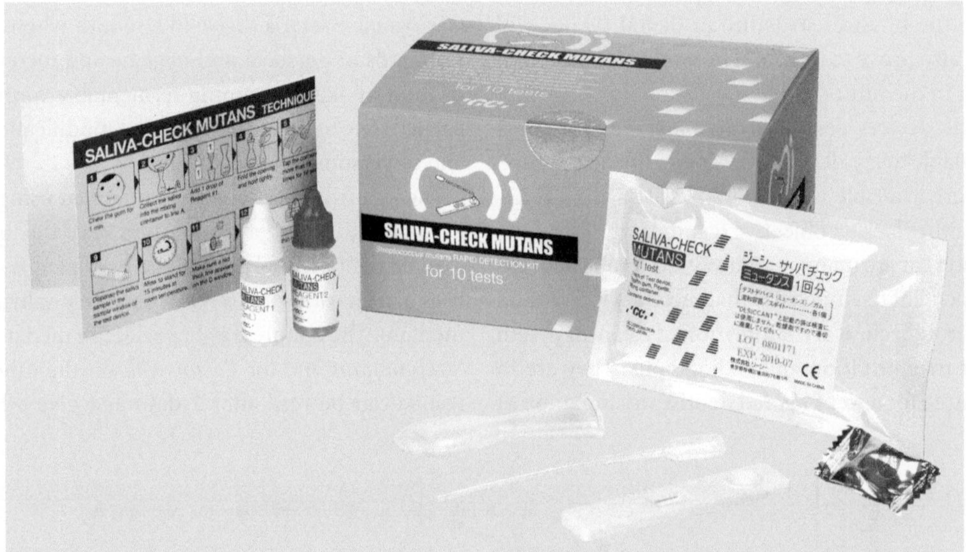

Figure 15.6 Saliva-check mutans from GC; this kit uses a monoclonal antibody to *Strep mutans* with reagents undergoing a colour change when the microorganism is present in saliva. *Source:* GC UK Ltd. Reproduced with permission of GC UK Ltd.

of microbiological load (Figure 15.5).[1] The alternative approach is to sample plaque on tooth surfaces and then test its acidogenicity by mixing the plaque sample with glucose and a pH-sensitive dye. This gives relatively rapid discrimination of areas where plaque is sufficiently mature to metabolize glucose to form acids.[2] One challenge with CRT is that they are relatively expensive and have a short shelf life. They are probably best used to identify components of caries risk in an at risk individual with increased caries activity or when screening patients who have other established caries risk variables, particularly periodontally compromised individuals with large amounts of root-surface exposure, or those with xerostomia either through medication or disease. Other more recent approaches, which are also more rapid in terms of the result, use monoclonal antibodies to identify *Strep mutans* in a saliva sample (Figure 15.6).[2]

Reduction in the levels of bacterial colonization can be achieved in a number of ways:

[1] CRT Bacteria Ivoclar Vivadent AG. Bendererstrasse 2. 9494 Schaan. Liechtenstein.

[2] GC Saliva Check Mutans GC EUROPE N.V. Interleuvenlaan 13, B - 3001 Leuven, Holland.

Personal oral hygiene. The physical removal of plaque on a regular basis will prevent caries from developing but can pose a significant challenge for older people. Plaque needs to be about 4-days old before the microbiological community is effective at metabolizing sugars to produce acid.

Modification to diet. Reducing the frequency and quantity of sugars intake will result in a decrease in cariogenic flora.

Chemical intervention. The use of topical antimicrobials agents can be beneficial, particularly to overcome acute problems. The most common agent used is chlorhexidine gluconate which is available in 0.1 and 0.2% concentrations; the specific concentration available in countries is governed by national prescribing law. Chlorhexidine has been shown to reduce levels of mutans streptococci but whether this leads to a reduction in caries is less conclusive, especially where coronal caries is concerned. It has been suggested that the antimicrobial effect on root caries may be different and a limited number of studies on high risk elderly patients have shown that chlorhexidine does have a beneficial effect, especially when applied as a varnish every three months.

There are a number of disadvantages of chlorhexidine. Firstly, prolonged use will result in stain accumulating on the surface of the teeth that can only be removed with professional intervention. Secondly, the majority of preparations that are currently available are in an alcohol base, which may be unpleasant for older people, particularly if they have a tendency towards having a dry mouth. Finally, it interacts with fluoride and sodium lauryl sulphate (a detergent commonly used in toothpastes). The interaction effectively negates the efficacy of the chlorhexidine and fluoride if it is involved. If both are used in a caries preventive regime, it is important to apply them independently on separate occasions.

Other antimicrobials are available in toothpaste (for example triclosan) but their efficacy in reducing bacterial load is unclear. The mixture of stannous and amine fluorides has been shown to have a synergistic effect as an antimicrobial combination over and above the effect of the fluoride alone.[3]

Vaccination. Vaccination against *Strep mutans* has been shown to be practical in primate models but there have been no clinical trials of immunization in man to date. The general decline in coronal caries levels seen in recent decades has probably rendered further development of caries vaccines unlikely, despite recent efforts to improve their effectiveness through genetic engineering techniques.

[3] Meridol GABA International AG, Emil Frey-Strasse 100, 4142 Münchenstein, Switzerland.

Genetic modification of bacteria. Recently, a genetically modified variant of *Strep mutans* has been described in which the lactate dehydrogenase enzyme system has been deactivated (thus rendering it incapable of metabolizing sugars to form acid). This strain survives and indeed displaces wild-type *Strep mutans* from the oral environment without any obvious detrimental effects as far as the oral environment is concerned. Furthermore it would be reasonable to assume that vertical transmission from mother to child would occur as it does with the current wild-type strains. Thus this replacement therapy would prevent the development of caries in successive generations of individuals and is effective in helping prevent decay even when patient compliance with other preventive strategies (diet, oral hygiene, fluoride) is poor.

This new technique may lead to the elimination of pathogenic variants of *Strep mutans* from the mouth; however, as far as root decay is concerned there are no data to support a suggestion that this would eliminate caries. *Lactobacilli* and the *Actinomyces* species would still be present and may result in a different pattern of decay if present alone on the root surface.

Diet

Bacteria metabolise sucrose and glucose into acids and also to a lesser extent fructose and lactose. Reduction and preferably elimination of added sugars from the diet would dramatically reduce caries activity in even the most high-risk subjects. It is not practical to eliminate sugars altogether because of the sugars contained within all foods.

Frequency

Frequency of sugars intake remains important. It should always be remembered that the pH for demineralization of dentine is about 6.0. Consequently, the Stephan curve will remain below the critical pH for demineralization of dentine for longer with each cariogenic challenge than it will for enamel.

Sugars replacement

The decision to suggest sugars replacement with artificial sweetening agents is often taken. Sugars in drinks are usually substituted with intense sweeteners like saccharine, aspartame or acesulfame-K. Bulk sugars replacement in foods and confectionery is more difficult as sugar has a number of roles in foods preparation which include not only sweetening, but also adding physical bulk (for example in candies) and as a preservative. Foods designed and manufactured for people with diabetes can be of benefit to this end.

Sugars are often present in large quantities in items that are apparently savoury (for example baked beans) and such *hidden sugars* add to the sugars intake burden. They are also widely used as sweetening agents and preservatives in syrup medicines used for older individuals. Liquid medicines (and those with prolonged oral clearance which are sucked) are used in large part in young and in old people. There has long been an effective campaign to eliminate sugars from medicines in children but not for the adult formulation.

Care is required when advising sugars replacement with bulk artificial sweeteners. Sugar alcohols and modified forms of sucrose (like sucralose) which are sweet but are not metabolized by either oral or gut flora remain within the bowel rather than being absorbed in the small intestine. This can result in fluid retention in the large bowel as much of the water uptake in the large bowel is through osmosis; the retention of osmotically active molecules in the bowel contents helps to retain water in the stool resulting in osmotic diarrhoea if taken in moderate quantity.

Much attention has been given to xylitol as a sugars replacement. This sugar alcohol not only has the benefit of a direct effect from sugars replacement, but it also causes an inhibition of the metabolic pathways in *Strep mutans* that results in reduced acid production. The evidence for a significant synergistic effect for the mouth when ingested in the quantities that would be part of a normal diet is limited but it may give an added benefit.

Malnourishment

One of the confounding problems in older people is that there can be problems getting them to eat a diet with sufficient calorific intake to meet their daily needs. Energy needs for older people are lower as a result of sarcopenia and lower levels of physical activity; paradoxically, calorific requirements are raised compared with younger individuals for a given level of activity as a consequence of a reduced efficiency within their gastrointestinal tract resulting in reduced efficiency of digestion and lower levels of absorption of digested food. Consequently, there can be competing demands in which achieving an adequate calorific intake to prevent malnourishment is balanced against an increased frequency and quantity of sugars intake raising caries risk. This is a particular problem in hospitalized people where high-energy foods supplements are often prescribed. These have very high sugars content and are often left by the individual's bed in a feeder cup to be sipped during the day between meals. There is an obvious analogy here to the use of sugars containing drinks in a comforter in children and the high caries rates that are associated with that practice.

Chewing efficiency

Reductions in chewing efficiency as a consequence of tooth loss make it more difficult for people to chew foods that are more challenging to chew. This can result in a self-selection away from foods high in complex carbohydrates and dietary fibre towards more highly processed foods containing finely milled starches and sugars.

There is a particular tendency in residential care homes for the diet to be targeted towards high calorific intake and the lowest common denominator in terms of chewing efficiency, the edentulous subject. Such diets tend to be rich in added sugars and hence increase both plaque accumulation and caries risk. The increased risk of caries seen in individuals in long-stay care has already been noted above; this dietary pattern is likely to be part of the cause.

Starches

Whilst sucrose is the sugar most often associated with caries activity, as a consequence of both acid and glucan production by *Strep mutans* during its metabolism, other sugars and highly refined, finely milled starches can also be metabolized to produce acid and hence may be associated with caries intake. Fruit sugars may have a lesser cariogenic activity but they will still result in decay if consumed in great enough quantity and frequency.

Oral hygiene

Mechanical

Caries cannot occur in the absence of plaque. However, there are few data linking plaque accumulation specifically to root caries activity in older people. Data from the *UK National Diet and Nutrition Survey* demonstrated a relationship between new carious lesions and a combination of partial denture wear (which is a risk variable for plaque accumulation) and high levels of plaque (Table 15.3). Furthermore, the same study showed high rates of decay in residents from residential care homes who have diets high in sugars and large quantities of plaque in their mouths (Table 15.1). Others showed that oral hygiene status is related to clinical indicators of mucosal and dental diseases, particularly in residential care settings and there are a number of studies that relate oral hygiene practices (like reported flossing) as negatively correlated with caries (the assumption here is that reported flossing is indicative of good oral hygiene habits).

It would therefore be reasonable to surmise that removal of plaque should result in reduction in caries risk for all.

Strategies for the older person should include assistance with the mechanical aspect of plaque removal, particularly for patients who have significant arthritic changes in their hands, as well as facilitating care by reducing the oral hygiene tasks into small activities undertaken throughout the day rather than expecting everything to be achieved at once. There are remarkably few data to help guide oral hygiene instruction

Table 15.3 The outcome of a logistic regression model for root caries risk for a representative sample of older people in the UK (Steele *et al.*, 2001)

Variable	OR
Sugars rich foods[a] – 9 or more intakes daily	2.1
Reports cleaning teeth less than once daily	3.4
Severe plaque deposits in combination with an RPD	2.5
Any teeth with 9 mm+ loss of attachment	2.2
Number of vulnerable (exposed) roots	1.5[b]
Number of vulnerable (exposed) but sound roots	0.7[b]
Number of teeth with restored but sound crowns	0.9[b]

[a]This is a compound variable comprising all foods and drinks that contain added (extrinsic) sugars or high levels of naturally occurring (intrinsic) sugars. It includes the use of sucrose to sweeten tea and coffee.
[b]This odds ratio is per tooth present; to calculate the risk in a patient the odds ratio should be raised by the power of the number of teeth that comply with the variable. Thus, if there were 10 vulnerable roots the odds of finding a new carious lesion would be 1.5^{10} or 57.6, if they were all sound however the odds ratio would be 0.7^{10} or 0.02. Odds ratios of less than 1 in this model indicate variables that are associated with reduced caries risk.

and techniques for older people. Studies have mainly been undertaken in younger age groups where some of the problems of both manual dexterity and vision are not apparent.

Intuitively the use of a mechanical brush should be beneficial as its action will replace some of the fine motor activity required for conventional brushing and the physical bulk of the motor and battery unit in the handle will make holding the brush easier for people with limited grip strength. There are some limited data that support the use of mechanical brushes by individuals who are providing oral hygiene advice for others, but no data in relation to self-care specifically among an older population.

Fluoride

As with many aspects of root caries, little work has been carried out on the effects of fluoride, compared to that on coronal caries in enamel and dentine. However, extrapolation of results and the evidence that is available on root caries supports the preventive use of fluoride in its many formats.

Water

Fluoridating the water supply has met strong opposition due to issues over mass medication, freedom of choice and possible side effects. In a systematic review of the literature it was found that water fluoridation does lead to a reduction in caries prevalence, but the level to which this reduction takes place is less clear. This will obviously depend partly upon the level of caries risk within the target population. In areas where water fluoridation has been withdrawn a clear increase in caries prevalence has been documented.

In the elderly, a link between the prevalence of root caries and water fluoridation has been identified. Life-long residents in a water fluoridated area were shown to have up to 77% fewer lesions compared to residents in a non-fluoridated area. Whilst many of the concerns and negative effects of water fluoridation pertain to children (in particular fluorosis) and young adults (possible links with congenital defects and IQ), some are more relevant to the elderly. It has been claimed there is an association between water fluoridation and bone effects, mainly bone fracture and in particular hip fracture. A systematic review of the literature revealed 29 papers investigating this and found no clear evidence for an association with fluoridation. Another concern is the effect of water fluoridation on cancer. Systematic review of the literature provides evidence from 26 studies: some suggesting fewer cancers (11), some more cancers (9) and some no effect (2). Only two, which were diametrically opposed, found a statistically significant link between fluoridation and cancer. A major confounding factor for such studies in the elderly is the general increased risk of cancer. Therefore, whilst the findings were mixed from these 26 studies, no clear pattern of association between fluoride and cancer has been shown.

Gels pastes and rinses

There have been a number of studies looking at professional applications of fluoride in a variety of formats (solution, gel, varnish, mousse). Once again there are tangible benefits in terms of reduced caries activity. There is some evidence that amine/stannous fluoride combination preparations are more effective than sodium fluoride preparations in terms of caries prevention. This may be because of the acidity of the amine/stannous fluoride preparations.

Where fluoride toothpastes are concerned there is a clear dose response to caries reduction. In addition it has been suggested that more fluoride is required to remineralize root dentine than enamel and it has been suggested that the fluoride concentration needs to be ten times higher. There are now a variety of higher concentration toothpastes available on the market, although their availability is limited by national prescribing law. These products are an additional benefit if helping to prevent caries in at risk elderly groups and also in helping with the remineralization of early lesions.

Care should be taken if using acidulated phosphate fluoride (APF) gels in adults as the gel can damage the glazed surface of porcelain (effectively it contains hydrofluoric acid which is capable of etching the porcelain surface, removing the glaze). APF products should not be used in people with impaired salivary flow because of the prolonged oral clearance associated with hyposalivation.

Varnishes have the benefit of targeted or generalized application. Using a varnish containing 2.6% fluoride (Duraphat[4]) application every three months has been shown to significantly affect remineralization or arrest of root caries lesions.

Milk

There is some evidence that the addition of 2% fluoride to milk may be of benefit from *in vitro* studies but there are no longer term clinical trials.

Rice

The fluoridation of rice has been explored as a method for delivery of fluoride in developing countries. The technique showed promise in initial studies but again, as yet, there are no data from the use of this approach in the field.

Other preventative/non-operative strategies

Casein phosphopeptide-amorphous calcium phosphate

Whilst topical fluoride does have an antibacterial effect, by virtue of its ability to inhibit the enolase enzyme in the glycolytic pathway, its main anticaries effect is to promote remineralization of early lesions so that they may never become clinically detectable or may simply arrest and regress. More recently a water soluble, sugar-free cream (Tooth Mousse, GC International, Tokyo Japan) has been produced, based upon the known anticariogenic effect of milk and milk-based products such as cheese. It consists of a nanocomplex of the milk protein casein phosphopeptide and amorphous calcium phosphate (CPP-ACP) which also promotes remineralization by maintaining calcium and phosphate in a supersaturated state and at the optimum ratio close to the tooth surface within the plaque. It has potential beneficial effects in relation to caries, erosion and dentine hypersensitivity.

Where caries activity is concerned there appears to be a dose response; with 0.1% w/v CPP-ACP a 14% reduction in caries activity can be expected but at 1% w/v a 55% reduction can be expected. In the laboratory there is emerging evidence that CPP-ACP may also be of benefit in improving the resistance of root surfaces to carious attack. When added to chewing gum, lozenges and sports drinks it has been shown to lead to better remineralization of tooth tissue and better resistance to further acid attack. Surprisingly, the elderly in residential/nursing homes and their carers' attitudes to medicated chewing gum has been found to be satisfactory, both from a perceived oral health gain and stimulated saliva flow in those with a dry mouth. Whilst the evidence at present is relatively limited, CPP-ACP, in a number of presentations, does appear to have potential in the management of caries in the elderly.

Ozone

It has been reported in laboratory studies that ozone is able to rupture the cell membranes of microorganisms and, as such, its antibacterial effect has been described as a potential method for pain-free preventive caries management. Ozone is delivered to the tooth and lesion via a delivery cup which is closely adapted to the tooth. After application of the ozone, any remaining gas is removed via a suction system with the delivery cup still in contact with the tooth. This is important as ozone has a number of side effects including headache, respiratory irritation and lung damage and it is an environmental pollutant. Two commercially available products, namely Healozone[5] and Ozi-cure,[6] have been tested for safety. Whilst the former was found to be safe to use the latter did lead to unacceptable levels of ozone.

Limited clinical data are available on the effectiveness of ozone in the management of caries with a Cochrane systematic review and a Health Technology Assessment by NICE both concluding that there was a lack of evidence to support its use for occlusal caries at present and limited data to support its use in root caries. This is not to say that ozone does not work in preventing/arresting caries, but further prospective randomized controlled trials of rigorous quality, following CONSORT criteria, are required before it can be advocated for clinical use.

Chlorhexidine

Chlorhexidine can be used to assist with plaque control, however there are few data to support its benefit in helping to reduce caries incidence when used as a rinse. There are two methods of delivery of chlorhexidine that have been shown to have some benefit in terms of reducing caries activity. Simons *et al.* have shown that the use of a chlorhexidine and fluoride-containing chewing gum on a regular basis helps control plaque in nursing home populations, reducing both gingivitis and caries incidence. There has also been a series of studies of a 4% chlorhexidine acetate varnish, which has to be applied topically to tooth surfaces on a weekly basis for 5 weeks. This approach has been shown to result in a 46–80% reduction in caries incidence in various groups.

Operative management

It is thought that the demineralization and remineralization process in relation to root dentine is similar to that of enamel and, to that end, the simplest form of operative intervention simply involves recontouring of cavitated lesions to facilitate improved oral hygiene and remineralization of the lesion. Recontouring must be accompanied by an appropriate preventative/remineralizing regime to maximize the chances of success. Early remineralizing strategies involved the use of

[4] Colgate Duraphat Varnish, Colgate-Palmolive (UK) Limited, Guildford, Surrey, UK.

[5] Healozone, Kavo Dental, GmbH, Biberach, Germany

[6] Ozi-cure, PO Box 68992, Centurion, South Africa

customized calcium phosphate solutions alongside an appropriate fluoride regime. The availability of calcium phosphate in its amorphous form in Tooth Mousse (also known as MI paste)[7] or as a calcium phosphosilicate glass (Novamin®) in either a prophylaxis paste (Nupro[8]) or as part of a toothpaste (Sensodyne Repair and Protect[9]) have the potential to make effective remineralization of root lesions more practicable.

Caries removal and restoration of root caries are notoriously difficult when the lesions are extensive. The restorative materials most commonly used are composite resins and glass ionomer cements (GICs). However there is still a place for more traditional restorative materials, particularly dental amalgam, in managing this condition. Root caries lesions often extend beneath the gingival margin and result in a cavity where moisture control is a challenge and as a consequence modern adhesive restorative techniques can be difficult to use effectively. Dental amalgam is less affected by moisture being present during its placement than these adhesive materials and remains a sensible treatment choice when aesthetics are not critical.

The choice between composite resin and GIC is not simple, both have advantages and disadvantages. Undoubtedly the aesthetics of composite resins are better than those of GICs although the appearance of GICs improves with time as they absorb water from the oral environment. Both are capable of bonding to dentine and enamel; the published data for composites would suggest their bond strength is higher, however, bonding resins to caries affected or sclerotic dentine is less predictable and results in lower attachment strengths than to 'fresh' dentine surfaces.

Much of the literature in relation to glass ionomer cement discusses fluoride uptake and release and its potential effect on the inhibition of secondary caries. However, a systematic review of clinical studies by Randal and Wilson on the incidence of secondary caries around GIC restorations suggests no demonstrable effect in terms of caries reduction. There is however one clinical study of the use of glass ionomer, light-activated glass ionomer and composite resin restorations in subjects with radiation induced xerostomia that showed that, while all subjects continued to develop caries in this very high risk population, those restored with either of the GIC forms developed significantly less caries than those restored with composite resins. This would suggest that in high caries risk populations a GIC, either light-activated or a conventional chemically setting material, would be the material of choice.

Complete caries removal in extensive root carious lesions runs the risk of pulpal exposure. If the pulp is still vital a direct pulp cap with calcium hydroxide could be considered, but this should be done with great caution as calcific bridge formation in relation to the root leads to restriction of the blood supply to the coronal pulp with eventual loss of vitality in this region. Subsequent bacterial infection of the necrotic pulp tissue could ensue, necessitating the need for root canal treatment that is also made more difficult by the calcific bridge formed. Careful consideration should therefore be given to the strategic importance of the tooth in the overall management of the patient's dentition and whether root canal treatment should be instituted. The same principles of removing caries infected dentine and leaving demineralized caries affected dentine to which the restorative material can be bonded are appropriate when managing root caries as they are when managing coronal disease. This approach is challenging when using hand or rotary instrumentation but is relatively straightforward if chemo-mechanical caries removal is undertaken using Carisolv®.[10]

[7] Tooth Mousse, GC UNITED KINGDOM Ltd. Newport Pagnell Bucks.

[8] Nupro, Dentsply Ltd., Aviator Park, Addlestone, Surrey.

[9] Sensodyne Repair and Protect, GSK Consumer Health Care, Weybridge, Surrey UK

[10] Carisolv MediTeam Dental Medicinaregatan 8B 413 46 Göteborg

Summary

Caries, as a clinical problem, forms a significant part of the oral disease burden in older people. As in younger populations, most of the disease is present in a relatively small number of individuals. Careful risk assessment should be used to identify those at most risk and to effectively target prevention using a mixture of fluorides and antimicrobials. Caries risk assessment can be assisted by monitoring the presence of cariogenic organisms in the saliva of at risk individuals.

Further reading

Baqir, W. & Maguire, A. (2000) Consumption of prescribed and over-the-counter medicines with prolonged oral clearance used by the elderly in the Northern Region of England, with special regard to generic prescribing, dose form and sugars content. *Public Health*, **114**(5), 367–373.

Brazzelli, M., McKenzie, L., Fielding, S., Fraser, C., Clarkson, J., Kilonzo, M. *et al.* (2006) *Systematic review of the effectiveness and cost-effectiveness of HealOzone® for the treatment of occlusal pit/fissure caries and root caries, Health Technology Assessment*, **10**(16).

Brustman, B.A. (1986) Impact of exposure to fluoride-adequate water on root surface caries in elderly. *Gerodontics*, **2**(6), 203–207.

Chalmers, J.M., Carter, K.D. & Spencer, A.J. (2005) Caries incidence and increments in Adelaide nursing home residents. *Special Care in Dentistry*, **25**(2), 96–105.

Cullinan, M.P., Ford, P.J. & Seymour, G.J. (2009) Periodontal disease and systemic health: current status. *Australian Dental Journal*, **54**(Suppl 1), S62–69.

Doherty, T.J. (2003) Invited review: Aging and sarcopenia. *Journal of Applied Physiology*, **95**(4), 1717–1727.

Drake, C.W., Beck, J.D., Lawrence, H.P. & Koch, G.G. (1997) Three-year coronal caries incidence and risk factors in North Carolina elderly. *Caries Research*, **31**(1), 1–7.

Ekstrand, K., Martignon, S. & Holm-Pedersen, P. (2008). Development and evaluation of two root caries controlling programmes for home-based frail people older than 75 years. *Gerodontology*, **25**(2), 67–75.

Featherstone, J.D., White, J.M., Hoover, C.I., Rapozo-Hilo, M., Weintraub, J.A, Wilson, R.S. *et al.* (2012) A Randomized Clinical Trial of Anticaries Therapies Targeted according to Risk Assessment (Caries Management by Risk Assessment). *Caries Research*, **46**(2), 118–129.

Fox, P.C. (2004). Salivary enhancement therapies. *Caries Research*, **38**(3), 241–246.

Fuller, E., Steele, J.G., Watt, W. & Nuttall, N. (2011) *1: Oral health and function - a report from the Adult Dental Health Survey 2009*. The Health and Social Care Information Centre, England.

Fure, S. (2003) Ten-year incidence of tooth loss and dental caries in elderly Swedish individuals. *Caries Research*, **37**(6), 462–469.

Fure, S. & Zickert, I. (1997) Incidence of tooth loss and dental caries in 60-, 70- and 80-year-old Swedish individuals, *Community Dentistry and Oral Epidemiology*, **25**(2), 137–142.

Graves, R.C., Beck, J.D., Disney, J.A. & Drake, C.W. (1992) Root caries prevalence in black and white North Carolina adults over age 65. *Journal of Public Health Dentistry*, **52**(2), 94–101.

Griffin, S.O., Regnier, E., Griffin, P.M. & Huntley, V. (2007) Effectiveness of fluoride in preventing caries in adults. *Journal of Dental Research*, **86**(5), 410–415.

Hamasha, A.A., Warren, J.J., Hand, J.S. & Levy, S.M. (2005) Coronal and root caries in the older Iowans: 9- to 11-year incidence. *Special Care in Dentistry*, **25**(2), 106–110.

Hand, J.S., Hunt, R.J. & Beck, J.D. (1988) Incidence of coronal and root caries in an older adult population. *Journal of Public Health Dentistry*, **48**(1), 14–19.

Jensen, M.E. & Kohout, F. (1988) The effect of a fluoridated dentifrice on root and coronal caries in an older adult population. *Journal of the American Dental Association*, **117**(7), 829–832.

Jepson, N.J., Moynihan, P.J., Kelly, P.J., Watson, G.W. & Thomason, J.M. (2001) Caries incidence following restoration of shortened lower dental arches in a randomized controlled trial. *British Dental Journal*, **191**(3), 140–144.

Longbottom, C. & Huysmans, M.C. (2004) Electrical measurements for use in caries clinical trials. *Journal of Dental Research*, **83**(Spec No C), C76–79.

Lundgren, M., Emilson, C.G., Osterberg, T., Steen, G., Birkhed, D. & Steen, B. (1997) Dental caries and related factors in 88- and 92-year-olds. Cross-sectional and longitudinal comparisons. *Acta Odontologica Scandinavica*, **55**(5), 282–291.

Makinen, K.K. (1984). Effect of long-term, peroral administration of sugar alcohols on man. *Swedish Dental Journal*, **8**(3), 113–124.

McComb, D., Erickson, R.L., Maxymiw, W.G. & Wood, R.E. (2002) A clinical comparison of glass ionomer, resin-modified glass ionomer and resin composite restorations in the treatment of cervical caries in xerostomic head and neck radiation patients. *Operative Dentistry*, **27**(5), 430–437.

McDonagh, M.S., Whiting, P.F., Wilson, P.M., Sutton, A.J., Chestnutt, I., Cooper, J. *et al.* (2000) Systematic review of water fluoridation, *British Medical Journal*, **321**(7265), 855–859.

Meurman, J.H. & Gronroos, L. (2010) Oral and dental health care of oral cancer patients: hyposalivation, caries and infections. *Oral Oncology*, **46**(6), 464–467.

Mjor, I.A. (2005) Clinical diagnosis of recurrent caries. *Journal of the American Dental Association*, **136**(10) 1426–1433.

Närhi, T.O., Meurman, J.H. & Ainamo, A. (1999) Xerostomia and hyposalivation: causes, consequences and treatment in the elderly. *Drugs & Aging*, **15**(2), 103–116.

Oeppen, J. & Vaupel, J.W. (2002) Demography. Broken limits to life expectancy. *Science*, **296**(5570), 1029–1031.

ONS (2011) 2010-based national population projections - principal projection and key variants. London.

Papas, A.S., Vollmer, W.M., Gullion, C.M., Bader, J., Laws, R., Fellows, J. *et al.* (2012) Efficacy of chlorhexidine varnish for the prevention of adult caries: a randomized trial. *Journal of Dental Research*, **91**(2), 150–155.

Petersson, L.G., Hakestam, U., Baigi, A. & Lynch, E. (2007) Remineralization of primary root caries lesions using an amine fluoride rinse and dentifrice twice a day. *American Journal of Dentistry*, **20**(2), 93–96.

Randall, R.C. & Wilson, N.H. (1999) Glass-ionomer restoratives: a systematic review of a secondary caries treatment effect. *Journal of Dental Research*, **78**(2), 628–637.

Rickard, G.D., Richardson, R.J., Johnson, T.M., McColl, D.C. & Hooper, L. (2008) Ozone therapy for the treatment of dental caries, *Cochrane Oral Health Library* On-line publication, http://onlinelibrary.wiley.com/doi/10.1002/14651858.CD004153.pub2/abstract;jsessionid=88F451184B4E9616001701B5DCBFFA5C.d01t04

Ship, J.A., Pillemer, S.R. & Baum, B.J. (2002) Xerostomia and the geriatric patient. *Journal of the American Geriatrics Society*, **50**(3), 535–543.

Simons, D., Brailsford, S., Kidd, E.A. & Beighton, D. (2001) Relationship between oral hygiene practices and oral status in dentate elderly people living in residential homes. *Community Dentistry and Oral Epidemiology*, **29**(6), 464–470.

Slot, D.E., Vaandrager, N.C., Van Loveren, C., Van Palenstein Helderman, W.H. & Van der Weijden, G.A. (2011) The effect of chlorhexidine varnish on root caries: a systematic review. *Caries Research*, **45**(2), 162–173.

Steele, J.G., Sheiham, A., Marcenes, W., Fay, N. & Walls, A.W. (2001) Clinical and behavioural risk indicators for root caries in older people. *Gerodontology*, **18**(2), 95–101.

Takano, N., Ando, Y., Yoshihara, A. & Miyazaki, H. (2003) Factors associated with root caries incidence in an elderly population. *Community Dental Health*, **20**(4), 217–222.

Tan, H.P., Lo, E.C., Dyson, J.E., Luo, Y. & Corbet, E.F. (2010) A randomized trial on root caries prevention in elders. *Journal of Dental Research*, **89**(10), 1086–1090.

Topping, G.V. & Pitts, N.B. (2009) International caries detection and assessment system committee. *Monogr Oral Sci.*, **21**, 15–41.

Vale, G.C., Tabchoury, C.P., Del Bel Cury, A.A., Tenuta, L.M., ten Cate, J.M. & Cury, J.A. (2011) APF and dentifrice effect on root dentin demineralization and biofilm. *Journal of Dental Research*, **90**(1), 77–81.

Walls, A.W., Silver, P.T. & Steele, J.G. (2000) Impact of treatment provision on the epidemiological recording of root caries. *European Journal of Oral Science*, **108**(1), 3–8

CHAPTER 16

Pathology and treatment of diseases of the pulp

John Whitworth
Newcastle University, UK

Introduction

Teeth perform daily function in a harsh environment and cannot be expected to pass through life unchanged. Some of these changes may be seen as physiological, affecting each of us as we age healthily, while others may be triggered or accelerated by episodes of trauma, dental disease and treatment. Reactions may be further modulated by the capacity of aging and previously injured tissues to respond, and by the effects of systemic disease and therapy. Endodontic disease is increasing in many heavily restored populations and the challenges created by changes such as pulp 'calcification' can be significant for dentists as they seek to preserve the teeth of their aging patients in practice.

This chapter will explore some of the age-associated changes in the dentine/pulp complex, with special emphasis on their clinical implications and management.

Age-related changes in the dentine/pulp complex

Before considering any features of aging dentine and pulp, it is important to emphasize their close anatomical and functional relationship (Figure 16.1). Dentine and pulp should not be viewed as discreet entities, but as an interrelated complex, where changes affecting one may have significant influence on the other. Few age-related changes are possible without a functioning pulp whose fluid and cellular components extend into dentine and orchestrate its responses. Dentine in return offers support and physical protection to the soft tissue of the pulp which would otherwise be extremely painful, fragile and vulnerable to injury.

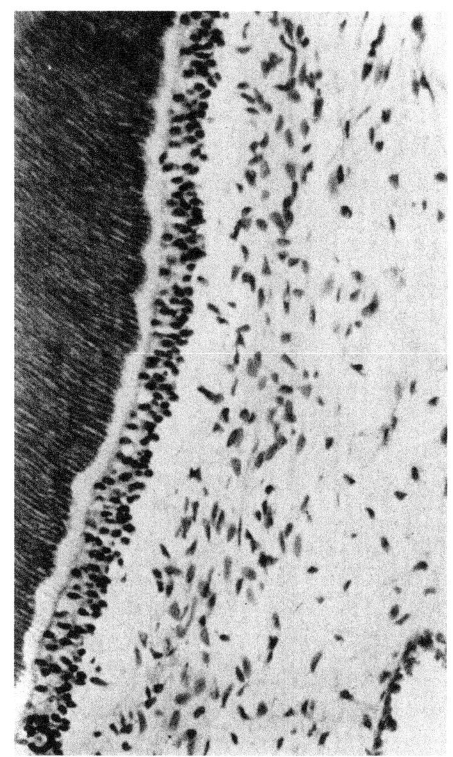

Figure 16.1 Paraffin section of coronal dentine–pulp interface. Dentine, predentine (unstained), odontoblast layer, cell-free zone and cell-rich zone (possibly containing undifferentiated cells) can be recognized (×100).

Physiological age-changes

Tooth formation

Teeth erupt into the mouth before they are fully formed. Deposition of primary dentine continues throughout the first 2–3 post-eruptive years, culminating in a tooth with

Textbook of Geriatric Dentistry, Third Edition. Edited by Poul Holm-Pedersen, Angus W. G. Walls and Jonathan A. Ship.

mature root length, apical architecture and wall thickness. The precise moment at which teeth are 'fully formed' is difficult to define clinically, but histologically, a demarcation between primary and subsequently-deposited secondary and tertiary dentine may be marked by changes in tubular alignment, density and organization [1, 2].

Secondary dentine deposition

The primary odontoblasts responsible for tooth formation have the capacity for continued dentine deposition throughout life, retreating concentrically and diminishing pulp volume as they do so. Secondary dentine is the term given to dentine laid down in continuity with primary dentine after tooth formation is complete. Athough the rate and extent of deposition may differ considerably from person to person, its acquisition is regarded as a physiological age change [3], rather than a response to external stimuli.

Accelerated secretion has been noted in some groups, such as renal transplant patients taking high doses of corticosteroids [4], though the mechanism has not been fully elucidated.

Secondary dentine is not laid down uniformly, and is usually thickest on the roof and floor of molar pulp chambers (Figure 16.2). In anterior teeth, the coronal pulp chamber may be completely obliterated as odontoblasts migrate apically and centrally. Changes may be least pronounced in the apical reaches of root canals, where root canals may remain wide into old age [5].

The deposition of secondary dentine may be beneficial, reducing the vulnerability of pulp-horns to pathological, traumatic and iatrogenic injury. However, thicker dentine and reduced pulp volume may complicate pulp diagnosis and access for root canal treatment if this becomes necessary.

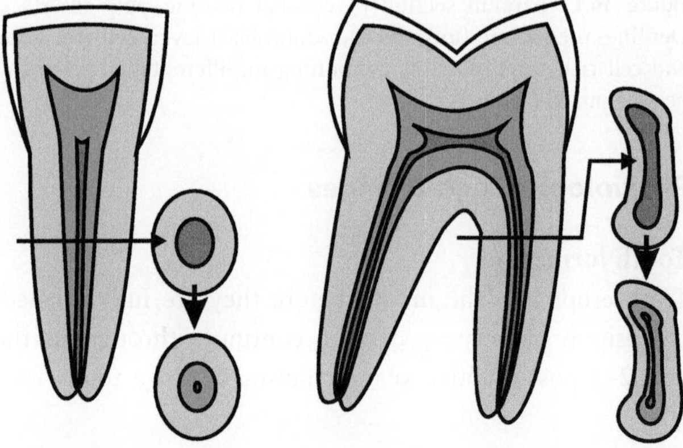

Figure 16.2 Diagrammatic illustration of secondary dentine deposition in anterior and posterior teeth. Sections show the concentric deposition of secondary dentine in roots.

Physiological peritubular dentine

Odontoblast processes extend approximately one third of the distance from the pulp chamber to the amelo/cemeno-dentinal junction [6]. More peripherally, the dentinal tubules of aging teeth are progressively obliterated by hypermineralized, peritubular dentine, referred to by some as 'intratubular' dentine [7]. Coronal dentine does acquire peritubular dentine, but changes are most pronounced in the apical third of the root. The resultant translucent dentine advances coronally with age and the examination of ground tooth sections is one method employed by forensic scientists to age human remains [8]. Complete obliteration of tubules in the crown is not seen until old age.

It is unclear whether physiological changes have any significant effect on the toughness of dentine and its age-related fracture resistance. However, if combined with large and undermining cavity preparations and stress-concentrating restorations, old, hypermineralized dentine may be more brittle and vulnerable to crack propagation than younger tissue [9].

Physiological changes in pulp

It is less easy to define age-changes in the pulp which are entirely physiological in nature. One notable example is the programmed loss (apoptosis) of odontoblasts during tooth development, presumably to prevent overcrowding of cells as they converge into an ever decreasing area [10, 11].

Age-related deterioration results from the intrinsic processes of living, the impact of external factors and age-associated diseases [12]. In the dental pulp, reduced cellularity and vascularity, with a concomitant increase in fibrosis, may be key features. All of these may diminish the capacity of the aging dentine/pulp complex to defend itself and repair after injury. Consideration will be given later to the aging effects of pulp injury and response.

Responses of the dentine/pulp complex to injury

Tertiary dentine deposition

As life progresses, dentine may be exposed to the mouth by gingival recession, caries, tooth wear, fracture or operative dentistry. The dentinal tubules opened by these processes connect directly with the pulp and leave it vulnerable to irritation and injury; microbial challenges are by far the most serious [13]. Tertiary dentine is laid down at the pulpal ends of opened tubules, and unlike secondary dentine, is a localized response to external insult. Tertiary dentine is less organized and less tubular than secondary dentine, and its relative impermeability may be a key feature of its defensive role.

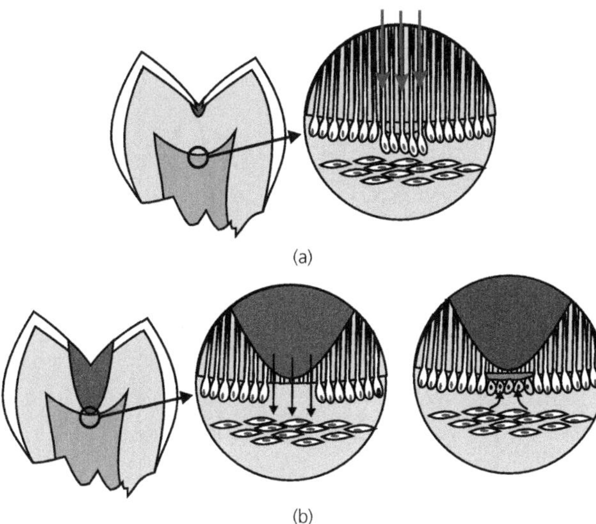

Figure 16.3 Tertiary dentine deposition. **a)** Upregulation of primary odontoblasts by dentine matrix components released by dental caries results in tertiary *reactionary* dentine deposition. **b)** Killing of odontoblasts by a deep carious lesion results in the migration and differentiation of stem cells into odontoblast-like cells with the deposition of tertiary *reparative* dentine.

If the injury is mild (e.g. early carious lesion), with large numbers of primary odontoblasts surviving, the deposition of tertiary dentine is described as *reactionary* [Figure 16.3(a)]. Here, primary odontoblasts are upregulated, for example, by dentine matrix components liberated by the carious process [14] to secrete tertiary, *reactionary* dentine. If, on the other hand, the insult is severe (e.g. frank pulp exposure) and kills a large number of primary odontoblasts, undifferentiated cells, probably from reserves of adult pulp stem cells [15, 16], must migrate to the pulp periphery and form odontoblast-like cells for the deposition of tertiary *reparative* dentine [Figure 16.3(b)].

Although the deposition of tertiary dentine is not chronological, the teeth of older people are likely to have endured more episodes of insult than those of younger people, and the accumulation of such deposits is likely to be more pronounced in the elderly.

The accumulation of mineralized deposits may also increase within dentinal tubules exposed to the mouth or affected by caries. Not only may the deposition of peritubular dentine be increased, but the deposition of hydroxyapatite and whitlockite crystals [17] may be noted, in the case of caries from reprecipitation of dissolved minerals. These are rarely sufficient to render the affected dentine totally impervious and the pulp totally protected.

Aging pulp tissue

Dental pulp is a well-perfused, richly innervated soft connective tissue, containing collagen bundles, fibroblasts, immunocompetent and undifferentiated cells [2]. The odontoblasts arranged at its periphery are post-mitotic and incapable of renewal [2, 16], but provided they remain viable, retain their secretory activity throughout life. Without these cells, dentine is unable to mount the responses described previously which above all seek to prevent the access of microorganisms and their toxins to the pulp. Additional responses include the outflow of dentine tubular fluid to dilute irritants and the concentration of IgG and other serum-derived proteins such as albumin and fibrinogen within dentinal tubules to decrease the inward flow of irritants and foreign antigens [18].

The entry of microorganisms and their toxins to the dentine/pulp complex elicits protective inflammatory and local immune responses [19], but these responses and any subsequent tissue organization after injury may result in cellular death and soft-tissue scarring. Intrapulpal haemorrhage following trauma may also result in cellular damage and scarring.

Key changes associated with age include an overall reduction in vascularity, cellularity and innervation [20], with a concomitant increase in fibrosis.

A reduction in vascularity is likely to compromise all functions of the dentine/pulp complex, including its ability to respond to injury and engage in effective maintenance. This may be compromised further by the circulatory impairments of unstable diabetes [21], though smoking-related changes in pulp vascularity and susceptibility to breakdown have not been established [22].

Reduced cellularity may include both the loss of odontoblasts and reduced stem cell number and activity, compromising the ability of the pulp to engage in tertiary dentine deposition after significant injury [16]. Equally, reduced innervation may not only diminish pulp symptoms and complicate diagnosis but impair defensive responses, many of which are believed to be mediated at least in part by neurogenic mechanisms [23].

In short, the reparative capacity of the dentine/pulp complex appears to be age-dependent [24].

Although very rare, both primary and metastatic cancers have been reported in the dental pulp [25, 26]. It has been postulated that such tumours expanding in a confined space usually result in signs and symptoms of pulpitis, which will sooner or later be treated by root canal treatment or extraction [25].

Internal calcification of the pulp

Aging pulps frequently contain mineralized inclusions. In the coronal pulp chamber, these denticles or 'pulp stones' are usually spheroidal in shape, sitting entirely within soft

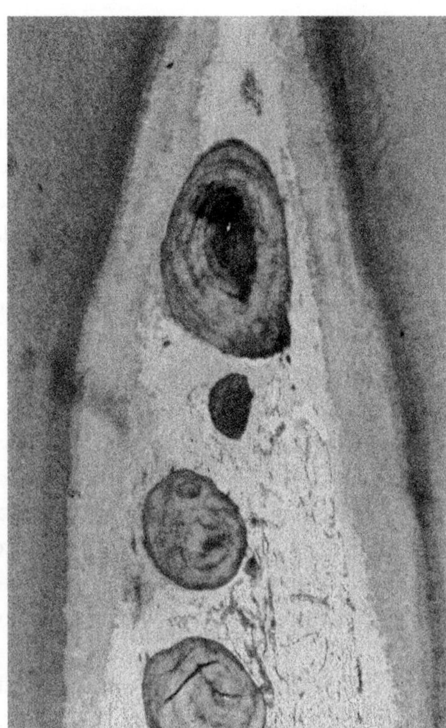

Figure 16.4 Paraffin section of the coronal pulp of an incisor from a 54-year old individual showing the development of pulp stones.

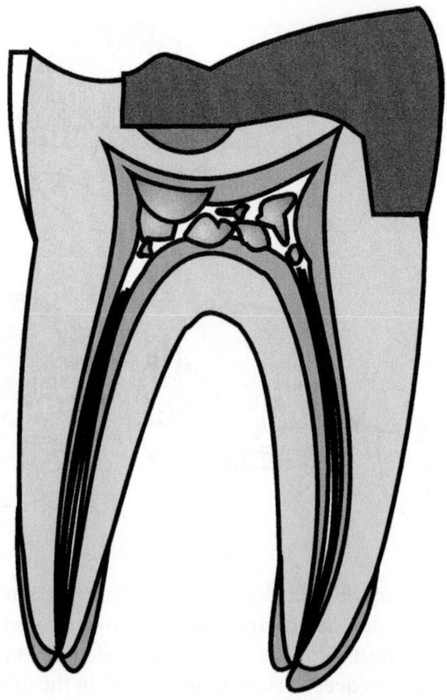

Figure 16.5 The composite aged tooth, displaying physiological age changes and changes in response to external insults, including tooth wear and coronal restoration. Changes illustrated include secondary and tertiary dentine deposition, pulp stones, linear calcifications within root canals and hypercementosis.

tissue or attached by secondary or tertiary dentine to the pulp chamber floor or walls (Figure 16.4). True denticles are composed of dentine-like tissue, while false denticles are often glassy translucent, with a lamellated structure created by successive layers of mineralization and may be seeded around degenerating cells, fibres and blood vessels in aging pulps [2].

Pulp stones of this sort extend to variable distances into root canals where mineralized inclusions usually take on a linear distribution, with areas of longitudinal calcification believed again to be seeded around degenerating cells, fibres and vessels.

The pathogenesis of such mineralized inclusions remains unclear. While they have traditionally been regarded as features of old, degenerating pulps, their presence can be noted in as many as 46% of 17–35 year olds [27]. Reports have also suggested a hereditary, non-pathological basis for their development [10]. A correlation with calcified atheromas and cardiovascular disease risk has even been postulated [28].

The presence of pulp stones is of no proven pathological significance, and mineralization of the pulp space is certainly no justification for elective root canal treatment. If extensive, their presence may however alert the clinician to difficulties of pulp diagnosis and entry to the pulp space for root canal treatment should this become necessary.

Cementum changes

Although cemental changes are of no direct relevance to the aging pulp, cementum does thicken around the apices of aging teeth [29], presenting challenges for accurate working length determination during root canal treatment.

The composite aged tooth is shown in Figure 16.5.

Clinical challenges of the aged tooth

Having outlined major age-associated changes in the dentine/pulp complex, consideration will now be given to how these may impact on clinical practice.

In doing so, it must be noted that the endodontic challenges of 'old' teeth are not necessarily chronological; accelerated and advanced mineralization can be seen in young teeth after trauma [30], while some pulps remain large and youthful into advanced years (Figure 16.6).

Pulp symptoms and reaction patterns

Textbooks of endodontics contain descriptions of classic symptoms associated with pulp injury and breakdown [31]. These range from the thermally provoked, transient, sharp pain of cervical hypersensitivity and reversible pulpitis to the unprovoked, lingering, heavy pain of irreversible pulpitis. It seems, however, that many pulps which succumb

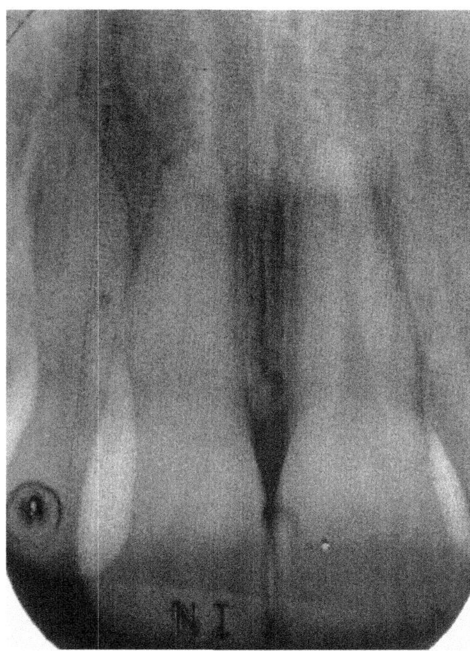

Figure 16.6 Old and young pulps in adjacent teeth following trauma. The pulp in the right central incisor appears totally obliterated with mineralized deposits while the tooth on the patient's left appears unaffected.

after a lifetime of small, cumulative insults give few if any symptoms [32].

Equally, the process of pulp diagnosis by provoking responses to thermal or electrical challenge may be compromised in the mineralized, poorly innervated and fibrosed pulps of old teeth. Problems are frequently compounded by large, non-metalic restorations or full coverage ceramic crowns. Failure to elicit a pulp sensibility response must never be seen in isolation as evidence of pulp necrosis, and equally, the absence of reported pulp symptoms should not lull clinicians into the complacent belief that all is well. More significant thermal challenge, such as the use of dry ice at −56 to −98°C may help in cases of uncertainty [31]. Even with such methods, non-uniform changes in the pulps of compromised teeth can give deceiving responses. Vigilance is always required, acknowledging that pulp diagnosis in the aging dentition may be as much an art as a science.

Cracked teeth are common in heavily restored populations [33] and should always be considered in cases of unusual chewing-related or thermally-induced pain. In addition to the usual pulp sensibility tests, potentially cracked teeth should receive careful periodontal examination to identify localized deep probing defects and examination of the occlusion, including differential wedging of cusps, classically eliciting pain on release of chewing pressure. Other strategies include restoration removal and staining or transillumination (Figure 16.7) to identify hitherto unseen fractures [31].

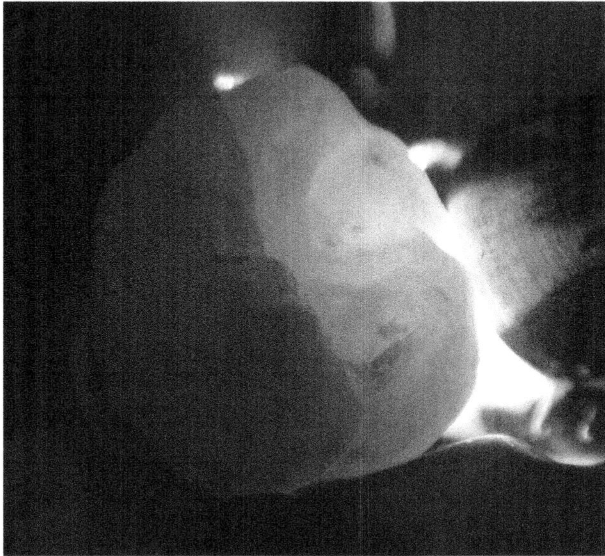

Figure 16.7 Transillumination with a simple light-curing unit identifies a mesiodistal fracture in a previously unrestored lower molar.

Operative dental procedures

Well-perfused tissues are often capable of healing themselves after injury. After a lifetime of injury and repair, poorly-perfused, fibrosed pulps with reduced cellularity may have reduced healing capacity and may not respond well if too much is expected of them. Surveys suggest that up to 20% of crowned teeth will undergo pulp breakdown in the decades after crown cementation [34], and the concept of the 'stressed pulp' has long been recognized [35]. This is not justification to electively devitalize all heavily restored or 'old' teeth before they are prepared for crown and bridgework but caution is required, especially if later entry for root canal treatment will catastrophically weaken the remaining tooth or restoration, or present real risks of iatrogenic complications such as perforation.

Late pulp breakdown may not be announced by acute symptoms, and the response may be slow and asymptomatic until the appearance of a chronic discharging sinus or discomfort on biting.

Caries management

Few studies have reported on the relative merits of complete or partial caries excavation in the elderly, though there does appear to be a movement towards partial caries excavation and the recognition of remaining dentine thickness as a key determinant of pulp survival [36]. It is conceivable that the upregulation of primary odontoblasts to create *reactionary* tertiary dentine may be a more realistic prospect than relying on stem-cell differentiation and *reparative* tertiary dentinogenesis in old teeth. Many questions remain unanswered, but challenges remain in the management of old teeth which display extensive recurrent, root-surface or radiation-associated caries. Whether the quality and volume of dentine tubular fluid is sufficient to remineralize altered dentine left in the depths of a cavity to avoid pulp exposure is not known. Work does, however, continue on methods of disinfecting deep layers of infected carious dentine, promoting remineralization or artificially hardening affected dentine with materials such as antimicrobial-containing resins [37].

Pulp capping and pulpotomy

Direct pulp capping following deep caries excavation remains controversial [38] and should not be regarded as a predictable procedure in the elderly [39]. Other vital pulp therapies such as pulpotomy have no established evidence base in the elderly and should be considered experimental. They can be justified to avoid root canal treatment or extraction only with proper discussion of the risks and with informed consent.

For the future, intense research activity surrounds the potential for tissue engineering in the injured pulp, seeding cells or upregulating stem cell activity [16], enhancing angiogenesis and perfusion and promoting the activities of other pulp-cell groups by molecular means [40]. At the same time, efforts continue to develop 'smart' materials capable of promoting cellular activity, or creating a sealed, microbe-free environment in which even compromised old pulps may be able to take care of themselves. Calcium silicate cements based on Mineral Trioxide Aggregate offer some justifiable hope in this regard [41].

Pulp breakdown and old teeth

The sad reality is that dental disease and its customary treatment continues to kill pulps, with pulp breakdown and apical periodontitis increasing in heavily restored, aging populations [42]. Estimates suggest that as many as 62% of people over the age of 60 have at least one tooth with apical periodontitis of pulpal origin [43]. The risks of pulp infection and apical periodontitis may be acute, in terms of unpredictable flare-up or chronic, with the potential threat of systemic consequences under renewed debate [44].

Although many older people are harbouring non-vital and infected pulps without apparent compromise, these conditions and their possible consequences should not be trivialized or ignored.

Root canal treatment

Root canal treatment is a legitimate, predictable way of helping aging patients to preserve pulpally compromised teeth. The emerging risks of tooth extraction in patients taking bisphosphonate drugs [45] add a further dimension to the case for tooth preservation by root canal treatment.

Successful root canal treatment restores the affected periradicular tissues to health and should be the first step in managing teeth with significant periodontal lesions where the pulp is found to be non-vital [46].

Sometimes the elective root canal treatment of a tooth with a healthy pulp is indicated within a broader framework of restorative care. Examples include the preparation of teeth as overdenture abutments or prior to root amputation in a tooth with localized, advanced periodontal destruction (Figure 16.8).

Many dentists dread the prospect of root canal treatment on 'old', 'calcified' teeth. The basic aetiology of endodontic disease is microbial infection of the pulp system, whether the patient is 9 or 90. Equally, the principles of successful treatment are the same, and healing should be anticipated if treatment is conducted with attention to infection control.

Access to the pulp chamber

Key dangers include failure to uncover the pulp space, leaving untreated infection or causing iatrogenic damage such as grossly weakening or perforating the tooth.

Tooth alignment and rotation should be examined clinically, especially in teeth with large plastic restorations or crowns which may be poorly contoured, or deliberately built to compensate for drift, tipping or rotation of the underlying tooth. Serious consideration should be given to the routine removal of coronal restorations in order to properly evaluate restorability, cracks, caries or other compromises [47].

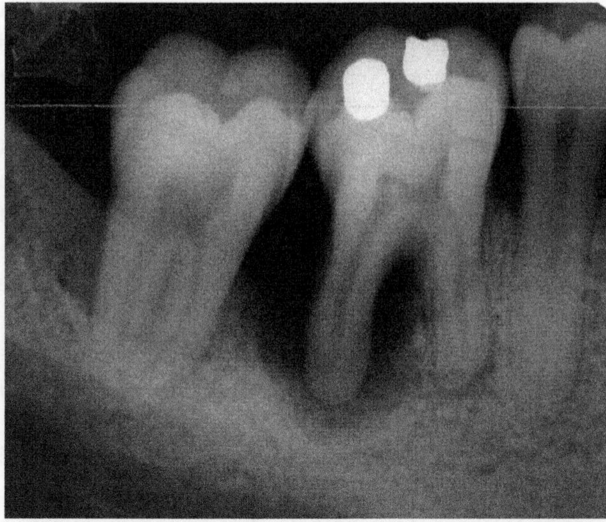

Figure 16.8 Periodontally compromised lower molar scheduled for elective root canal treatment prior to distal root amputation. *Source*: Dr Geoffrey Sharpe, Dubai London Clinic. Reproduced with permission of Dr Geoffrey Sharpe.

Weakened teeth may benefit from cusp reduction and the application of an orthodontic band or copper ring to provide support and facilitate rubber dam isolation.

Good quality radiographs should be inspected with magnification to assess pulp chamber volume, location, shape, mineralized inclusions and the number and location of root canals. Pulps which appear to suddenly disappear at mid-root level are usually dividing into two or more canals rather than vanishing due to calcific obliteration.

It is a common mistake to think that access cavities in general, and those in 'old', 'calcified' teeth, will require the use of long burs for pulp location. In reality, the pulp chamber can usually be reached with standard-length burs, and orientation against an undistorted radiograph shows when entry should be expected (Figure 16.9). If the chamber is small or filled with pulp stones, the satisfying 'drop' of the bur will not be noted as the chamber is entered, and constant checks are required to control depth and alignment of cut.

Pulp access should be outlined according to classic textbook designs [48], though the lateral extention can be more conservative if the pulp has retreated centrally. While the preservation of tooth tissue is an important principle, it is folly to over-react and prepare through a 'mouse-hole' which prevents good visualization of the anatomical clues which may guide the operator to safe entry.

Magnification tools, ranging from the simplest of loupes to the operating microscope are essential for safe, conservative entry; a front-silvered mirror also improves image quality.

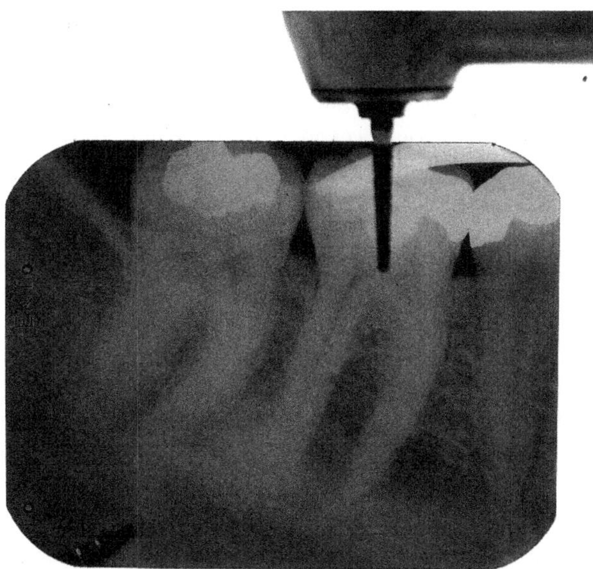

Figure 16.9 Orientation of a standard-length bur against the undistorted image of a 'calcified' molar shows it able to reach the chamber. The use of a longer bur may risk over-cutting and perforation.

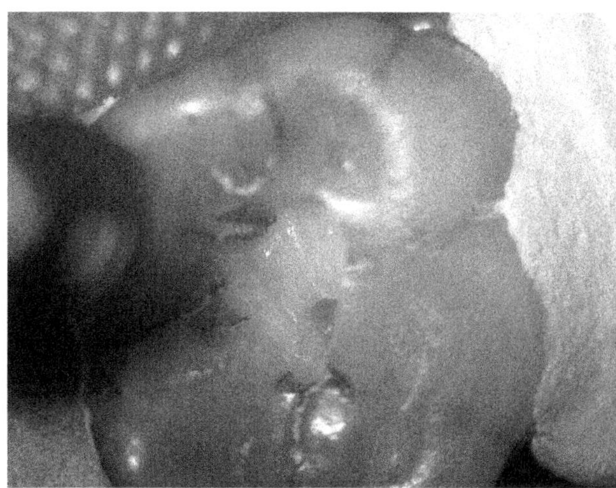

Figure 16.10 Endodontic file entering a puncture through the pulp chamber roof. Pulp chamber floors are generally darker than the walls of the access cavity and have developmental lines connecting canal entrances. The pulp chamber roof should be removed with a suitable bur or ultrasonic tip.

The interior of any pulp chamber is relatively dark compared to the overlying and surrounding dentine, and punctures through the pulp chamber roof should not be confused with root canal entrances (Figure 16.10). Pulp chamber roofs can be safely removed with long-shanked round burs, non end-cutting burs or cutting tips driven by powerful piezoelectric ultrasonic units. Care should be taken with such devices to avoid overheating or burning the tissues [49].

Pulp stones often have a glassy translucency and grey/green colouration quite distinct from the chamber walls or floor [Figure 16.11(a)]. They are often separated by bands of soft tissue which allow them to be broken-up and removed with a probe or excavator. The most efficient tool is with a well-irrigated ultrasonic tip, which fragments the material and washes it free before it has the opportunity to fall into canals and block them.

The chamber floor is usually identified as a dark, domed structure with a series of developmental lines, which act like a 'road map' to guide the observant operator to canal entrances [Figure 16.11(b)]. All efforts should be made to avoid damaging the helpful contour of the chamber floor.

Sometimes, masses of firmly attached material remain on the chamber floor. If they are securely attached and do not compromise location of the internal anatomy, they can remain.

Canal identification

In multi-rooted teeth, canal entrances lie at the extremities of the pulp chamber, at the point where the dark floor meets the lighter walls. In many teeth, such as mandibular molars and

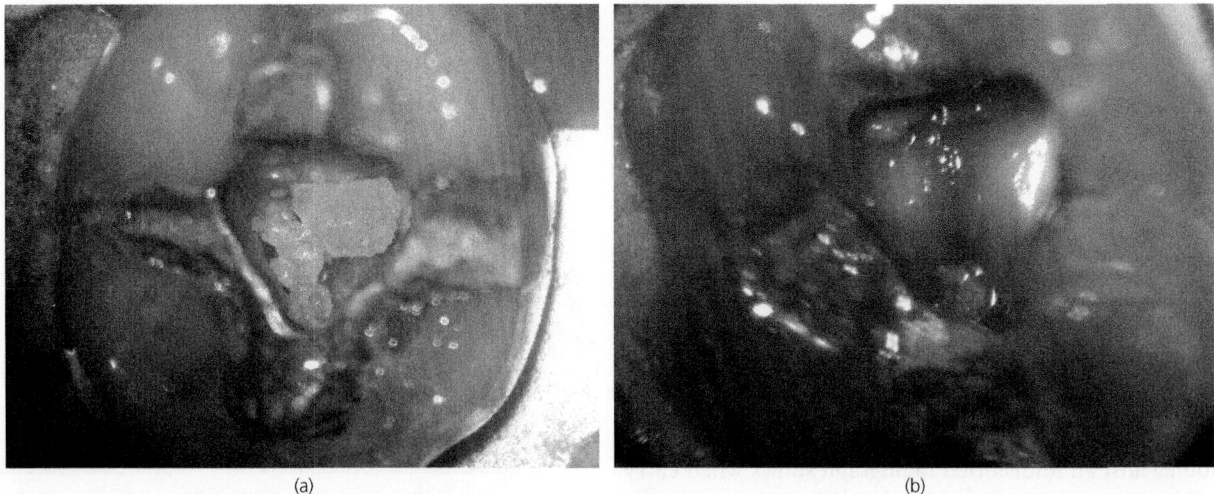

(a) (b)

Figure 16.11 a) Removing pulp stones from a molar pulp chamber. **b)** Pulp stone removal reveals a dark, domed, fissured pulp chamber floor. Canal entrances will be confirmed by probing firmly with a DG16 canal probe before walking-in with small files.

maxillary premolars, canal entrances lie equidistantly from a line drawn mesiodistally through the chamber floor [50].

In single-rooted teeth, the only place the root canal can be located is in the centre of the root. It is important to maintain long-axis orientation buccolingually and mesiodistally. Good light and magnification are again invaluable to identify features such as the junction between primary and secondary/tertiary dentine which can be followed from pulp horns apically as canal entrances are chased. In masses of dentine, clues may be presented by subtle differences in tissue colour or translucency.

Suspected canal entrances should be probed firmly with a strong, sharp-tipped probe such as a DG16 endodontic explorer. Unless the probe sticks positively, with resistance to withdrawal, there is no path to be followed with files of any size, and any effort to 'fight' in with hand or rotary instruments will result at best in frustrating instrument damage as they bend on an impregnable wall of dentine or mineralized deposits.

If no 'stick' is observed, hard tissue should be carefully removed under magnification with a long, narrow-shanked goose-neck bur or with a fine ultrasonic cutting tip. Excavation should be punctuated by further probing to detect sticking points which can be followed with files. Excavations may progress deeply before a negotiable canal is found, and orientation should be constantly checked, both visually and radiographically. Sometimes there is wisdom in abandoning excavations and referring to a specialist if early efforts are not successful.

Canal negotiation and enlargement

Canals are best negotiated with small (size 06-15) stainless steel hand files, which are progressively advanced with 'watch-winding' and 'picking' motions. Watch-winding involves clockwise/anticlockwise rotation of the file handle between first finger and thumb with very little apical pressure. This motion allows the instrument to advance into the canal, but care should be taken to prevent it from embedding so deeply that it may be damaged or fracture on withdrawal. Watch-winding is therefore punctuated by picking motions, which involve a periodic pull on the instrument to free it from the canal, removing debris as it does so. The process is eased by the accompanying use of a lubricant paste such as medicated soap or an EDTA-based product. Other aids include periodic, low-amplitude rasping motions around the canal walls or early flaring of canal entrances by stepping-back with small instruments or the judicious use of tapered rotary instruments to remove interferences at the coronal end of the canal. Canals often negotiate quickly when coronal interferences are removed (Figure 16.12).

Files for negotiation often need some degree of 'drive' and many have relatively sharp tips and more rigid steel shafts than usual. Shorter, 21 mm files are generally stiffer than 25 or 31 mm instruments and advance with greater ease.

Resistance to further apical advance may be felt as 'tight' or 'loose'. Tight resistance is where watch-winding results in the sticky sense of resistance to withdrawal. This usually means that the instrument is binding in some part of the canal and that there is still progress to be made. Early flaring of the coronal part of the canal can be helpful to facilitate deeper progress.

Loose resistance is when the instrument advances to a solid obstruction and no sticky sensation is noted on withdrawal. Dentists usually rationalize this as 'apical calcification'. Build up of debris it may be, but often the cause is a deep canal

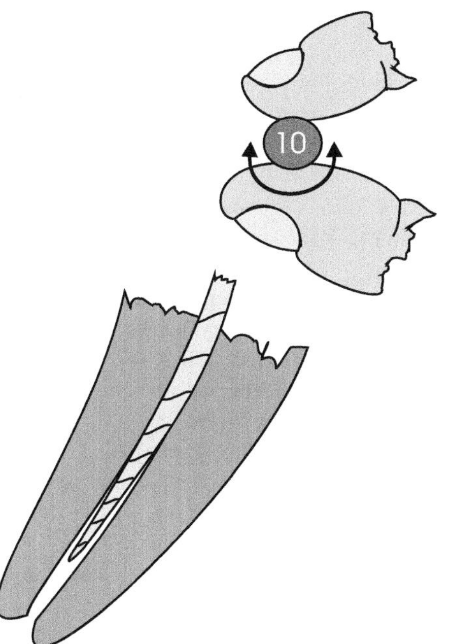

Figure 16.12 Watch-winding motion for canal negotiation. Often the interference is more coronal than expected as the tapered instrument hangs-up in a narrow canal. Patient coronal enlargement often frees the interference and allows rapid apical progress.

curvature. Files should be carefully curved in their apical 2–3 mm and walked around the canal walls to scout for a path to follow. This may again be a tight, sticky point which is negotiated as before, or an open canal which is easily followed. The true path should be consolidated by making light, low amplitude up–down filing motions for several seconds before removing the instrument. Contemporary electronic apex locators are reported to be safe in patients with cardiac pacemakers/cardioverters/defibrillators [51] and invaluable tools for indicating progress and alerting to the presence of perforations at any stage of the process. Perforations, especially those in the pulp chamber or coronal part of the canal, should be sealed without delay, ideally with a calcium silicate cement such as Mineral Trioxide Aggregate [52].

Challenges are not confined to 'calcified' canals. Obstructions just as significant can occur in the apparently wide canals of 'old' teeth as the insertion of instruments compresses fibrosed pulp tissue apically. Lubricants are again indicated to prevent this by allowing small files to glide between fibre bundles and large masses of pulp tissue should be removed with barbed broaches before file entry.

Canal enlargement

Having negotiated canals to full length with the help of the electronic apex locator and confirmatory radiographs, it is usual to create a free glide path to instrument size 15 or 20 before the work of canal shaping. This initial opening can be challenging, especially in the apical part of the canal whose walls may be hypermineralized by the progress of peritubular dentine deposition (translucent dentine). Problems may be compounded by the fact that the increase in instrument diameter is least helpful for small file sizes, with the tip of the size 15 file, for example, being 50% wider than that of the size 10. Many manufacturers now produce half sizes, i.e. 10, 12.5, 15, 17.5, 20, to overcome this problem. Small file sizes should be considered disposable and should never be reinserted if they show signs of damage.

Ongoing treatment

Following the development of a smooth glide-path, root canal treatment can proceed by standard protocols [53]. Outcomes should be predictable if treatment has adequately managed pulp-space infection. The management of post-treatment disease is beyond the scope of this account.

Well planned and executed restorations are critical to the survival of root canal treated teeth, especially those with previous large restorations and evidence of craze or crack lines. Restorations must seal and provide adequate cuspal/ferrule protection. These can range from cuspal coverage composite or amalgam restorations to partial or full coverage crowns.

Conclusions

- Age changes in the dentine/pulp complex may be physiological or pathological, resulting from dental or systemic disease and its treatment.
- Age changes may complicate the diagnosis of pulp conditions and compromise the ability of the pulp to defend itself in the face of new insult. As in all teeth, the chief threats to pulp survival are microbial.
- The presence of pulp calcification and the absence of response to sensibility testing are not justification to perform root canal treatment without further evidence of disease.
- Old teeth are generally not good candidates for vital pulp treatments.
- Root canal treatment may present technical challenges in old teeth, but developments in magnification and instrumentation have simplified care.
- Root canal treatment and adequate restoration can predictably save many old teeth from loss.

References

1 Berkovitz, B.K.B., Holland, G.R. and Moxham, B.J. (2002) Dentin. In: B.K.B. Berkovitz, G.R. Holland & B.J. Moxham (eds), *Oral Anatomy, Histology and Embryology*, 3rd edn, Ch. 9, pp. 125–148, Mosby, St Louis, MO.

2 Nanci, A. (2003) Dentin-pulp Complex. in: Nanci A (ed) *Ten Cate's Oral Histology*, 6th edn, Ch. 8, pp. 192–239, Mosby, St Louis, MO.

3 Solheim, T. (1992) Amount of secondary dentin as an indicator of age. *Scandinavian Journal of Dental Research*, **100**, 193–199.

4 Nasstrom, K., Moller, B. & Petersson, A. (1993) Effect on human teeth of renal transplantation: a post-mortem study. *Scandinavian Journal of Dental Research*, **101**, 202–209.

5 Gani, O. & Visvisian, C. (1999) Apical canal diameter in the first upper molar at various ages. *Journal of Endodontics*, **25**, 689–691.

6 Goracci, G., Mori, G. & Baldi, M. (1999) Terminal end of the odontoblast process: a study using SEM and confocal microscopy. *Clinical Oral Investigations*, **3**, 126–132.

7 Pashley, D. (2002) Pulpodentin Complex. In: K.M. Hargreaves & H.E. Goodis (eds), *Seltzer and Bender's Dental Pulp*, Ch. 4, pp. 63–93, Quintessence Publishing Co. Ltd, Chicago.

8 Amariti, M.L., Restori, M., De Ferrari, F., Paganelli, C., Faglia R. & Regani, G. (2000) A histological procedure to determine dental age. *Journal of Forensic Odonto-Stomatology*, **18**, 1–5.

9 Kinney, J.H., Nalla, R.K., Pople, J.A., Breunig, T.M. & Ritchie, R.O. (2005) Age-related transparent root dentin: mineral concentration, crystallite size, and mechanical properties. *Biomaterials*, **26**, 3363–3376.

10 Trowbridge, H.O. (2003) Pulp biology: progress during the past 25 years. *Australian Endodontic Journal*, **29**, 5–12.

11 Franquin, J.C., Remasut, M., Abou Hashien, I. & Dejou, J. (1998) Immunohistochemical detection of apoptosis in human odontoblasts. *European Journal of Oral Science*, **106**(Suppl. 1), 384–387.

12 Masoro, E.J. (2003) Physiology of Aging. In: R.C. Tallis & H.M. Fillit (eds), Brocklehurst's textbook of Geriatric medicine and Gerontology, 6th edn, Ch. 9, pp. 91–100, Churchill Livingstone, Edinburgh.

13 Bergenholtz, G. (2000) Evidence for bacterial causation of adverse pulpal responses in resin-based dental restorations. *Critical Reviews in Oral Biology & Medicine*, **11**, 467–480.

14 Smith, A.J., Cassidy, N., Perry, H., Begue-Kirn C., Ruch J.V. & Lesot H. (1995) Reactionary dentinogenesis. *International Journal of Developmental Biology*, **39**, 273–280.

15 Smith, A.J., Tobias, R.S., Plant, G.C., Browne, R.M., Lesot, H. & Ruch, J.V. (1990) *In vivo* morphogenic activity of dentin matrix proteins. *Journal de Biologie Buccale*, **18**, 123–129.

16 Sloan, A.J. & Smith, A.J. (2007) Stem cells and the dental pulp: potential roles in dentin degeneration and repair. *Oral Diseases*, **13**, 151–157.

17 Nicholson, J.W. (2006) Biologic Considerations. In: J.B. Summitt, J.W. Robbins, T.J. Hilton & R.S. Schwartz (eds), *Fundamentals of Operative Dentistry, A Contemporary Approach*, 3rd edn, Ch. **1**, pp. 1–36, Quintessence Publishing Co. Ltd, Chicago, IL.

18 Hahn, C.-L. & Liewehr, F.R. (2007) Innate immune responses of the dental pulp to caries. *Journal of Endodontics*, **33**, 643–651.

19 Trowbridge, H.O. (2002) Histology of pulpal inflammation. In: K.M. Hargreaves & H.E. Goodis (eds), *Seltzer and Bender's Dental Pulp*, Ch. 10, pp. 227–245, Quintessence Publishing Co. Ltd, Chicago, IL.

20 Fried, K. (1992) Changes in pulp nerves with aging. *Proceedings of the Finnish Dental Society*, **88**(Suppl. 1), 517–528.

21 Bender, I.B. & Bender, A.B. (2003) Diabetes mellitus and the dental pulp. *Journal of Endodontics*, **29**, 383–389.

22 Duncan, H.F. & Pitt Ford, T.R. (2006) The potential association between smoking and endodontic disease. *International Endodontic Journal*, **39**, 843–854.

23 Byers, M.R. & Närhi, M.V.O. (1999) Dental injury models: experimental tools for understanding neuroinflammatory interactions and polymodal nociceptor functions. *Critical Reviews in Oral Biology & Medicine*, **10**, 4–39.

24 Murray, P.E., About, I., Lumley, P.J., Franquin, J.C., Remusat, M. & Smith A.J. (2000) Human odontoblast cell numbers after dental injury. *Journal of Dentistry*, **28**, 277–285.

25 Neuhaus, K.W. (2007) Teeth: malignant neoplasms in the dental pulp? *Lancet Oncology*, **8**, 75–78.

26 Stefani, M. & Angiero, F. (2006) Dental pulp metastasis from oral squamous cell carcinoma: a case report and review of the literature. *Pathologica*, **98**, 48–52 (Italian).

27 Ranjitkar, S., Taylor, J.A. & Townsend G.C. (2002) A radiographic assessment of the prevalence of pulp stones in Australians. *Australian Dental Journal*, **47**, 36–40.

28 Edds, A.C., Walden, J.E., Scheetz, J.P., Goldsmith, L.J., Drisko, C.L. & Eleazor, P.D. (2005) Pilot study of the correlation of pulp stones with cardiovascular disease. *Journal of Endodontics*, **31**, 504–506.

29 Stein, T.J. & Corcoran, J.F. (1990) Anatomy of the root apex and its histologic changes with age. *Oral Surgery, Oral Medicine, Oral Pathology*, **69**, 238–242.

30 Amir, F.A., Gutmann, J.L. & Witherspoon, D.E. (2001) Calcific metamorphosis: a challenge in endodontic diagnosis and treatment. *Quintessence International*, **32**, 447–455.

31 Berman, L.H. & Hartwell, G.R. (2011) Diagnosis. In: K.M. Hargreaves & S. Cohen (eds), *Cohen's Pathways of the Pulp*, 10th edn, Ch. 1, pp. 2–39, Mosby/Elsevier, St Louis, MO.

32 Michaelson, P.L. & Holland G.R. (2002) Is pulpitis painful? *International Endodontics Journal*, **35**, 829–832.

33 Roh, B.D. & Lee, Y.E. (2006) Analysis of 154 cases of teeth with cracks. *Dental Traumatology*, **22**, 118–123.

34 Valderhaug, J., Jokstad, A., Ambjornsen, E. & Norheim, P.W. (1997) Assessment of the periapical and clinical status of crowned teeth over 25 years. *Journal of Dentistry*, **25**, 97–105.

35 Abou-Rass, M. (1982) The stressed pulp condition: an endodontic-restorative diagnostic concept. *Journal of Prosthetic Dentistry*, **48**, 264–267.

36 Ricketts, D.N., Kidd, E.A., Innes, N. & Clarkson J. (2006) Complete or ultraconservative removal of decayed tissue in unfilled teeth. *Cochrane Database of Systematic Reviews*, **9**, 3:CD003808.

37 Imazato, S., Tay, F.R., Kaneshiro, A.V., Takahashi, Y. & Ebisu, S. (2007) An in vivo evaluation of bonding ability of comprehensive antibacterial adhesive system incorporating MDPB. *Dental Materials*, **23**, 170–176.

38 Bergenholtz, G. & Spångberg, L. (2004) Controversies in Endodontics. *Critical Reviews in Oral Biology & Medicine*, **15**, 99–114.

39 Auschill, T.M., Arweiler, N.B., Hellwig, E., Zamani-Alaeei, A. & Sculean A. (2003) Success rate of direct pulp capping with calcium hydroxide. *Schweizer Monatsschrift für Zahnmedizin*, **113**, 946–952.

40 Bergenholtz, G. (2005) Advances since the paper by Zander and Glass (1949) on the pursuit of healing methods for pulpal exposures: historical perspectives. *Oral Surgery, Oral Medicine, Oral Pathology, Oral Radiology and Endodontology*, **100**(2 Suppl.), S102–S108.
41 Parirokh, M. & Torabinejad, M. (2010) Mineral trioxide aggregate: a comprehensive literature review – Part III: Clinical applications, drawbacks, and mechanism of action. *Journal of Endodontics*, **36**, 400–413.
42 Bjørndal, L. & Reit, C. (2004) The annual frequency of root fillings, tooth extractions and pulp-related procedures in Danish adults during 1977-2003. *International Endodontic Journal*, **37**, 782–788.
43 Eriksen, H.M., Kirkevang, L.-L. & Petersson, K. (2002) Endodontic epidemiology and treatment outcome: general considerations. *Endodontic Topics*, **2**, 1–9.
44 Wu, M.-K., Dummer, P.M.H. & Wesselink, P.R. (2006) Consequences and strategies to deal with residual post-treatment root canal infection. *International Endodontic Journal*, **39**, 343–356.
45 Woo, S.B., Hellstein, J.W. & Kalmar, J.R. (2006) Narrative [corrected] review: bisphosphonates and osteonecrosis of the jaws. *Annals of Internal Medicine*, **144**, 753–761.
46 Chen, S.Y., Wang, H.L. & Glickman, G.N. (1997) The influence of endodontic treatment upon periodontal wound healing. *Journal of Clinical Periodontology*, **24**, 449–456.
47 Abbott, P.V. (2004) Assessing restored teeth with pulp and periapical diseases for the presence of cracks, caries and marginal breakdown. *Australian Dental Journal*, **49**, 33–39.
48 Vertucci, F.J. & Haddix, J.E. (2011) Tooth Morphology and access cavity preparation. In: K.M. Hargreaves & S. Cohen (eds), *Cohen's Pathways of the Pulp*, 10th edn, Ch. 7, pp. 136–222, Mosby/Elsevier, St Louis, MO.
49 Gluskin, A.H., Ruddle, C.J. & Zinman, E.J. (2005) Thermal injury through intraradicular heat transfer using ultrasonic devices: precautions and practical preventive strategies. *Journal of the American Dental Association*, **136**, 1286–1293.
50 Vertucci, F.J. (2005) Root canal morphology and its relationship to endodontic procedures. *Endodontic Topics*, **10**, 3–29.
51 Wilson, B.L., Broberg, C., Baumgartner, J.C., Harris, C. & Kron, J. (2006) Safety of electronic apex locators and pulp testers in patients with implanted cardiac pacemakers or cardioverter/defibrillators. *Journal of Endodontics*, **32**, 847–852.
52 Main, C., Mirzayan, N., Shabahang, S. & Torabinejad, M. (2004) Repair of root perforations using mineral trioxide aggregate: a long-term study. *Journal of Endodontics*, **30**, 80–83.
53 Peters, O.A. & Peters, C.I. (2011) Cleaning and shaping of the root canal system. In: K.M. Hargreaves & S. Cohen (eds), *Cohen's Pathways of the Pulp*, 10th edn, Ch. 9, pp. 283–348, Mosby/Elsevier, St Louis, MO.

CHAPTER 17

Pathology and treatment of gingivitis and periodontitis in the aging individual

Poul Holm-Pedersen[1], **Frauke Müller**[2] **and Niklaus P. Lang**[3]
[1]Copenhagen Gerontological Oral Health Research Center, Department of Odontology, University of Copenhagen, Copenhagen, Denmark
[2]School of Dental Medicine, University of Geneva, Geneva, Switzerland
[3]School of Dental Medicine, University of Berne, Berne, Switzerland

Gingivitis and periodontitis

Etiology

It is well established that gingivitis and periodontitis are triggered by pathogenic bacteria in the biofilm, or dental plaque that forms on all hard, non-shedding surfaces such as tooth surfaces in a fluid environment as complex, mixed, interdependent colonies. Extensive population studies have demonstrated a strong correlation between the presence of microbial plaque and the frequency and severity of chronic periodontitis. The original studies of experimental gingivitis by Löe *et al.* [1] showed that gingivitis can be induced experimentally in humans when bacterial plaque is allowed to accumulate and that gingival inflammation resolves rapidly, restoring gingival health, when the microbial accumulations are removed from the teeth and effective oral hygiene is implemented. These studies were followed by a rapid series of experiments that analyzed the causality between bacteria and periodontal diseases. The efficacy of antimicrobial agents in controlling gingivitis provided further proof that gingivitis and chronic periodontitis are initiated and perpetuated by microorganisms.

Additional evidence for the role of bacterial plaque in the etiology of periodontitis has been derived from longitudinal clinical trials investigating the effect of various types of periodontal treatment. Taken together, these studies have shown that the progression of chronic periodontitis can be retarded or practically arrested by the introduction of meticulous and regularly performed oral hygiene procedures and control of other risk factors.

Pathogenesis of periodontal disease

The fundamental tissue reaction in gingivitis and periodontitis is inflammation. Clinically, gingivitis is characterized by redness and swelling of the gingiva and an increased tendency to bleed on gentle probing. If left untreated, the inflammatory process may spread in the lateral and apical directions and eventually result in loss of periodontal attachment, loss of alveolar bone and deepened periodontal pockets. Other manifestations of periodontitis may include gingival recession and, in the advanced stages of the disease, increased tooth mobility, impaired mastication and even tooth loss.

Chronic periodontitis is insidious and the early stages are often overlooked or ignored because patients do not associate the innocuous symptoms with initiation of a potentially serious condition. This lack of awareness may account, in part, for not seeking periodontal treatment among dentate elderly people.

Histologically, gingivitis is evidenced by a transformation of the junctional epithelium into a pocket epithelium, which is ulcerated, infiltrated by lymphocytes and plasma cells and transmigrated by polymorphonuclear leukocytes. In the subjacent connective tissue, a dense inflammatory cell infiltrate comprising of inflammatory cells such as polymorphonuclear leukocytes, lymphocytes, plasma cells and macrophages is observed. The collagen content of the inflamed connective tissue is significantly reduced as a result of enzymatic degradation. As these changes occur, the coronal portion of the junctional epithelium (pocket epithelium) loses its contact with the tooth surface, allowing for subgingival bacterial

Textbook of Geriatric Dentistry, Third Edition. Edited by Poul Holm-Pedersen, Angus W. G. Walls and Jonathan A. Ship.

colonization of the gingival sulcus and further propagation of the inflammatory lesion.

At the stage when the collagen fibres invested into the root surface immediately apical to the cemento-enamel junction are degraded, the pocket epithelium proliferates onto cementum and osteoclastic alveolar bone resorption may be induced. This represents a significant change in the periodontal condition. A pathologically deepened pocket is formed and a corresponding loss of attachment has taken place. The extension of the pocket epithelium apical to the cemento-enamel junction along the root surface marks the transition of the disease from gingivitis to periodontitis.

Although microorganisms are the cause of gingivitis and periodontitis, a susceptible host is another prerequisite for the development of the disease. The inflammatory responses to the bacteria and their products are important features of the pathogenesis of periodontal disease. A vast number of microbial antigens evoke both humoral antibody-mediated and cell-mediated immune responses. Thus, gingivitis and periodontitis reflect the combined results of the interaction between the invading bacteria and the response of the host defence systems.

The progression of periodontitis depends on a variety of factors, including the virulence of the infecting bacteria and the response of the immune system evoked by the microbial challenge. The host defence systems, which on the one hand protect the tissues by destroying and removing, or neutralizing, invading microorganisms and their products, are also responsible for the tissue destruction characteristic of periodontitis. Thus, much of the tissue destruction appears to be caused by tissue enzymes, including matrix metalloproteinases released from fibroblasts and leukocytes in the response to the release of cytokines and other mediators involved in the inflammatory process. The defence systems are ineffective against the metabolic activity of plaque bacteria residing on the tooth surface and cannot restore established periodontal pockets. Gingival recession may reduce the depth of periodontal pockets, but the arrest and reversal of the lesions require treatment.

The progression of the periodontal lesion is a logical sequence of events initiated and perpetuated by bacterial activity. There is general consensus that periodontitis always starts as gingivitis, but gingivitis does not necessarily proceed to periodontitis. The rate of progression of periodontal lesions varies between individuals and also from one local area to another in the same dentition. In addition, periodontal lesions may progress at different rates at varying times during life. The individual differences in disease distribution and progression have led to much confusion about the nature of the disease. However, the general consensus now is that the progression of chronic periodontitis is a continuous process that undergoes episodes of acute exacerbation and remission. The recognition that there are different clinical types of periodontitis has been linked to differences in both the nature and pathogenicity of the (subgingival) microbiota and the quality of the host response, especially the immune system and the polymorphonuclear leukocyte-antibody-complement system. For example, neutrophil chemotactic defects seem to be associated with severe, rapidly progressive periodontitis. As far as the role of microorganisms is concerned, there is some evidence to support the hypothesis that periodontitis may develop and progress in response to certain types of bacterial species rather than to the entire biomass. These suspected periodontal pathogens first of all include *Porphyromonas gingivalis, Tannerella forsythensis* and the spirochaete *Treponema denticola*. Thus, periodontitis may represent an opportunistic bacterial infection with a range of gram-negative bacteria that may invade superficial and deeper gingival tissues.

The mechanisms leading to progression or stability of a periodontal lesion are incompletely understood. Chronic periodontitis is a complex infection in which interactions between the aggression of the microflora and the local host responses contribute to the breakdown of the attachment apparatus. Much research is still required to adequately explain the basis for active periodontal destruction. Nevertheless, as pointed out by Löe and co-workers, there is a commonality to the cause of both the initial and the progressive lesion, and there is a degree of continuity to the progression from the incipient to the advanced lesion. So far, there are no reliable predictors of progressing lesions.

Aging and periodontal disease

Epidemiology

Periodontitis is among the most prevalent chronic inflammatory conditions in dentate older populations. Several epidemiological surveys have found that the prevalence and severity of chronic periodontitis increase with chronological age. One of these studies, the 1985–1986 national survey of oral health in United States adults, found that periodontal attachment loss increased progressively with age, whereas the proportion of individuals with gingival bleeding remained relatively constant for each decade of adult life [2]. Only a weak correlation between pocket depth and ascending age was observed. Comparable data have been reported in other studies. One of these, also conducted in the United States, described the prevalence of periodontitis in a well-defined, selected, population of 22- to 90-year-old healthy individuals who were nonsmokers and not taking prescription medications [3]. The results revealed higher percentages of tooth surfaces (sites) with dental plaque, gingival bleeding, calculus, recession and attachment loss in the oldest age group as compared with the young and middle-aged groups. Mean periodontal pocket depths increased slightly with age, but only the youngest and the oldest age groups differed significantly.

Other studies, however, found that the proportion of individuals with advanced periodontitis (defined as pockets greater than 5 mm) decreased in the oldest age groups. This observation may be associated with selective tooth survival, that is, that teeth with advanced attachment loss have been lost in the oldest age cohorts, or periodontal pockets may have been reduced as a result of gingival recession. A study of older adults attending senior activity centres in Florida found that sites with severe attachment loss were typically not accompanied by severe pockets, but rather by substantial gingival recession [4]. Use of pocket depth alone would have considerably underestimated the degree of periodontal breakdown in this elderly sample.

Although the findings of these studies, and others not referred to, may not provide a complete picture of the pattern of periodontal disease in elderly populations, several epidemiological surveys strongly document that the prevalence of mild to moderate periodontitis is high in dentate elderly populations and the prevalence of more advanced periodontal conditions is somewhat lower. In general, most dentate older subjects have a relatively small number of teeth with serious periodontal conditions, and a minority has many teeth affected. Since the rates of edentulism and tooth loss in the new cohorts of older adults are now declining, periodontal disease patterns may change. People who survive into old age with natural dentition may retain more teeth susceptible to periodontitis. If this is true, the prevalence of the more advanced forms of periodontitis may increase in the future. A recent cross-sectional study compared changes in the periodontal status in a Swedish population living in Jönköping over a period of 20 years (1973, 1983, 1993) [5]. The proportion of 60- and 70-year-old persons in the group with healthy periodontium without signs of alveolar bone loss increased, and the proportion of 60- and 70-year-old persons in the group with moderate bone loss decreased between 1973 and 1983. However, the proportion of 60- and 70-year-old persons in the group with severe bone loss increased between 1973 and 1983, but was unchanged between 1983 and 1993, despite persons in this group exhibiting a further significant increase in tooth retention. Another cross-sectional study of periodontal conditions in Switzerland included 1224 dentate subjects from 20 to 89 years of age [6]. The results showed that periodontal pockets increased slightly from age 20 to approximately 50 years. Thereafter, the mean pocket depth remained approximately 3 mm. However, the loss of periodontal attachment increased dramatically after age 50, indicating that chronic periodontitis is a disease that primarily affects many subjects 50 years of age and older. Another recent study of community-dwelling, generally healthy persons over the age of 80 years living in Stockholm, Sweden, revealed that more than 50% of all study participants met the criteria used for 'serious' periodontitis [7].

Cross-sectional findings of age-related increases in loss of periodontal attachment have not been corroborated by longitudinal results, however, and it has been suggested that perhaps the relationship of increasing attachment loss with age group may be because of a cohort effect [8].

A 10-year longitudinal study of periodontitis incidence and progression in adult and elderly Chinese found that baseline periodontal disease experience was predictive for future periodontal breakdown and that age was a significant predictor of progressing disease, but not of new disease [9]. It was suggested that the age-associated increased risk of disease progression might result from a decline with age in the capacity to mount a sufficient host response to pre-existing local periodontal infections. According to the authors, the observation that age was not a predictor of new disease would indicate that such a decline in the host response may be more pronounced for sites with periodontitis, possibly because periodontal inflammation might in itself result in exhaustion of the local host response.

In summary, findings may suggest there will be an increase in the prevalence and severity of periodontitis among older populations in the future, because more people are surviving into old age with natural teeth, which may be susceptible to periodontitis. The increase in life expectancy further implies that these teeth have to be cared for for several more years than in the past. In addition, there is an association between periodontal diseases and systemic diseases and other medical conditions that become more prevalent with increasing age, and which may compromise periodontal health. Persons that are socially and economically disadvantaged or in poor health are at particular risk of serious periodontal conditions.

Risk indicators and risk populations

Several studies have found that periodontal diseases are also influenced by complex sociodemographic factors, including age, sex, ethnicity, education and income, by behavioral factors, including poor oral hygiene, smoking, irregular use of dental services, low physical activity and stress-producing life changes, and by systemic conditions, including diabetes. Several of these factors are probably interrelated.

Not everyone is equally susceptible to periodontitis. Several epidemiological studies have been conducted for subgroups of elderly people such as those who are frail or institutionalized. Overall, these studies have found that the periodontal health of frail and functionally dependent elderly persons is extremely poor, and that older persons living in institutions have more unmet oral health care needs than do their peers in the community. Institutionalized elderly persons have higher rates of edentulism, more missing teeth, poorer oral hygiene and more severe gingivitis and periodontitis than age-matched, non-institutionalized dentate elderly people.

A study conducted on old-age pensioners living in a medium-sized municipality near Oslo, Norway found that institutionalized elderly people had higher levels of plaque and gingival inflammation than did the non-institutionalized older adults. Only minor differences were observed, however, in the degree of periodontal breakdown between the two residential groups. It was speculated that the teeth most resistant to periodontal breakdown had remained, thus masking the possible influence of differences in oral hygiene earlier in life [10]. Another study of periodontal health among dentate nursing home residents in Denmark found that two thirds of the subjects had abundant plaque. Twenty-five per cent had severe gingivitis with ulceration and/or tended to bleed spontaneously. Sixty per cent had periodontal pockets between 4 and 5.5 mm and 17% had periodontal pockets greater than 6 mm. Nursing home residents older than 85 years had a higher prevalence of deep pockets than those younger than 75, and nursing home residents who regularly used dental services had fewer deep pockets than those who had not seen a dentist since the time of admission. Interestingly, this study revealed that elderly people who received assistance from the nursing staff in maintaining oral hygiene had a significantly higher prevalence of abundant plaque and more severe gingivitis than did those who cleaned their own teeth. Elderly who received assistance generally were in poor health, which may have complicated the maintenance of adequate oral hygiene. In addition, nursing staff untrained in oral hygiene therapy were often responsible for providing oral hygiene procedures for the residents [11].

A survey of elderly patients admitted to a geriatric hospital in Switzerland found that the single highest treatment need was for periodontal disease [12]. Of the natural teeth present, 45% had advanced periodontitis. Oral cleanliness was extremely poor. Another study of institutionalized elderly people in Connecticut, United States, reported a mean periodontal attachment loss of 5.7 mm, Gingival Index of 2.1 and Plaque Index of 2.2 [13]. This study also found that the duration of institutionalization did not significantly alter the periodontal findings. These observations suggest that, on admission to nursing homes, many elderly people already have advanced periodontal disease, which may persist at that level throughout their stay in the institution. The poor periodontal health of institutionalized elderly may therefore, in part, reflect oral neglect and oral problems that accumulated prior to admission, when they were still living at home with deteriorating general health. A follow-up study of the residents who were still present in the nursing home 5 years later (45% of the residents) revealed that periodontitis had progressed, as evidenced by a statistically significant increase in loss of periodontal attachment [14]. These findings clearly emphasize that conclusions on the progression of disease cannot be based on cross-sectional data such as those reported above. The observation of the first study that the periodontal disease parameters were unrelated to the length of stay in the institution, therefore, may reflect the fact that the residents who were in poor health and survived for only a limited period of time after admission to the nursing home may also have been more susceptible to periodontal breakdown than those who lived longer, thus masking the accumulated loss of periodontal attachment that occurred over time.

Recent evidence has also substantiated a link between the oral microflora/periodontitis and aspiration pneumonia in high-risk individuals such as the very frail elderly nursing home resident [15, 16]. Although more studies are needed to establish a direct causal relationship, these findings underscore the importance of oral hygiene in the care of these subjects.

When comparing data from different studies it should be taken into consideration that there is a lack of uniformity in the literature with regard to how a periodontitis case was defined [17]. Several studies have used different combinations of clinical attachment loss and periodontal pocket depths to establish a case definition. The rationale behind periodontal pocket depths and clinical attachment loss combinations is that periodontal pocket depths is considered to indicate the presence of current disease, whereas clinical attachment loss represents a cumulative measure of periodontal tissue destruction over the life course. In addition, the findings of different studies are dependent upon the thresholds used to define a periodontitis case. Furthermore, some studies have used a full-mouth design with probing measurements at several sites on each remaining tooth, whereas other studies have used a half-mouth design or only scored index teeth. The latter methods may cause an underestimation of the severity of disease. It has been recognized that a full-mouth design with probing measurements at four or more sites on each remaining tooth more correctly detects an individual with periodontitis.

In summary, the evidence indicates that elderly people living in nursing homes have more severe periodontal conditions and poorer oral hygiene than do non-institutionalized elderly people. This trend may be explained by the higher degree of helplessness among nursing home residents. In addition, oral health often assumes a lower priority among the frail elderly people than do other aspects of their physical health. Other barriers may be the mobility status of the patient, the availability of dental services and the accessibility of a dental office. Financial constraints may also play a role. Furthermore, systemic diseases, frailty, functional disability, medications and such conditions as drug-induced salivary hypofunction may further complicate oral hygiene and make the tissues more vulnerable to periodontal infections (see Chapters 19 and 25).

Susceptibility to periodontal disease

Enhanced severity of periodontitis with age has been related to the length of time the periodontal tissues have been exposed to the dentogingival bacterial plaque and is considered to reflect the individual's cumulative oral history. However, the susceptibility of the periodontium to plaque-induced periodontal breakdown may be influenced by the aging process or by the specific health problems of the aging patient. Knowledge of the tissue changes that occur during aging is therefore not only essential for understanding the basic pathophysiological features of aging but is also of great clinical significance in planning treatment and in evaluating the prognosis of the treatment chosen for the elderly patient.

Age has been suggested to be a predisposing factor for the development of periodontal inflammation. The background of this phenomenon, however, is not completely understood. Aging reduces the ability of the individual to adapt to environmental stress. At the biological level, aging is associated with changes that lead to a progressive, irreversible deterioration of the functional capacities of several tissues and organs. As mentioned in the previous section, changes in structure and function during aging may affect the host response to plaque microorganisms and may influence the rate of periodontal destruction in older people. Although age changes in the periodontal tissues have been investigated extensively, there is less information on the response of the periodontium of older humans to microbial infection.

A controlled study of experimental gingivitis in 20- to 24-year-old and 65- to 78-year-old healthy human volunteers who abstained from oral hygiene procedures for 21 days showed that gingival inflammation developed more rapidly and was more intense in the elderly subjects than in the young subjects (Figures 17.1–17.3) [18]. Plaque accumulation was also enhanced in the older people. However, when oral hygiene measures were resumed after three weeks, gingivitis decreased rapidly and there were no differences in the rate of healing of the inflamed gingiva and restitution of gingival health in the two groups [Figures 17.1, 17.2(a),(b), 17.3(a),(b)].

Variations in the development and metabolism of plaque may be related to changes in the oral environment with age. The greater amount of plaque recovered in the elderly subjects could be due, in part, to a larger area for plaque retention because of gingival recession. Further, exposed cementum of the root surface and dental enamel constitute two unlike types of hard dental tissue with distinct surface

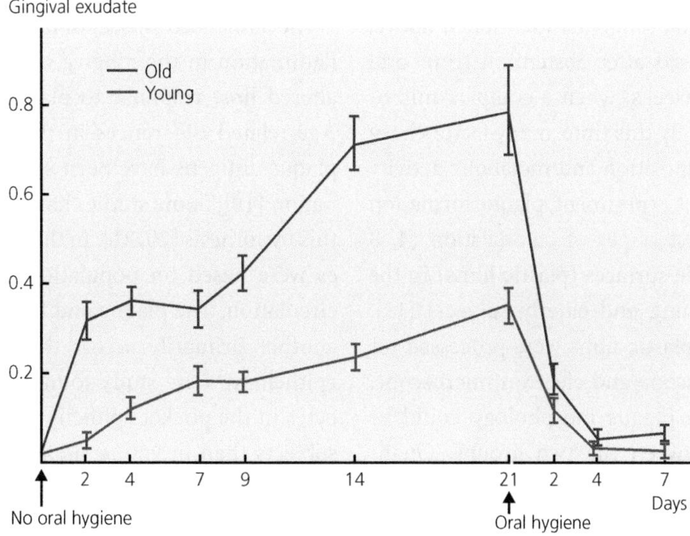

Figure 17.1 Experimental gingivitis. Mean amounts of gingival exudate collected from buccal gingival sulci in young and elderly individuals during a 21-day oral hygiene abstention period and during a subsequent period of controlled oral hygiene.

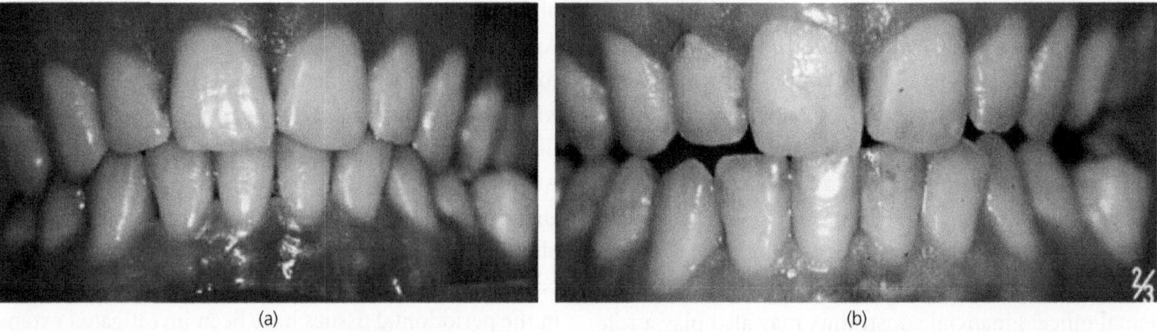

(a) (b)

Figure 17.2 **a**) Clinically normal gingiva and clean teeth in a young individual at the start of a 21-day period of oral hygiene abstention. **b**) Plaque accumulation at the end of the 21-day period of oral hygiene abstention (same individual as shown in Figure 17.2(a).

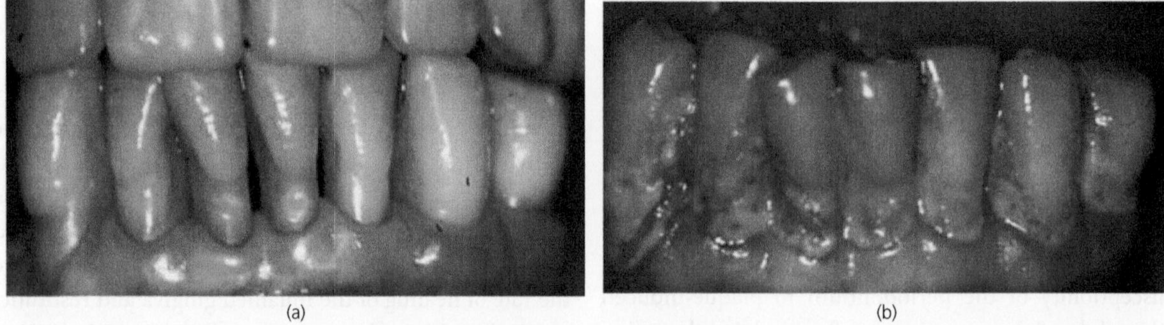

(a) (b)

Figure 17.3 **a**) Clinically normal gingiva and clean teeth in an elderly individual at the start of a 21-day period of oral hygiene abstention. **b**) Plaque accumulation and gingival inflammation at the end of the 21-day period of oral hygiene abstention (same individual as shown in Figure 17.3(a).

characteristics, which may influence the plaque formation rate differently. Differences in dietary habits, increased flow of gingival exudate from the inflamed gingiva and the presence of salivary hypofunction may similarly alter the conditions for growth and multiplication of the plaque microorganisms.

In the study of experimental gingivitis mentioned above, plaque formation was assessed after abstention from oral hygiene for several days or weeks, when a complex microbiota had already developed. By this time, many factors have influenced the bacterial composition and metabolic activity of the biofilm. In a subsequent experiment, plaque formation was studied from the earliest stages of colonization (4, 8 and 24 hours) on comparable surfaces (plastic films) in the dento-gingival region of young and elderly subjects [19]. The plaque deposits on the plastic films were processed for examination by light microscope and electron microscope. No consistent differences in plaque morphology could be ascertained qualitatively between the two groups. Quantitatively, however, the 4-hour samples obtained from the older group had significantly fewer bacteria than did similar samples from the younger subjects. This difference decreased in the 8-hour samples and was no longer evident at the last examination period of 24 hours. Thus, although the initial rates of plaque formation in elderly individuals are lower, once bacterial accumulation starts, it seems to occur faster than in the younger subjects. These results are in line with the previous studies showing that more plaque was formed in older subjects after three weeks of plaque development.

The enhanced susceptibility to microbially induced inflammation in the gingiva of elderly people may reflect an altered host response to plaque microorganisms with age. Age-related differences in the immune response to dental plaque antigens have been suggested as one possible explanation [18]. Some studies have provided evidence to support this hypothesis [20, 21]. In these studies, the cellular responses were based on populations of leukocytes in peripheral circulation. The plaque and the host, however, confront one another primarily across the gingival junctional (pocket) epithelium. One study found that the number of lymphocytes in the pocket epithelium was slightly higher in elderly subjects than in young subjects, but the difference was not statistically significant and could not explain the difference in clinical inflammation score between the two age groups. Also, ultrastructural differences were not observed among lymphocytes from young and elderly subjects [22].

A Dutch study reported apparently conflicting results: a group of younger adults (mean age 34 years) developed experimental gingivitis more rapidly than a group of middle-aged individuals (mean age 48 years) [23]. Both groups had the same amounts of attachment loss. This was considered to reflect differing susceptibility to periodontal breakdown. Thus, it was suggested that the individuals who had suffered from a more rapid form of periodontal disease (the younger group) also developed gingivitis more rapidly. According to this hypothesis, the susceptibility of the periodontium to periodontal disease prevails over the age factor. In subsequent studies from the same laboratory, carried out with the same subjects who participated in the former investigation, it was reported that supragingival plaque samples from the older subjects had higher proportions of motile microorganisms than did samples from the younger subjects. No differences were observed in the composition of the inflammatory cell infiltrate in gingival biopsies from the two age groups. It was concluded that age is of minor importance in the development of experimentally induced gingival inflammation in subjects resistant to periodontal destruction. Since these studies were confined to groups of younger and middle-aged adults, it is not clear whether their observations are inconsistent with the results discussed before or how they would be influenced by the aging process.

A Swedish group from Göteborg reported on the development of experimental gingivitis in young (1 year) and old (8–9 years) Beagle dogs [24]. The dogs were selected from the same Beagle colony and had been given professional tooth cleaning every 3 months to maintain periodontal health and prevent plaque formation. Prior to the study, a 6-week period of daily plaque control was initiated. Samples of subgingival plaque were harvested and gingival biopsies were obtained at the start of the experiment (day 0) and after 3 weeks of plaque formation (day 21). Histological analysis of the inflamed gingiva (obtained on day 21) revealed that the inflammatory cell infiltrate in the gingival connective tissue was significantly larger and extended more laterally and apically in old dogs than in young dogs. Morphometric assessments further showed that the inflammatory lesion in the old dogs harboured a significantly larger volume of plasma cells and smaller volumes of macrophages, lymphocytes and polymorphonuclear leukocytes than in the young dogs. In the electron microscope, many of the plasma cells in the old dogs showed signs of degeneration. Based on these findings it was suggested that the observed difference in plasma cell density might be related to aging. The morphometric measurements also showed that the volume fraction of the junctional epithelium of normal gingiva (day 0) that was occupied by leukocytes was similar in young and old dogs. At the end of the plaque formation period (day 21), the volume of leukocytes in the young dogs had increased by a factor of three, whereas in the old dogs the increase was less conspicuous. According to the authors, this difference in leukocyte migration may indicate that young dogs respond to plaque formation with an inflammatory reaction, the acute component of which seems to be more pronounced than in old dogs, or that the different response may be related to differences in the subgingival microbiota.

A subsequent study of experimental gingivitis in young and elderly humans conducted by same group in Sweden found that the inflammatory cell infiltrates of day 21 biopsies were larger in the older group and harboured a higher proportion of B-cells and a lower density of PMN cells compared to infiltrates in the young group of subjects [25]. The finding that elderly individuals during experimental gingivitis exhibit a different inflammatory response to plaque antigens compared to young individuals corroborates the results from the Danish clinical trails in humans and from the experiment in dogs but the data are not consistent with the findings reported by the Dutch group. As previously mentioned, the discrepancy between these findings may be due to the different age of the subject samples. The Swedish study also showed that the level of IgG3 measured in the gingival exudate was consistently higher in the old than in the young subjects. According to the authors, the difference in IgG3 levels may be interpreted as an age-related altered response to plaque antigens but could also reflect an increased aged-dependent serum immunoglobulin level.

Thus, most of the investigations concerned with determining the influence of aging on the development of gingival inflammation have shown that the host response to plaque microorganisms changes with increasing age, manifested by a more pronounced inflammatory reaction in the gingiva.

The aging of the immune system is manifested by an increased susceptibility to infections. Age-related changes in the levels of many pro- and anti-inflammatory cytokines have been documented, but the course or source of this altered cytokine production have not been clearly identified. Since cytokines and matrix metalloproteinases, as well as the NADPH-oxidase NOX2 [26], play a major role in the breakdown of tissue associated with periodontitis, it is possible that age changes in the stimulation and synthesis of these inflammatory mediators may be significant factors for increased susceptibility to periodontal disease with age. Combined effects of altered innate and acquired immune function paired with slower cell metabolism and healing capacity increase the risk of disease. This suggests that an age-associated increased susceptibility might result from an altered capacity to mount a sufficient host response to periodontal infection [27].

Studies are still needed to determine whether the rate of progression of periodontitis involving the deeper parts of the periodontium is different in young and old subjects. Periodontitis is usually considered to progress slowly in elderly subjects. The increased intensity of the inflammatory reaction in the gingiva of older people during the course of experimental gingivitis may, therefore, reflect a local defence mechanism by which the host attempts to compensate for a less effective immune response.

Periodontal inflammation, systemic diseases and aging

Often researchers differentiate between primary (natural, unavoidable) aging processes, governed by the inherent properties of the genotype, and secondary aging processes, which refer to acceleration of the normal aging processes derived from diseases and environmental influences. It has been increasingly recognized that the aging process is shaped throughout the entire life course, not only in old age. Strain in childhood, youth and early adulthood (e.g. diseases, poverty, low education, stressful working environment) increases the risk of early occurrence of chronic disease and comorbidity, which in turn increases the risk of premature disability. Generally, adverse health-related outcomes usually occur late in life, but the biology leading to these events begins much earlier. Consequently, it is important to identify early signs of accelerated aging.

Inflammatory processes have been implicated as predictors of, or contributors to, several chronic diseases and conditions of aging [28], including cardiovascular diseases, osteoarthritis, muscle wasting, physical performance, frailty, disability and mortality. These associations have been proposed to be caused by altered cytokine profiles due to aging of the innate immune system and/or non-immune cell types, and/or to age-related changes in body composition.

There is also strong evidence from several large, longitudinal population studies and prospective intervention trails that periodontal inflammation and tooth loss are associated with an increased risk of artherosclerosis, coronary heart disease and stroke. These relationships are biologically possible and supported by data on systemic markers of inflammation. An alternative explanation for the periodontal-cardiovascular relationship is that these diseases share common risk factors.

Three recent meta-analyses showed that periodontitis was found to increase the risk of coronary heart disease [29–31]. Another recent meta-analysis found that periodontitis associated with elevated levels of systemic markers of bacterial exposure was associated with coronary heart disease and carotid intima-medial thickening as a measure of early atherosclerosis, with an effect stronger than previous meta-analyses have shown for clinical periodontitis [32]. It was suggested that the level of systemic bacterial exposure from the infected periodontium may be the biological pertinent exposure with regard to atherosclerosis risk.

In most studies reporting an association between oral infections and cardiovascular events, the majority of participants have been middle-aged or young-old adults, and the risk of periodontitis-associated coronary heart disease is considerably higher in younger than in older individuals. Few studies have included the oldest segments of the population, those over the age of 80 years. A recent study found that severe periodontal inflammation in nondisabled 70-year-old individuals tended to be associated with mortality during 21-year follow-up [33].

The role of genetic factors predisposing people to greater or lesser age-related changes in inflammatory processes and chronic disease is not well understood. However, cytokines do not exist in a vacuum, but they participate in a complex matrix of genetic, biological, behavioral, socioeconomic and environmental factors including comorbidity.

It is unclear to what extent periodontal inflammation is an unrecognized source of inflammatory stress leading to increased morbidity, disability and mortality in aging.

Prognosis

Prognosis is a prediction of the probable course of a disease and of the prospect for recovery. It includes evaluation of the natural history of the disease without treatment as well as assessment of the anticipated response to treatment.

The prognosis for periodontal therapy is generally considered to be better for elderly than for younger individuals if an equal amount of periodontal attachment loss has occurred, because periodontal destruction may have progressed at a much slower rate in the older person. Therefore, the past history, that is, the duration of the disease, or the length of time during which the periodontal tissues have been exposed to plaque in the dento-gingival region, may be important in estimating the prognosis. In principle, a moderate attachment loss in a young subject should be regarded as a rather serious situation, whereas a corresponding severity of periodontal destruction in an elderly patient may be considered as being less serious.

Despite these general guidelines, it should not be overlooked that periodontitis is often very selective. Substantial destruction may occur at some teeth and little or none at others. The overall prognosis of the dentition depends on, but may differ from, that of individual teeth.

Good oral hygiene is crucial to all periodontal therapy regardless of age. The presence of a variety of dental restorations and gingival recessions, offering additional retention sites for plaque accumulation, frequently requires a higher level of manual dexterity and effort to maintain good oral hygiene.

Longitudinal studies have shown that successful therapeutic results can be obtained and maintained for years in elderly subjects. In a clinical trial comprising 75 patients 26–79 years old with advanced periodontal disease, Lindhe and Nyman [34] studied the long-term effect of periodontal therapy. Following completion of periodontal treatment, which included surgical elimination of pathologically deepened pockets, the patients were recalled for maintenance care every 3–6 months for the following 5 years. At these periodic recalls, the patients were instructed in effective oral hygiene methods and given thorough dental prophylaxis. The results demonstrated that advanced periodontitis can be treated successfully in young as well as in old patients and that periodontal health and attachment levels can be maintained over an observation period of five years.

In a subsequent study the same group reported on the effect of age on the outcome of periodontal therapy [35]. Two groups of patients with different degrees of periodontal disease were included in the study. One group (sample A) consisted of 62 patients with moderately advanced periodontitis. Thirteen subjects were less than 40 years of age, 26 subjects were 40–49 years old and 23 subjects were more than 49 years old. The second group (sample B) consisted of the six youngest and the 15 oldest of the patients treated for advanced periodontitis 14 years earlier and presented above. Six of these patients were between 26 and 29 years of age and 15 were at least 60 years old at the time they entered the first study (14 years earlier).

In sample A, the younger and older groups responded to active therapy with the same degree of gingivitis resolution, probing pocket depth reduction and attachment level change. These observations were further supported by the 14-year follow-up examination of the subjects in sample B. During the 14 years of maintenance, the younger and the old patients demonstrated a similar but very low tendency to develop recurrent periodontal disease. These results are in accordance with the findings of the first study demonstrating that successful therapeutic results can be sustained for years following optimum plaque control in young as well as in old subjects. A similar conclusion was reached in a 30-year longitudinal study by Axelsson and co-workers [36]. Lindhe and co-workers also found that young individuals who were considered to be susceptible to periodontitis healed following therapy equally well or better than older patients who were supposedly less susceptible. On that basis, it was concluded that the concept that a young subject with moderate to advanced periodontitis has a poorer prognosis than an older patient with a similar severity of disease is more likely related to the risk of reinfection over a longer period of time than to the healing capacity of the tissues.

Longitudinal periodontal tissue changes following periodontal therapy of advanced periodontitis and during a 12-year period of maintenance has revealed that approximately two thirds of the patients maintained stable conditions with only an occasional loss of a tooth (0.3 tooth per patient in 12 years) [37]. However, this study by Rosling and co-workers also identified a group of approximately one third of the patients that lost a six times higher number of teeth (1.9 teeth per patient in 12 years) despite better oral hygiene practices. These high susceptibility patients were characterized by a significantly higher loss of alveolar bone after active therapy (mean of 6.5 mm versus 3.4 mm) and a significantly greater pocket probing depth (3.3 mm versus 2.6 mm) than the 'normal susceptibility' group. Hence, it is evident that prognosis for reinfection may already be suspected at the end of active therapy irrespective of the age of the patients.

It has been well documented that the rate of wound healing in the skin and gingiva is slower in older than in younger subjects [38]. However, the studies of experimental gingivitis referred to above demonstrated rather clearly that the gingiva of elderly people healed rapidly and completely after removal of microbial plaque and reinstitution of effective oral hygiene.

Thus, these findings indicate that the altered host response and the reduced healing capacity in elderly subjects can be compensated for by reducing the bacterial impact. The ability of the elderly patient to heal so well suggests that the healing capacity is far in excess of what is needed for normal tissue healing. Adequate plaque control is of paramount importance and can be achieved. However, in patients who are not proficient in oral hygiene, the altered biological responses may imply an increased risk for complications and progression of periodontitis.

Periodontal treatment and prophylaxis

Treatment considerations

Clinical experience and the results from clinical and experimental studies demonstrate that periodontal disease can be treated successfully in old individuals and that the prognosis

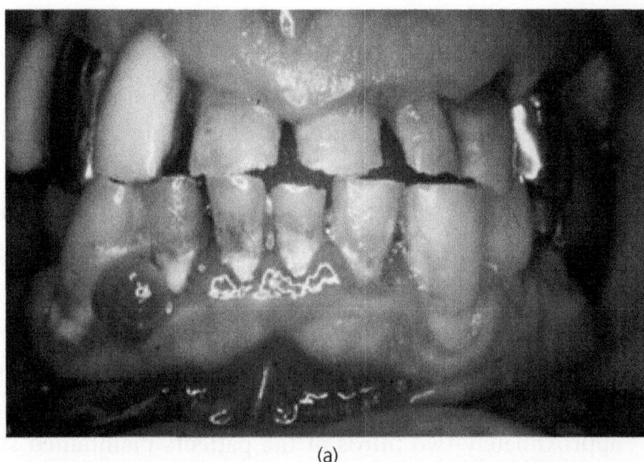

(a)

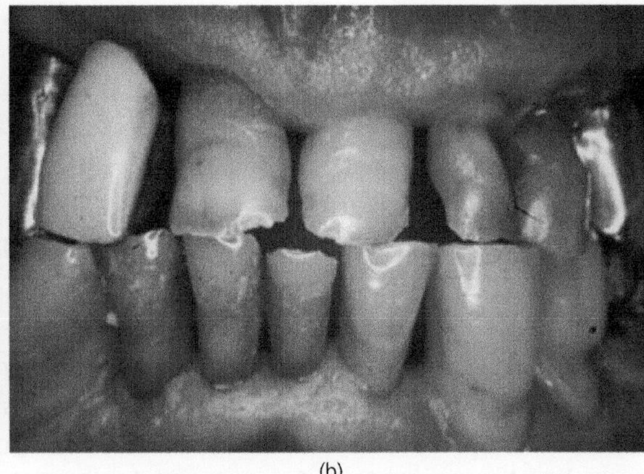

(b)

Figure 17.4 a) A 70-year-old patient consults a new dentist because a fixed bridge in the right side of the upper jaw is loose. Most teeth have 6–8 mm deep pockets, heavy amounts of plaque and pronounced gingival inflammation. The patient expressed a sincere wish to maintain all his teeth. He has never been offered preventively oriented dental care. **b)** The same patient 6 months following completion of periodontal treatment, which included periodontal surgery. The outcome of treatment has been successful and the patient has learned an effective method of oral hygiene.

is generally good [Figure 17.4(a),(b)]. However, when decisions on the choice of treatment in elderly patients are made, it should be remembered that the 65 and over population is far from homogeneous. Many are healthy and vigorous; others are disabled and ill. Most live in the community, but some live in institutions. For this reason it is useful to divide this patient population into three groups, as suggested by Ettinger [39] and by the American Association of Dental Schools [40] (see also Chapter 25):

- *Functionally independent elderly people living in their own home*
  This is the largest group of people over 65 years of age. Their social functioning is not impaired by general health problems. Some of these subjects have chronic ailments or slight disabilities, but they are mobile and are able to live independently in the community.
- *Frail elderly people*
  The frail elderly are individuals who have more serious physical, medical and/or emotional problems along with loss of social independence. The majority of these people live in the community with support services; a small minority live in institutions. Some are homebound; others are ambulatory and can come to the dental office if helped.
- *Functionally dependent elderly people*
  This is the smallest group and is estimated to make up less than 10% of the population over 65 years of age in several industrialized countries. These people's functional capacities are so impaired by debilitating physical, medical and/or emotional problems that they are unable to maintain independence. They are either homebound or institutionalized (Figure 17.5). For further definitions of frailty and disability, see Chapter 10.

Obviously, these groups are not distinct entities, as each one blends with the others. The terms for providing dental care, including periodontal therapy, differ both between these groups and within them. When decisions are being made as to what treatment should be given to individual elderly patients, their oral health status, their attitudes, previous dental experiences and expectations should be carefully considered. Similarly, their physical and emotional

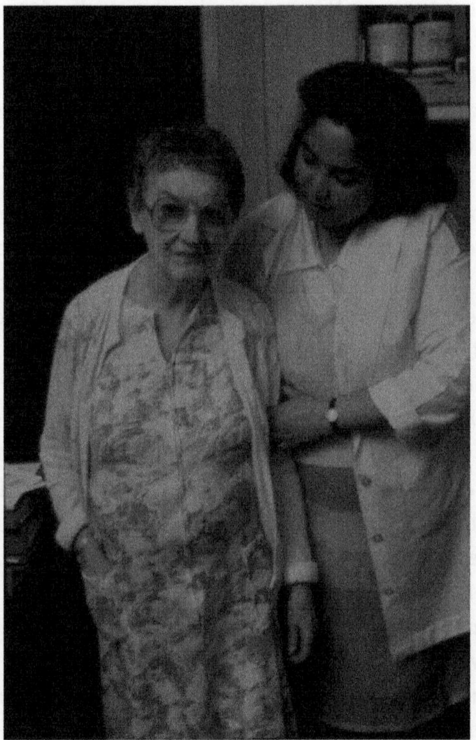

Figure 17.5 An 83-year-old functionally dependent resident of a nursing home being accompanied to the dental clinic by an assistant nurse.

status, mobility status, and social support systems need to be assessed. Accumulated oral problems and periodontal breakdown, as well as potential complications due to medical conditions or medications, may modify the treatment plan and necessitate a more holistic approach (see Chapter 14 and 22).

The age of the patient is also a factor in treatment planning. Although, in many studies, and often in the community, 'old' is defined as age 65 years and over, it must be borne in mind that this chronological age is arbitrary and may differ significantly from the individual's biological age. The arithmetic interval between 65 to 95 years corresponds to that between 35 to 65 years. It stands to reason that the basis for treatment may change over such a span of 30 years or more. In fact, the vast majority of 65-year-old people are physically vital, relatively healthy and function well mentally. Several epidemiological studies have given some support to the division of the elderly population into young-old (age 65–74), medium-old (75–84) and oldest-old (85+ years), as impairment, disability and handicap become more prevalent in the oldest age groups. Nevertheless, age *per se* should not be a major factor in limiting certain types of dental treatment and should not influence the decision to treat or not to treat.

As discussed previously, the healing capacity of the periodontal tissues is not lost even in very old individuals, and biological aging processes do not *per se* limit the opportunities for periodontal therapy. Nevertheless, old age may influence the treatment decision. Is the patient strong enough to tolerate the treatment? What prognosis may be anticipated? What are the short- and long-term outcomes without treatment or of a more conservative therapy? What are the risks of treatment?

In periodontal care for elderly people, the usual practice before the late 1950s was to postpone treatment and adopt a holding pattern until the patient was considered ready for complete dentures. Old patients were looked at with reluctance by many dentists, and periodontal treatment and more complex restorations were often not considered. This attitude to treatment of older people was based on the idea that the elderly patient could not endure periodontal treatment which included surgery, that the prognosis for the treatment was poor or simply that complex therapy was unwarranted, since the person had only a few years left to live. It was not based on the range of the therapeutic options afforded to other patients.

Postponing treatment until the patient has grown older may seriously limit the possibilities for treatment or make the implementation of necessary dental care difficult. The life expectancy of a 65-year-old man is more than 15 years and more than 20 years for a 65-year-old woman in several of the developed countries, and the goal of all dental care must be to maintain the dentition in a good functional condition throughout life. Therefore, postponing treatment is not the paradigm of choice if any other conservative approach is feasible. On the contrary, major dental procedures should be carried out as early as possible and subsequent care should concentrate on maintaining periodontal health and preventing the recurrence of disease (Figure 17.6).

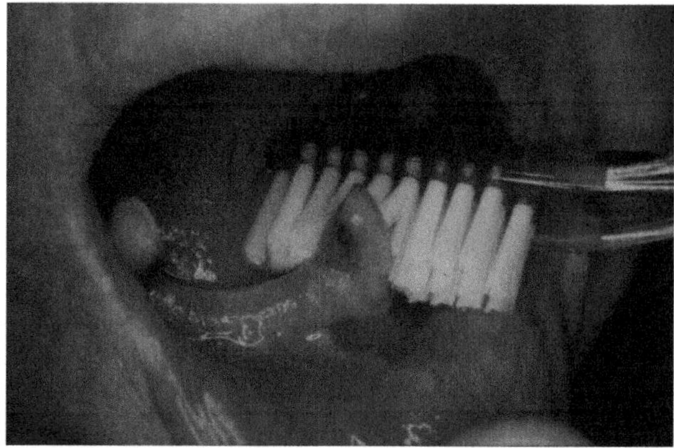

Figure 17.6 Mechanical plaque removal is the basic oral home care procedure. This should be stressed even if the patient has only a few natural teeth left. These may serve an important function as, for example, abutment teeth for a removable partial denture.

Older people are increasingly likely to have chronic impairments or even more serious disabilities or diseases that may adversely affect periodontal health. As mentioned previously, frail and functionally dependent elderly people constitute a high-risk population based on complex health problems and functional status, which may seriously influence oral health and related treatment. This group also includes patients who are unable to carry out adequate oral hygiene [Figure 17.7(a),(b)] and anyone taking medications that produce salivary hypofunction as a side effect (see Chapters 12 and 19). Therefore, these subgroups of older adults need to be especially targeted for preventive procedures.

Approaches to treatment

Both gingivitis and periodontitis are opportunistic infections initiated and maintained by bacteria colonizing the teeth and periodontal tissues. The aim of periodontal treatment is to eliminate or control gingivitis and to arrest the progression of periodontitis by removing the microbial plaque. Conservative therapy consisting of frequent tooth cleaning and repeated individualized instruction in oral hygiene techniques constitutes an appropriate therapeutic approach. In cases in which the clinician considers it unlikely that complete removal of (subgingival) soft and hard bacterial deposits from infected root surfaces will be achieved by scaling and root planing alone, periodontal surgery may be

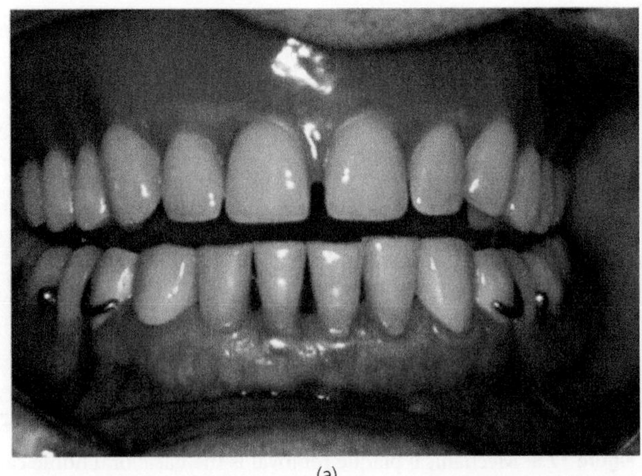
(a)

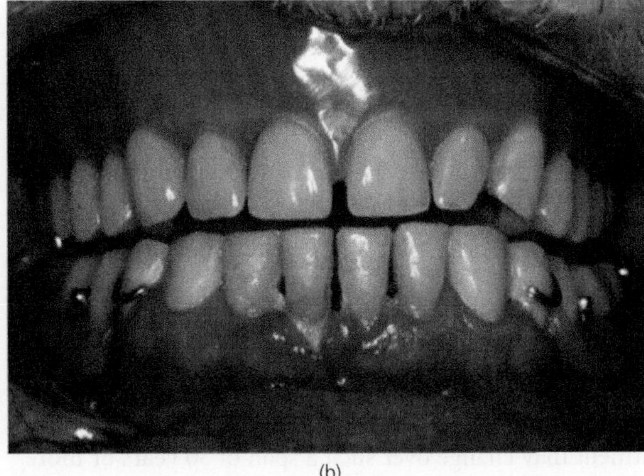
(b)

Figure 17.7 Periodontal breakdown may appear within a very short time. **a**) This 88-year-old patient meticulously cleaned his teeth until the age of 91 years, **b**) when he appeared for his recall appointment badly shaved and dressed in sneakers and a jogging costume.

necessary to create access for proper debridement. A second indication for periodontal surgery is to establish a gingival morphology that facilitates the patient's self-performed postoperative plaque control.

The age of the patient is no contraindication to periodontal surgery. For instance, a robust 80-year-old may be an excellent candidate for maximum treatment. On the other hand, the outcome in terms of tooth longevity may not outweigh the trauma of surgical treatment to a frail elderly patient.

Complicated surgical management requires knowledge of, and deference to, the general health status of the patient, the altered tissue responses and healing. The principles for periodontal surgery are basically the same for adults of any age, and there are no real differences between the surgical procedures used in young and old people. To minimize patient discomfort and reduce the risk of postoperative complications, surgery should be performed as atraumatically as possible. Available evidence clearly demonstrates that excellent wound healing can be obtained in elderly people, provided that the tissues are handled properly.

Several clinical trials have compared the effect of surgical and nonsurgical periodontal therapy in patients with moderate or advanced periodontitis (for review, see Kieser [41]). The results of these studies did not find marked differences in the outcome of the surgical and nonsurgical methods. Both treatment modalities resulted in resolution of inflammation (e.g. bleeding on probing), pocket depth reduction and maintenance or gain of clinical attachment levels. In deep periodontal lesions, the surgical methods resulted in greater reduction of probing pocket depths than did the nonsurgical methods. However, no differences have been revealed between the surgical and nonsurgical methods in terms of patterns of recolonization of pockets by microorganisms [42]. The results of these and other clinical trials demonstrate that subgingival instrumentation is an effective method for eliminating the subgingival infection and arresting the progression of chronic periodontitis.

Complete removal of subgingival plaque and calculus is extremely difficult in deep periodontal pockets. Studies have found that failure to remove all plaque and calculus is common. Therefore, if pockets bleed on gentle probing or produce suppuration at the evaluation after initial therapy, renewed treatment should be considered. If bleeding on probing is caused by inadequate oral hygiene, the patient should be given renewed instruction in proper oral hygiene techniques. If the patient is unable to perform effective home care, supportive treatment, including regular visits for professional tooth cleaning, may be appropriate.

Even though the value of proper and regular personal plaque control is undisputed, it has to be realized that patients present with a different susceptibility to periodontitis. Especially in the elderly, the periodontal health status may be indicative of the patient's history and susceptibility to periodontal breakdown. Obviously, the amount of plaque presents a poor predictor for the risk assessment of future disease. This, in turn, does not mean that abundant plaque should be accepted in an elderly patient provided that the loss of periodontal attachment appears rather limited, but it also points to the fact that the very ambitious goal of regular and complete plaque removal can, indeed, be modified and personal oral hygiene programs made more 'realistic', since this patient population is most likely going to maintain a functional dentition for the rest of their lives, provided that some preventive services are rendered.

Consultation with the elderly patient's physician is often necessary prior to treatment to clarify specific aspects of his or her medical problems and/or medications. Patients with certain types of valvular heart disease should receive antibiotic prophylaxis prior to scaling and surgery to prevent infection by haematogenous spread (see Chapter 8).

In medically and/or mentally compromised elderly patients, nonsurgical periodontal therapy may be the best approach to treatment. In old individuals who are in poor health, the aims of treatment should be to keep the patient free of pain and infection and to maintain the dentition in a functional condition for life. Subjective oral well-being should be the leading concept in treatment planning. A primary goal must be that the trauma of treatment does not exceed the gains of treatment. Therefore, in individual cases the clinician may have to modify the treatment plan to include procedures appropriate for that specific patient.

Maintenance

The key word in geriatric dentistry is maintenance. Dental auxiliaries such as dental hygienists play a key role in maintaining periodontal health in frail and functionally dependent elderly individuals. The dental hygienist is able to perform most types of uncomplicated periodontal therapy and assist nursing staff, or a family member, in performing oral hygiene for individual patients. The dental hygienist is also able to develop educational programmes for nursing and allied health professionals, deliver in-service education and develop oral health care plans for individual patients and at community levels. Assuming this role, the dental hygienist must work closely with the dentist as a member of the dental or interdisciplinary health care team (see Chapter 25). Because of the complexity of the problems encountered in frail and functionally dependent elderly patients, the dental hygienist needs to develop specific skills and to acquire additional knowledge in geriatric dentistry, including geriatric medicine and pharmacology (see Chapter 25).

Conclusion

The rates of edentulism and tooth loss are rapidly declining. Therefore, the number of old individuals requiring periodontal treatment will most likely increase. Prevention and treatment of periodontal disease in elderly subjects require dental services based on improved knowledge of the biology and pathology of the periodontium. Periodontal care for elderly people involves a complete analysis of the physical and emotional status of the patient. Age changes may affect the assessment of the periodontal problem, the treatment plan, its prognosis and the risk of complications following therapy. Available evidence clearly demonstrates that periodontitis can be treated successfully in the elderly and that periodontal health can be sustained.

References

1 Löe, H., Theilade, E. & Jensen, S.B. (1965) Experimental gingivitis in man. *Journal of Periodontology*, **36**, 177–187.

2 Miller, A.J., Brunelle, J.A., Carlos, J.P., Brown, L.J. & Löe, H. (1987) *Oral health of United States adults. The national survey of oral health in U.S. employed adults and seniors: 1985-1986*. NIH publication no. 87-2868, US Department of Health and Human Services, Washington, DC.

3 Ship, J.A. & Wolf, A. (1988) Gingival and periodontal parameters in a population of healthy adults, 22-90 years of age. *Gerondotology*, **7**, 55–60.

4 Gilbert, G.H. & Heft, M.W. (1992) Periodontal status of older Floridians attending senior activity centers. *Journal of Clinical Periodontology*, **19**, 249–255.

5 Hugoson, A., Norderyd, O., Slotte, C. & Thorstensson, H. (1998) Distribution of periodontal disease in a Swedish adult population 1973, 1983 and 1993. *Journal of Clinical Periodontology*, **25**, 542–548.

6 Schürch, E. Jr & Lang, N.P. (2004) Periodontal conditions in Switzerland at the end of the 20th century. *Oral Health & Preventive Dentistry*, **2**, 359–368.

7 Holm-Pedersen, P., Russell, S.L., Avlund, K., Viitanen, M. & Winblad, B. (2006) Periodontal disease in the oldest-old living in Kungsholmen, Sweden: findings from the KEOHS project. *Journal of Clinical Periodontology*, **33**, 376–384.

8 Ship, J.A. & Beck, J.D. (1996) Ten-year longitudinal study of periodontal attachment loss in healthy adults. *Oral Surgery, Oral Medicine, Oral Pathology*, **81**, 281–290.

9 Baelum, V., Luan, W.-M., Chen, X. & Fejerskov, O. (1997) Predictors of destructive periodontal disease incidence and progression in adult and elderly Chinese. *Community Dentistry and Oral Epidemiology*, **25**, 265–272.

10 Ambjørnsen, E. (1986) Remaining teeth, periodontal condition, oral hygiene and tooth cleaning habits in dentate old-age subjects. *Journal of Clinical Periodontology*, **13**, 583–589.

11 Vigild, M. (1988) Oral hygiene and periodontal conditions among 201 dentate institutionalized elderly. *Gerodontics*, **4**, 140–145.

12 Stuck, A.E., Chappuis, C., Flury, H. & Lang, N.P. (1989) Dental treatment needs in an elderly population referred to a geriatric hospital in Switzerland. *Community Dentistry and Oral Epidemiology*, **17**, 267–272.

13 Holm-Pedersen, P., Neely, A. & Katz, R.V. (1991) Periodontal disease in an institutionalized elderly population. *Journal of Dental Research*, **70**, (Special Issue), Abstract 1192.

14 Neely, A. & Holm-Pedersen, P. (1994) Progression of periodontal disease in an institutionalized elderly population. *Journal of Dental Research*, **73**, (Special Issue), Abstract 2610.

15 Yoneyhama, T., Yoshida, M., Ohrui, T., Mukaiyama, H., Okamoto, H., Hoshiba, K. *et al.* (2002) Oral care reduces pneumonia in older patients in nursing homes. *Journal of the American Geriatrics Society*, **50**, 430–433.

16 Taylor, G.W., Loesche, W.J. & Terpenning, M.S. (2000) Impact of oral diseases on systemic health in the elderly: diabetes mellitus and aspiration pneumonia. *Journal of Public Health Dentistry*, **60**, 313–320.

17 Page, R.C. & Eke, P.I. (2007) Case definitions for use in population-based surveillance of periodontitis. *Journal of Periodontology*, **78**, 1387–1399.

18 Holm-Pedersen, P., Agerbæk, N. & Theilade, E. (1975) Experimental gingivitis in young and elderly individuals. *Journal of Clinical Periodontology*, **2**, 14–24.

19 Brecx, M., Holm-Pedersen, P. & Theilade, J. (1985) Early plaque formation in young and elderly individuals. *Gerodontics*, **1**, 8–13.

20 Gaumer, H.R., Holm-Pedersen, P. & Folke, L.E.A. (1976) Indirect blastogenesis of peripheral blood leukocytes in experimental gingivitis. *Infection and Immunity*, **13**, 1347–1353.

21 Holm-Pedersen, P, Gaumer, H.R. & Folke, L.E.A. (1979) Aberrant blastogenic response to LPS in experimental gingivitis of elderly subjects. *Scandinavian Journal of Dental Research*, **87**, 431–434.

22 Holthuis, A.F., Holm-Pedersen, P. & Folke, L.E.A. (1977) Interepithelial lymphocytes in experimental gingivitis in young and elderly individuals. *Journal of Periodontal Research*, **12**, 166–178.

23 Van der Velden, U., Abbas, F. & Hart, A.A.M. (1985) Experimental gingivitis in relation to susceptibility to periodontal disease. *I. Clinical observations. Journal of Clinical Periodontology*, **12**, 61–68.

24 Berglundh, T. & Lindhe. J. (1993) Gingivitis in young and old dogs. *Journal of Clinical Periodontology*, **20**, 1–7.

25 Fransson, C., Mooney, J., Kinane, D.F. & Berglundh, T. (1999) Differences in the inflammatory response in young and old human subjects during the course of experimental gingivitis. *Journal of Clinical Periodontology*, **26**, 453–460.

26 Giannopoulou, C., Krause, K.H. & Müller, F. (2008) The NADPH oxidase NOX2 plays a role in periodontal pathologies. *Seminars in Immunopathology*, **30**, 273–278.

27 Persson, G.R. (2006) What has ageing to do with periodontal health and disease? *International Dental Journal*, **56**(Suppl. 1), 240–249.

28 National Institute of Aging. (2005) *Workshop on Inflammation, Inflammatory Mediators, and Aging*. Workshop Summary. National Institute of Aging, Bethesda, MD.

29 Janket, S.-J., Baird, A.E., Chuang, S.-K. & Jones, J.A. (2003) Meta-analysis of periodontal disease and risk of coronary heart disease and stroke. *Oral Surgery, Oral Medicine, Oral Pathology, Oral Radiology and Endodontology*, **95**, 559–569.

30 Khader, Y.S., Albasharireh, Z.S.M. & Alomari, M.A. (2004) Periodontal diseases and the risk of coronary heart and cerebrovascular diseases: a meta-analysis. *Journal of Periodontology*, **75**, 1046–1053.

31 Bahekar, A.A., Singh, S., Saha, S., Molnar, J. & Arora, R. (2007) The prevalence and incidence of coronary heart disease is significantly increased in periodontitis: a meta-analysis. *American Heart Journal*, **154**, 830–837.

32 Mustapha, I.Z., Debrey, S., Oladubu, M. & Ugarte, R. (2007) Markers of systemic bacterial exposure in periodontal disease and cardiovascular disease risk: a systematic review and meta-analysis. *Journal of Periodontology*, **78**, 2289–2302.

33 Avlund, K., Schultz-Larsen, K., Krustrup, U., Christiansen, N. & Holm-Pedersen, P. (2009) The role of inflammation in the periodontium in early old age on mortality at 21-year follow-up. *Journal of American Geriatrics Society*, **57**, 1206–1212.

34 Lindhe, J. & Nyman, S. (1975) The effect of plaque control and surgical pocket elimination on the establishment and maintenance of periodontal health. A longitudinal study of periodontal therapy in cases of advanced disease. *Journal of Clinical Periodontology*, **2**, 67–79.

35 Lindhe, J., Socransky, S.S., Nyman, S., Westfelt, E. & Haffajee, A. (1985) Effect of age on healing following periodontal therapy. *Journal of Clinical Periodontology*, **12**, 774–784.

36 Axelsson, P., Nyström, B. & Lindhe, J. (2004) The long-term effect of a plaque control program on tooth mortality, caries and periodontal disease in adults. Results after 30 years of maintenance. *Journal of Clinical Periodontology*, **31**, 749–757.

37 Rosling, B., Serino, G., Hellström, M.-K., Socransky, S.S. & Lindhe, J. (2001) Longitudinal periodontal tissue alterations during supportive therapy. Findings from subjects with normal and high susceptibility to periodontal disease. *Journal of Clinical Periodontology*, **28**, 241–249.

38 Holm-Pedersen, P. (1992) Influence of age on tissue healing. In: P. Worthington & P.-I. Brånemark (ed) *Advanced osseointegration surgery. Applications in the maxillofacial region*. pp. 47–56, Quintessence, Chicago, IL.

39 Ettinger, R.L. (1985) Geriatric dental curricula and the needs of the elderly. In: H.H. Chauncey, S. Epstein, C.L. Rose & J.J. Hefferen (eds) *Clinical Geriatric Dentistry. Biomedical and Psychosocial Aspects*. pp. 193–204, American Dental Association, Chicago, IL.

40 American Association of Dental Schools. (1988) *Special report: curriculum guidelines in geriatric dentistry. Appendix. Geriatric dentistry curriculum resource book*. American Association of Dental Schools, Washington, DC.

41 Kieser, J.B. (1994) Non-surgical periodontal therapy. In: N.P. Lang & T. Karring (eds) *Proceedings of the 1st European Workshop on Periodontology*. pp. 130–158, Quintessence, London.

42 Pedrazzoli, V., Kilian, M., Karring, T. & Kirkegaard, E. (1991) Effect of surgical and non-surgical periodontal treatment on periodontal status and subgingival microbiota. *Journal of Clinical Periodontology*, **18**, 598–604.

CHAPTER 18
Pathology and treatment of oral mucosal diseases

Palle Holmstrup[1], Jesper Reibel[1] and Ian C. Mackenzie[2]
[1]Department of Odontology, University of Copenhagen, Copenhagen, Denmark
[2]Centre for Cutaneous Research, Blizard Institute of Cell and Molecular Science, Barts and the London School of Medicine and Dentistry, London, UK

Functional aspects of normal oral mucosa

The mucosal lining of the oral cavity may be classified into three broad types: (a) the masticatory mucosa of the gingivae and hard palate; (b) the lining mucosa of the cheek, soft palate, floor of mouth and ventral surface of the tongue; and (c) specialized mucosae of the dorsum of the tongue, gingivae and the lips.[1–3] In all regions the oral mucosa consists of two main components, an epithelium and an underlying lamina propria and both of these components show marked regional differences in their structure, rates of regeneration and patterns of macromolecular synthesis. Such differences appear to be related mainly to the need to form flexible or fixed tissues, and the density of collagen, the size and organization of collagen fibre bundles and the proportion of elastic fibres in the lamina propria vary regionally in relation to such functions [4]. Lining mucosae need to adapt to changing shapes during opening and closing of the mouth and distention of the oral cavity with food to permit movement and stretching. The lamina propria of lining mucosae is therefore loose with a high proportion of elastic fibres [4]. Masticatory mucosae are bound down to form an almost immoveable surface and, in order to provide resistance against physical forces to which they are exposed, they have a densely collagenous lamina propria with larger and straighter collagen fibrils. Firm attachment of masticatory mucosae serves several purposes. For example, the bound-down gingival mucosa protects the dento-gingival junction from undue movement and the firm palatal surface, together with the rugae, enable fine comminution of food between the tongue and the palate.

In humans and other mammals the surface layer of the mucosa is formed by a stratified squamous epithelium which has a basic pattern of organization similar to that of the epidermis [1]. As for skin, the primary function of the epithelium is to act as a barrier between the internal and external environments and so protect against mechanical damage, entry of noxious substances and organisms and loss of fluid out of the underlying tissues. The epithelial component of the mucosa shows regional variation in its rates of cell replacement, density and size of its cells and in the degree of its surface keratinization and patterns of arrangement of the superficial cells [5, 6] The permeability of oral mucosa differs somewhat from region to region [1] but the marked regional variations found in epithelial structure are, like those of the lamina propria, primarily associated with regional differences in distensibility and the ability to resist mechanical stresses. Bound-down mucosae, being immobile, need an epithelial surface with greater resistance to abrasion and this is provided by extensive interdigitation of the epithelial-connective tissue interface and a greater degree of keratinization to form a more massive and inflexible stratum corneum [7]. The stretchy epithelium of lining mucosae is non-keratinized and has large cells with pleated cell walls and larger amounts of intercellular glycoprotein that allow its distension. Adding to the basic lining/masticatory classification, oral epithelia also show other regionally-related functional adaptations. For example, the epithelia of the lips, dorsum of tongue and gingival margin each has special physiological or structural properties in order to provide for intermittent dehydration, taste, masticatory functions or specialized attachment [1, 3].

In all regions the epithelial surface is subject to abrasion and an intact epithelial structure is maintained by quite rapid cell proliferation. The continuous replacement of the epithelial surface resulting from cell proliferation has the important additional function of providing a self-cleansing mechanism

Textbook of Geriatric Dentistry, Third Edition. Edited by Poul Holm-Pedersen, Angus W. G. Walls and Jonathan A. Ship.

that prevents build up of bacteria or fungi on the epithelial surface and resists penetration of microorganisms into the deeper tissue [8]. Marked regional variation in the rates at which the epithelial surface is replaced are produced by the combined effects of regional differences in rates of cell proliferation and the size of surface cells [9].

Although mucosal epithelia can respond to functional stresses by thickening, for example in response to friction [10], their regionally-differing functional requirements tend to be anticipated by developmentally-determined patterns of structure and kinetics [11]. Post-developmentally, the differing phenotypes expressed by mucosal epithelia are largely determined by mechanisms that are intrinsic to the epithelium itself rather than in response to external factors [12]. For example, regionally-specific rates of cell proliferation and differentiation are maintained when mucosae are transplanted to protected sites where they are not exposed to mechanical stimuli [4, 11]. Although the differing phenotypes expressed by adult epithelia are normally stable they can be altered by recombination with foreign connective tissues, indicating that epithelia maintain responsiveness to developmental signals throughout life [13–15]. Such interactions are continuously involved in maintenance of adult epithelia and 'organotypic' cell cultures, in which the effects of various connective tissues can be evaluated, indicating that epithelial maintenance involves reciprocal interactive signalling between the epithelial and connective tissue components [16]. In summary, regionally-diverse properties of the oral mucosa have been selected to provide optimal functional performance and significant age-associated changes in these properties would be expected to lead to some loss of function. However, evidence for marked age changes is not strong and the mucosa usually performs its normal functions quite adequately, even at advanced ages. As discussed below, some changes in structure and function can be detected but their causes are uncertain.

Clinical and histological changes occurring in aging oral mucosa

Changes with age are found in many tissues of the body and similar age-related changes are perhaps to be expected for the oral mucosa [17]. However, although clinical examination of the mucosae of the elderly often suggests subtle changes in mucosal texture and colouration, such changes may not be directly related to age itself [18]. Several studies have reported that the oral mucosa becomes increasingly thin, smooth and dry with age [19, 20] and that it acquires a satin-like, oedematous appearance with loss of elasticity and stippling [21]. The tongue in particular is reported to show marked clinical changes with a tendency for the development of sublingual varices [22, 23] and a smoother surface with loss of filiform papillae [24]. An increasing susceptibility to pathological conditions such as candidal infections could reflect a reduced epithelial turnover and a decreased rate of wound healing has been reported [25, 26]. Although such observations suggest an age-associated tendency to epithelial atrophy, data from kinetic studies have not clearly or consistently indicated loss of regenerative abilities [27–30]. Possibly mucosae may become more susceptible to minor injury with age and also become more permeable to noxious substances [22]. However, with the exception of permeability [31], few direct measurements of the mechanical properties of a normal or aging mucosa have been made that can be related to its structural or kinetic functions [7, 19, 32]. Quantitative data are few but clinical experience suggests that advancing age is associated with reduced levels of taste, loss of other forms of sensory perception and perhaps a reduced or altered control of immune defences.

Age-associated changes in skin [33, 34] have been investigated more extensively than changes in oral mucosa and the appearance and texture of the skin of the elderly clearly differ from the skin of the young. Underlying these clinical changes are various changes in the structure and function of the epidermis and dermis including simplification of the contour of the dermo-epidermal junction and greater variation in the thickness of the epidermis and in the size and shape of keratinocytes [34–36]. Structural changes are reported to be accompanied by kinetic changes such as reduced rates of epidermal desquamation [37], reduced thymidine labelling [38] and up to a 50% reduction in the rate of growth of appendages such as nail and hair [39]. Age-associated dermal changes, which may be the main cause of the altered appearance of 'old' skin [40], include decreased synthesis of dermal collagen and increased intermolecular cross-linking with a decreased proportion of soluble collagen [41]. There is also a loss of dermal volume and a reduction in the number of fibroblasts, mast cells and capillaries and good evidence for a markedly reduced rate of wound healing [42]. There is considerable evidence, from both clinical and animal investigations, that skin aging is also characterized by a dysregulated immune state [43, 44]. Although information about age changes in skin may be relevant to age changes occurring in oral mucosa, a major caveat is that most of the changes occurring in skin are related to damage from ultraviolet light [45], an environmental effect with little relevance to the oral cavity.

Age-associated histological changes reported for human oral mucosa include thinning [46, 47] changes of the epithelial-connective tissue interface and loss of keratinization [48, 49]. A 30% reduction in the thickness of the lingual epithelium and atrophy of the lingual papillae in old individuals has been reported [49] but others have found no age-related differences in the thickness of the gingival epithelium [48] and exfoliative cytology has not detected consistent age-related differences in the size or form of human oral epithelial cells [50]. Whether there are age-associated changes in the rate of cell renewal in oral epithelia remains uncertain and investigations of rates of cell proliferation have produced inconsistent data [51–56]. It has been suggested that aging may lead to loss of the stability of the mechanisms controlling epithelial homeostasis and thus be associated with a greater variation in tissue properties [56]. It is now apparent that mucosal renewal, like that of skin, depends on the presence of a sub-population of somatic stem cells [57] whose function includes protecting the tissues from malignant change [58]. Rates of malignancy increase greatly with age but whether there is loss of stem cell functions is uncertain. Evidence from mice suggests that epidermal stem cells change little with age [59].

To what extent any of the changes reported to occur in human mucosae with advancing age actually result from intrinsic (i.e. developmentally-determined) patterns of aging of the tissue itself is uncertain. The potential importance of other non-intrinsic environmental factors is suggested by aged rodents whose exposure to damaging environmental agents can be controlled and who do not show consistent age-related changes of the oral mucosa [8, 27–30]. Human mucosal changes may therefore result primarily from accumulation of extrinsic environmental insults with the passage of time. Mucosal exposure to tobacco and alcohol can produce overt pathological changes but whether lesser responses can masquerade as age changes is unclear. It is also possible that many of the changes detected are responses secondary to systemic changes produced by age changes or disease in other systems. Mucosal change might also be related to dietary deficiencies of iron or B vitamins and atrophic changes could follow reduced oestrogen levels in older women [20, 46, 60]. The reportedly high prevalence of mucosal lesions in the elderly [61, 62] may be associated with denture-wearing habits, general medical status or use of medications, factors which differ in the elderly [63, 64]. Examination of healthy persons between the ages of 20 and 95 years found no significant age-associated differences in subjective complaints about the oral mucosa or its clinical status. However, another study found that the age-corrected prevalence of a range of mucosal disorders was much higher in the elderly particularly for the frequency of malignant and premalignant disease [18], a finding in keeping with many clinical reports.

Common diseases of the oral mucosa

Prevalence of mucosal lesions

Oral mucosal lesions are common among the elderly. An epidemiological health investigation in Helsinki, Finland, revealed one or more lesions in as much as 38% of the examined 338 home-living individuals: 91 men and 247 women, aged 76, 81 or 86 years [65]. Among complete denture wearers the prevalence of mucosal lesions was 51% while in elderly with some natural teeth the prevalence was 31%. These findings were consistent with the results of a large study of elderly people in Santiago, Chile [66]. The most common finding of both studies was denture stomatitis, which occurred alone or combined with other lesions in 22–25% of denture wearers. In the Finnish study the most common changes unrelated to denture wearing were coating of the tongue (7%), angular cheilitis (6%) and varicose veins under the tongue (4%). Leukoplakia and inflammation of the buccal mucosa were both seen in 3% of the examined individuals. Interestingly, the total number of mucosal lesions correlated positively with the number of daily medications.

Another investigation of 255 independent elderly with equal numbers of men and women showed that almost half of them had mucosal lesions [67]. The lesions were significantly associated with the use of dentures and tobacco. Not surprisingly, stomatitis, angular cheilitis and denture-related hyperplasia were significantly associated with male gender and the use of defective dentures. Whereas a regression analysis demonstrated that neither age alone or quality of dentures predisposed to mucosal lesions, the odds of presence of stomatitis, hyperplasia and angular cheilitis increased threefold in denture users, and almost doubled in men.

Diseases of infectious origin

Candidosis

Yeast infections are rather common in elderly individuals. This may be due to smoking habits, medications and impaired resistance related to general diseases. Moreover, a study has demonstrated a number of additional factors important for the susceptibility to oral candidosis of the elderly [68]. These include increased numbers of *Candida* adhering to oral keratinocytes from elderly than to those from young controls. Also, decrease of salivary flow rate and of salivary anti-candidal factors, as well as suppression of salivary neutrophil function, predispose the elderly to oral candidosis.

A classification of candidosis has been proposed based on the clinical appearance of the lesions [69]:

Acute types

Pseudomembranous
Erythematous

Chronic types

Pseudomembranous
Erythematous
Plaque-like
Nodular

Lesions with a pathogenesis involving both *Candida* strains and other factors are entitled *Candida*-associated lesions. These lesions comprise denture stomatitis, angular cheilitis and median rhomboid glossitis. Whereas the first two of these lesions are described below, the latter condition will not be dealt with in this chapter. In the case of widespread chronic oral candidosis presenting with lesions of the above-mentioned types, the term chronic oral multifocal candidosis may be used as a supplementary description.

Pseudomembranous lesions are characterized by whitish, creamy patches that can be scraped off, leaving an erythematous mucosal surface. The acute pseudomembranous form is frequently seen in patients treated with antibiotics, corticosteroids or cytostatics. Acute erythematous lesions, which may have a similar background, appear as red, sometimes fiery red, areas often with ill-defined borders. The lesions are always accompanied by pain.

Pseudomembranous and erythematous lesions may sometimes show a chronic course, persisting for months. The clinical manifestations of such lesions are not essentially different from those of the acute forms except for milder symptoms. Antimycotic therapy of these types of chronic lesions results in a normal mucosal surface.

The chronic plaque-like lesions are characterized by the presence of patchy, whitish, often frayed plaques surrounded by erythema, whereas the nodular lesions show whitish papules or nodules on an erythematous background. Some of the plaque-like lesions disappear after antimycotic treatment, whereas others show residual lesions with white plaques. Nodular lesions demonstrate homogeneous white plaques after antimycotic treatment [70]. Residual lesions are commonly reinfected after cessation of antimycotic treatment. Candidal infections may play a role in the development of oral epithelial neoplasia [71]. This may be related to a catalytic potential of *Candida albicans* in the production of nitrosamine [72]. Consequently, chronic forms of oral candidosis should always be treated and, if possible, preventive measures should be established to avoid recurrence. Quitting of tobacco smoking is important to prevent such recurrence. Identification of other background factors may be necessary [73]. Commonly used antimycotics for topical use are amphotericin B, nystatin and miconazole. For systemic treatment, amphotericin B, ketoconazole and fluconazole can be used, but possible side effects must be considered [74].

Denture stomatitis

The inflammatory changes seen beneath a denture have been denoted stomatitis prothetica, denture sore mouth or denture stomatitis. The latter term seems to have gained universal acceptance.

The inflammatory changes are characterized mainly by erythema and are found under complete or partial dentures in both jaws, but more frequently in the maxilla. Denture stomatitis can be graded into three types [75, 76]: type I shows localized inflammation or pin-point hyperaemia; type II shows more diffuse erythema, and type III is a non-neoplastic granular hyperplasia with inflammation to a varying degree. The granular hyperplasia is usually located in the central part of the hard palate and may be either nodular or mossy in appearance.

As denture-wearing is mostly confined to elderly people, denture stomatitis is a problem of older age groups. Table 18.1 [77–83, 85] gives information on the prevalence of the three types of denture stomatitis in different groups of elderly individuals. The table only includes investigations where a distinction has been made between the three types.

Type I denture stomatitis is due to trauma from the dentures, whereas type II and III in addition to trauma from an ill-fitting denture are associated with candidal and/or bacterial infection. The infection is primarily due to a contamination of the surface of dentures by yeasts and bacteria, and *Candida hyphae* are always present on the denture in cases of denture stomatitis.

With regard to treatment, type I denture stomatitis should be treated by correcting the denture and establishing proper occlusal relations. Treatment of type II denture stomatitis consists first of all of instructing the patient to maintain rigid hygiene of the denture: mechanical cleaning twice a day, removal of the denture during the night and adjusting the denture as the oedema of the mucosa resolves. If the denture stomatitis has not regressed after 3–4 weeks on this regime, mycostatic treatment may be instituted, preferably in the form of antimycotic ointment or gel applied on the denture. Treatment of type III denture stomatitis depends on the intensity of the granular hyperplasia. In mild cases the treatment is the same as for type II. In patients with a marked degree of papillary hyperplasia, surgery is most often necessary as the first step of the treatment. To reduce bleeding the removal of papillary hyperplasia may be carried out by electrosurgery.

Angular cheilitis

The lateral lip fissures, well known among elderly denture wearers, have been called by a variety of names, such as rhagades, perlèche, angular cheilitis and angular cheilosis. It is

Table 18.1 Prevalence of denture stomatitis in selected studies

Investigators	Year	Size and type of material	Age in years	% with denture stomatitis	
Grabowski & Bertram [77]	1976	560 rural individuals in Denmark	>65	Type I	41
				Type II	10
				Type III	14
Vigild [80]	1987	413 denture wearers in nursing homes in Denmark	>64	Type I	10
				Type II	13
				Type III	12
Kuc et al. [82]	1999	63 residents of long-term care facility in Canada	Mean 83,4	Type I	16
				Type II	3
				Type III	2
Figueiral et al. [83]	2007	70 patients recruited from a dental school in Portugal	>18	Type I	41
				Type II	34
				Type III	24
Kossioni [85]	2011	106 patients with dentures treated in a Dental School in Greece	Mean 67,7	Type I	17
				Type II	16
				Type III	7

generally recognized that the most important causal factor is infection with *Candida albicans*, usually coming from a denture stomatitis. Sometimes the infecting organism is *Staphylococcus aureus*. Predisposing factors may be flaccid, sagging cheeks, deepened labial angles constantly moistened by saliva and decreased vertical dimension of the occlusion. Among 463 people older than 65 years in Denmark, 19% had angular cheilosis [84]. Among 2277 people aged 65–74 years in Sweden, the prevalence was 10% [86]. The lesions are treated with antimycotic ointment or gel and in cases of *Staphylococcus aureus infection*, fusidin ointment is the treatment of choice.

Manifestations of mucocutaneous diseases

Lichen planus

Lichen planus is a mucocutaneous disorder with frequent oral manifestations. It is found predominantly in older age groups and is characterized by white striations and papules. Sometimes the lesions are atrophic-ulcerative, plaque-like or bullous [87]. The etiology of the disease is unknown. Any part of the oral mucosa may be affected, and fluctuations between the various clinical types of lichen planus are common. There is an increased tendency for oral lichen planus lesions to develop cancer. Despite differences in experimental design, it is striking that the majority of studies have reported a rate of malignant transformation in the range of 0.5–2% over a 5-year period [88–90]. When the gingiva is affected oral hygiene procedures may become painful. Plaque accumulation aggravates the lesions and their symptoms. Hence frequent professional oral hygiene is recommended at short intervals: every 2–3 months [91]. Lesions that are resistant to improved oral hygiene can usually be treated with supplemental topical steroids [92] eventually combined with antimycotics, but recurrence is common after cessation of therapy. Topical tacrolimus may be beneficial in recalcitrant cases [93]. Drug induced-stomatitis, for instance, due to antirheumatics, may show clinical manifestations similar to lichen planus, i.e. lichenoid lesions. Thus, information on drug intake is very important. Altered medication may be necessary. Due to contact allergy, lichenoid lesions may also be found in mucosal areas of contact with amalgam fillings [94, 95]. In such cases, replacing the fillings with alternative materials causes the contact lesions to regress.

Benign mucous membrane pemphigoid

Pemphigoid is subdivided into bullous pemphigoid and benign mucous membrane pemphigoid. Only benign mucous membrane pemphigoid is discussed here, as bullous pemphigoid is rare and seldom has oral manifestations.

Benign mucous membrane pemphigoid is an autoimmune bullous disorder. Most of the patients have deposition of gammaglobulins at the epithelium-connective tissue interface. Benign mucous membrane pemphigoid is a disease of elderly people, and many of the patients are over 70 years of age at the onset of the disease. The disease is much more frequent in women than in men.

Whereas the oral mucosa is almost always affected, skin lesions are not routinely seen [96]. Not only do oral bullae often precede lesions in other mucous membranes and skin, but they are often the only manifestation of the disease. The initial oral changes consist of a yellow or, more rarely, a haemorrhagic bulla originating from an erythematous background. Because of the moist environment, the bullae burst, leaving a fibrin-covered ulceration. The predominant oral locations are the palate, the buccal mucosa, the gingiva and the alveolar ridge. Figure 18.1 shows a characteristic palatal lesion in a 76-year-old woman.

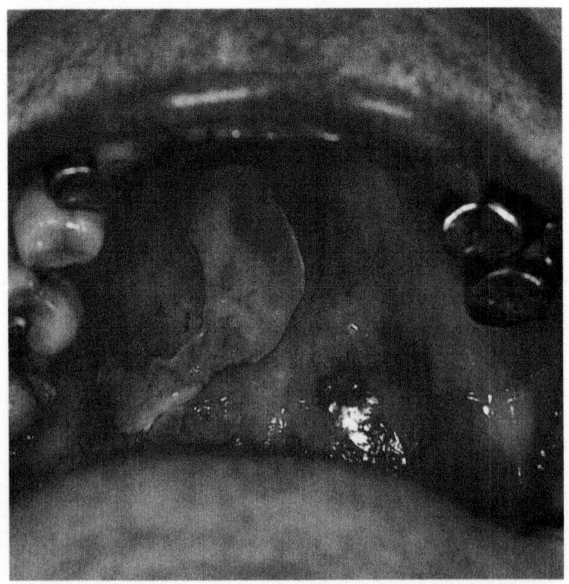

Figure 18.1 Benign mucous membrane pemphigoid-bulla in the soft palate of a 76-year-old woman.

Another characteristic clinical aspect of benign mucous membrane pemphigoid is a diffuse gingival involvement. The gingiva becomes fiery red and tags of desquamating epithelium can be seen in several areas. Previously, these gingival changes were called desquamative gingivitis.

Histologically, benign mucous membrane pemphigoid is characterized by a subepithelial bulla formation. The basal layer of the oral epithelium becomes separated from the underlying connective tissue and fluid accumulates, whereby a vesicle or a bulla is formed.

The treatment of benign mucous membrane pemphigoid is symptomatic. Systemic corticosteroids have been reported to alleviate the disease. If the oral lesions are painful, topical use of, for example, betamethasone cream or ointment provides some relief. Patients should be examined by an ophthalmologist as ocular involvement can lead to blindness.

Professional supervision of oral hygiene is necessary to develop an individual programme that enables plaque removal without damaging the gingival tissue. The tendency to develop new benign mucous membrane pemphigoid lesions seems to decrease with improved oral hygiene.

Denture irritation hyperplasia

Denture hyperplasia is usually seen in patients who have worn ill-fitting dentures over a rather long period of time. It is therefore observed more frequently in elderly people. In one of the largest studies of denture hyperplasia, 71% were found in persons above 50 years [97]. Table 18.2 [79, 80, 84, 86, 98–103, 65, 99, 100] shows the prevalence of denture irritation hyperplasia in elderly people. The range varies from 3 to 26%, but most materials have a prevalence of less than 10%. The irritation may come from overextended flanges or from sharp margins of the denture.

Diseases of the nervous system

Burning mouth syndrome

Burning mouth includes glossodynia (painful tongue) or glossopyrosis (burning tongue). Although the symptoms may be located anywhere in the mouth a painful burning tongue is the most common type of oral dysaesthesia [104]. In a study of 292 patients in a general dental practice in England, 5.1% had or had had a burning sensation of the tongue. The highest prevalence was found among the 40- to 49-year-olds [105]. In a study of 72 patients with glossodynia in Germany, 76% were women, with an average age of 60 years [106].

The term glossodynia should be confined to patients who clinically do not show any pathological changes. It is interesting that the symptoms are often absent in the morning but build up during the day. Whereas the symptoms are often described by the patients as unbearable, the symptoms are usually present over periods of months or years. Often the patients establish a background in dental treatment as the cause of the symptoms by referring to the symptoms arising after a dental treatment procedure. However, such a relation is almost never reliable. It is important to exclude possible lesions of the oral mucosa as the cause of the symptoms, which is why

Table 18.2 Prevalence of denture irritation hyperplasia in elderly denture wearers (selected studies)

Investigator	Year	Country	Size of material	Age in years	% affected
Pape et al. [98]	1970	Germany	1502	average 77	4
Ritchie [101]	1973	UK	206	>65	3
Grabowski [84]	1974	Denmark	463	>65	26
Axéll [86]	1976	Sweden	2277	>65	12
Vigil [80]	1987	Denmark	413	>64	9
Nevalainen et al. [65]	1997	Finland	260	>76	3
Jainkittivong et al. [99]	2010	Thailand	380	average 65	5
Rabiei et al. [100]	2010	Iran	121	>65	33

meticulous examination to exclude such lesions is mandatory. Abnormal blood values including iron and vitamin deficiency, primarily vitamin B-group deficiency, are other causes of sensation disturbances to exclude in the patients.

The cause of burning mouth is poorly understood, and often the patients are circulating in the health care system. The condition is probably of multifactorial origin and in a large number of patients probably involves interactions among local, systemic and/or psychogenic factors. In other cases, associations have emerged between burning mouth and either peripheral nerve damage or dopaminergic system disorders, emphasizing a neuropathic background. Patience and understanding is important and since many of the patients suffer from cancerophobia, it is essential to explain to the patients that the symptoms are not due to cancer. In some patients this may result in relief. A step by step approach is outlined by van der Waal [104] and Scala *et al.* [107].

Premalignant lesions

Leukoplakia

Leukoplakia is defined as a predominantly white lesion of the oral mucosa that cannot be characterized as any other definable lesion [108]. Leukoplakia is the most common premalignant lesion of the oral mucosa. This means that it is associated with an increased risk of malignant development. The lesions can be subdivided into homogeneous and non-homogeneous types, homogeneous lesions showing whitish, smooth or corrugated changes of the oral mucosa, whereas non-homogeneous lesions are whitish–reddish, sometimes nodular, speckled or verrucous changes. The non-homogeneous leukoplakias are associated with the highest potential for malignant development, which was also increased for lesions sized 200 mm^2 or more [109–111].

The age distribution in a large study of oral leukoplakia is given in Figure 18.2 [112]. The majority of oral leukoplakias are found among people aged 40–70 years. Women tend to develop leukoplakia later than men. Burkhardt [113] has explained the increasing frequency in higher age groups by the fact that leukoplakia may be caused by agents requiring a long period of action. An extensive study of 20 333 adults in Sweden found that idiopathic leukoplakia had the highest prevalence rate in individuals aged 55–75+ years [114].

Leukoplakia in the various sites of the oral mucosa does not have the same age and sex distribution. Leukoplakia in the floor of the mouth is 2.4 times more frequent among women than among men. The age distribution also reveals a difference by a shift to older age groups for leukoplakia in the floor of the mouth (Figure 18.3) [115]. Figure 18.4 illustrates a leukoplakia in the floor of the mouth in a 70-year-old Danish woman who smokes cheroots. Figure 18.5 shows an idiopathic leukoplakia in a 71-year-old woman. Among 55 cases of leukoplakia in the floor of the mouth recorded in London, 50% were above the age of 60 years [116]. In the same material it was demonstrated that leukoplakia

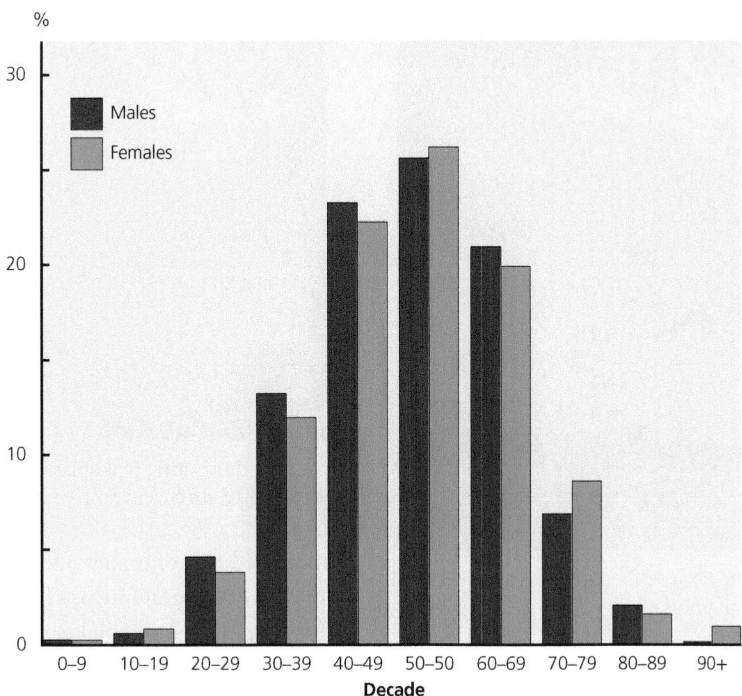

Figure 18.2 Age distribution of 3256 cases of oral leukoplakia. Prepared on the basis of figures from Waldron and Shafer [112].

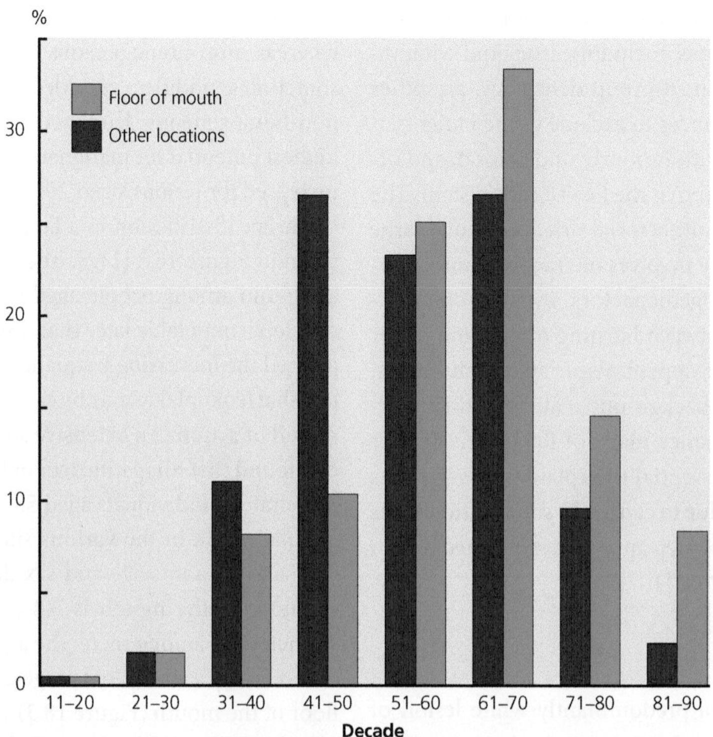

Figure 18.3 Age distribution of 368 cases of leukoplakia in the floor of the mouth and in other locations. Prepared on the basis of figures from Pindborg *et al.* [115].

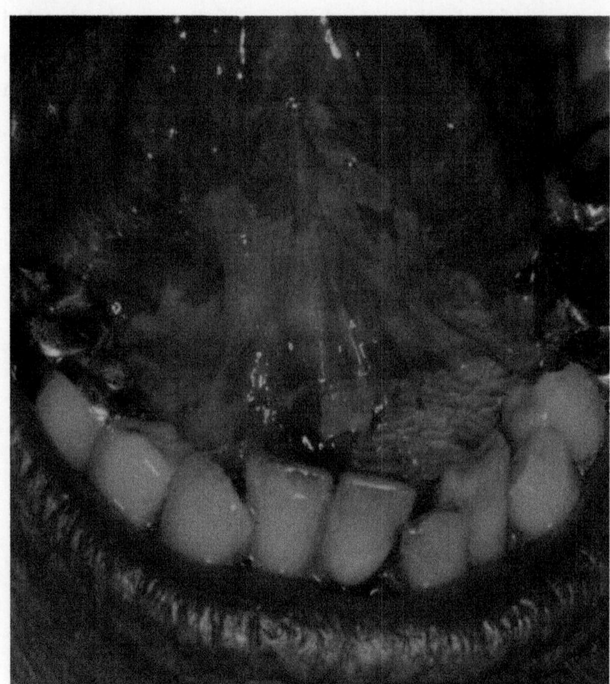

Figure 18.4 Leukoplakia in the floor of the mouth in a 70-year-old Danish woman who smokes cheroots.

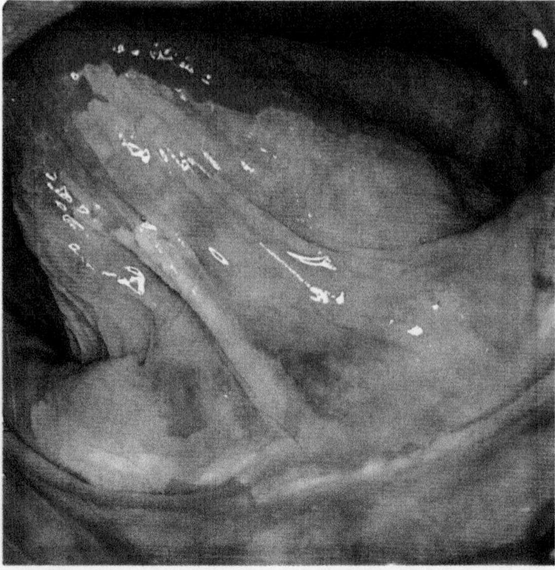

Figure 18.5 Idiopathic leukoplakia in the floor of the mouth and inferior lingual surface in a 71-year-old Danish woman.

in the floor of the mouth carries a high risk of malignant transformation. However, more recent studies have not been able to confirm that certain areas of the oral mucosa exhibit an increased risk of malignant development compared with other sites of the oral mucosa [111, 117].

Most types of leukoplakia associated with tobacco are reversible. Figure 18.6(a) and (b) illustrate the regression of a lesion of this type in a 60-year-old man two months after he had stopped smoking. Leukoplakia is a clinical diagnosis and

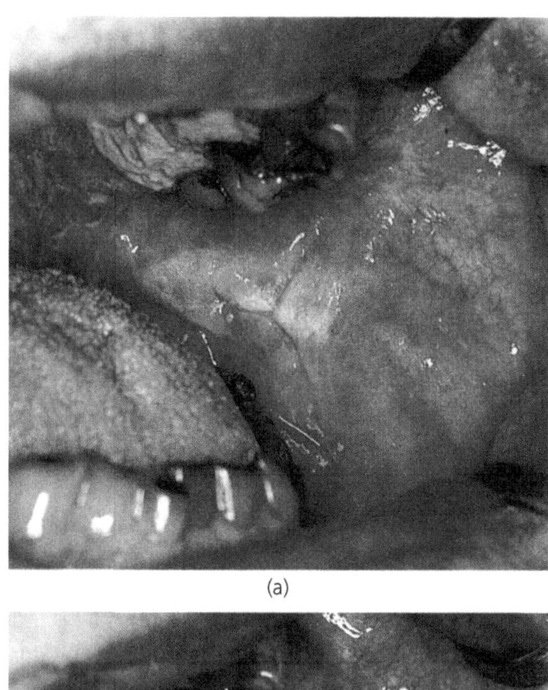

(a)

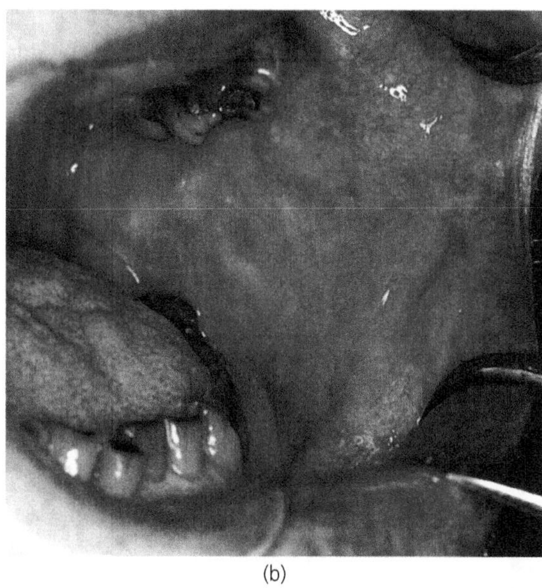

(b)

Figure 18.6 a) Leukoplakia of the buccal mucosa in a 60-year-old man. b) Two months later after the patient quit smoking.

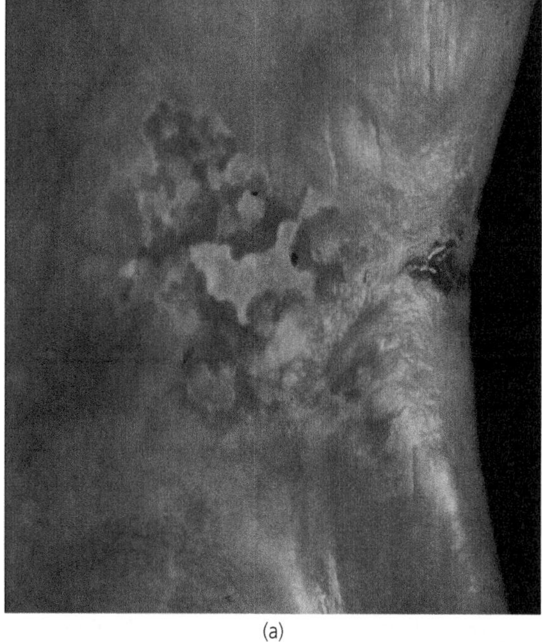

(a)

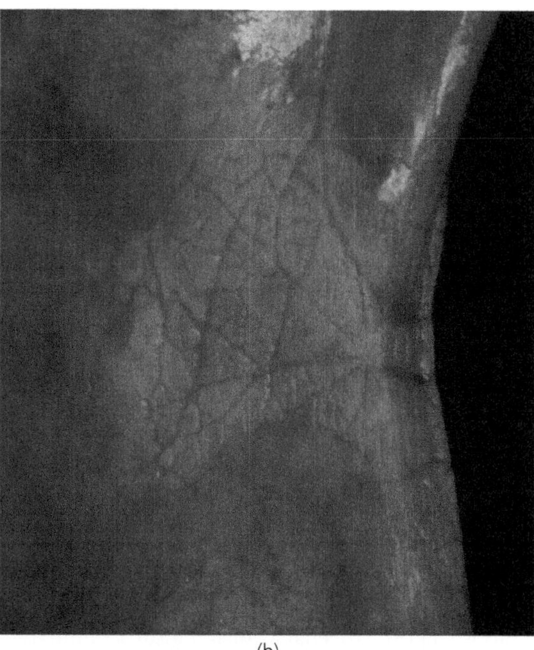

(b)

Figure 18.7 a) *Candida*-infected leukoplakia in the commissure of a 64-year-old man. b) Six weeks later after antimycotic treatment.

there is no uniform histopathology of leukoplakia, which usually shows hyperkeratosis, atrophy or hyperplasia and sometimes varying degrees of epithelial dysplasia. Dysplasia has been regarded as a sign of increased risk of malignant development, but a recent study did not show such an association [118], probably because genetically altered epithelial cells may be left unrevealed by routine histological examination and even include areas with normal histology [119]. The use of molecular markers, including TP53-mutated DNA, as supplementary indicators of a lesion's prognosis may be valuable for an improved result of treatment and follow-up of the lesions [120].

Twenty to forty per cent of all cases of leukoplakia are infected by *Candida*. In some instances, these lesions have a nodular or speckled appearance. Following antimycotic treatment, the nodular or speckled lesions may change to the homogeneous type of leukoplakia [Figure 18.7(a) and (b)].

In India, leukoplakia is more common in younger age groups than it is in the West [121]. This phenomenon is related to the widespread habit of bidi smoking in India. A bidi is

Table 18.3 Bidi smoking and oral leukoplakia among 10,000 inhabitants of Mumbai [122]

	Age (years)	Percentage with leukoplakia
Bidi smoking ± other habits	20–39	9
	40–59	16
	60+	20
No habits	20–39	0.2
	40–59	0.3
	60+	1.0

Roed-Peterson *et al.*, 1972. Reproduced with permission from the World Health Organization.

a cheap smoking stick that is a strong leukoplakia-producing agent. Table 18.3 [122] clearly demonstrates this relationship and also shows an increasing prevalence with age. Above the age of 60, 20% of bidi smokers have leukoplakia, which is one of the highest leukoplakia rates on record [122].

As leukoplakia is a premalignant lesion, it would be interesting to study the relationship between leukoplakia and carcinoma with age. Figures published by Bánóczy [123] on malignant transformation of leukoplakia in Hungary demonstrate that the carcinomatous transformation exhibits a shift towards higher age groups compared with the distribution of leukoplakia that has not yet become malignant.

Treatment

Patients with tobacco-associated leukoplakia should quit smoking permanently. Sometimes it has been recommended to remove persistent lesions if histological examination shows any grade of epithelial dysplasia. Since surgical removal has been questioned as a treatment to reduce risk of malignancy [111] it is debatable to recommend this type of treatment irrespective of degree of epithelial dysplasia. In cases of surgery meticulous histological examination of the removed tissue is important due to possible underdiagnosis by the biopsy [124]. Thus 7% of lesions have been shown to harbour a carcinoma, which was not revealed in the presurgical biopsy [118]. To enable histological examination of the entire lesion including the borders, a surgical procedure with knife is recommended [125]. Moreover, irrespective of treatment undertaken, follow-up examination at short intervals is mandatory.

Erythroplakia

Much less frequent but more dangerous than leukoplakia is erythroplakia, a lesion that presents bright red patches that cannot be characterized clinically or histopathologically as any other condition [108]. Sharp demarcation is a characteristic feature of erythroplakia. The lesion is most common in the sixth and seventh decades of life [126].

Erythroplakia is usually associated with epithelial dysplasia, carcinoma *in situ* or frank squamous cell carcinoma, and the lesions should be surgically removed or observed at short intervals. The above considerations on surgical removal mentioned for leukoplakia may also apply to erythroplakia.

In a sample of 800 patients with oral lichen planus, it was found that 1% had an erythroplakic lesion, often in close association with striae of Wickham [127]. In eight such patients with a median age of 68 years, two had a simultaneous squamous cell carcinoma and a third developed a carcinoma after 3.6 years.

Verrucous hyperplasia

In 1980, Shear and Pindborg [128] described the verrucous hyperplasia of the oral mucosa, characterized by either sharp or blunt verrucous processes (Figure 18.8). The lesion is often

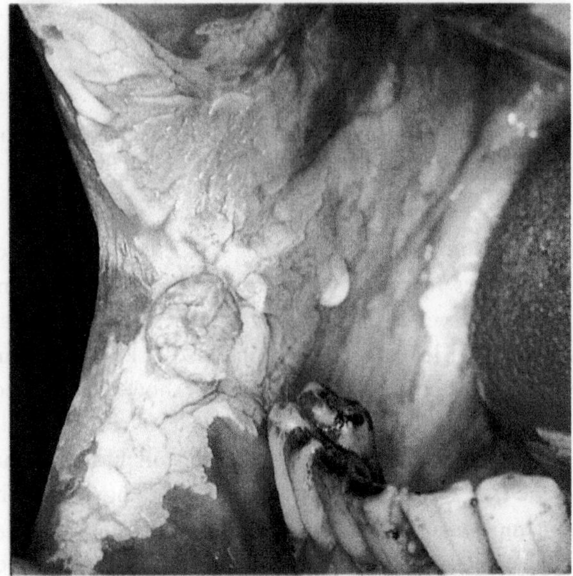

Figure 18.8 Verrucous hyperplasia of the buccal mucosa in a 73-year-old man.

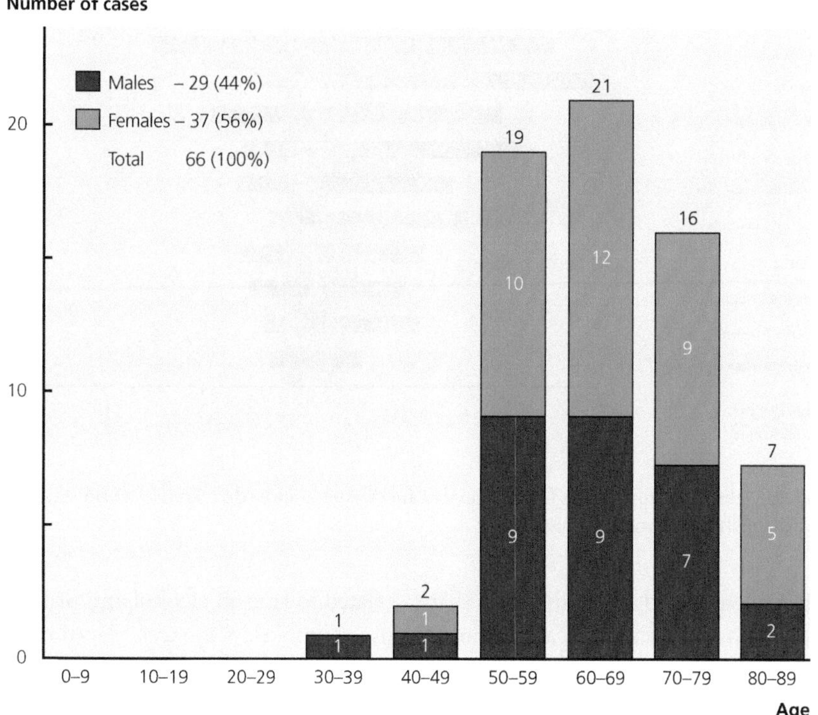

Figure 18.9 Age distribution of 66 cases of verrucous hyperplasia. Reproduced from Shear and Pindborg [128].

associated with leukoplakia. Figure 18.9 [128] demonstrates clearly that the lesion is found predominantly in old people. Verrucous hyperplasia should be regarded as potentially precancerous, often becoming, with time, verrucous carcinoma or squamous cell carcinoma. Surgical intervention is therefore necessary.

Solar lip damage

Elderly men, especially those with an outdoor occupation and a history of extensive sun exposure, sometimes show a narrowing of the lower vermilion border. The border assumes a pale, slightly bluish or grayish colour, and the demarcation between the skin of the lip and the vermilion border, which is normally sharp, becomes blurred (Figure 18.10). Sometimes interspersed red areas are seen.

This condition is referred to as solar or actinic elastosis reflecting the aetiology and the histological finding of amorphous, acellular, basophilic changes in the connective tissue possibly representing transformation of the collagenous tissue into elastic fibres and/or increased deposition of elastic fibres. The condition is irreversible, however, patients should be encouraged to use lip balm with ultraviolet light protection to prevent further development.

The condition is premalignant and can progress to solar or actinic keratosis in which crusty areas develop as a result of hyperkeratinization. Epithelial dysplasia is almost invariably present in actinic keratosis. The term solar/actinic cheilitis is possibly synonomous with the spectrum of actinic elastosis and keratosis [129, 130].

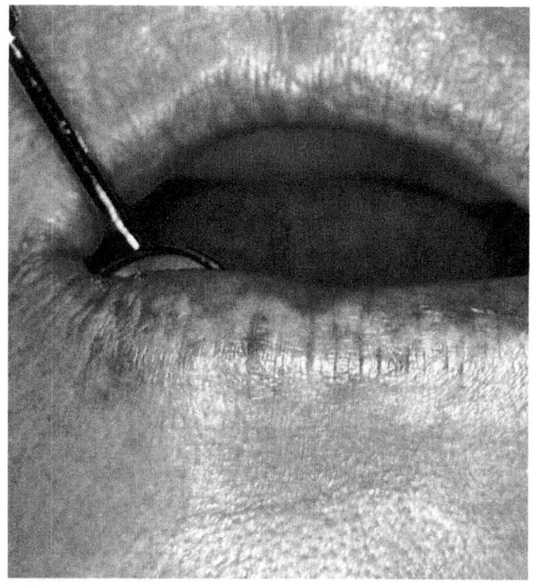

Figure 18.10 Actinic elastosis of the lower lip in a 60-year-old man.

Cancer of the vermilion border is often preceded by actinic elastosis and not rarely a clinical diagnosis of actinic keratosis reveals squamous cell carcinoma histologically. A connection between elastotic changes and development of squamous

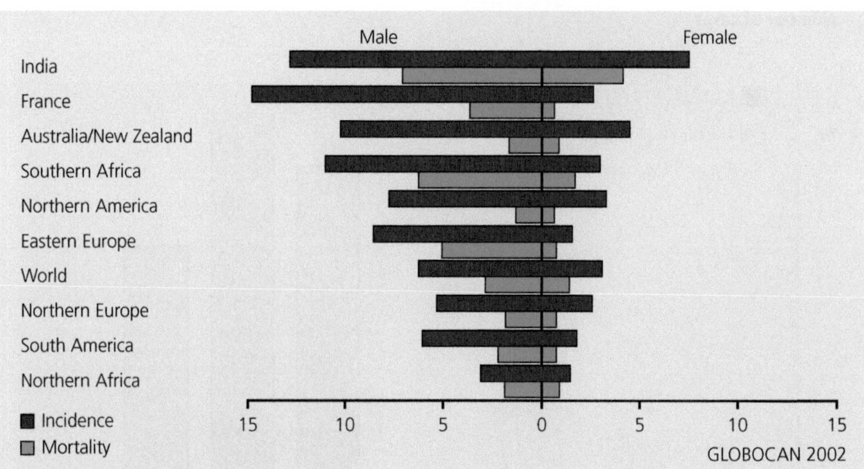

Figure 18.11 Incidence and mortality rates for all ages for oral cavity cancer. Age-standardized rates (world standard population) per 100 000 population per year. Reproduced from reference [133].

cell carcinoma of the lip was suggested a long time ago as in 1951 Bernier and Clark [131] reported an increased amount of elastotic tissue in 84% of lip carcinomas.

Oral cancer

The term oral cancer comprises several types of malignancies; however, squamous cell carcinomas (SCC) are by far the most prevalent type, accounting for more than 90% of malignant neoplasms of the oral cavity and oropharynx [132]. Non-Hodgkin lymphomas are rare in the oral cavity although the second most prevalent type. Sarcomas, e.g. fibrosarcomas and liposarcomas primarily seen in younger age groups, and malignant melanomas are very rare.

Epidemiology and aetiology of oral cancer

Globally some 300 000 cancers of the oral cavity occur and oral cancer causes some 145 000 deaths [133]. The incidence and morbidity rates vary considerably worldwide (Figure 18.11) reflecting cultural and social practices and, possibly of minor importance, genetic predisposition [134]. It also appears from Figure 18.11 that men are affected much more often than women possibly reflecting, at least in industrialized countries, the greater use of tobacco and alcohol among men. The global incidence and mortality rates for oral cancer increase sharply with age (Figure 18.12), even more clearly illustrated for lip cancer alone in Denmark [135] (Figure 18.13). It should be mentioned that increases in incidence have been seen in younger subjects in recent decades [136].

The primary risk factors are tobacco and excessive alcohol use. Furthermore, numerous studies have shown a synergistic effect of these agents [137]. In many European countries a significant rise in incidence of intraoral cancer has been related to rises in alcohol and/or tobacco consumption. The use of smokeless tobacco placed intraorally is a major cause of oral cancer in several countries e.g. India; however, other smokeless tobacco types are less carcinogenic, e.g. those used in parts of Scandinavia. Recent studies have indicated that human papillomavirus infection possibly plays a role in a small subgroup of cancers of the oral cavity [138]. Also, inadequate consumption of fresh fruit and vegetables contributes to the risk of developing oral cancer [139]. As mentioned earlier extensive sun exposure is a risk factor for lip cancer although tobacco habits also seem to be involved. Furthermore, patients who are immunosuppressed, e.g. renal transplant recipients, have a higher risk of cancer development of the lower lip [140]. Possible factors that may contribute to malignant transformation in the elderly are decreased cellular immunity and malnutrition. When etiological factors are considered among women with tongue cancer, the average age among those who use tobacco and alcohol is 11 years lower (60 years) than for those who do not use tobacco and alcohol (71 years). The implication is obvious: exposure accelerates the carcinogenic process [141].

Clinical features

Cancers may arise anywhere in the oral cavity; cancer of the upper lip, however, is rare. Symptoms have often been present for four to five months, ranging from a few weeks up to one year. The delay in diagnosis, attributable to patients ('patient's delay') as well as health professionals ('professional delay'), is poorly understood and seems difficult to overcome [142, 143].

Small carcinomas may be completely asymptomatic, whereas patients with large tumours may have varying complaints such as discomfort and irritation, pain, reduced

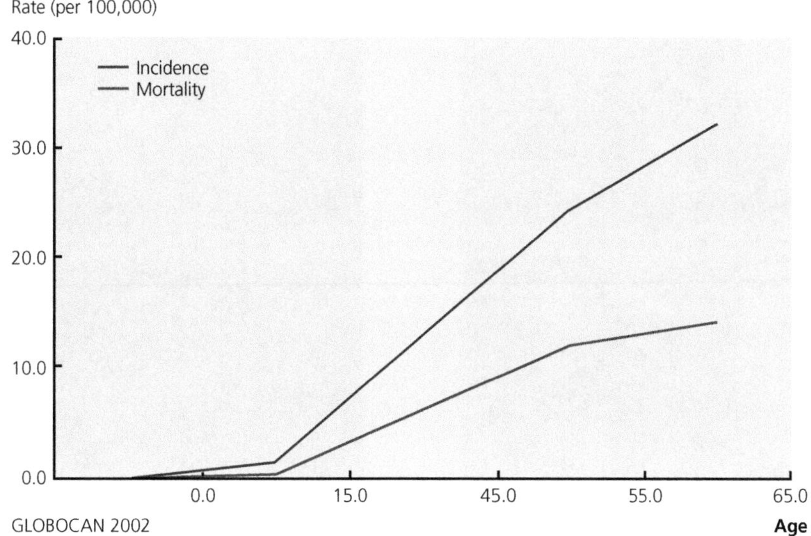

Figure 18.12 Age-specific incidence rates for oral cancer worldwide for males. Reproduced from reference [133].

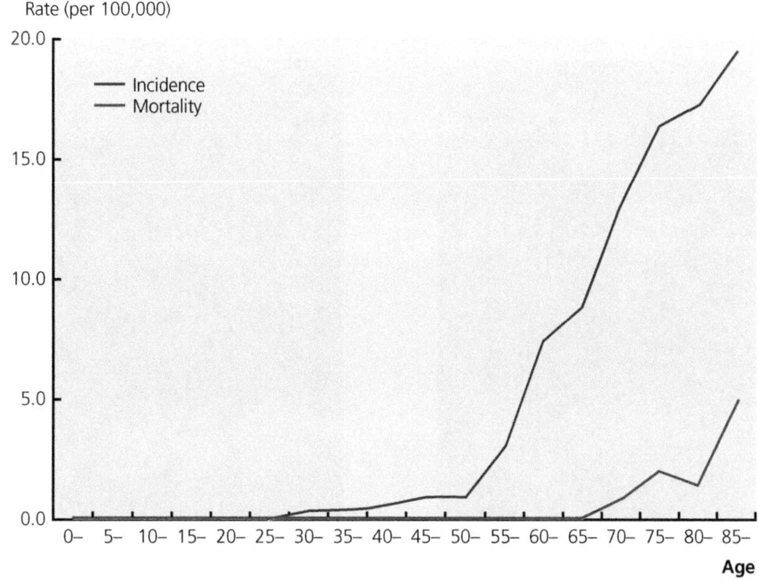

Figure 18.13 Age-specific incidence rates for lip cancer in Denmark 1997–2001 for males. Reproduced from reference [135].

mobility of the tongue and, in carcinomas of the alveolar ridge and the palate, some discomfort in denture wearing.

Oral SCC may present a varied clinical picture from white, erythematous and mixed white and erythematous lesions often containing small nodules to similar changes with ulcerations with raised borders, swelling and even overtly exophytic growths (Figures 18.14 and 18.15). As mentioned earlier, crusty lesions on the vermillon border of the lip not resolving within a week or two are always suspicious (Figure 18.16). A most important feature, and this applies to all cancers of the oral mucosa, is the induration that can be palpated at the periphery of the tumour.

Cancer in the floor of the mouth is usually an ulcerated lesion with raised and indurated margins located in the anterior part (Figure 18.17), while cancers of the tongue are most often located at the borders. Cancer of the tongue rarely develops on the dorsum.

The risk of lymphatic spread is primarily influenced by the site and size of the primary tumour. Cancers of the tongue and floor of the mouth show a much higher tendency to regional metastasis than cancers of the lower lip.

Diagnosis and referral

It is recognized that recommendations differ globally on how to manage suspicious lesions. In some parts of the world,

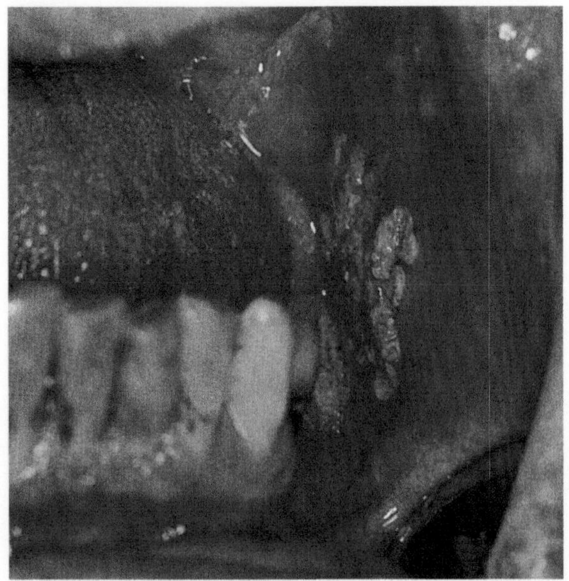

Figure 18.14 Cancer of the buccal mucosa in a 62-year-old man.

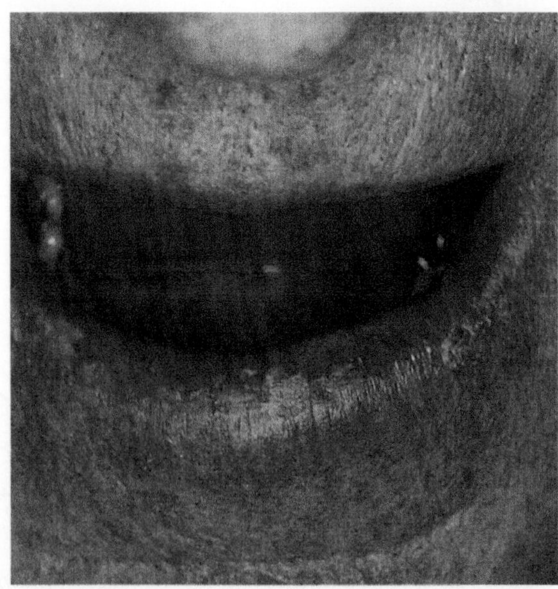

Figure 18.16 Cancer of the vermilion border in a 71-year-old man.

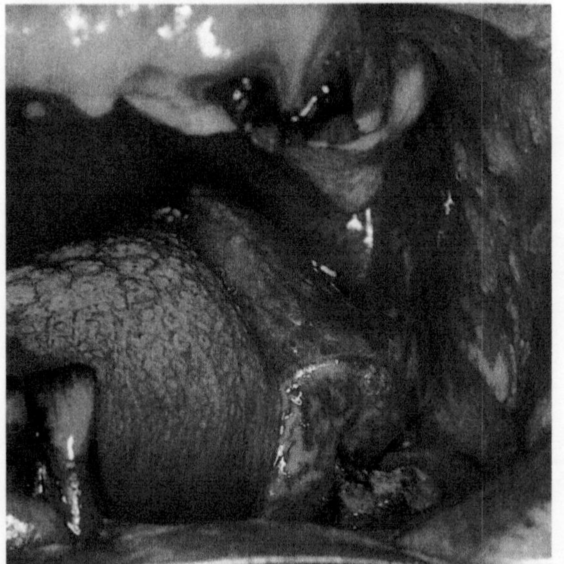

Figure 18.15 Exophytic cancer of the tongue in a 68-year-old man.

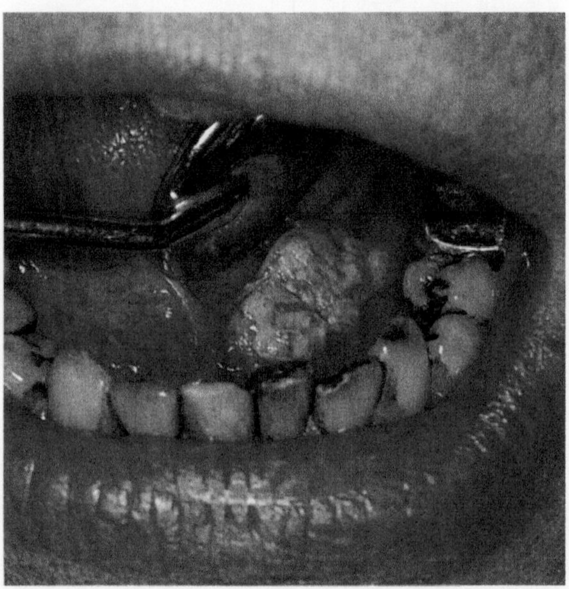

Figure 18.17 Cancer in the floor of the mouth in a 75-year-old man.

dentists are taught to take biopsies from any suspicious lesion, while in other countries they are advised to refer a patient with a suspicious lesion immediately for biopsy. Small oral cancers may mimic reactive lesions, such as irritation caused by a broken down tooth. In some parts of the world it is acceptable to wait for a period of up to two weeks to observe the result of the elimination of possible causative factors. If the lesion does not disappear, biopsy or referral should be done without delay. Sometimes a diagnostic delay is the result of short term improvement of the lesion due to the use of antibiotics, antifungal drugs or mouth rinses.

Treatment and prognosis

It is not the purpose of this chapter to discuss the treatment of oral cancer in any detail. The primary treatment modalities are surgery or radiotherapy or a combination of the two. In most centres the choice of treatment depends on the staging of the tumour according to the TNM-classification [144], i.e. the size of the tumour and the presence or absence of regional and distant metastases. The presence of regional metastases at time of presentation varies from one intraoral cancer site to another from about 10 to 65%. Chemotherapy is not generally being used as the treatment of first choice in oral SCC.

Morgan *et al.* [145] studied the influence of age on the outcome of major head and neck surgery and found a perioperative mortality (death within 30 days of the operation) of 3.5% (29 of 810) in patients over the age of 65. This rate is relatively low compared with perioperative mortality in patients below 65 years. The authors conclude that advanced age alone should not be a deterrent to surgical therapy for head and neck cancer, a point of view supported by Jun *et al.* [146] based on a study of 159 patients above the age of 80.

The prognosis for cancer of the lower lip is good. A five-year survival rate of more than 90% can be expected in small non-metastatic lip cancers. The prognosis for intraoral cancer depends largely on the size of the primary growth and the presence or absence of metastatic nodes. Five-year survival rates vary from almost 80% in small non-metastatic cancers to about 15% in large cancers with metastatic spread.

Other malignancies

Non-Hodgkin's lymphomas (NHL) account for 3–4% of oral cancers and most patients are in the 6th and 7th decades [147]. Hodgkin's lymphoma is seen primarily in patients below middle age and is not dealt with here. The aetiology of NHL is unknown. In the head and neck region the tonsils are the most prevalent site followed by the parotid gland, palate, gingiva (Figure 18.18) and tongue [147]. Patients usually present with an ulcer and swelling and/or loose teeth. The feeling of sore throat often is a complaint in patients with tonsillar NHL. The current WHO classification of tumours of lymphoid tissues is complicated [148] and will not be dealt with here. Since differentiation between reactive and neoplastic lesions may be difficult with standard hematoxylin and eosin stained sections, advanced techniques are used for classification of NHL. Radiotherapy and chemotherapy, or a combination of the two, are the treatments of choice.

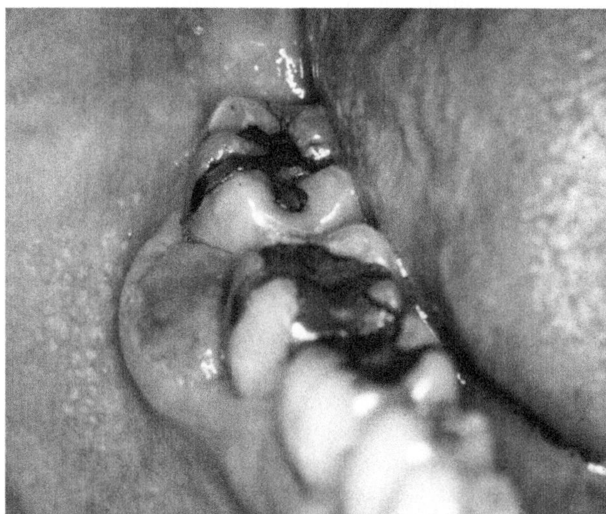

Figure 18.18 Lymphoma of the gingiva in a 61-year-old man.

Oral malignant melanoma is very rare. The aetiology is unknown although chronic trauma (e.g. from ill-fitting dentures) has been suggested. The vast majority of oral malignant melanomas arise on the palate, maxillary alveolar process or gingiva [149, 150] Oral malignant melanomas are usually irregular growths with black, grayish or reddish colour. Satellite foci may surround the primary tumour. Sometimes they are even amelanotic (pigmentation is absent). They can present as flat or swollen lesions and pain is a frequent complaint. It is an aggressive malignancy with a low 5-year survival rate [150].

Metastases are uncommon in the oral region and are often a sign of widespread disease. In an analysis of 673 cases, 25% of oral metastases were found to be the first sign of the metastatic spread and in 23% it was the first indication of an undiscovered malignancy at a distant site [151]. The jawbones are more frequently affected than the oral soft tissues. In the oral soft tissues the gingiva is the most commonly affected site (Figure 18.19). An analysis of 396 metastases from the literature [152] revealed that oral metastases in middle-aged and old people originate from the lungs (mean age 58 years), stomach (mean age 56 years) and liver (mean age 61 years). Metastases from melanomas appear in middle-aged people (mean age 51 years). Metastases from hypernephromas also occur late in life (mean age 60 years).

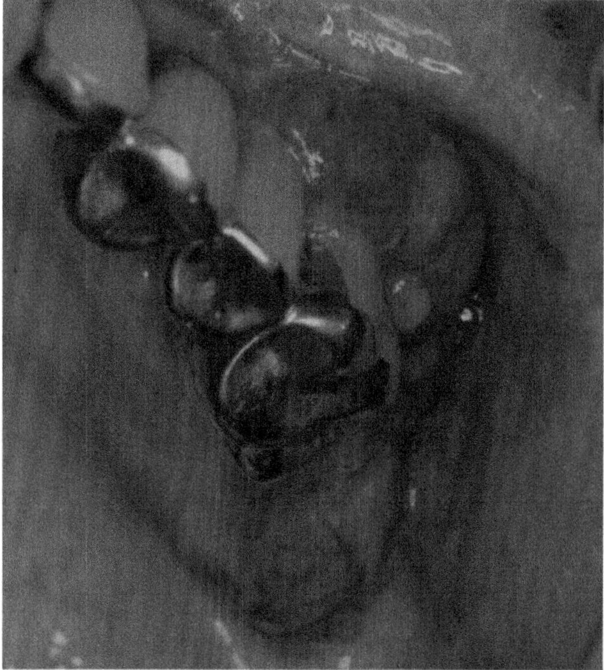

Figure 18.19 Metastasis to the gingiva from a breast carcinoma in a 56-year-old woman.

Calonius *et al.* [153] reported on 13 oral metastases with a mean age at diagnosis of 60 years; the mean age for carcinomas was 62 years and for the sarcomas 54 years.

References

1 Squier, C.A., Johnson, N.W. & Hackemann, M. (1975) Structure and function of normal human oral mucosa. In: A.E. Dolby (ed), *Oral mucosa in health and disease*. pp. 1–112, Blackwell Scientific Publications, Oxford.

2 Schroeder, H.E. (1981) *Differentiation of human oral epithelia*. Karger, Basel.

3 Mackenzie, I.C., Rittman, G., Gao, Z., Leigh, I. & Lane, E.B. (1991) Patterns of cytokeratin expression in human gingival epithelia. *Journal of Periodontal Research*, **26**, 468–478.

4 Melcher, A.H. & Eastoe, J.E. (1969) The connective tissue of the periodontium. In: A.H. Melcher & W.H. Bowen (ed), *Biology of the periodontium*. pp. 167–344, Academic Press, London.

5 Alvares, O.F. & Meyer, J. (1971) Variable features and regional differences in oral epithelium. In: C.A. Squier & J. Meyer (ed) *Current concepts of the histology of oral mucosa*. pp. 97–113, Charles C. Thomas, Springfield, IL.

6 Thilander, H. (1968) An electron microscope study of normal human palatal epithelium. *Acta Odontologica Scandinavica*, **26**, 191–212.

7 Scapino, R.P. Biomechanics of masticating and lining mucosa. (1971) In: C.A. Squier & J. Meyer (ed), *Current concepts of the histology of oral mucosa*. pp. 181–202, Charles C. Thomas, Springfield, IL.

8 Karring, T. & Löe, H. (1973) The effect of age on mitotic activity in rat oral epithelium. *Journal of Periodontal Research*, **8**, 164–170.

9 Kvidera, A. & Mackenzie, I.C. (1994) Rates of clearance of the epithelial surfaces of mouse oral mucosa and skin. *Epithelial Cell Biology*, **3**, 175–180.

10 Mackenzie, I.C. & Ettinger, R.L. (1975) Differences in the response of rodent oral mucosa and skin to repeated surface trauma. *Journal of Prosthetic Dentistry*, **34**, 666–674.

11 Mackenzie, I.C. & Hill, M.W. (1981) Connective tissue influences on patterns of epithelial architecture and keratinization in skin and oral mucosa of the mouse. *Cell Tissue Research*, **219**, 597–607.

12 Gibbs, S. & Ponec, M. (2000) Intrinsic regulation of differentiation markers in human epidermis, hard palate and buccal mucosa. *Archives of Oral Biology*, **45**, 149–158.

13 Hill, M.W. & Mackenzie, I.C. (1989) The influence of subepithelial connective tissues on epithelial proliferation in the adult mouse. *Cell Tissue Research*, **255**, 179–182.

14 Hill, M.W. & Mackenzie, I.C. (1984) The influence of differing connective tissue substrates on the maintenance of adult stratified squamous epithelia. *Cell Tissue Research*, **237**, 473–478.

15 Mackenzie, I.C. & Hill, M.W. (1981) Maintenance of regionally specific patterns of cell proliferation and differentiation in transplanted skin and oral mucosa. *Cell Tissue Research*, **219**, 597–607.

16 Costea, D.E., Loro, L.L., Dimba, E.A., Vintermyr, O.K. & Johannessen, A.C. (2003) Crucial effects of fibroblasts and keratinocyte growth factor on morphogenesis of reconstituted human oral epithelium. *Journal of Investigative Dermatology*, **121**, 1479–1486.

17 Ship, J.A. & Baum, B.J. (1993) Old age in health and disease. Lessons from the oral cavity. *Oral Surgery, Oral Medicine, Oral Pathology*, **76**, 40–44.

18 Wolff, A., Ship, J.A., Tylenda, C.A., Fox, P.C. & Baum, B.J. (1991) Oral mucosal appearance is unchanged in healthy, different-aged persons. *Oral Surgery, Oral Medicine, Oral Pathology*, **71**, 569–572.

19 Kydd, W.L. & Daly, C.H. (1982) The biologic and mechanical effects of stress on oral mucosa. *Journal of Prosthetic Dentistry*, **47**, 317–329.

20 Bottomly, W.K. (1979) Physiology of the oral mucosa. *Otolaryngologic Clinics of North America*, **12**, 15–20.

21 Pickett, H.G., Appleby, R.G. & Osborn, M.O. (1972) Changes in denture supported tissues associated with aging. *Journal of Prosthetic Dentistry*, **27**, 35–42.

22 Miles, A.E.W. (1972) Sans teeth: changes in oral tissues with advancing age. *Proceedings of the Royal Society of Medicine*, **65**, 801–806.

23 Ettinger, R.L. & Manderson, R.D. (1974) A clinical study of sublingual varices. *Oral Surgery, Oral Medicine, Oral Pathology*, **38**, 540–45.

24 Frantzell, A., Törnquist, R. & Waldenström, J. (1945) Examination of the tongue: a clinical and photographic study. *Acta Medica Scandinavica*, **122**, 207–237.

25 Holm-Pedersen, P. & Löe, H. (1971) Wound healing in the gingiva of young and old individuals. *Scandinavian Journal of Dental Research*, **79**, 40–53.

26 Southam, J.C. (1974) Retention mucoceles of the oral mucosa. *Journal of Oral Pathology*, **3**, 197–202.

27 Cameron, I.L. (1972) Cell proliferation and renewal in aging mice. *Journal of Gerontology*, **27**, 162–172.

28 Ryan, E.J., Toto, P.D. & Garguilo, A.W. (1974) Aging in human attached gingival epithelium. *Journal of Dental Research*, **53**, 74–75.

29 Toto, P.D., Rubinstein, A.S. & Garguilo, A.W. (1975) Labelling index and cell density of aging rat oral tissues. *Journal of Dental Research*, **54**, 553–556.

30 Hill, M.W. (1988) Influence of age on the morphology and transit time of murine stratified squamous epithelia. *Archives of Oral Biology*, **33**, 221–229.

31 Lesch, C.A., Squier, C.A., Cruchley, A., Williams, D.M. & Speight, P. (1989) The permeability of human oral mucosa and skin to water. *Journal of Dental Research*, **68**, 1345–1349.

32 Picton, D.C.A. & Wills, D.J. (1978) Viscoelastic properties of the periodontal ligament and mucous membrane. *Journal of Prosthetic Dentistry*, **40**, 263–672.

33 Kligman, A.M. & Takase, Y. (ed) (1988) *Cutaneous aging*. University of Tokyo Press, Tokyo.

34 Hurley, H.J. (1993) Skin in senescence: a summation. *Journal of Geriatric Dermatology*, **1**, 55–61.

35 Cerimele, D., Celleno, L. & Serri, F. (1990) Physiological changes in aging skin. *British Journal of Dermatology*, **122**(Suppl. 35), 13–20.

36 Lavker, R.M. (1979) Structural alterations in exposed and unexposed aged skin. *Journal of Investigative Dermatology*, **73**, 59–66.

37 Leyden, J.J., McGinley, K.J. & Grove, G.L. (1978) Age-related difference in the rate of desquamation of skin surface cells. In: R.D. Aldeman, J. Roberts & V.J. Cristofalo (eds) *Pharmacological intervention in the aging process*, p. 297, Plenum Press, New York, NY.

38 Grove, G.L. & Kligman, A.M. (1983) Age-associated changes in human epidermal cell renewal. *Journal of Gerontology*, **38**, 137–142.

39 Orentreich, N., Markofsky, J. & Vogelman, J.H. (1979) The effect of aging on the rate of linear nail growth. *Journal of Investigative Dermatology*, **73**, 126–132.

40 Lapière, C.M. (1990) The aging dermis: the main cause for the appearance of "old" skin. *British Journal of Dermatology*, **122**(Suppl. 35), 5–11.

41 Marks, R. (1988) Alterations of the physical function of skin with aging. In: A.M. Kligman & Y. Takase (eds), *Cutaneous aging*. pp. 56–72, University of Tokyo Press, Tokyo.

42 Grove, G.L. (1982) Age-related differences in healing of superficial skin wounds in humans. *Archives of Dermatological Research*, **272**, 381.

43 Hirokawa, K. (1988) Aging and the immune system. In: A.M. Kligman & Y. Takase (eds), *Cutaneous aging*. pp. 103–115, University of Tokyo Press, Tokyo.

44 Ben-Yehuda, A & Weksler, M.E. (1993) Immune senescence: mechanisms and clinical implications. *Journal of Geriatric Dermatology*, **1**, 77–84.

45 Baumann, L. (2007) Skin ageing and its treatment. *Journal of Pathology*, **211**(2), 241–251.

46 Richman, M.J. & Arbarbanel, A.R. (1943) Effects of estradiol upon the atrophic human buccal mucosa with a preliminary report on the use of estrogens in the management of senile gingivitis. *Journal of Clinical Endocrinology*, **3**, 224–226.

47 Shklar, G. (1966) The effects of aging upon oral mucosa. *Journal of Investigative Dermatology*, **47**, 115–120.

48 Löe, H. & Karring, T. (1971) The three dimensional morphology of the epithelium connective tissue interface of the gingiva as related to age and sex. *Scandinavian Journal of Dental Research*, **79**, 315–326.

49 Scott, J., Valentine, J.A., Hill, C.A. & Balasooriya, B.A.W. (1983) A quantitative histologic analysis of the effects of age and sex on human lingual epithelium. *Journal de Biologie Buccale*, **11**, 303–315.

50 Plewig, G. (1970) Regional differences of cell sizes in the human stratum corneum. *Journal of Investigative Dermatology*, **54**, 19–23.

51 Toto, P.D. & Dhawan, A.S. (1966) Generation cycle of oral epithelium in 400-day old mice. *Journal of Dental Research*, **45**, 948–950.

52 Sharav, Y. & Massler, M. (1967) Age changes in oral epithelia: progenitor population, synthesis index and tissue turnover. *Experimental Cell Research*, **47**, 132–138.

53 Barakat, N.J., Toto, P.D. & Choukas, N.C. (1969) Aging and cell renewal of oral epithelium. *Journal of Periodontology*, **40**, 599–602.

54 Thrasher, J.D. (1971) Age and cell cycle of the mouse esophageal epithelium. *Experimental Gerontology*, **6**, 19–25.

55 Hansen, E.R. (1966) Mitotic activity in the oral epithelium of the rat. Variations according to age and time of the day. *Swedish Dental Journal*, **74**, 196–201.

56 Ettinger, R.L. & Mackenzie, I.C. (1986) Epithelial thickness and labelling index in young and old mice. *Gerodontology*, **5**, 183–189.

57 Tudor, D., Locke, M., Owen-Jones, E. & Mackenzie, I.C. (2004) Intrinsic patterns of behavior of epithelial stem cells. *Journal of Investigative Dermatology Symposium Proceedings*, **9**(3), 208–214.

58 Mackenzie, I.C. (2006) Stem cell properties and epithelial malignancies. *European Journal of Cancer*, **42**, 1204–1212.

59 Stern, M.M. & Bickenbach, J.R. (2007) Epidermal stem cells are resistant to cellular aging. *Aging Cell*, **6**(4), 439–452.

60 Belding, J.H. & Tade, W.H. (1978) Evaluation of epithelial maturity in hormonally related stomatitis. *Journal of Oral Medicine*, **33**, 17–19.

61 Österberg, T., Ohman, A., Heyden, G. & Svanborg, A. (1985) The condition of the oral mucosa at age 70: a population study. *Gerodontology*, **4**, 71–75.

62 Hand, J.S. & Whitehill, J.M. (1986) The prevalence of oral mucosal lesions in an elderly population. *Journal of the American Dental Association*, **112**, 73–76.

63 Budtz-Jörgensen, E. (1981) Oral mucosal lesions associated with the wearing of removable dentures. *Journal of Oral Pathology*, **10**, 65–80.

64 Cottone, J.A. & Kafrawy, A.H. (1979) Medications and health histories: a survey of 4,365 dental patients. *Journal of the American Dental Association*, **98**, 713–718.

65 Nevalainen, M.J., Närhi, T.O. & Ainamo, A. (1997) Oral mucosal lesions and oral hygiene habits in the home-living elderly. *Journal of Oral Rehabilitation*, **24**, 332–337.

66 Espinoza, I., Rojas, R., Aranda, W. & Gamonal, J. (2003) Prevalence of oral mucosal lesions in elderly people in Santiago, Chile. *Journal of Oral Pathology & Medicine*, **32**, 571–575.

67 MacEntee, M.I., Glick, N. & Stolar, E. (1998) Age, gender, dentures and oral mucosal disorder. *Oral Diseases*, **4**, 32–36.

68 Tanida, T., Ueta, E., Tobiume, A., Hameda, T., Rao, F. & Osaki, T. (2001) Influence of aging on candidal growth and adhesion regulatory agents in saliva. *Journal of Oral Pathology & Medicine*, **30**, 328–335.

69 Holmstrup, P. & Axéll, T. (1990) Classification and clinical manifestations of oral yeast infections. *Acta Odontologica Scandinavica*, **48**, 57–59.

70 Holmstrup, P. & Besserman, M. (1983) Clinical, therapeutic and pathogenic aspects of chronic multifocal candidiasis. *Oral Surgery, Oral Medicine, Oral Pathology*, **56**, 388–395.

71 Field, E.A., Field, J.K. & Martin, M.V. (1989) Does *Candida* have a role in oral epithelial neoplasia? *Journal of Medical and Veterinary Mycology*, **27**, 277–294.

72 Krogh, P., Hald, B. & Holmstrup, P. (1987) Possible mycological etiology of oral mucosal cancer: catalytic potential of infecting *Candida albicans* and other yeasts in production of N-nitrosobenzylmethylamine. *Carcinogenesis*, **8**, 1543–1548.

73 Samaranayake, L.P. (1990) Host factors and oral candidosis. In: L.P. Samaranayake & T.W. MacFarlane (ed), *Oral candidosis*, pp. 66–103, Wright, London.

74 Martin, M.V. (1990) Antifungal agents. In: L.P. Samaranayake & T.W. MacFarlane (ed), *Oral candidosis*, pp. 238–251, Wright, London.

75 Newton, A.V. (1962) Denture sore mouth. *British Dental Journal*, **112**, 357–360.

76 Budtz-Jørgensen, E. (1981) Oral mucosal lesions associated with the wearing of removable dentures. *Journal of Oral Pathology*, **10**, 65–80.

77 Grabowski, M. & Bertram, U. (1976) Den aeldre befolknings oralstatus og odontologiske behandlings behov i Vestsjaellands amt (in Danish with English summary). *Danish Dental Journal*, **80**, 1–7.

78 Pindborg, J.J. & Sørensen, N.A. (1983) The condition of the oral mucosa and dentures in a Danish nursing home population (in Danish with English summary). *Danish Dental Journal*, **87**, 307–311.

79 Pindborg, J.J., Glenert, U., Andreasen, J.O., Holmstrup, P., Schiodt, M. & Hansen, H.J. (1985) Condition of the oral mucosa in 478 inhabitants in a Danish old age home (in Danish with English summary). *Danish Dental Journal*, **89**, 223–227.

80 Vigild, M. (1987) Oral mucosal lesions among institutionalized elderly in Denmark. *Community Dentistry and Oral Epidemiology*, **15**, 309–313.

81 Cumming, C.G., Wight. C., Blackwell. C.L. & Wray, D. (1990) Denture stomatitis in elderly. *Oral Microbiology & Immunology*, **5**, 82–85.

82 Kuc, I.M., Samaranayake L.P., van Heyst E.N. (1999) Oral health and microflora in an institutionalised elderly population in Canada. *Int. Dent. J.*, **49**, 33–40.

83 Figueiral M.H., Azul A., Pinto E., Fonseca P.A., Branco P.M., Scully C. (2007) Denture-related stomatitis: identification of aetiological and predisposing factors – a large cohort. *J Oral Rahab*, **34**, 448–455.

84 Grabowski, M. (1974) Den aeldre befolknings oralstatus og odontologiske behandlingsbehov. Thesis. Royal Dental College, Aarhus.

85 Kossioni A.E. (2011) The prevalence of denture stomatitis and its predisposing conditions in an older Greek population. *Gerodontology*, **28**, 85–90.

86 Axéll, T. (1976) A prevalence study of oral mucosal lesions in an adult Swedish population. Thesis. *Odontologisk Revy*, **27**(Suppl. 36).

87 Thorn, J.J., Holmstrup, P., Rindum, J. & Pindborg, J.J. (1988) Course of various clinical forms of oral lichen planus. A prospective follow-up study of 611 patients. *Journal of Oral Pathology*, **17**, 213–218.

88 Mattson, U., Jontell, M. & Holmstrup, P. (2002) Oral lichen planus and malignant transformation: is a recall of patients justified? *Critical Reviews in Oral Biology & Medicine*, **13**, 390–396.

89 Ingafou, M., Leao, J.C., Porter, S.R. & Scully, C. (2006) Oral lichen planus: a retrospective study of 690 British patients. *Oral Diseases*, **12**, 463–468.

90 Hsue, S.S., Wang, W.C., Chen, C.H., Lin, C.C., Chen, Y.K. & Lin, L.M. (2007) Malignant transformation in 1458 patients with potentially malignant oral mucosal disorders: a follow-up study based in a Taiwanese hospital. *Journal of Oral Pathology & Medicine*, **36**, 25–29.

91 Holmstrup, P., Schiøtz, A.W. & Westergaard, J. (1990) Effect of dental plaque control on gingvial lichen planus. *Oral Surgery, Oral Medicine, Oral Pathology*, **69**, 585–590.

92 Guiglia, R., Di Liberto, C., Pizzo, G., Picone, L., Lo Muzio, L., Gallo, P.D. *et al.* (2007) A combined treatment regimen for desquamative gingivitis in patients with oral lichen planus. *Journal of Oral Pathology & Medicine*, **36**, 110–116.

93 Kaliakatsou, F., Hodgson, T.A., Lewsey, J.D., Hegarty, A.M., Murphy, A.G. & Porter, S.R. (2002) Management of recalcitrant ulcerative oral lichen planus with topical tacrolismus. *Journal of the American Academy of Dermatology*, **46**, 35–41.

94 Bolewska, J., Hansen, A.J., Holmstrup, P., Pindborg, J.J. & Stangerup, M. (1990) Oral mucosal lesions related to silver amalgam restorations. *Oral Surgery, Oral Medicine, Oral Pathology*, **70**, 55–58.

95 Holmstrup, P. (1991) Reactions of the oral mucosa related to silver amalgam: a review. *Journal of Oral Pathology & Medicine*, **20**, 1–7.

96 Chiou, S., Gobetti, J.P. & D'Silva, N.J. (2007) Mucous membrane pemphigoid: a retrospective study. *Journal of Michigan Dental Association*, **89**, 46–52.

97 Nordenram, Å. & Landt, H. (1969) Hyperplasia of the oral tissues in denture cases. *Acta Odontologica Scandinavica*, **27**, 481–491.

98 Pape, H.D., Hausamen, J.E. & Neumann, D. (1970) Stomatologische Erhebungen bei 1970 Altersheim- und Trinkerheilanstalt insassen. *Deutsche Zahnaerztliche Zeitschrift*, **25**, 103–105.

99 Jainkittivong A., Aneksuk V., Langlais R.P. (2010) Oral mucosal lesions in denture wearers. *Gerondotology*, **27**, 26–32.

100 Rabiei M., Kasemnezhad E., Masoudi H., Shakiba M., Pourkay H. (2010) Prevalence of oral end dental disorders in institutionalised elderly people in Rasht, Iran. *Gerodontology*, **27**, 174–177.

101 Ritchie, G.M. (1973) A report of dental findings in a survey of geriatric patients. *Journal of Dentistry*, **1**, 106–112.

102 Manderson, R.D. & Ettinger, R.L. (1975) Dental status of the institutionalized elderly population of Edinburgh. *Community Dentistry and Oral Epidemiology*, **3**, 100–107.

103 Jorge, J. Jr, de Almeida, O.P., Bozzo, L., Scully, C. & Craner, E. (1991) Oral mucosal health and disease in institutionalized elderly in Brazil. *Community Dentistry and Oral Epidemiology*, **19**, 173–175.

104 van der Waal, I. (1990) *The burning mouth syndrome*. Munksgaard. Copenhagen.

105 Basker, R.M., Sturdee, D.W. & Davenport, J.C. (1978) Patients with burning mouths. A clinical investigation of causative factors, including the climacteric and diabetes. *British Dental Journal*, **145**, 9–16.

106 Haneke, E. (1980) *Zungen- und Mundschleimhautbrennen*. Carl Hansen Verlag, München.

107 Scala, A., Checchi, L., Montevecchi, M., Marini, I., Giamberardino, M.A. (2003) Update on burning mouth syndrome: overview and patient management. *Critical Reviews in Oral Biology & Medicine*, **14**, 275–291.

108 Pindborg, J.J., Reichart, P., Smith, C.J. & van der Waal, J. (1997) *WHO: Histological typing of cancer and precancer of the oral mucosa*, 2nd edn, Springer-Verlag, Berlin.

109 Lind, P.O. (1987) Malignant transformation in oral leukoplakia. *Scandinavian Journal of Dental Research*, **95**, 449–455.

110 Napier, S.S., Cowan, C.G., Gregg, T.A., Stevenson, M., Lamey, P.J. & Toner, P.G. Potentially malignant oral lesions in Northern Ireland: size (extent) matters. *Oral Diseases*, **9**, 129–137.

111 Holmstrup, P., Vedtofte, P., Reibel, J. & Stoltze, K. (2006) Long-term treatment outcome of oral premalignant lesions. *Oral Oncology*, **42**, 461–474.

112 Waldron, C.A., Shafer, W.G. (1975) Leukoplakia revisited. A clinicopathologic study of 3256 leukoplakias. *Cancer*, **36**, 1386–1392.

113 Burkhardt, A. (1980) Der Mundhöhlenkrebs und seine Vorstadien. Ultrastrukturelle und immunpathologische Aspekte, Gustav Fisher Verlag, Stuttgart.

114 Axéll, T. (1987) Occurrence of leukoplakia and some other white lesions among 20333 adult Swedish people. *Community Dentistry and Oral Epidemiology*, **15**, 46–51.

115 Pindborg, J.J., Roed-Petersen, B. & Renstrup, G. (1972) Role of smoking in floor of the mouth leukoplakias. *Journal of Oral Pathology*, **1**, 22–29.

116 Kramer, I.R.H., El-Labban, N. & Lee, K.W. (1978) The clinical features and disk of malignant transformation in sublingual keratosis. *British Dental Journal*, **144**, 171–180.

117 Schepman, K.P., van der Meij, E.H., Smeele, L.E. & van der Waal, I. (1998) Malignant transformation of oral leukoplakia: a follow-up study of a hospital-based population of 166 patients with oral leukoplakia from the Netherlands. *Oral Oncology*, **34**, 270–275.

118 Holmstrup, P., Vedtofte, P., Reibel, J. & Stoltze, K. (2007) Oral premalignant lesions: is a biopsy reliable? *Journal of Oral Pathology & Medicine*, **36**, 262–266.

119 Tabor, M.P., Braakhuis, B.J., van der Wal, J.E., van Diest, P.J., Leemans, C.R., Brakenhoff, R.H. *et al.* (2003) Comparative molecular and histological grading of epithelial dysplasia of the oral cavity and the oropharynx. *Journal of Pathology*, **199**, 354–360.

120 Van Houten, V., Leemans, C.R., Kummer, J.A., Dijkstra, J., Kuik, D.J., van den Brekel, M.W. *et al.* (2004) Molecular diagnosis of surgical margins and local recurrence in head and neck cancer patients: a prospective study. *Clinical Cancer Research*, **10**, 3614–3620.

121 Pindborg, J.J. (1978) Oral cancer and precancer as diseases of the aged. *Community Dentistry and Oral Epidemiology*, **6**, 300–307.

122 Roed-Petersen, B., Gupta, P.C., Pindborg, J.J. & Singh, B. (1972) Association between oral leukoplakia and sex, age, and tobacco habits. *Bulletin of the World Health Organization*, **47**, 13–19.

123 Bánóczy, J. (1977) Follow-up studies in oral leukoplakia. *Journal of Maxillofacial Surgery*, **5**, 69–75.

124 Pentenero, M., Carrozzo, M., Pagano, M., Galliano, D., Broccoletti, R., Scully, C. *et al.* (2003) Oral mucosal dysplastic lesions and early squamous cell carcinomas: underdiagnosis from incisional biopsy. *Oral Diseases*, **9**, 68–72.

125 Vedtofte, P., Holmstrup, P., Hjørting-Hansen, E. & Pindborg, J.J. (1987) Surgical treatment of premalignant lesions of the oral mucosa. *International Journal of Oral and Maxillofacial Surgery*, **16**, 656–664.

126 Shafer, W.G. & Waldron, C.A. Erythroplakia of the oral cavity. *Cancer*, **36**, 1021–1028.

127 Holmstrup, P., Pindborg, J.J. (1976) Erythroplakic lesions in relation to oral lichen planus. *Acta Dermato-Venerologica*, **59**(Suppl. 85): 77–84.

128 Shear, M. & Pindborg, J.J. (1980) Verrucous hyperplasia of the oral mucosa. *Cancer*, **46**, 1855–1862.

129 Kaugars, G.E., Pillion, T., Svirsky, J.A., Page, D.G., Burns, J.C. & Abbey, L.M. (1999) Actinic cheilitis: a review of 152 cases. *Oral Surgery, Oral Medicine, Oral Pathology, Oral Radiology and Endodontology*, **88**(2), 181–186.

130 Markopoulos, A., Albanidou-Farmaki, E. & Kayavis, I. (2004) Actinic cheilitis: clinical and pathologic characteristics in 65 cases. *Oral Diseases*, **10**(4), 212–216.

131 Bernier, J.L. & Clark, M.L. (1951) Squamous cell carcinoma of the lip. A critical statistical and morphological analysis of 835 cases. *Military Surgeon*, **109**, 379–405.

132 Barnes, L,, Eveson, J.W., Reichart, P. & Sidransky, D. (eds) (2005) *World Health Organization Classification of Tumours. Pathology and Genetics of Head and Neck Tumours.* IARC Press, Lyon.

133 Ferlay, J., Soerjomataram, I., Ervik, M., Dikshit, R., Eser, S., Mathers, C., Rebelo, M., Parkin, D.M., Forman, D. & Bray F. (2013) GLOBOCAN 2012 v1.0, Cancer Incidence and Mortality Worldwide. *IARC CancerBase No. 11*, International Agency for Research on Cancer, Lyon. Accessed January 2015 from http://globocan.iarc.fr.

134 Shah, J.P., Johnson, N.W. & Batsakis, J.G. (eds) (2003) *Oral Cancer*. Martin Dunitz, London.

135 Engholm, G., Storm, H.H., Ferlay, J., Christensen, N., Bray, F., Ólafsdóttir, E. *et al.* (2006) *NORDCAN. Cancer Incidence and Mortality in the Nordic Countries*, Version 2.2., Danish Cancer Society.

136 Llewellyn, C.D., Linklater, K., Bell, J., Johnson, N.W. & Warnakulasuriya, K.A. (2003) Squamous cell carcinoma of the oral cavity in patients aged 45 years and under: a descriptive analysis of 116 cases diagnosed in the South East of England from 1990 to 1997. *Oral Oncology*, **39**(2), 106–114.

137 Blot, W.J., McLaughlin, J.K., Winn, D.M., Austin, D.F., Greenberg, R.S., Preston-Martin, S. *et al.* (1998) Smoking and drinking in relation to oral and pharyngeal cancer. *Cancer Research*, **48**, 3282–3287.

138 Herrero, R., Castellsagué, X., Pawlita, M., Lissowska, J., Kee, F., Balaram, P. *et al.* (2003) Human Papillomavirus and Oral Cancer: The International Agency for Research on Cancer Multicenter Study. *Journal of the National Cancer Institute*, **95**: 1772–1783.

139 Tavani, A., Gallus, S., La Vecchia, C., Talamini, R., Barbone, F., Herrero, R. *et al.* (2001) Diet and risk of oral and pharyngeal cancer. An Italian case-control study. *European Journal of Cancer Prevention*, **10**, 191–195.

140 de Visscher, J.G., Bouwes Bavinck, J.N. & van der Waal, I. (1997) Squamous cell carcinoma of the lower lip in renal-transplant recipients. Report of six cases. *International Journal of Oral and Maxillofacial Surgery*, **26**(2), 120–123.

141 Wey, P.D., Lotz, M.J. & Trideman, L.J. (1987) Oral cancer in women nonusers of tobacco and alcohol. *Cancer*, **60**, 1644–1650.
142 McLeod, N.M., Saeed, N.R., Ali, E.A. (2005) Oral cancer: delays in referral and diagnosis persist. *British Dental Journal*, **198**(11), 681–684.
143 Scott, S.E., Grunfeld, E.A. & McGurk, M. (2006) Patient's delay in oral cancer: A systematic review. *Community Dentistry and Oral Epidemiology*, **34**(5), 337–343.
144 Sobin, L.H. & Wittekind, C. (eds) (1977) Union Internationale Centre Le Cancer. TNM Classification of malignant tumours, 5th edn, Wiley-Liss, Inc, New York, NY.
145 Morgan, R.F., Hirata, R.M., Jaques, D.A. & Hoopes, J.E. (1982) Head and neck surgery in the aged. *American Journal of Surgery*, **144**, 449–451.
146 Jun, M.Y., Strong, E.W., Saltzman, E.I. & Gerould, F.P. (1983) Head and neck cancer in the elderly. *Head & Neck Surgery*, **5**, 376–382.
147 Epstein, J.B., Epstein, J.D., Le, N.D. & Gorsky, M. (2001) Characteristics of oral and paraoral malignant lymphoma: a population-based review of 361 cases. *Oral Surgery, Oral Medicine, Oral Pathology, Oral Radiology and Endodontology*, **92**(5), 519–525.
148 Swerdlow, S.H., Campo, E., Harris, N.L., Jaffe, E.S., Pileri, S.A., Stein, H., Thiele, J. & Vardiman, J.W. (2008) *WHO Classification of Tumours of Haematopoietic and Lymphoid Tissues*, 4th edn, IARC Press, Lyon.
149 Hicks, M.J. & Flaitz, C.M. (2000) Oral mucosal melanoma: epidemiology and pathobiology. *Oral Oncology*, **36**, 152–169.
150 Meleti, M., Leemans, C.R., Mooi, W.J. & van der Waal, I. (2007) Oral malignant melanoma: the Amsterdam experience. *Journal of Oral and Maxillofacial Surgery*, **65**(11), 2181–2186.
151 Hirshberg, A., Shnaiderman-Shapiro, A., Kaplan, I. & Berger, R. (2008) Metastatic tumours to the oral cavity – Pathogenesis and analysis of 673 cases. *Oral Oncology*, **44**, 743–752.
152 Oikarinen, V.J., Calonius, P.E.B. & Sainio, P. (1975) Metastatic tumours to the oral region I. An analysis of cases in the literature. *Proceedings of the Finnish Dental Society*, **71**, 58–65.
153 Calonius, P.E.B., Sainio, P. & Oikarinen, V.J. (1975) Metastatic tumours to the oral region. II. Report on 13 cases. *Proceedings of the Finnish Dental Society*, **71**, 66–71.

CHAPTER 19

Salivary function and disorders in the older adult

Jonathan A. Ship†

Bluestone Center for Clinical Research, New York University (NYU) College of Dentistry, New York, NY, USA

Introduction

Saliva is critical for the maintenance of oral and pharyngeal health and assists in three essential functions: host defence, nutritional intake and communication. Salivary gland function is remarkably intact in very healthy older adults, but the majority of the elderly experience some level of xerostomia (complaints of mouth dryness) and/or salivary hypofunction (diminished salivary secretions). This chapter will review the normal physiology of salivary secretion, disorders of salivation in the elderly, their diagnosis and treatment.

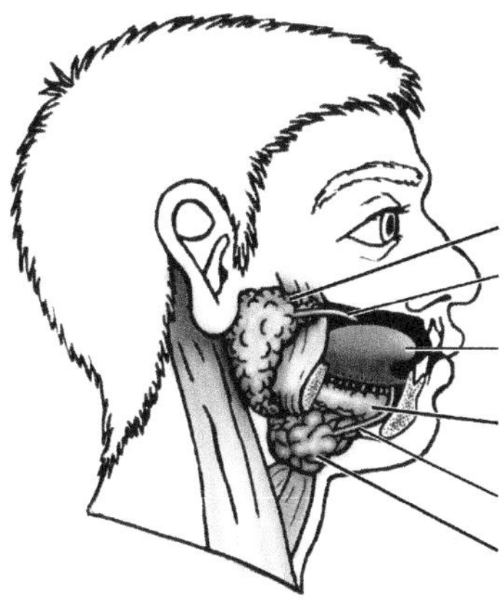

Figure 19.1 Anatomic location of the three major salivary glands. In: Greenberg MS, Glick M, Ship JA (eds) Burket's Oral Medicine, 11th edn, BC Decker, Hamilton, Ontario, Canada. 2008. *Source*: Fox and Ship (2008). Reproduced with permission of PMPH USA.

Formation of saliva

Three major paired salivary glands (parotid, submandibular and sublingual) secrete a complex, protein-rich saliva. Initial water transport (from the serum) is through the acinar cells, and then saliva is modified as it is carried via a branching duct system into the oral cavity. There are also hundreds of minor salivary glands (labial, palatal, buccal) throughout the mouth and extending down the tracheo-bronchial tree. These minor glands are located just below the mucosal surface and secrete onto the mucosa through short ducts. At rest (basal or unstimulated function), it is estimated that the minor glands may produce up to half of the saliva in the oral cavity. With stimulation, however, the major glands predominate and produce over 90% of all saliva.

Saliva is the product of the major and minor salivary glands dispersed throughout the oral cavity (Figure 19.1). It is a highly complex mixture of water and organic and non-organic components. The three major salivary glands are composed of acinar and ductal cells (Figure 19.2). Acinar cells make up the secretory endpieces. Parotid acinar cells are serous, those of the sublingual and minor glands are mucous, while the submandibular gland is composed of mixed mucous and serous types. The duct cells form a branching system that carries the saliva from the acini into the oral cavity. While fluid secretion occurs only through the acini, proteins are produced and transported into the saliva through both acinar and ductal cells. The primary saliva within the acinar endpieces is isotonic with serum but undergoes extensive resorption of sodium and chloride and secretion of potassium within the duct system. The saliva, as it enters the oral cavity, is a protein-rich hypotonic fluid.

The secretion of saliva is controlled by sympathetic and parasympathetic neural input. Fluid secretion stimulation is primarily via muscarinic-cholinergic receptors, while the stimulus for protein release occurs largely through β-adrenergic receptors. Activation of these and other receptors induces a complex signalling and signal transduction

† Author is deceased.

Textbook of Geriatric Dentistry, Third Edition. Edited by Poul Holm-Pedersen, Angus W. G. Walls and Jonathan A. Ship.

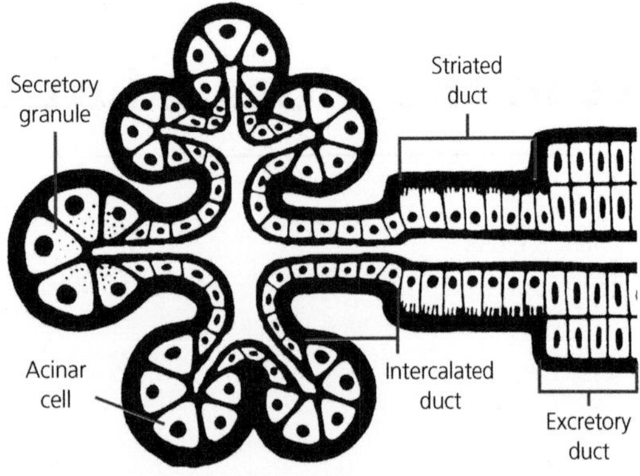

Figure 19.2 Diagram of the basic histologic organization of the acinar and ductal components of a major salivary gland. In: Greenberg MS, Glick M, Ship JA (eds) Burket's Oral Medicine, 11th edn, BC Decker, Hamilton, Ontario, Canada. 2008. *Source*: Fox and Ship (2008). Reproduced with permission of PMPH USA.

pathway within the cells, involving numerous transport systems, resulting in a tightly regulated secretion process. There are aspects of salivary physiology that have implications for the treatment of salivary gland disorders. Acinar cell loss (e.g. from high doses of external beam radiotherapy for head and neck cancer, or the autoimmune exocrinopathy Sjögren's syndrome) will limit the ability of the gland to transport fluid and therefore to produce saliva. Many drugs taken by older adults have anti-muscarinic or anti-adrenergic side effects, which could limit the ability to stimulate these cells. Alternatively, muscarinic agonists (parasympathomimetics) are efficacious as secretagogues and can be used effectively to stimulate salivary output.

Salivary gland function with aging

It was previously thought that salivary output diminishes with increasing age. This was based on the clinical observation that older individuals frequently have a dry mouth and complain of xerostomia. However, investigations reveal that, in general, there is no substantial diminution in salivary production across the human life span in healthy adults. Thus, in the absence of complicating factors (e.g. certain systemic diseases, medications), there is no generalized age-related perturbation in the production of salivary fluid. In addition, there appear to be no significant clinical alterations in the composition of saliva in older, healthy persons.

These physiological findings contrast with the morphological changes seen in aging salivary glands. Major salivary glands lose ~30 per cent of their parenchymal tissue over the adult life span. The loss primarily involves acinar or fluid-producing components, while proportional increases are seen in ductal cells and in fat, vascular and connective tissues. Because acinar components are primarily responsible for the secretion of saliva, it is not known why, in the presence of a significant reduction in the gland acinar volume, total fluid production does not diminish with increasing age. It has thus been deduced that salivary glands possess a functional reserve capacity that enables them to maintain fluid output throughout the human adult life span. There is evidence that with a reduced reserve capacity, additional burdens placed on aging salivary glands (e.g. anticholinergic medications, systemic diseases such as Sjögren's syndrome) increase their vulnerability to functional decline. Therefore, salivary hypofunction and complaints of a dry mouth (xerostomia) should not be considered to be normal sequelae of aging but instead are indicative of a host of conditions and their treatments.

The most common etiology of salivary gland hypofunction is iatrogenic. Many medications taken by older persons reduce or alter salivary gland performance (Box 19.1). A host of medical disorders, as well as radiation for head and neck neoplasms and cytotoxic chemotherapy, can have direct and dramatic deleterious effects on salivary glands (Table 19.1). Older adults are also vulnerable to salivary gland infections, obstructions and neoplasms that will affect salivary output.

Box 19.1 Common medication categories associated with salivary hypofunction.

Anticholinergics
Antihistamines
Antihypertensives
Anti-Parkinson's disease
Anti-seizure
Cytotoxic agents
Sedatives and tranquilizers
Skeletal muscle relaxants
Tricyclic antidepressants

Table 19.1 Oral and systemic conditions associated with salivary hypofunction in older adults

Category	Examples
Oncological therapy	Cytotoxic chemotherapy
	Head and neck radiotherapy
Oral conditions	Bacterial and viral infections
	Salivary gland obstructions
	Traumatic lesions
	Neoplasms
Other conditions	Alzheimer's disease
	Cerebrovascular accidents
	Dehydration
	Diabetes mellitus
	Late-stage liver disease
	Sjögren's syndrome
	Systemic lupus erythematosus
	Thyroid disorders (hyper and hypo)

Etiology of salivary hypofunction in the older adult

The evaluation of salivary disorders in the older adult is no different than for a person of any age (see above). Overall, salivary problems are caused by local as well as systemic conditions. Oral sources of salivary gland pathology are infectious (bacterial and viral), non-infectious (obstructions – sialolith, mucocele, ranula) and neoplastic (benign – pleomorphic adenoma; malignant – mucoepidermoid carcinoma, adenoid cystic carcinoma). However, the most common cause of salivary disorders in the elderly is systemic conditions, which are divided into systemic diseases, medications and head and neck radiotherapy.

The most common systemic disease that causes a dry mouth in middle-aged and older-aged adults is Sjögren's syndrome, an autoimmune exocrinopathy producing dry eyes and a dry mouth. Sjögren's syndrome is a chronic autoimmune disease characterized by symptoms of oral and ocular dryness, exocrine dysfunction and lymphocytic infiltration and destruction of the exocrine glands. The etiology of Sjögren's syndrome is unknown and there is no cure. The salivary and lacrimal glands are primarily affected, but Sjögren's syndrome is a systemic disorder and dryness may affect other mucosal areas (nose, throat, trachea, vagina), skin and many organ systems (thyroid, lung, kidney, etc.).

Sjögren's syndrome primarily affects peri- and postmenopausal women (the female to-male ratio is 9 : 1) and is classified as primary or secondary. Primary Sjögren's syndrome is a systemic disorder that includes both lacrimal and salivary gland dysfunctions without another autoimmune condition. Secondary Sjögren's syndrome patients have salivary and/or lacrimal gland dysfunction with another connective tissue disease (e.g. systemic lupus erythematosus, rheumatoid arthritis, scleroderma, primary biliary cirrhosis).

Patients with Sjögren's syndrome may experience intermittent or chronic salivary gland enlargement. They are also susceptible to salivary gland infections and/or gland obstructions that present as acute exacerbations of chronically enlarged glands. Patients have an increased risk of developing malignant lymphoma, most typically mucosal-associated B cell lymphomas (MALT lymphomas) involving the salivary glands. For example, patients with primary Sjögren's syndrome have an estimated 20- to 40-fold increased risk of lymphoma. Sjögren's syndrome patients also frequently experience arthralgias, myalgias, peripheral neuropathies and rashes.

Other systemic conditions that inhibit salivary function include rheumatoid arthritis, HIV+ infection, diabetes, Alzheimer's disease, dehydration and strokes. In addition to medical conditions, a common cause of salivary disorders in the elderly is prescription and non-prescription medications. This is due to anticholinergic and anti-adrenergic effects, which inhibit the production of saliva and its constituents and can affect adversely the transport of saliva from the acinar cells till the major excretory ducts and ultimately the mouth. For example, 80% of the most commonly prescribed medications have been reported to cause xerostomia, with over 400 medications causing a side effect of salivary gland hypofunction. These medications include tricyclic antidepressants, sedatives and tranquilizers, antihistamines, antihypertensives, cytotoxic agents, anti-Parkinsonian, and anti-seizure drugs (Box 19.1).

Chemotherapeutic agents have also been associated with salivary disorders. After completion of chemotherapy, most patients experience return of salivary function to pre-chemotherapy levels, yet long-term changes have been reported. Radioactive iodine (I-131) used for thyroid tumours will also cause salivary disorders, yet only in the parotid gland in a dose-dependent fashion.

A common therapeutic modality for head and neck cancers is external beam radiation, which causes severe and permanent salivary hypofunction and persistent complaints of xerostomia. Since 95% of these cancers occur in individuals greater than 50 years of age, this phenomenon is of concern for middle- and older-aged adults. The cause is radiation-induced destruction of the serous-producing salivary cells via a process termed apoptosis (programmed cell cell). Within one week of the start of irradiation (after 10 Gy have been delivered) salivary output declines by 60–90%, with no recovery unless the total dose to salivary tissue is <25 Gy. Most patients receive therapeutic dosages that exceed 60 Gy and their salivary glands undergo atrophy and become fibrotic. Patients experience a plethora of oral and pharyngeal side effects from the salivary dysfunction.

Clinical evaluation

The most common presentation of salivary gland disease is the complaint of dry mouth. The subjective report of oral dryness is termed xerostomia, which is a symptom, not a diagnosis or disease. Since individuals with salivary gland hypofunction are at risk for a variety of oral and systemic complications due to alterations in normal salivation, patients need a careful objective examination. The differential diagnosis of xerostomia, salivary masses and salivary gland dysfunction is lengthy. The optimal diagnostic evaluation should include a detailed evaluation of symptoms, a past and present medical history and a head/neck/oral examination.

Symptoms of xerostomia

Symptoms in the patient with salivary gland hypofunction are related to decreased fluid in the oral cavity and the effects this has on mucosal hydration and oral functions. Patients complain of dryness of all oral/pharyngeal mucosal surfaces, including the lips and throat and also of difficulty chewing, swallowing, tasting, and speaking. Oral pain is common. The mucosa may be sensitive to spicy or coarse foods, which limits the patient's enjoyment of meals and may compromise nutrition.

Past and present medical history

The past and present medical history may reveal medical conditions or medications that are known to be associated with salivary gland disorders (Box 19.1, Table 19.1). Examples would be a patient who has received radiotherapy for a head and neck malignancy or an individual who has recently started taking a tricyclic antidepressant. Over 400 drugs are reported to have dry mouth as a side effect. A complete history of all medications being taken (including over-the-counter medications, supplements and herbal preparations) is critical. Often the temporal association of symptom onset with the treatment is a valuable clue. When the history does not suggest an obvious diagnosis, further exploration of the complaint should be undertaken. A patient's report of eye, throat, nasal, skin or vaginal dryness, in addition to xerostomia, may be a significant indication of the most common systemic condition with salivary gland sequelae: Sjögren's syndrome.

Clinical examination

Most patients with advanced salivary gland hypofunction have obvious signs of mucosal dryness with cracked, peeling and atrophic lips. The buccal mucosa may be pale and corrugated in appearance (Figure 19.3) and the tongue may be smooth and erythemic, with evidence of depapillation (Figure 19.4). Patients may report that their lips stick to the teeth and the oral mucosa may adhere to the dry enamel. There is often a marked increase in erosion and caries, particularly decay on root surfaces (Figure 19.5). The decay may be progressive, even in the presence of vigilant oral hygiene. With diminished salivary output, there is a tendency for greater accumulations of food debris in interproximal regions, especially where gingival recession has occurred.

Candidiasis is a frequent finding in patients with salivary hypofunction. It can occur as red patches on the mucosa (erythematous), as well as pseudomembraneous removable plaques on all mucosal surfaces (Figure 19.6). Angular cheilitis is common, as is denture stomatitis, an asymptomatic fungal infection of the dental prosthesis as well as the denture-bearing mucosa.

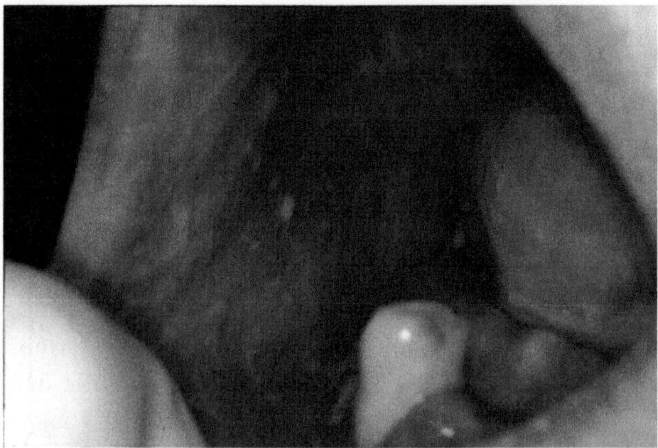

Figure 19.3 Dessicated buccal mucosa in a patient with salivary gland hypofunction.

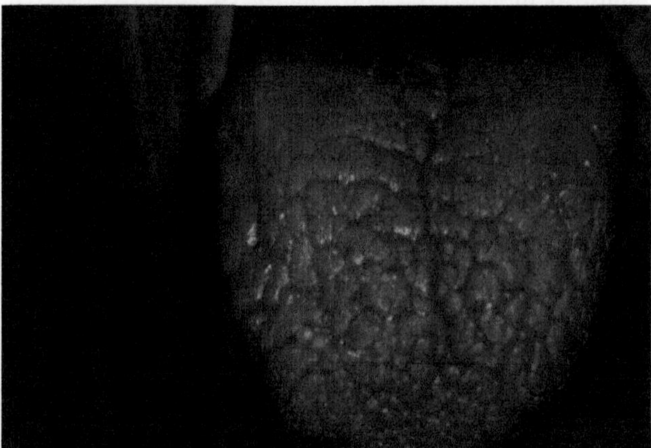

Figure 19.4 Dry and depapillated tongue dorsum secondary to salivary gland hypofunction.

Enlargement of the salivary glands can be visualized, requiring distinction between inflammatory, infectious or neoplastic etiologies. The major salivary glands should be palpated to detect masses and also to determine if saliva can be expressed via the main excretory ducts. The expressed saliva should be clear, watery and copious. Viscous or scant secretions suggest chronically reduced function. A cloudy exudate may be a sign of bacterial infection. Enlarged glands that are painful on palpation are indicative of infection or acute inflammation. If distinct masses within the body of the major salivary gland are palpated, an obstruction (e.g. sialolith), benign or malignant tumour should be considered.

Salivary gland imaging

A number of imaging techniques are useful in evaluation of the salivary glands. Since the salivary glands are located

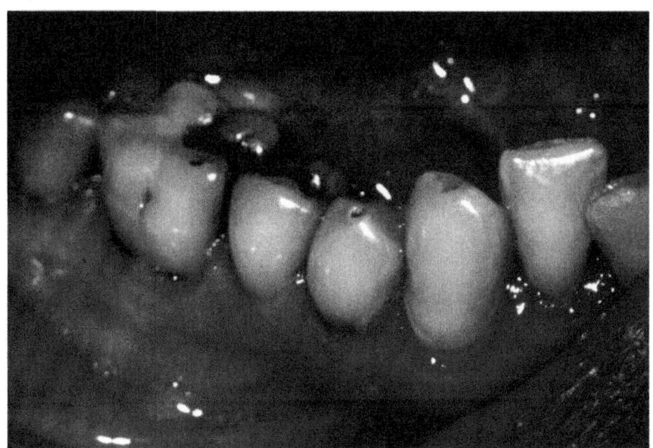

Figure 19.5 Root surface decay on the buccal cervical margins of the mandibular right teeth in a patient with chronic salivary gland hypofunction and complaints of xerostomia.

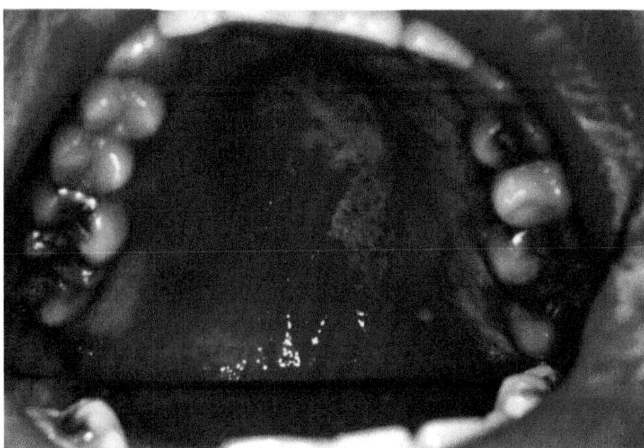

Figure 19.6 Pseudomembraneous candidiasis on the palate of a patient who has received head and neck radiotherapy for oral cancer and is experiencing severe salivary gland hypofunction.

relatively superficially, radiographic images may be obtained with standard dental radiographic techniques to help visualize possible radiopaque sialoliths (stones). Sialography is the radiographic visualization of the salivary gland following retrograde instillation of soluble contrast material into the ducts. Sialography is the recommended method for evaluating ductal obstruction, whether by a sialolith, tumour or stricture. Scintigraphy with technetium (Tc) 99m pertechnetate is a dynamic and minimally invasive diagnostic test to assess salivary gland function and to determine abnormalities in gland uptake and excretion. Scintigraphy provides quantitative information on the functional capabilities of the glands. It has been used to aid in the diagnosis of ductal obstruction, sialolithiasis, gland aplasia, Bell's palsy and Sjögren's syndrome. CT and MRI are useful for evaluating salivary gland pathology, adjacent structures and the proximity of salivary lesions to the facial nerve. Since calcified structures are better visualized by CT, this modality is especially useful for the evaluation of inflammatory conditions that are associated with sialoliths. Ultrafast CT and three-dimensional–image CT sialography have been reported to be an effective method of visualizing masses that are poorly defined on MRI. MRI has become the imaging modality of choice for preoperative evaluation of salivary gland tumours because of its excellent ability to differentiate soft tissues and its ability to provide multiplanar imaging. Positron emission tomography (PET) has been utilized recently for evaluation of the salivary glands. Preliminary reports suggest this may be a useful technique for measuring regional salivary gland function and recognizing inflammatory changes. Combination of PET with computed axial tomography may allow differentiation of salivary gland alterations in Sjögren's syndrome.

Salivary gland biopsy

Definitive diagnosis of salivary pathology may require tissue examination. When Sjögren's syndrome is suspected, the labial minor salivary gland is the most frequently sampled site. Biopsy of minor glands can also be used to diagnose amyloidosis, sarcoidosis and in diagnosing and monitoring chronic graft-versus-host disease. Minor gland biopsy is a minimal operative procedure that can be done with limited morbidity, using appropriate techniques.

When major gland biopsy is indicated for the evaluation of a distinct salivary mass, fine-needle aspiration (FNA) can be attempted. If this does not yield an adequate sample for diagnosis, an open biopsy procedure should be performed. Fine-needle aspiration biopsy is a simple and effective technique that aids the diagnosis of solid lesions. It may be particularly useful for elderly patients who cannot tolerate an excisional biopsy because of medical considerations. A preoperative surgical biopsy is rarely indicated for salivary masses. In almost all salivary gland tumours, the treatment of choice is an excisional biopsy.

Serological evaluation

Laboratory blood studies are helpful in the evaluation of dry mouth, particularly in suspected cases of Sjögren's syndrome. The presence of nonspecific markers of autoimmunity, such as antinuclear antibodies, rheumatoid factors, elevated immunoglobulins (particularly immunoglobulin G [IgG]) and erythrocyte sedimentation rate, or the presence of antibodies directed against the extractable nuclear antigens SS-A/Ro or SS-B/La are important contributors to the definitive diagnosis of Sjögren's syndrome. Approximately

80% of patients with Sjögren's syndrome will display antinuclear antibodies and about 60% will have antibodies against anti-SS-A/Ro. This latter autoantibody is considered the most specific marker for Sjögren's syndrome, although it may be found in a small percentage of patients with systemic lupus erythematosus or other autoimmune connective-tissue disorders.

Treatment strategies

There are five categories of treatment strategies for the older patient with salivary hypofunction: (1) preventive therapy, (2) symptomatic or palliative treatment, (3) local or topical salivary stimulation, (4) systemic salivary stimulation and (5) therapy directed at an underlying systemic disorder. In general, the overall strategy should include a combination of supplemental fluoride (for dentate individuals), topical palliative agents and a secretagogue (Table 19.2).

Preventive therapy

The dentate older adult with salivary gland hypofunction must be treated with fluoride to prevent and limit the development of dental caries. There are many different fluoride therapies available, from low concentration over-the-counter fluoride rinses, to more potent highly concentrated prescription fluorides (e.g. 1.0% sodium fluoride) that are applied by brush or in a custom carrier. Fluoride varnishes are also efficacious for caries prevention. The dosage chosen and the frequency of application (from daily to once per week) should be determined based on the severity of the dry mouth condition and the rate of caries development.

Patients with salivary hypofunction must also maintain meticulous oral hygiene. Visits to dental professionals should be more frequent (usually every 3–4 months) and patients must work closely with their dentist to maintain optimal dental health. Older patients and their caregivers should be counselled on their diet in order to avoid cariogenic foods and beverages and to perform oral hygiene immediately after meals.

Patients with dry mouth also experience an increase in oral infections, particularly mucosal candidiasis. There are multiple presentations, the most common being pseudomembraneous (white, easily removed plaques on any mucosal surface) and erythematous (mucosal erythema with complaints of a burning sensation of the tongue or other intraoral soft tissues). Denture stomatitis occurs frequently but is rarely symptomatic and therefore clinicians must examine denture-bearing surfaces at all visits. Dentures infected with fungal infections require immersion in solutions containing benzoic acid, 0.12% chlorhexidine or 1% sodium hypochlorite to eradicate the fungal organisms that have colonized the denture material. Daily denture hygiene and topical antifungal ointment is also helpful. Periodic re-examinations are important to ensure that the oral fungal infections have been eradicated.

Table 19.2 Treatment of dry mouth problems in the elderly

Dry mouth-associated problem	Treatment
Dental caries	Daily use of fluoridated dentifrice (0.05% sodium fluoride) Daily use of prescription fluoride gel (1.0% sodium fluoride, 0.4% stannous fluoride) Application of 0.5% sodium fluoride varnish to teeth Dental examinations at least every 6 months and bitewing radiographs for early diagnosis every 12 months
Dry mouth	Oral moisturizers/lubricants, mouthwashes and sprays Sugarfree gums, mints, lozenges Artificial saliva rinses and sprays Pilocarpine 5 mg tid and qhs; cevimeline 30 mg tid Lubricants on lips q2h Bedside humidifier during sleeping hours
Dysgeusia	Fluid use during eating
Dysphagia	Careful eating with frequent use of fluids during meals Avoid dry, hard, sticky and difficult to chew foods
Oral candidiasis	Nystatin oral suspension 100 000 units/mL, rinse qid Nystatin ointment applied qid Antifungal lozenges dissolved in mouth qid: nystatin pastilles 200 000 units; clotrimazole troches 10 mg; nystatin vaginal suppositories Denture antifungal treatment: daily hygiene, soak prosthesis for 30 min in benzoic acid, 0.12% chlorhexidine or 1% sodium hypochlorite
Salivary gland bacterial infections	Systemic antibiotics × 10 days: amoxicillin with clavulanate 500 mg q8h; clindamycin 300 mg tid; cephalexin 500 mg q6h Increase hydration Salivary stimulation with sugarfree gums, mints, lozenges
Poorly fitting prostheses	Soft and hard-tissue relines by dentist Denture adhesives

Symptomatic treatment

Water is the most readily available symptomatic treatment and patients should be encouraged to sip water throughout the day. Water will help to moisten the oral cavity, hydrate the mucosa and clear food debris from the teeth and mucosal tissues. Careful water drinking with meals is very important, since it will improve mastication, swallowing and taste perception. It will also help prevent choking and possible pulmonary aspiration. Dentate individuals should be advised to avoid the regular use of sugar-free carbonated drinks, as the acidic content of many of these beverages is high and may increase tooth demineralization.

Another symptomatic treatment to lessen xerostomia, particularly at night, is the use of room humidifiers. As part of the normal diurnal variation in salivary physiology, salivary output drops almost to zero during rest. Desiccation of the oral mucosa is particularly troublesome at night and frequent awakening due to mouth dryness may interfere with restorative sleep.

Oral rinses, mouthwashes and gels are available for dry mouth patients and can help reduce symptoms of dry mouth. Products containing aloe vera or vitamin E are also helpful. Persistent cracking and erythema at the corners of the mouth (angular cheilitis) should be investigated for a fungal or bacterial cause.

There are many commercially available salivary substitutes ('artificial salivas') that can help reduce complaints of dry mouth and provide some fluid to help hydrate oral hard and soft tissues. They come in many different formulations (rinse, spray, mist); however they are not well accepted long-term by some patients. Patients should be encouraged to try different brands and formulations to find an acceptable salivary replacement.

Salivary stimulation

Several approaches are available for stimulating salivary flow, from oral approaches to systemic strategies. Chewing will stimulate salivary flow effectively, as will sour and sweet tastes. The combination of chewing and taste, as provided by gums or mints, can be very effective in relieving symptoms for patients who have remaining salivary function. However, patients with dry mouth must be advised not to use products with sugar, due to the increased risk for dental caries. Electrical stimulation has been recently examined as a possible therapy for salivary hypofunction with an intraoral custom-fabricated removable device that delivers a very low-voltage electrical charge to the tongue and palate. Initial results have been modest using this device in patients with dry mouth. Finally, acupuncture, with application of needles in the peri-oral and other regions, has been proposed as a therapy for salivary gland hypofunction and xerostomia. Further well controlled trials are necessary to evaluate this treatment modality fully.

Systemic stimulation

Several systemic secretagogues have been proposed as possible efficacious agents for stimulating saliva in patients with salivary hypofunction. To date, however, only two agents have demonstrated consistent safety and efficacy in controlled clinical trials and have also been approved by the US Food and Drug Administration (FDA): pilocarpine hydrochloride and cevimeline hydrochloride.

Pilocarpine hydrochloride is FDA-approved specifically for the relief of xerostomia following radiotherapy for head and neck cancers and for those with Sjögren's syndrome. Pilocarpine hydrochloride functions as a muscarinic cholinergic agonist, which increases salivary output and stimulates any remaining gland function. The adverse effects of pilocarpine are common and usually mild, consistent with the known mechanism of action of the drug. Sweating is the most common side effect, with other frequently reported side effects including hot flashes, urinary frequency, diarrhoea and blurred vision.

After administration of pilocarpine, salivary output increases fairly rapidly, usually reaching a maximum within 1 hour. The best-tolerated doses are 5.0 to 7.5 mg, given three or four times daily. The duration of action is approximately 2 to 3 hours. Pilocarpine is contraindicated for patients with pulmonary disease, asthma, cardiovascular disease, glaucoma or urethral reflux. Patients do not appear to develop tolerance to pilocarpine following prolonged use. Pilocarpine has been shown to be a safe and effective therapy for patients with diminished salivation but who have some remaining secretory function that can be stimulated.

Cevimeline hydrochloride is another parasympathomimetic agonist that is FDA-approved for the treatment of symptoms of oral dryness in Sjögren's syndrome. Cevimeline is prescribed at 30 mg/three times daily. This medication reportedly selectively targets the M1 and M3 muscarinic receptors of the salivary and lacrimal glands. However, in clinical use, its side effects are similar to those of pilocarpine and it still must be used with caution in patients with a history of glaucoma or cardiovascular, respiratory or gall bladder disease and in patients who use various medications. The duration of secretagogue activity is longer than pilocarpine (3 to 4 hours) and the onset is somewhat slower.

Pilocarpine hydrochloride and cevimeline hydrochloride are the only systemic sialogogues that are available in the USA. Both are effective at transiently relieving symptoms of oral dryness and increasing salivary output. Consultation with the patient's physician prior to prescribing these drugs for patients with significant medical conditions may be indicated, although they have a good safety record in many years of use.

Two other drugs are used in Europe and the Middle East as systemic sialogogues (bromhexine, anetholetrithione) but have not demonstrated consistent benefit in patients with salivary hypofunction. Bromhexine is a mucolytic agent with an unknown mechanism of action for salivary stimulation. No proven benefit to salivary function has been shown in controlled clinical trials. Anethole trithione is a mucolytic agent that has been shown to increase salivary output in clinical trials with mild adverse effects. The mechanism of action is not known definitively, but it has been suggested that anethole trithione may upregulate muscarinic receptors.

Treatment of underlying systemic disorders

Most clinical work has been done in Sjögren's syndrome, which includes treatment with muscarinic agonists and immunomodulatory drugs. These techniques may also work with other systemic diseases, depending upon the etiopathogenesis of the salivary problem.

New approaches to head and neck radiotherapy are now accepted using salivary sparing techniques (intensity-modulated radiotherapy or IMRT) that minimize exposure of salivary gland glands to radiotherapy while providing therapeutic levels of radiotherapy to tumours and sites at risk for tumour spread. In addition to improvements in the planning and delivery of radiation therapy, radioprotective agents may help limit radiation therapy-induced salivary gland damage. Amifostine, a cytoprotective agent, is FDA approved for xerostomia prevention in patients undergoing radiation treatment for head and neck cancers when the radiation port includes a substantial portion of the parotid glands. The proposed mechanism of action involves the intracellular scavenging of free oxygen radicals. Amifostine is administered intravenously or subcutaneously 15–30 minutes prior to each fractionated radiation treatment. In combination with IMRT, amifostine may provide even more effectiveness in preventing permanent salivary gland destruction. Major side effects include hypotension, nausea, vomiting and dermatological reactions.

Polypharmacy is a common problem amongst the elderly, and with its attendant xerostomia side effects, it can significantly impair an older person's quality of life. Addressing this frequent problem requires collaborative and concomitant interactions by multiple health care providers. Occasionally, medications with xerostomic sequelae may no longer be required but the patient continues to take them. Other times multiple drugs are prescribed for similar medical conditions by different health care providers. Under these conditions, it is advisable to recommend critical review of all medications. Drug substitutions may help reduce the adverse side effects of medications associated with xerostomia if similar drugs are available with fewer xerostomic side effects. For example, selective serotonin specific reuptake inhibitors (SSRIs) have been reported to cause less dry mouth than tricyclic antidepressants.

If anticholinergic medications can be taken during the daytime, nocturnal xerostomia can be diminished since salivary output is lowest at night. If drug dosages can be divided, unwanted side effects from a large single dose can be avoided. Scrutiny of drug side effects can assist in diminishing the xerostomic potential of many pharmaceuticals used by the elderly.

Further reading

Anusavice, K.J. (2002) Dental caries: risk assessment and treatment solutions for an elderly population. *Compendium of Continuing Education in Dentistry*, **23**(10 Suppl), 12–20.

Arduino, P.G., Carrozzo, M., Pentenero, M., Bertolusso, G. & Gandolfo, S. (2006) Non-neoplastic salivary gland diseases. *Minerva Stomatologica*, **55**(5), 249–270.

Atkinson, J.C., Grisius, M. & Massey, W. (2005) Salivary hypofunction and xerostomia: diagnosis and treatment. *Dental Clinics of North America*, **49**(2), 309–326.

Brennan, M.T., Shariff, G., Lockhart, P.B. & Fox, P.C. (2002) Treatment of xerostomia: a systematic review of therapeutic trials. *Dental Clinics of North America*, **46**(4), 847–856.

Chao, K.S., Deasy, J.O., Markman, J., Haynie, J., Perez, C.A., Purdy, J.A. *et al.* (2001) A prospective study of salivary function sparing in patients with head-and-neck cancers receiving intensity-modulated or three-dimensional radiation therapy: initial results. *International Journal of Radiation Oncology, Biology, Physics*, **49**(4), 907–916.

Fife, R.S., Chase, W.F., Dore, R.K., Wiesenhutter, C.W., Lockhart, P.B., Tindall, E. *et al.* (2002) Cevimeline for the treatment of xerostomia in patients with Sjogren syndrome: a randomized trial. *Archives of Internal Medicine*, **162**(11), 1293–1300.

Fox, P.C. (2004) Salivary enhancement therapies. *Caries Research*, **38**(3), 241–246.

Ghezzi, E.M. & Ship, J.A. (2003) Aging and secretory reserve capacity of major salivary glands. *Journal of Dental Research*, **82**(10), 844–848.

Guggenheimer, J. & Moore, P.A. (2003) Xerostomia: etiology, recognition and treatment. *Journal of the American Dental Association*, **134**(1), 61–69.

Jensen, S.B., Pedersen, A.M., Reibel, J. & Nauntofte, B. (2003) Xerostomia and hypofunction of the salivary glands in cancer therapy. *Supportive Care in Cancer*, **11**(4), 207–225.

Kassan, S.S. & Moutsopoulos, H.M. (2004) Clinical manifestations and early diagnosis of Sjogren syndrome. *Archives of Internal Medicine*, **164**(12), 1275–1284.

Närhi, T.O., Meurman, J.H. & Ainamo, A. (1999) Xerostomia and hyposalivation: causes, consequences and treatment in the elderly. *Drugs & Aging*, **15**(2), 103–116.

Rabinov, J.D. (2000) Imaging of salivary gland pathology. *Radiologic Clinics of North America*, **38**(5), 1047–1057, x–xi.

Shiboski, C.H., Hodgson, T.A., Ship, J.A. & Schiodt, M. (2007) Management of salivary hypofunction during and after radiotherapy. *Oral Surgery, Oral Medicine, Oral Pathology, Oral Radiology and Endodontology*, **103**(Suppl 1), S66–S73.

Ship, J.A. & Fischer, D.J. (1997) The relationship between dehydration and parotid salivary gland function in young and older healthy adults. *Journals of Gerontology Series A, Biological Sciences & Medical Sciences*, **52A**(5), M310–M319.

Ship, J.A. & Hu, K. (2004) Radiotherapy-induced salivary dysfunction. *Seminars in Oncology*, **31**(6 Suppl 18), 29–36.

Ship, J.A. (2004) Xerostomia: aetiology, diagnosis, management and clinical implications. In: M. Edgar, C. Dawes, D. O'Mullane (eds) *Saliva and Oral Health*, 3rd edn, pp. 50–70, British Dental Association, London.

Speight, P.M. & Barrett, A.W. (2002) Salivary gland tumours. *Oral Diseases*, **8**(5), 229–240.

Sreebny, L.M. & Schwartz, S.S. (1997) A reference guide to drugs and dry mouth – 2nd edn. *Gerodontology*, **14**(1), 33–47.

Thomson, W.M., Chalmers, J.M., Spencer, A.J. & Slade, G.D. (2000) Medication and dry mouth: findings from a cohort study of older people. *Journal of Public Health Dentistry*, **60**(1), 12–20.

Turner, R.J. & Sugiya, H. (2002) Understanding salivary fluid and protein secretion. *Oral Diseases*, **8**(1), 3–11.

Vissink, A., Jansma, J., Spijkervet, F.K., Burlage, F.R. & Coppes, R.P. (2003) Oral sequelae of head and neck radiotherapy. *Critical Reviews in Oral Biology & Medicine*, **14**(3), 199–212.

Vitali, C., Bombardieri, S., Jonsson, R., Moutsopoulos, H.M., Alexander, E.L., Carsons, S.E. *et al.* (2002) Classification criteria for Sjogren's syndrome: a revised version of the European criteria proposed by the American-European Consensus Group. *Annals of the Rheumatic Diseases*, **61**(6), 554–558.

Vivino, F.B., Al-Hashimi, I., Khan, Z., LeVeque, F.G., Salisbury, P.L., 3rd,, Tran-Johnson, T.K. *et al.* (1999) Pilocarpine tablets for the treatment of dry mouth and dry eye symptoms in patients with Sjogren syndrome: a randomized, placebo-controlled, fixed-dose, multicenter trial. P92-01 Study Group. *Archives of Internal Medicine*, **159**(2), 174–181.

von Bultzingslowen, I., Sollecito, T.P., Fox, P.C., Daniels, T., Jonsson, R., Lockhart, P.B. *et al.* (2007) Salivary dysfunction associated with systemic diseases: systematic review and clinical management recommendations. *Oral Surgery, Oral Medicine, Oral Pathology, Oral Radiology and Endodontology*, **103**(Suppl. 1), S57–S65.

CHAPTER 20

Oral and maxillofacial surgery for the geriatric patient

Michael Turner[1] and Mark Greenwood[2]
[1]Department of Otolarygnology, Mount Sinai Beth Israel, New York, USA
[2]School of Dental Sciences, Newcastle University, UK

Introduction

Due to significant advances in medicine and surgery, the percentage of people living to older ages is increasing. The portion of the population older than age 65 years in the USA is estimated to increase in size from 12.4% to approximately 20.7% by the year 2050 [1]. As this section of the population increases, it is important prior to undergoing surgery, maxillofacial or otherwise, to understand the factors that influence life expectancy, the actual life expectancy of the individual patient based on their overall health and the quality of life postoperatively.

Anaesthesia

In the last twenty years, the number of patients in the USA over the age of 65 who had surgery of the maxillofacial and pharyngeal area increased from 488 000 to 680 000. This increase in the amount of operations is not entirely due to the increase in the number of older patients. It is also a shift in the medical and dental professions to offer more invasive treatments to the elderly. With the advancement of anaesthetic techniques and monitoring, the chance of encountering an anaesthetic complication secondary to the surgery has decreased. Although there is a definite age-related increase in mortality, studies have shown that chronological age has minimal effect on overall outcome and that it is the coexistence of various disease processes that actually have the most importance in adverse outcomes [2]. Prior to initiating therapy, a thorough history and physical should be obtained. If there is any question as to the accuracy of the medical history, a consultation with the patient's physician should be obtained. If the patient does not have a physician, an appropriate referral should be made.

Local anaesthesia

In the geriatric population, careful monitoring of the dosage amount being administered is one of the most important factors in preventing anaesthetic overdose. The two most susceptible populations to local anaesthesia overdose are the paediatric and geriatric populations, mostly due to their low body mass. In the elderly, the nerve axon function deteriorates, nerve morphology changes and the surrounding fatty tissue disappears leading to an increased sensitivity to the local anaesthetics, necessitating smaller doses. Cardiovascular disease comorbidity can also make the geriatric patient susceptible to hypertensive crises, congestive heart failure, angina and arrhythmias [3]. For patients with pre-existing cardiac and cardiopulmonary diseases, it has been suggested that the maximum amount of epinephrine that should be administered is 0.4 mg (the approximate amount in two 1.7–2.0 mL carpules), although multiple studies have shown an increase in plasma epinephrine levels without concurrent haemodynamic response [4]. The total amount of local anaesthetic agent that can be administered is dependent on the patient's weight, the volume in each carpule and the per cent volume of the anaesthetic. A relatively safe amount of anaesthetic agent that can be administered to the geriatric patient is approximately 70% of the maximum dose reported by the manufacturer. Note, each local anaesthetic agent has a slightly different maximum dose and the practitioner should know the maximum daily dose for each agent they are administering.

Textbook of Geriatric Dentistry, Third Edition. Edited by Poul Holm-Pedersen, Angus W. G. Walls and Jonathan A. Ship.

Table 20.1 ASA classification system and associated mortality rate

Class	Definition	Mortality rate
I	Normal healthy patient	–0.3%
II	Patient with mild systemic disease	0.3–1.4%
III	Patient with severe systemic disease that limits activity, but is not incapacitating	1.8–4.5%
IV	Patient that has incapacitating disease that is a constant threat to life	7.8–25.9%
V	Moribund patient not expected to survive 24 hours with or without an operation	9.4–57.8%

Sedation and general anaesthesia techniques

Before engaging in sedation and general anaesthetic use, a thorough appropriate history and physical should be taken for the determining coexistence of systemic diseases. In 2002, the American Society of Anesthesiologists (ASA) published a guide for preoperative preparation of the patient prior to operative and non-operative procedures [5] (Table 20.1).

Surgical risk and outcome in patients aged 65 and older depend mostly on four important factors: (1) age, (2) the patient's physiological status and coexisting disease (ASA class), (3) whether the surgery is elective or urgent and (4) the type of procedure. The most important factor in preventing complications was a preoperative review by the patient's physician [6].

Anaesthetic agents

Nitrous oxide

Inhalation sedation and analgesia utilizing nitrous oxide is generally considered a safe method for pain and anxiety management in the elderly because of its rapid elimination and minimum effect on the cardiovascular system. It is noninvasive, easily adjustable, and quickly reversible. Nitrous oxide is a colourless, odourless, tasteless, nonflammable, nonirritating, inorganic gas. The exact mechanism by which it functions is not known. A preoperative mental evaluation should be done to assess cognitive function because of the commonly occurring episodic dementia.

Oral sedation

The use of oral sedation in the elderly can often be difficult due to the difficulty in titration of an effective but safe dose. Polypharmacy in the elderly is very common and can make it difficult to accurately assess the patient's metabolism and their current medical regimens. Complications that occur can result in hypotension, apnea and unconsciousness resulting from cardiovascular compromise and respiratory depression. The pharmacological agents used most commonly include antihistamines, benzodiazepines and opioids.

Antihistamines are generally a safe medication that can be prescribed. The two most common are diphenhydramine (Benadryl©) and hydroxyzine (Vistaril©). Although they do cause some drowsiness, they do not have an anxiolytic effect. The patient will also have hyposalivation that can exacerbate their pre-existing polypharmacy-induced xerostomia.

The benzodiazepines are appropriate medications for the elderly and have been found to be safe and effective in the medically compromised and cognitively challenged. These medications should be given in lower doses for the elderly because of decreased metabolism and delayed clearance of the agents. Shorter acting benzodiazepine, like triazolam (Halcion©) or lorazepam (Ativan©), are a better choices for these reasons. Contraindications for triazolam use occur in patients who have a history of depression, glaucoma, who are on phenytoin for seizures and depression, on erythromycin antibiotics and who have degenerative neurological disorders (see Table 20.2).

Intravenous sedation

Intravenous sedation is a generally safe and effective procedure for both the healthy and frail elderly. As with any sedation, the patient should not have anything to eat or drink after midnight the night before surgery. At the consultation appointment, the patient should be counselled to continue their normal medical regimen and that it is acceptable to have a small sip of water to swallow their medication. Monitoring is required before, during and after procedures. Essential monitoring includes pulse-oximeter, ECG, blood

Table 20.2 Oral and intravenous sedation medications

Agent	Class	Route of administration	Dosage
Diphenhydramine (Benadryl©)	Antihistamine	Oral	25–50 mg
Hydroxyzine (Vistaril©)	Antihistamine	Oral	50–100 mg
Lorazepam (Ativan©)	Benzodiazepine	Oral	0.5–2.0 mg
Oxazepam (Serax©)	Benzodiazepine	Oral	10–30 mg
Triazolam (Halcion©)	Benzodiazepine	Oral	0.0625–0.125 mg
Midazolam	Benzodiazepine	IV	0.5–4.0 mg titrated to effect
Diazepam (Valium©)	Opioid	IV	5–10 mg titrated to effect
Fentanyl (Sublimaze©)	Opioid	IV	25 mcg IV every 3 minutes as needed up to 100 mcg

pressure monitoring and a continuous recording of vital signs. Additional padding should be available to be placed in the cervical region secondary to kyphosis. When placing the intravenous angiocatheter, particular care must be taken due to the fragility of the skin. Adhesive tape to stabilize the site must be positioned carefully so as to not abrade the skin.

As with many medications, titration of the sedative agents is recommended, allowing more time for peak effect under lower doses. Medications that are generally used are benzodiazepines, specifically midazolam. Midazolam is a short acting, water soluble benzodiazepine, which is a safe and effective anxiolytic, with the added benefit of retrograde amnesia. There are many other agents that can be given intravenously, although, as mentioned previously, cardiac and pulmonary suppression should be avoided in patients with coexisting cardiovascular diseases. Postoperative monitoring must be administered during recovery time because of the risk of postoperative delirium and increased risk of falls.

Medical management of common surgical comorbidities

Anticoagulant therapy

The uses of oral anticoagulants are very common in the treatment of thromboembolic disorders secondary to cardiovascular insufficiency in the elderly. The anticoagulant effect of these medications must be evaluated prior to surgical procedures. The three major classes of anticoagulants are warfarin, prostaglandin induced platelet inhibition and adenosine diphosphate (ADP) antagonist platelet inhibition.

Warfarin

Warfarin is the prototypical oral anticoagulant and by far the most frequently prescribed [4]. It binds to the enzyme vitamin K 2,3-epoxide reductase in liver and antagonizes the vitamin K-dependent synthesis of several coagulation factors, especially factors II, VII, IX and X and proteins C, S and Z, so that the prothrombin time (PT) is prolonged. In the past, the recommendation to discontinue warfarin three days prior to treatment had been suggested. Multiple studies have shown that most patients who are within their therapeutic range, measured by the international normalized ratio (INR) [2.0 to 3.0 for most conditions and 2.5 to 3.5 for mechanical heart valves], can have most dentoalveolar procedures with local haemostatic measures, without changing the anticoagulation therapy regimen. This can consist of biting on gauze, sutures, oxidized cellulose, topical thrombin and tranexamic acid as a mouthwash or on gauze.

Cyclooxygenase inhibitors

Cyclooxygenase (COX) is responsible for the conversion of arachidonic acid to prostaglandin G_2 (PGG_2), the first step in prostaglandin synthesis and precursor to prostaglandins of the E and F series. COX induced inhibition of thromboxane A_2 (TXA_2) and prostacyclin (PGI_2) has opposing effects on haemostasis. Thromboxane A_2 is a potent vasoconstrictor and platelet agonist, while PGI_2 inhibits platelet aggregation and vasodilation. The two types of medications that are commonly used in the geriatric patients are aspirin, which causes a permanent COX inhibition in the platelets, and the family of medications called non-steroidal anti-inflammatories (NSAIDs), which cause a reversible inhibition of platelet aggregation that resolves 24 hours after NSAID discontinuation. In general NSAIDs are utilized for their anti-inflammatory and analgesic properties.

Aspirin is utilized in many different ways. It can be used a prophylactic medication for patients with atherosclerosis or in the management of acute myocardial infarction, arterial thromboembolism prophylaxis, myocardial infarction prophylaxis, percutaneous coronary intervention (PCI), stroke prophylaxis, thrombosis prophylaxis, transient ischaemic attack (TIA) and unstable angina. It is also used, like the NSAIDs for its anti-inflammatory and analgesic properties. Discontinuing aspirin in patients who are taking it for its prophylactic, analgesic or anti-inflammatory properties is acceptable prior to surgery but is usually not necessary. Generally, since it is a permanent inhibitor of platelet aggregation and the platelets have a life span of approximately 10 days, if it is discontinued 5 days prior to the surgery no haemorrhagic increase will generally be noticed. If the patient is taking it for the management of a severe thromboembolic disease, discontinuation is not recommended. Use of haemostatic techniques like biting on gauze, sutures, oxidized cellulose, topical thrombin and tranexamic acid as a mouthwash or on gauze is suggested.

Adenosine diphosphate antagonist platelet inhibitor

Adenosine diphosphate (ADP) antagonist inhibitors are class of anticoagulants that are used in the management of acute myocardial infarction, arterial thromboembolism prophylaxis, myocardial infarction prophylaxis, PCI, stroke prophylaxis, thrombosis prophylaxis, TIA, and unstable angina. These medications irreversibly inhibit ADP-induced platelet aggregation. They prevent the binding of ADP to its platelet receptor, and through a cascade effect, fibrinogen formation is impaired. Without the fibrinogen, platelet aggregation is inhibited. Due to the morbidity of the diseases that are managed with these medications, it is not recommended that they be halted for most dentoalveolar procedures.

Bisphosphonate therapy

The therapeutic use of a group of drugs known as bisphosphonates has been associated with a destructive outcome termed osteonecrosis of the jaws (also osteonecrosis of the mandible/osteonecrosis of the maxilla). The majority of reported cases of medication-related osteonecrosis are associated with higher potency intravenous forms that are administered adjunctively for chemotherapy. These case series and case reports have attempted to describe this phenomenon, which has mostly been observed in patients taking intravenous bisphosphonates for the treatment of certain types of cancer (multiple myeloma, breast cancer and other cancers with osseous metastases) and bone disorders such as Paget's disease of bone. Treatment with oral Fosamax (alendronate), which is also a bisphosphonate, has resulted in a few documented cases of osteonecrosis of the jaws. Most cases of osteonecrosis were observed after tooth extractions in patients taking bisphosphonates, though some cases were apparently spontaneous as there was no precipitating dentoalveolar surgery/trauma.

It is important to avoid dental extractions wherever possible in patients taking bisphosphonates. If possible, patients should be rendered dentally fit prior to commencement of bisphosphonate therapy.

Mucosal fragility and impaired healing

Common factors that impair healing in older patients include a decrease in the rate of cell proliferation, wound tensile strength, collagen deposition and wound contraction. The aging process causes a change in the dermis and mucosa that consists of a decreased glycoaminoglycanes with escalated amounts of hydrophobic ground substance, decreased fibronectin synthesis and type I binding of collagen; and decreased immune competence specifically T-cell mediated immunity and antibody-mediated functions. Clinically, this causes an increase in tissue fragility. Other coexisting factors that contribute to delayed healing are: poor nutrition, dehydration, decreased vascular perfusion and the use of multiple medication [7].

Dentoalveolar surgery in elderly patients

Excluding coexisting disease process in elderly patients is difficult, but generally, extractions are considered a relatively safe procedure. As discussed above, patients with bleeding disorders must have preoperative evaluations prior to surgery. Other anatomical considerations to take into account are bone density, bone resorption patterns and change in the blood supply to the mandible.

In many elderly patients, the intermaxillary distance will be increased due to alveolar bone loss. In such cases, the simplest and most effective treatment may be to avoid surgery in the posterior region and use a removable prosthesis for oral rehabilitation. If a fixed prosthesis is used, the crown length will be long and generally not acceptable aesthetically to contemporary patients.

It is important that both the quantity and quality of hard and soft tissue are taken into account when evaluating the geriatric patient. If dental implants are being considered, there needs to be adequate bone volume. In elderly patients, there is an increased likelihood of osteoporosis and, when dental extractions were carried out several years previously, the alveolar bone will have resorbed to leave an atrophic alveolar ridge. The soft tissue quality may also be inferior intraorally, with a lack of keratinized gingival. This can lead to a less than optimal result.

Anatomical considerations are paramount for safe surgical practice. Structures to be considered include the inferior alveolar nerve and vessels, the mental nerve, the maxillary sinus and floor of nose. These structures may come to lie more superficially as the alveolar bone reabsorbs. In many cases, plain radiography is adequate to make these assessments but increasingly CT scans are used to provide more accurate visualization of important structures (Figure 20.1). Three-dimensional CT reconstructions not only provide a clearer picture of the position of anatomical structures, they also facilitate the construction of accurate surgical stents.

It should be remembered that in the mandible of elderly patients the blood supply is diminished compared to younger patients. This occurs as a result of the fact that the blood supply is much less derived from the inferior dental artery with increasing age. As a result, it is important that bone is attached to viable periosteum as loss of bone vitality is more likely to occur otherwise [8].

Planning for dental alveolar surgery

It is clearly critical that the patient and clinician communicate effectively. Surgical goals must be set and the patients must have a realistic expectation on what their outcomes are. This is good practice in most cases, but even more so with geriatric patients. A team approach is indicated, which will include the surgeons, the restorative dentists, and in frail elderly patients, the primary physicians or cardiologists.

Preprosthetic surgery

It is important that the future need for replacement of teeth is remembered prior to the extraction(s). If this is not done,

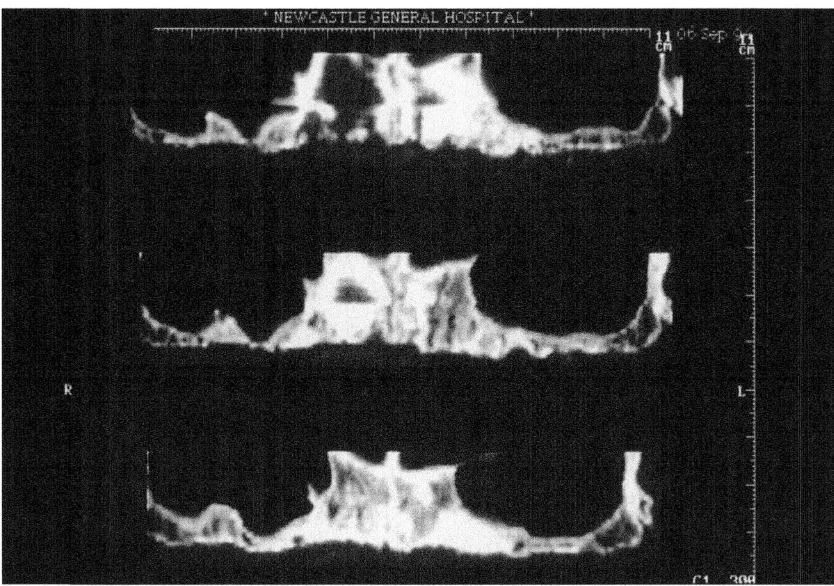

Figure 20.1 A CT scan showing atrophy in bone in the region of the maxillary sinuses.

the excessive loss of bone during a minor oral surgical procedure may necessitate future ridge augmentation which could have been avoided. When making these considerations, the two most important factors to consider are future form (aesthetics) and function.

Clearly it is important to be conservative in surgery to smooth sharp ridges to maintain the maximum amount of bone. In some cases, the use of soft linings in the prosthesis will obviate the need for surgery in these cases.

A relatively simple procedure can remove undercuts on the alveolar ridges but it is important that the soft tissues are replaced accurately and are well supported to avoid loss of sulcus depth postoperatively. The act of raising the flap itself will induce a degree of resorption and this should be done as atraumatically as possible.

Dental extractions

Attrition and brittleness of teeth (particularly if root filled) may complicate exodontia. Endodontic treatment itself may be complicated due to the deposition of secondary dentine. Other factors complicating surgical procedures include brittle dentine, low bone density and hypercementosis. Many elderly patients have frail, atrophic mucosa and a dry mouth which complicates soft tissue healing.

The extraction of multiple teeth is by no means confined to the geriatric patient. It is still true, however, that proportionately more elderly patients will require multiple extractions to facilitate oral rehabilitation compared to younger patients. It is important that liaison is carried out between surgeon and restorative dental surgeons so that the appropriate teeth are removed. The possibility of overdentures should be borne in mind and therefore teeth which may be coronally unrestorable may still be of some use. In the longer term perspective some prosthodontists prefer to start with a partial replacement prosthesis in order to facilitate the adaptation process which may be prolonged in elderly patients.

The patient's ability to withstand the planned surgical procedure should be estimated. Concomitant medical conditions should also be considered. If necessary, the procedures should be staged over more than one appointment.

As mentioned earlier, when dental extractions are carried out, they should be done in a manner which recognizes the need for future dental unit replacement. If a transalveolar approach becomes unavoidable, any bone removal should be kept to a minimum. Endodontically treated teeth tend to be brittle and sometimes require a transalveolar approach to facilitate their removal. With improvements in endodontic techniques and instrumentation, it is frequently possible to save non-vital teeth. Although apical surgery is still carried out, current thinking is that well executed orthograde root fillings are the treatment of choice. Apical surgery is often still required when associated periapical pathology is significant, for example a radiolucency exceeding 1 cm in diameter.

Dental implants in the elderly patient

Multiple studies have failed to correlate age with implant failure, after adjusting for confounding coexisting medical conditions. Failing implants related to patients' age happens rarely and is not a contraindication for placement. A success rate of 90–96% was found in the geriatric patients, equivalent to the corresponding population at large [9].

A successful dental implant is defined as a direct functional and structural connection between ordered living bone and the surface of a load-carrying implant and is termed osseointegration. Primary stability, also called initial stability, is the degree of tightness on an implant after placement. This can be difficult in the elderly patient due to the coexistence of osteoporosis. Patients with osteoporosis may exhibit longer healing times and therefore consideration needs to be given to this with respect to implant loading.

Other examples that can reflect upon the success of the implant are sclerotic bone, irradiated bone, diabetes or any pre-existing soft tissue pathology. As mentioned above, the soft tissues in an elderly patient's mouth may be frail and atrophic which can lead to impaired healing compared to younger counterparts.

Relevant local factors include the quality of oral hygiene, the presence of active periodontal disease and dental caries. Active soft tissue disease such as vesiculobullous disorders or erosive lichen planus is also a contraindication. Smoking, and along with it severe systemic effects, also adversely affects the implant success rate. Patients should be encouraged to stop a minimum of 10 weeks prior to implant placement. If the patients do not discontinue smoking, they should be made fully aware of the detrimental effects of smoking and the decrease in the implant success rate as part of the informed consent [10].

Indications for implants in the edentulous patient are shown in Box 20.1. Examples of cases treated using dental implants and implant-borne prostheses are shown in Figures 20.2, 20.3 and 20.4.

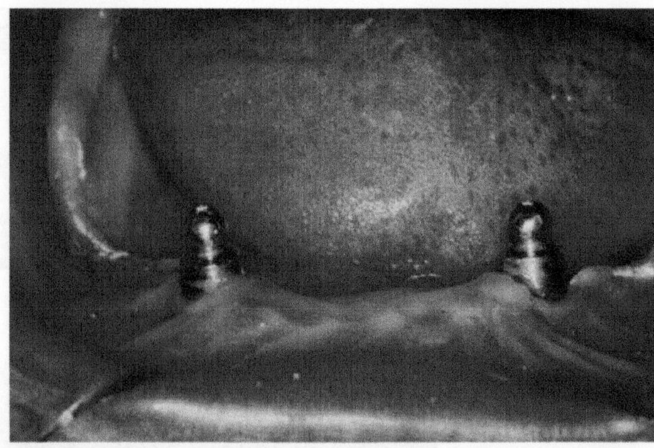

Figure 20.2 Two mandibular implants for overdenture retention.

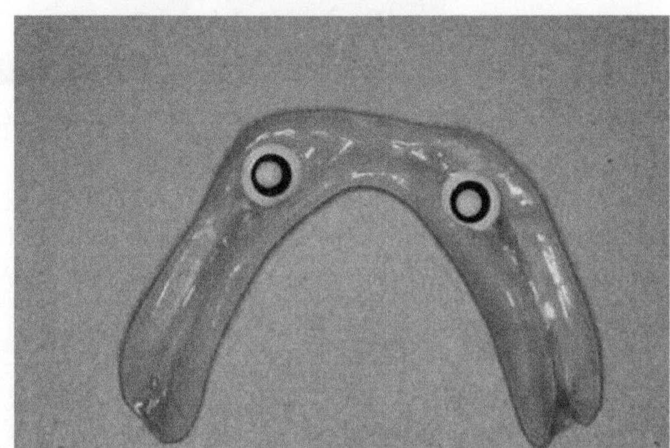

Figure 20.3 Implant retained overdenture.

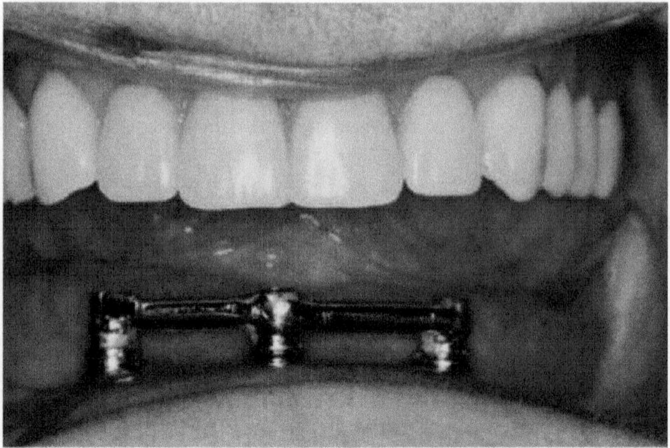

Figure 20.4 Mandibular implants with a Dolder bar.

Implants in the partially dentate

The partially dentate patient also requires thorough evaluation to ensure that there is sufficient bone in all dimensions (width and height) for correct implant placement. If there is insufficient bone, augmentation needs to be planned either as a separate procedure prior to implant placement or augmentation of the ridge at the time of implant placement or prior to implant placement.

Box 20.1 Indications for implant placement in the edentulous patient.

- Mobility of dentures/poor retention
- Mucosal intolerance
- Difficulties with nerve compression (usually the mental nerve)
- A strong gag reflex
- Poor muscular co-ordination
- Psychosocial reasons

A good example of consideration with regard to future prosthetic replacement of the dentition involves the preservation of the soft tissue profile by temporary support. This could include using socket fitted dentures or placement of appropriately contoured bridge pontics, placing immediate implants or even retaining tooth roots so long as they do not have any associated pathology.

The hard tissue profile may also be maintained by retaining roots without associated pathology and the immediate placement of dental implants. Relatively simple measures such as avoiding over-zealous socket compression post extraction and the use of osteoplastic flaps can all contribute to maintaining bone as much as possible.

Bone grafting

The optimum material for grafting is autogenous bone, which has both osteoconductive and osteoinductive qualities. Autogenous bone does have the disadvantage, however, of creating a donor site with the associated morbidity. Donor sites include the symphysis of the mandible, the ramus of the mandible or a distant site such as the iliac crest. In the elderly patient the same problems may arise with regard to vascularity, quantity and quality of bone. In addition, the temporary restriction in mobility which can be produced by iliac crest bone grafts may be particularly problematic in the elderly. Onlay grafts (Figure 20.5) can be used to increase the height and width of an atrophic ridge but it is important that once the graft has taken that it is stimulated to prevent resorption by placing dental implants. This is usually carried out between three and six months after grafting. The grafts are usually fixed to the alveolus using screws and may be supplemented with a particulate bone substitute [11].

Several bone graft substitutes have been developed. They can be divided into osteoconductive and osteoinductive types. Osteoconduction implies bone apposition onto and into a material from existing bone progenitor or bone cells. Osteoinduction implies the conversion of undifferentiated cells into osteoblasts or chondroblasts [12].

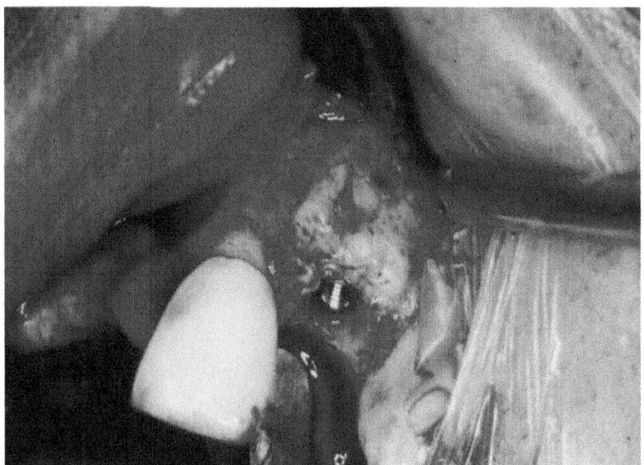

Figure 20.5 An onlay bone graft.

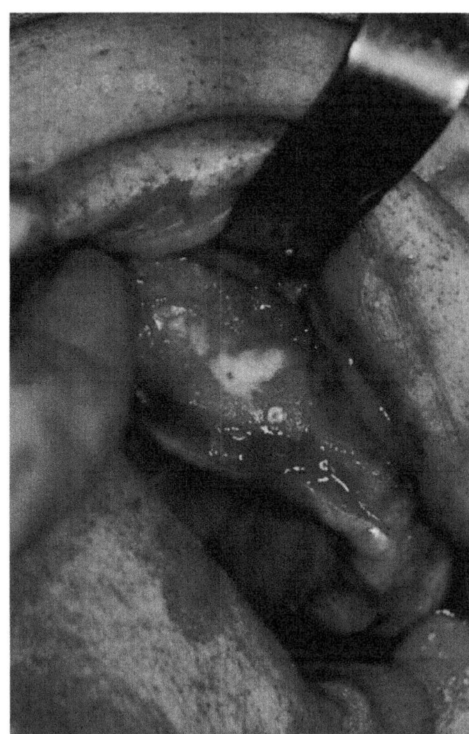

Figure 20.6 A membrane placed over a bone graft (GBR technique).

The technique of guided bone regeneration (GBR) uses a membrane which acts as a barrier preventing the ingrowth of soft tissue, thereby facilitating the formation of new bone in bony defects. Membranes may be resorbable or non-resorbable. The disadvantage of the latter is that a further procedure is required to remove them when the bone has stabilized as a result of the fact that non-resorbable membranes remain in the wound and thus act as a nidus of infection. An example of GBR is shown in Figure 20.6. Wherever possible, the membranes are left *in situ* for nine months to facilitate bony regeneration and maturation. The latter is particularly important as early removal leads to less mature bone being present which is more prone to resorption.

Fraenectomy

Prominent fraenal attachments can prevent the prosthesis sitting correctly and in some cases fraenectomy may be required. With increasing ridge resorption, the fraenal attachments become relatively more prominent with increasing age. In many cases such surgery can be avoided by generously relieving the prosthesis in the relevant area.

Many techniques of fraenectomy are described but the use of a carbon dioxide laser can be beneficial to minimize soft tissue shrinkage.

Maxillary tuberosity reduction

The carbon dioxide laser can also be useful in this situation. One technique described is the use of a double ellipse technique. In this technique, an ellipse of mucosa is removed on the surface mucosa on the ridge crest to remove excess tissue together with an underlying ellipse of deeper tissue to allow a tension-free closure.

Atrophic mandible and denture mental nerve compression

As the alveolar bone resorbs, the inferior dental nerve, particularly as it emerges from the mental foramen as the mental nerve, comes to lie more superficially. It can come to lie so superficially that in the mental region it is not covered by bone at all. Clearly a prosthesis lying on such a nerve can cause significant pain and discomfort. The principal methods of dealing with this include: relief of the denture in the relevant area, soft lining of the denture and the use of implants to bear the denture and nerve repositioning. This latter procedure is rarely carried out and runs the risk of postoperative sensibility disturbance [13].

Vestibuloplasty

Various vestibuloplasty techniques have been described with the intention of effectively increasing the height of alveolar ridge available for prosthesis placement. This technique will only be successful if there is sufficient underlying bone and therefore augmentation of the alveolus may be necessary.

All vestibuloplasty techniques require muscle attachments to be surgically displaced apically. The alveolus left without soft tissue support post vestibuloplasty can either be left to granulate or covered with a split-thickness mucosal or skin graft. These techniques have met with varying degrees of success and also introduce the problem of a second surgical site from where the graft is derived. One alternative to grafting is laser vestibuloplasty and submucous vestibuloplasty. Both of these techniques are not in common use today.

Denture-induced hyperplasia

Denture-induced hyperplasia is precipitated by long-term, ill-fitting dentures stimulating soft tissue overgrowth. Excess tissue can be removed using a scalpel but the superior healing properties of the carbon dioxide laser make this a useful mode of excision. It is important to try and minimize the amount of surgical reduction required whenever possible and this is facilitated by the use of a tissue conditioner or other prosthesis modification. In some cases, if acceptable to the patient, leaving the prosthesis out altogether for a short period can be very useful.

Biopsies

Biopsy is the process of providing a tissue sample that can be subjected to histopathological examination. It is important that the possibility of malignancy is borne in mind with all patients, but particularly so with the elderly. The incidence of malignancy increases with age. Unless a lesion is clearly clinically benign, it is safest to carry out an incisional biopsy to determine the nature of the lesion. Excisional biopsy should only be carried out for clinically benign lesions. Local analgesia will facilitate biopsy but consideration may need to be given to general anaesthesia if the lesion is in an inaccessible part of the oral cavity. It is important that local anaesthetic solution is not infiltrated directly into the tissue to be removed as tissue distortion may be produced.

Basic biopsy techniques

Both incisional and excisional biopsy should be carried out using sharp dissection so that any artifact introduced by the crushing of tissue is minimized. Likewise, manipulation of the specimen should be kept to the minimum and toothed forceps should be used carefully at the periphery. Some surgeons place a suture through the specimen to minimize damage to other areas. This also has the advantage of facilitating orientation of the specimen. The principles of good biopsy technique are given in Box 20.2.

Box 20.2 The principles of good biopsy technique.

- Biopsy the most suspicious looking area (incisional biopsies).
- Do not inject local anaesthetic solution into the future specimen.
- The specimen should be of adequate size (2 mm depth) and adequate surface dimension.
- If the lesion is large, more than one incisional biopsy may be required as the sample may not be representative – remember that the clinical appearance does not always correlate with the microscopic.
- It is important that the specimen does not taper to a point on the deep surface.
- If an incisional biopsy is carried out and the histopathological report appears incongruous with the clinical appearance, consideration should be given to a repeat biopsy.

It is important that anatomical structures are considered so as to minimize the risk of damage. Intraoral examples include the mental, lingual and greater palatine nerves and the parotid and submandibular ducts.

Difficult situations can arise with very small lesions with regard to incisional biopsy. One example is minor salivary gland lesions. In these cases an excisional biopsy can be considered but the patient must be informed that additional treatment may need to be carried out depending on the results obtained from histopathological analysis. Lesions such as this are clearly best treated by a specialist in oral and maxillofacial surgery.

It is sometimes necessary to perform a bone biopsy. Such biopsies can be facilitated by raising a mucoperiosteal flap to gain access to the lesion. The lesion can then be delineated using a fissure bur and an osteotome used to remove the specimen.

Where soft tissues have been incised, clearly the wound edges should be closed with the aim in most cases of achieving healing by primary intention. Resorbable sutures are commonly used. Occasionally primary closure is not possible and some lesions will heal by secondary intention, which may be facilitated by the placement of a surgical pack.

The biopsy sample, if it is soft tissue in origin, will usually be sent as a fixed specimen in 10% neutral buffered formalin and the volume of solution should be at least ten times that of the specimen. If a vesiculobullous lesion is suspected, the specimen should be sent fresh to the laboratory and it is wise to liaise closely with laboratory staff so that receipt of the specimen is expected.

Fine needle aspiration biopsy

The technique of fine needle aspiration biopsy (FNAB) is invaluable for obtaining cells from a lump which are then subjected to cytological examination. It is particularly useful in the aspiration of lymph nodes and major salivary gland lesions. The technique is carried out using a 20 mL syringe with a 21 gauge needle attached. About 1–2 mL of air is retained in the syringe and the needle placed in the lump to be aspirated. Suction is then applied manually to the syringe and several passes are made within the lesion. The suction is then released and the needle removed, first from the patient and then from the syringe. About 10 mL of air is drawn into the syringe, the needle replaced and the plunger of the syringe depressed so as to expel any aspirate obtained onto a microscope slide which can be sent to the laboratory either air dried or fixed.

It is important to remember that, if the correct size of needle is used, seeding will not occur, even if the lump being aspirated is malignant. The procedure of the FNAB is best carried out by an appropriate specialist in hospital practice.

The technique of FNAB can also be used for the aspiration of a cystic lesion whose nature is not known. Due consideration should be given to the possibility that this procedure can introduce infection and such aspiration is therefore usually reserved for lesions which are atypical in nature and where malignancy may be expected. Aspiration of radiolucent lesions immediately prior to surgery also has a place to exclude an unexpected vascular lesion.

Key points

1 Geriatric patients generally have comorbidities and, because of this, the provider must be aware of the necessary modification of treatment.
2 Polypharmacy is common in the elderly so drug interaction and potential hazards should be recognized and accounted for.
3 Because of polypharmacy, hypersalivation can be present in the elderly, which can increase caries rate and mucosal fragility.
4 Although it is safe to operate on the elderly, appropriate consultations should be obtained prior to surgery.

References

1 Martini, E.M., Garrett, N., Lindquist, T. & Isham, G.J. (2007) The boomers are coming: a total cost of care model of the impact of population aging on health care costs in the United States by Major Practice Category. *Health Services Research*, **42**(1 Pt 1), 201–218.
2 Seymour, D.G. & Vaz, F.G. (1989) A prospective study of elderly general surgical patients: II. Post-operative complications. *Age Ageing*, **18**(5), 316–326.
3 Helgeson, M.J., Smith, B.J., Johnsen, M. & Ebert, C. (2002) Dental considerations for the frail elderly. *Special Care in Dentistry*, **22**(3 Suppl), 40S–55S.
4 Brand, H.S., Gortzak, R.A., Palmer-Bouva, C.C., Abraham, R.E. & Abraham-Inpijn, L. (1995) Cardiovascular and neuroendocrine responses during acute stress induced by different types of dental treatment. *International Dental Journal*, **45**(1), 45–48.
5 American Society of Anesthesiologists Task Force on Preanesthesia (2002) Evaluation Practice advisory for preanesthesia evaluation: a report by the American Society of Anesthesiologists Task Force on Preanesthesia Evaluation. *Anesthesiology*, **96**(2), 485–496.
6 Schein, O.D., Katz, J., Bass, E.B., Tielsch, J.M., Lubomski, L.H., Feldman, M.A. *et al.* (2000) The value of routine preoperative medical testing before cataract surgery. Study of Medical Testing for Cataract Surgery. *New England Journal of Medicine*, **342**(3), 168–175.
7 Ashcroft, G.S., Horan, M.A. & Ferguson, M.W. (1998) Aging alters the inflammatory and endothelial cell adhesion molecule profiles during human cutaneous wound healing. *Laboratory Investigation*, **78**(1), 47–58.

8 Eiseman, B., Johnson, L.R. & Coll, J.R. (2005) Ultrasound measurement of mandibular arterial blood supply: techniques for defining ischemia in the pathogenesis of alveolar ridge atrophy and tooth loss in the elderly? *Journal of Oral Maxillofacial Surgery*, **63**(1), 28–35.

9 Bryant, S.R. & Zarb, G.A. (1998) Osseointegration of oral implants in older and younger adults. *International Journal of Oral & Maxillofacial Implants*, **13**(4), 492–499.

10 Strietzel, F.P., Reichart, P.A., Kale, A., Kulkarni, M., Wegner, B. & Kuchler, I. (2007) Smoking interferes with the prognosis of dental implant treatment: a systematic review and meta-analysis. *Journal of Clinical Periodontology*, **34**(6), 523–544.

11 Nowzari, H. & Aalam, A.A. (2007) Mandibular cortical bone graft part 2: surgical technique, applications, and morbidity. *Compendium of Continuing Education in Dentistry*, **28**(5), 274–280, quiz 81–2.

12 Jalbout, Z. & Tabourian, G. (1995) *Glossary of Implant Dentistry*. ICOI, Upper Montclair, NJ.

13 Louis, P.J. (2001) Inferior alveolar nerve repositioning. *Atlas of Oral & Maxillofacial Surgery Clinics of North America*, **9**(2), 93–128.

CHAPTER 21

Orofacial pain in older adults

Dena J. Fischer[1] and Joel B. Epstein[1,2]
[1]Department of Oral Medicine and Diagnostic Sciences, College of Dentistry, University of Illinois at Chicago, USA
[2]Chicago Cancer Center, College of Medicine, USA

Age-related change in pain perception/reporting

The aging population in the USA has been expanding for several decades and will continue to do so in the foreseeable future. The United States population of adults aged 65 and older is projected to grow from 35 million in 2000 (12.4% of the total population) to 70 million in 2030 (20.6% of the population). As a result, dentists and other health care professionals will care for a larger number of individuals living to an advanced age.

Pain is a common symptom and significant problem for older adults. Up to one half of community-dwelling adults aged ≥65 years have pain that interferes with normal function. Self-reports of chronic pain seem to increase up to, but not beyond, the seventh decade of life, despite the increasing burden of pain-associated diseases in old age. Declines in both reports and severity of pain are associated with age ≥85 years. Evidence indicates that older adults do not experience less pain than younger cohorts, but there is an underreporting of pain, perhaps because of a modified experience of pain as well as an expectation that pain is a natural part of the aging process.

Age-related neuronal changes may contribute to alterations in pain sensation in older adults. Evidence suggests that there is a loss of unmyelinated and myelinated peripheral nerve fibres, with a reduction of about 50% of unmyelinated fibres compared with a 35% loss in myelinated afferent fibres in older adults aged 65 to 75 years. Furthermore, biochemical studies have documented a marked reduction in the content of substance P and calcitonin gene-related peptide (CGRP), major neurotransmitters of primary afferent nociceptive fibres. These age-related findings may reflect a decrease in peripheral nerve fibres of all types (e.g. motor, sensory, sympathetic and nociceptive), contributing to a decrease in pain transmission from afferent peripheral nerves. Similar findings have also been reported in the central nervous system, where loss of myelin, evidence of axonal involution and decreases in neurochemical transmission systems have been reported. These age-related changes may affect pain perception in older adults.

It is difficult to ascertain the functional consequences of age-related structural changes given the multifaceted nature of pain processing. It appears that older people have a higher pain threshold for thermal stimuli than younger people, while mechanical and electrical pain thresholds seem to be constant across the age spectrum. The threshold for pain is more likely to be increased when stimuli are of short duration and are delivered to the distal extent of the limbs or to the viscera. There is also limited evidence for slower central processing of noxious stimuli in older compared with younger adults. These altered pain responses in older adults may be due to disproportionate fibre loss with age and may result in an increased risk of injury from thermal stimuli.

Reaction/adaptation to pain in older adults

Underreporting of pain in older adults may be due to an adaptation to pain with aging or a belief that pain is a natural part of the aging process. In acute postsurgical patients, older adults seem to report less pain intensity compared with younger cohorts. However, the duration of postoperative pain may be greater in older compared with younger adults. Evidence also suggests that wound healing, hyperalgesia (increased sensation or sensitivity to a painful stimulus)

Textbook of Geriatric Dentistry, Third Edition. Edited by Poul Holm-Pedersen, Angus W. G. Walls and Jonathan A. Ship.

and inflammation are prolonged in older subjects, possibly contributing to the extended duration of acute pain in older patients. The literature is inconsistent with regards to whether or not sensory changes are part of the normal aging process. Older adults with chronic pain conditions appear to have a decreased tolerance for pain, though there may be a reduced tendency for the elderly to report and seek treatment for pain.

Dementia

Age-related mental decline such as cognitive impairment and dementia makes pain evaluation more difficult. The perception of pain intensity appears to be independent of cognitive status, as the somatosensory cortical areas are preserved in Alzheimer's disease, thus maintaining a person's ability to experience acute painful stimuli. In the clinical setting, when questions are phrased simply and straightforwardly and when health care providers allow time for patients with dementia to assimilate their thoughts, individuals with moderate dementia can give valid and reliable information about their pain experience. In non-communicative patients, behaviours such as facial expressions, patient sounds and heavy breathing may correspond with physical and emotional pain. However, cognitively impaired individuals appear less precise in describing the location of their acute and chronic pains, suggesting sensory changes or reporting difficulties associated with dementia. Furthermore, the expectation of pain may be altered in patients with dementia. Patients with severe dementia may have a decrease in emotions associated with the experience of pain, possibly because of memory loss and/or the functional loss in the prefrontal cortex and limbic structures, which are associated with emotion and expectation.

Dementia is related to a lower prevalence of reported pain in older adults. It has been difficult to determine if decreased pain reports in cognitively impaired individuals are due to altered pain sensations or lessened ability to report such pain. A recent study suggests that changes in facial expression are sensitive measures of pain assessment during intraoral anaesthetic injections in cognitively impaired patients, though these individuals demonstrate fewer facial movements in anticipation of pain stimuli, suggesting a reduced expectation of pain. There is a considerable risk that disorders causing pain may not always be recognized in patients with dementia, and it is well reported that individuals with reduced cognitive abilities receive less analgesic pain medications for their chronic pain conditions compared with elderly persons without dementia. As a result, cognitively impaired individuals may experience a significant amount of untreated pain, which may contribute to behavioural problems.

Treatment of pain in the elderly

Treatment for pain in elderly persons is underutilized. As many as 30% of community-dwelling older adults who report daily pain do not take over-the-counter analgesics or prescription pain medications to decrease symptoms. Self-management pain strategies are very limited in scope, despite evidence that straightforward measures such as physical exercise have been shown to significantly decrease pain in older persons. Based upon health care utilization practices, older individuals tend to seek care early in the course of their pain conditions and then resign themselves to the symptoms and make emotional or physical adjustments to them.

Pain has a substantial impact upon quality of life in older adults, related to functional limitations, fatigue, sleeping problems and depressed mood. Epidemiological studies have shown that the presence of pain on a daily basis has a great impact on perceived health status among home-dwelling elderly people. Chronicity of pain may have an additional negative influence on emotional and functional status in older patients, complicated by multiple comorbidities and considerable functional impairments.

Common causes of orofacial pain (Table 21.1)

The prevalence of orofacial pain appears to progressively decrease with age. Compared with an overall prevalence of about 40% in the general population, orofacial pain is reported in one-quarter of those aged 65–75 years and 17% of those aged 75+ years. Lipton *et al.* (1993) found that prevalence of toothache, oral sores and jaw joint pain decreased across the age groups, while face pain and burning mouth were highest in the 75+ years age group. Other studies have suggested that oral sores are the most commonly reported orofacial pain in older adults, followed by toothache, jaw joint pain, face pain and burning mouth. Older females report a higher prevalence of jaw joint pain and facial pain than males, while complaints of toothache, mouth sores and burning mouth are similar in older males and females. It has been proposed that females may be more sensitive to pain than males and these sex differences may not change with age. Severity of orofacial pain, but not recency of onset, has been associated with visiting a health care provider amongst older adults.

Table 21.1 Categories of orofacial pain in older adults

Category	Condition	Symptoms
Neoplasm	Primary head and neck cancer, intracranial tumour, metastatic disease, systemic cancer, distant non-metastasized cancer	• Mass due to benign or neoplastic tumour • Pain due to tissue damage • Numbness
Infection	Dento-alveolar Infections/Abscesses	• Pain • Swelling • Inflammation • Difficulty chewing • Malodour, halitosis
	Candidiasis	• Pseudomembraneous, erythematous, or hyperplastic presentation • Inflammation • Burning sensation • Taste change
	Osteomyelitis	• Facial pain • Numbness • Tenderness • Swelling if acute
	Salivary gland infection	• Salivary gland enlargement • Tenderness • Cloudy exudate from gland
Musculoskeletal	Temporomandibular disorder	• Facial pain • Jaw joint pain
	Headache (muscular origin)	• Bilateral facial pain
Vascular	Cranial arteritis	• Severe headache • Tenderness in temporal region • Visual disturbance • Jaw claudication
	Migraine headache	• Unilateral, severe facial pain • May be associated with aura
Cardiac	Angina pectoris or myocardial infarction	• Pain radiating to mandible or sometimes maxilla
Cerebrovascular	Cerebrovascular accident (CVA)	• Headache • Unilateral numbness • Dysphagia • Slurred speech
Neurological	Trigeminal neuralgia	• Severe, paroxysmal, unilateral pain
	Postherpetic neuralgia	• History of herpes zoster • Constant pain
	Chronic trigeminal neuropathy	• Persistent pain, varies in intensity • No odontogenic pathology
Traumatic	Oral ulceration	• Soft tissue inflammation, ulceration

Orofacial pain complaints may cause older adults to present to dental practices. The diagnostic process and time needed to investigate a pain complaint in an older patient will likely be more complex. Pain complaints may involve teeth and their supporting structures. However, orofacial pains may also be due to non-odontogenic causes, particularly in older adults taking multiple medications with concomitant medically complex conditions. It is important for the dental professional to have an understanding of various orofacial pain presentations and their etiologies. Pain management may be particularly challenging since it is often multifactorial, the differential diagnosis is complex and the achievement of pain relief may be difficult. Non-odontogenic pain conditions often require referral to pain specialists, and a timely and appropriate referral can improve quality of life and associated morbidity.

Dentofacial pain

When assessing the cause of orofacial pain in older adults, the dental practitioner must first rule out odontogenic etiology. The risk for caries continues into old age, particularly when hyposalivation occurs secondary to multiple medications with xerostomic effects. Age-related atrophy to acinar cells may also contribute to salivary dysfunction due to reduced secretory reserve of salivary glands. Consequently, the protective effects of saliva are diminished, and coronal and root surface caries are prevalent, especially if oral hygiene is poor. Further, in older adults pulp space diminishes due to the deposition of secondary and reparative dentine with pulp fibrosis, resulting in diminished nociceptive pain complaints. Whereas classic acute symptoms of pulpal and periapical pathology are commonly reported by older adults, periapical pathology may also develop without the patient being aware. Consequently, it may be beneficial for dental practitioners to consider taking intraoral radiographs in the absence of symptoms since radiographic appearances of periapical pathoses are similar in young and old patients.

It is estimated that 20% of older adults have experienced chronic severe periodontitis, and the rates are much higher in certain minority racial groups. While some level of attachment loss is found in most elderly individuals, this appears to occur as a function of time related to the aging process. Nevertheless, older adults have an increased risk of developing acute periodontal infections; therefore, infections of periodontal origin should be considered when individuals present with orofacial pain complaints.

Another common sequela of reduced salivary flow is an increase in oral infections such as candidiasis. Saliva has antifungal properties, and saliva collected from elderly individuals has a reduced ability to inhibit attachment of *Candida* to mucosal surfaces. Oral fungal infections are associated with inflammation and erythema of oral mucosal tissues and may result in a sore, burning mouth and altered taste.

Oral mucosal inflammation (stomatitis), which may be accompanied by tissue atrophy and ulceration, is also common in older adults. Salivary hypofunction may decrease lubrication, making soft tissues more friable and likely to develop traumatic lesions, particularly in denture-wearing adults. In addition, an altered local immune response may contribute to a secondary infection. Importantly, stomatitis and ulcerations can be extremely painful and debilitating, leading to an impaired quality of life.

Osteomyelitis is an acute or chronic bone infection that can occur in older people secondary to mandible fractures, odontogenic or soft tissue infection or as a complication of a local or regional surgical procedure. The failure of microcirculation in the cancellous bone is a critical factor in the establishment of osteomyelitis. Symptoms include deep pain and tenderness, swelling, erythema and in acute cases fever. If osteomyelitis is suspected, expeditious referral is necessary. These patients often require a prolonged course of antimicrobial therapy, possibly with surgical debridement.

Osteoporosis is the most prevalent metabolic bone disease in the USA, characterized by compromised bone strength and predisposition to an increased risk of fracture. It is estimated that more than 10 million Americans over the age of 50 have osteoporosis, including 7.8 million women. Bisphosphonate medications are potent inhibitors of osteoclasts and angiogenesis, thereby causing a reduction in bone resorption and maintenance of mineralization. Oral bisphosphonates, such as alendronate (Fosomax), risedronate (Actonel) and ibandronate (Boniva), are commonly used in the management of osteoporosis, and high potency intravenous bisphosphonates are important agents in cancer treatment. Recently, osteonecrosis and osteomyelitis of the jaws have been observed in patients treated with bisphosphonate medications, particularly those on intravenous therapy. Bisphosphonate-associated osteonecrosis (BON) or osteonecrosis of the jaws (ONJ) appear to occur only in the oral and maxillofacial region and not elsewhere in the skeleton.

Prior to initiation of bisphosphonate therapy, patients should have a dental examination, and therapy should not be initiated until all dental treatment is completed. For patients receiving bisphosphonate therapy, management should include avoidance of surgical procedures, including tooth removal, if at all possible. For patients with ONJ, treatment should be directed at eliminating or controlling pain, managing infection with topical antimicrobial agents (e.g. 0.12% chlorhexidine) and systemic antibiotics, with a goal of preventing progression of the exposed bone.

Salivary disorders

The most common complaints for salivary gland pathology are pain and swelling (see also Chapter 19 on saliva). These presenting symptoms may be confused with odontogenic infections, making diagnosis difficult. Careful history and examination is mandatory. Inflammatory disease of the salivary glands is usually accompanied by visible enlargement of the major salivary glands and often, but not always, involves obstruction of the salivary gland. A swollen gland may or may not be tender, and swelling is often recurrent. Salivary gland obstruction has a classic history of acute pain and swelling on eating with a tender enlarged gland. Eighty to ninety per cent of sialoliths occur in the submandibular gland. Etiologies for salivary gland inflammatory disease include salivary hypofunction, long periods of dehydration and/or systemic disease which affects the salivary glands. Systemic disease that causes inflammation of the salivary glands is associated with persistent pain and tenderness and usually involves more than one gland.

Sjögren's syndrome (SS) is an autoimmune condition that primarily affects salivary and lacrimal glands. SS may be primary, in which only salivary and lacrimal glands are involved, or secondary in association with other autoimmune diseases. The hallmarks of SS are lymphocytic infiltrates of the minor salivary glands, serum autoantibodies to Ro (SSA) or La (SSB) or both, and objective evidence of salivary gland and ocular involvement. Severe oral dryness may be accompanied by burning or itching of the mouth. Swollen major salivary glands are a frequent finding due to salivary hypofunction, ductal inflammation and acinar destruction. The prevalence of SS ranges between 0.5 and 4.8% worldwide. Over 90% of patients with primary SS are female, often in their fifth decade of life when diagnosed. However, SS may be diagnosed in adults aged 65 to 80 years old.

Bacterial infections of the salivary glands occur when bacteria colonizing in the oral cavity invade the salivary duct(s) and cause an acute bacterial infection. This occurs more frequently in patients with salivary gland hypofunction and/or chronic obstructions, and the parotid gland is the most commonly affected gland. Infections of the salivary glands present with a sudden onset of pain, salivary gland enlargement and tenderness to palpation of the involved gland. A cloudy exudate may be expressed from the duct orifice and should be cultured to guide treatment.

If a distinct mass is noted within the body of a salivary gland, a neoplastic growth must be considered. Salivary gland neoplasms are usually painless until the late stages as a result of neural involvement. Facial nerve paralysis may be an indicator of parotid gland malignancy. Diagnosis of salivary gland pathology is difficult, so the dental practitioner must always consider a neoplastic condition and refer appropriately when a patient presents with a salivary gland enlargement without signs of acute infection (e.g. suppuration).

Temporomandibular disorders

Temporomandibular disorders (TMD) are conditions affecting the temporomandibular joint (TMJ) and the muscles of mastication. The clinical signs and symptoms of TMD can be classified as muscular disorders, internal derangements of the TMJ and degenerative changes to the bony components of the joints. The prevalence of TMD pain (myofascial pain, arthritis and/or arthralgia) and internal derangements of the TMJ (e.g. clicking, locking) appear to be stable across adulthood, then decrease in older adults aged more than 65 years. However, osteoarthrosis (crepitus without joint pain) has a higher prevalence in older adults compared with younger cohorts. In cadaver studies of the TMJs of older adults, ~60% of joints exhibited degenerative changes at the articular surfaces. Evidence suggests that, while aged TMJs show signs of bony deterioration, inflammation is less than in younger adults, thereby possibly contributing to the reduction in joint pain in elderly compared with younger subjects.

When older adults complain of jaw pain, the most likely cause is osteoarthritis of the TMJs. When the occasional disk derangement occurs, it is often secondary to degenerative changes of the TMJs. Treatment always begins with conservative modalities, including patient education, reducing stressful jaw function, eliminating aggravating factors and physical therapy. Short-term use of non-steroidal anti-inflammatory drugs (NSAIDs) may also be beneficial in older adults who have no obvious gastrointestinal problems and are not at an increased risk for bleeding problems. If muscle hyperactivity is suspected, an occlusal appliance such as a splint or night guard may be indicated to decrease the loading force on the joint structures. Osteoarthritis of the TMJ is often self-limiting in older adults and is usually managed well with conservative management.

Rheumatoid arthritis (RA) is a chronic inflammatory disease of the synovial membrane, characterized by formation of granulation tissue at the articular surfaces and erosion of the underlying bone. RA has a peak incidence between the ages of 40 and 60 years, and women are affected more than men. If the TMJs are affected, involvement is usual bilateral. Symptoms are typically transient and commonly include joint pain and limitation of opening; crepitus may also be evident. Pain usually occurs in the acute phases of the disease but is not a common complaint in later stages. Radiographic findings of the TMJ include loss of joint space, flattening of the condyle, osteophytes, (small bone projections) and erosion of the glenoid fossa. During acute flares of RA affecting the TMJs, conservative treatment and anti-inflammatory medications are recommended in coordination with the patient's rheumatologist.

Headache

Population-based studies have demonstrated that the overall prevalence of headaches declines with age. This trend may have a biological basis or may occur because headache sufferers develop strategies over time to prevent and manage their headaches and therefore lessen their impact. Alternatively, older adults may experience a change in perception of headache, deeming them less important and therefore less likely to be reported. When new headaches develop in the elderly, underlying etiologies such as central nervous system pathology or organic disease, such as intracranial mass, subdural haematoma, haemorrhagic or ischaemic stroke or giant cell arteritis, must be considered in the differential diagnosis.

Tension-type headache (TTHA) is the most common headache, with the annual prevalence peaking at about 45% in the fourth to fifth decade, then declining to 25% in the seventh decade. TTHA is divided into episodic and chronic subtypes, with the episodic subtype involving attacks fewer than 15 days per month or 180 days per year and chronic TTHA including those who experience headache more frequently. TTHAs are characterized by bilateral, steady and mild-to-moderate discomfort that is neither severe nor disabling. These headaches may last from 30 minutes to 7 days and may be associated with pericranial muscular tenderness that can be detected by manual palpation. Clinical assessment of headache pain in the elderly is more complex than in the younger adult due to complications of impaired memory, poor overall health, multiple medications and psychosocial concerns. Organic disease must be excluded before considering primary tension-type headache since intracranial disease or extracranial disorders seen among the elderly may present with symptoms of tension-type headaches.

Migraine headache is the result of neurological activity on intracranial vascular structures. Its prevalence progressively declines with age after 40 years, from a peak prevalence of about 20% in the third decade to a minimum of less than 5% in those older than 70 years. Approximately 2% of new onset migraines occur after the age of 50 years. A typical migraine episode will last from 4 to 72 hours and often is relieved by sleep. Migraine headaches are characterized by unilateral, throbbing or pulsating, moderate-to-severe pain that may be associated with an aura (prodrome) phase. They usually involve the presence of nausea, photophobia, phonophobia and/or pain worsening with activity. Evidence suggests that migraine attacks get shorter and less typical with advancing age. Migraine features such as pain intensity, throbbing pain and phonophobia also decrease with age, while the presence of aura increases in older adults. Importantly, it is not uncommon for older patients to get migraine headaches which present as an aura only with no pain. A subgroup of migraneurs may transform to chronic daily headaches with increasing age. With neurovascular headaches, the decrease in migraine prevalence may be due to age-related biochemical changes. There is an age-related decline in cerebral blood vessel dilatation, which could contribute to the reduction in headaches.

Managing headaches in older adults presents several challenges. Management with medications (e.g. NSAIDs, opioids, triptans) requires extra caution due to a reduced tolerance to medications and potential for increased contraindications due to concomitant disease or polypharmacy (see also Chapter 12 on pharmacology). Older adults who present with new onset of a headache should have a thorough work-up with a neurologist or pain specialist. Most patients with TTHA and episodic migraine may be successfully managed with stress management, trigger avoidance and simple analgesics such as NSAIDs or acetaminophen (paracetamol). For patients experiencing at least 2 to 3 headache days per week, abortive migraine medication (triptans: e.g. sumatriptan, rizatriptan, zolmitriptan) and preventive pharmacological therapy (e.g. anticonvulsants or antidepressants for TTHA; antidepressants or beta-blockers for migraine) may be beneficial. It is recommended to start preventive treatment at low dosages and increase slowly in older adults.

Giant cell arteritis

Giant cell arteritis (cranial arteritis, temporal arteritis) (GCA) is a chronic inflammatory disorder involving large and medium-sized vessels with a tendency to affect the extracranial branches of the carotid artery. The temporal artery is the most commonly involved branch. This condition develops in adults over 50 years, at an average age of 72 years, and women are affected two to six times more frequently than men. There is a high prevalence in individuals of Northern European descent. GCA has a strong association with polymyalgia rheumatica (PMR), as up to 40% of patients with GCA develop classic PMR, which involves accompanying joint and muscle pain.

GCA is an inflammatory process in which infiltrates consisting predominantly of T lymphocytes and macrophages affect the inner walls of arteries. Classic findings include granulomatous inflammation and multinucleated giant cells. Release of local inflammatory mediators leads to the destruction of components of the vessel wall. Numerous genetic and environmental factors, including infectious etiologies, have been suspected as the trigger of the inflammatory response.

Visual disturbances including blurred vision, diplopia and eye pain are often early manifestations of the disease. Complete visual loss in at least one eye may develop in up to 60% of patients and usually results in permanent deficit. Other symptoms include fever, malaise and weight loss as well as headache, tenderness in the temporal region and jaw claudication (fatigue or pain on function). Seventy per cent of individuals present with headache, most commonly localized to the temporal or occipital areas. Palpation of the involved superficial temporal arteries reveals a tender and thickened pulsating vessel. Jaw claudication may result from ischaemia of the muscles of mastication, seen in approximately half of cases of GCA. Vestibular dysfunction and/or hearing impairment may also occur. Long-term and severe complications of GCA include stroke and aortic aneurysm as a result of chronic vasculitis. Up to 15% experience permanent visual loss and 2% incur stroke despite therapy, but the majority of patients are symptom-free 3 years after treatment.

Diagnostic findings include an elevated erythrocyte sedimentation rate (ESR) above 50 mm/h (normal is 20 mm/h or under) and elevated C-reactive protein (CRP). Temporal artery biopsy remains the gold standard to confirm the diagnosis of GCA, demonstrating a chronic inflammatory infiltrate with destruction of the internal elastic lamina. An adequate length of biopsy tissue (>2 cm) is necessary since the entire vessel may not be involved, so a negative biopsy result does not rule out temporal arteritis. The role of imaging techniques, such as magnetic resonance imaging (MRI) or positron emission tomography (PET), is uncertain at this time.

Treatment with systemic corticosteroids must be initiated promptly to reduce the risk of blindness and stroke. Initial daily doses range from 40 to 60 mg prednisone (or an equivalent) in a single or divided dose. Divided dosing may provide greater anti-inflammatory properties but at the expense of greater risk of adverse effects. After attaining clinical remission, steroid doses are tapered to a lower maintenance dose. ESR and CRP are used to monitor disease status. Steroids may be carefully discontinued within 2 years of drug initiation since giant cell arteritis often runs a self-limited course. Immunosuppressive agents have also been considered for treatment due to their potential steroid-sparing effects. Treatment with methotrexate has been studied in clinical trials, but the results have been conflicting.

Referred cardiac pain

Pain may be referred from distant sites to orofacial structures and often presents a diagnostic challenge for the dentist. Angina pectoris is described as an aching, heavy, squeezing pressure or tightness in the mid-chest region that is brief (1–5 minutes), resulting from temporary ischaemia of the myocardium. Angina is occasionally referred to the orofacial structures, most commonly the mandible and mandibular molars, though cases of angina pain have been reported in the maxilla and soft palate. Angina presents a significant cardiac risk, as it may precede a myocardial infarction, particularly in older adults. Cardiac pain associated with myocardial infarction also arises in the chest and is similar to angina pain, though pain is prolonged (at least 15 minutes) and occasionally radiates to the left arm, shoulder, neck and/or face. Appropriate diagnosis includes obtaining a thorough history of ischaemic cardiac disease as well as symptoms that exacerbate and relieve the pain. Patients with a positive history of coronary disease, precipitating symptoms with exercise, eating or stress and alleviating pain with rest and nitroglycerin are indicators of cardiac etiology to the pain condition. An accurate history is necessary for proper diagnosis and appropriate, prompt referral.

Neuropathic pain conditions

Orofacial pain may be nociceptive, in which pain is transmitted by normal physiological pathways via peripheral nerves to the central nervous system in response to potentially tissue-damaging stimuli. Pain may also be classified as neuropathic (Box 21.1), in which pain is initiated or caused by a primary lesion or dysfunction in the nervous system. Neuropathic pain can be an extremely debilitating form of pain that occurs when peripheral, autonomic and/or central nerves are affected. This dysfunction in the nervous system may be exacerbated by persistent, unrelieved nociceptive (inflammatory) pain, trauma to neural tissue and/or changes that increase the sensitivity of nerves. These alterations in pain processing at the peripheral and central levels produce characteristic symptoms such as hyperalgesia (an increased response to a stimulus that is normally painful), allodynia (pain due to a stimulus that does not normally provoke pain) and paraesthesia (an abnormal sensation, whether spontaneous or evoked). These pains commonly present with an aching, persistent quality for which it may be difficult to obtain relief.

Box 21.1 Characteristics of neuropathic pain.

- Pain may be sharp, shooting, burning or may be a dull ache.
- Characteristic pain symptoms:
  - hyperalgesia: an increased response to a stimulus that is normally painful.
  - allodynia: pain due to a stimulus that does not normally provoke pain.
  - paraesthesia: an abnormal sensation, whether spontaneous or evoked.
- Pain is often constant or recurrent and remains unchanged for weeks to months.
- There is no obvious source of local pathology.
- Response to thermal and percussion testing does not consistently relate to the pain.
- Trigger areas may evoke severe pain.
- Response to local anaesthetic is equivocal.
- Similar pain complaints may be in multiple teeth or multiple areas in the mouth and may move from tooth to tooth or area to area.
- Dental treatment does not resolve the pain.
- There may be associated precipitating factors, such as trauma or disease.
- Management with pharmacotherapy.

Trigeminal neuralgia

Trigeminal neuralgia (TN) is a neuropathic pain syndrome that affects approximately 5 per 100 000 population, occurring more often in women, and the incidence gradually increases with age, beginning around 40 years old. However, in patients older than 80 years, males have a higher incidence than females. This condition is characterized by sudden, sharp, severe unilateral pain. It is often described as stabbing, electric, shooting and burning and follows one or more branches of the trigeminal nerve, typically the maxillary or mandibular branch. The sensation can last seconds to minutes, then disappearing, leaving pain-free intervals between attacks. Pain is often evoked by trigger areas around the nose and mouth and can include intraoral sites, including teeth. Upon presentation of TN, an MRI should be performed to rule out lesions which may be compressing the trigeminal nerve or plaques of multiple sclerosis. Intraoral compression of the mental nerve by an ill-fitting denture can also lead to trigeminal neuralgia-like symptoms. Increasing evidence suggests that 80–90% of TN cases may be caused by compression of the trigeminal nerve close to its exit from the brainstem by an aberrant loop of vessel(s), possibly (combined with) focal demyelination at the site of compression.

Many patients attribute pain to dental causes and will seek dental treatment as a first line of therapy. However, it is important for dentists to consider possible nondental causes of pain and not attempt irreversible procedures without a specific diagnosis and confidence that dental treatment will address an odontogenic or oral mucosal condition. TN may present exclusively intraorally, a manifestation that can make diagnosis confusing for patients and clinicians.

TN is a chronic disorder in which pain attacks will continue unless treated appropriately. Treatment involves anticonvulsant medications such as carbamazepine, baclofen and lamotrigine, all of which have reported results superior to placebo in controlled clinical trials. Sometimes multiple drug therapy is necessary to control pain. Elderly patients are more prone to certain central nervous system side effects of carbamazepine, so alternate drugs may be preferable (e.g. baclofen, lamotrigine, oxcarbazepine). If medical management does not alleviate symptoms, surgical intervention including stereotactic radiofrequency, gamma knife radiosurgery and microvascular decompression procedures may be considered.

Burning mouth syndrome

Burning mouth syndrome (BMS) is a chronic pain syndrome that is defined as burning pain in the tongue or other oral mucous membranes lasting at least 4–6 months and associated with normal signs and laboratory findings. Other synonyms for BMS include glossodynia, glossopyrosis, glossalgia, stomatodynia, stomatopyrosis, sore tongue, burning tongue, scalded mouth syndrome, oral dysesthesia and burning mouth condition. The prevalence of BMS ranges from 0.6 to 15% and primarily affects females in the fifth to seventh decade, with a female-to-male ratio of about 7 : 1. The burning sensation is typically bilateral, moderate in severity and may be constant, progressively increasing throughout the day, or intermittent. Unilateral symptoms require careful investigation to rule out underlying disease. Remission of burning usually occurs with sleeping and may be less severe or absent when eating, chewing gum or using an oral lozenge. Associated symptoms include xerostomia without measurable hyposalivation, paraesthesia and altered taste (e.g. bitter, metallic). Over half the patients with BMS may experience a spontaneous onset of symptoms, while 17–33% attribute onset to an identifiable triggering factor, suggesting the possibility of peripheral and/or central neurological alterations preceding burning.

BMS may be classified as primary (essential/idiopathic) BMS or secondary BMS in which symptoms are due to underlying local or systemic conditions. Diagnosis is made by obtaining a careful history and excluding possible causes, including local pathology of the mucosal tissues, salivary hypofunction, nutritional deficiencies, hormonal disturbances, psychological factors, medication side effects and systemic conditions which may cause oral burning (e.g. diabetes mellitus).

Secondary BMS requires appropriate diagnosis and treatment of the underlying condition to manage symptoms. In primary BMS, the etiology is unclear, so treatment options are based upon patients' symptomatology often yielding unsatisfactory results. Patients have shown some benefit from cognitive behavioural therapy. Topical and systemic clonazepam, gabapentin and alpha-lipoic acid have demonstrated efficacy in clinical trials. Further, patients require information and reassurance about their condition, since they are likely to have consulted numerous specialists and have had the condition for months to years prior to diagnosis.

Postherpetic neuralgia

Herpes zoster is a clinical manifestation of the reactivation of varicella zoster virus (VZV), which resides in latent form in sensory trigeminal and dorsal root ganglia after primary infection. The clinical presentation is a painful, usually unilateral, eruption of vesicular lesions in the dermatome supplied by that nerve. Healing of the lesions occurs after a period of 2 to 4 weeks. The most frequent sites of reactivation are the thoracic nerves followed by the ophthalmic division of the trigeminal nerve. Older adults and those with compromised immunity are at greater risk for developing herpes zoster. The incidence increases with age to affect 50% of those over 85 years.

Pain which persists after the rash has healed is known as postherpetic neuralgia (PHN) and is the most common complication of herpes zoster. PHN may present in the exact area of the lesions or may encompass larger or smaller zones. This neuropathic pain syndrome is described as constant, mild to severe and burning, deep aching, tingling, itching and/or stabbing pain. Epidemiological studies have shown that the degree of pain and severity of rash and inflammation during the herpes zoster attack are important predictors for the development and severity of PHN. Evidence points to the inflammatory process causing central and peripheral nerve injury to the dorsal root ganglion and adjacent neuronal tissues, resulting in a persistent neuropathic pain. More than 25% of individuals older than 55 years of age and two-thirds of patients over 70 years of age will suffer from PHN after an episode of herpes zoster. Because of its severity and chronicity, PHN is a considerable cause of orofacial pain in older adults.

Treatment of PHN consists of tricyclic antidepressants (TCAs; amitriptyline or nortriptyline), anticonvulsants (gabapentin, pregabalin) and opioids. Topical lidocaine and capsaicin creams have also shown some benefit in treatment of PHN. Combination therapy and a consultation with a pain management specialist are often required. There is evidence that the use of antiviral drugs, particularly famciclovir or valacyclovir, along with a short course of low dose TCA during the acute phase of the herpes zoster outbreak may decrease the incidence and severity of PHN. Regardless, the most effective future treatment of this disease may be focusing on prevention of VZV infection. A VZV vaccine has been developed and recently approved by the US Food Drug Administration (FDA) for the prevention of herpes zoster in individuals 60 years of age and older. A large randomized clinical trial has shown that adult vaccination (at age ≥60 years) reduces the incidence of herpes zoster by 51% and of PHN by 66% compared with placebo.

Chronic trigeminal neuropathy/non-odontogenic toothache

A number of terms have been commonly used to describe painful trigeminal neuropathies potentially associated with trauma, such as atypical facial pain and atypical odontalgia. This condition is classified as a form of neuropathic pain and is inconsistently presented in the literature. A chronic trigeminal neuropathy typically presents as prolonged periods of constant throbbing, sharp or burning pain in a tooth or tooth region in the absence of odontogenic etiology observed clinically or radiographically. It usually persists for months or years, being continuous and persistent but varying in intensity, with episodes when the pain is more acute and severe. Patients often have difficulty localizing the pain and the location may change. There is usually a variable response to local anaesthetic blocks. To further complicate diagnosis, the tooth or tooth region may exhibit hyperalgesia demonstrated by a positive response to percussion, sensitivity to cold or pain associated with chewing. Accurate identification depends on recognizing pain characteristics that indicate a neuropathic pain condition (see Table 21.1). Once a diagnosis is established, further dental procedures that could aggravate the pain must be avoided. While the literature suggests a predominance among women beginning in their mid-40s, people of all ages could be affected by chronic trigeminal neuropathies.

The pathophysiology of this pain condition is that it may be related to trauma, sensitization of nociceptive pain fibres, activation of afferent fibres and/or loss of inhibitory mechanisms. Currently, the most accepted theory is that trauma to the orofacial structures alters the neural continuity of the tissues, creating sensitization of the peripheral nociceptive nerves and resulting in a neuropathic pain syndrome.

Treatment is similar to other neuropathic pain syndromes. TCAs have been prescribed with good results. The primary alternative to TCAs is an anticonvulsant medication, such as gabapentin or clonazepam. Topical medications such as capsaicin may also provide some relief. Opioid analgesics are usually only moderately effective for neuropathic pain and produce unacceptable side effects in older adults.

Head and neck cancer

Head and neck cancer (HNC) is relatively common in older adults and must be considered in patients presenting with orofacial pain. Data obtained by the National Cancer Institute SEER (Surveillance, Epidemiology and End Results) programme from 1985 to 1996 reported 50% of newly diagnosed oral and pharyngeal cancer cases to be at least 65 years old and 32% were aged between 50 and 64 years. Orofacial pain may be a presenting symptom of primary tumours, metastatic disease of the jaw bones or systemic cancer such as lymphoma or leukaemia and may motivate patients to seek care from a dental professional. Rarely, orofacial pain may present in patients suffering from a distant non-metastasized cancer, most commonly from the lungs. In patients with a history of head and neck cancer, orofacial pain may be a presenting symptom of a recurrent or second primary cancer in the head and neck.

While undergoing treatment for HNC, cancer therapy protocols almost always cause acute pain. Oral mucositis is a common complication of chemotherapy (CT) and/or radiation therapy (RT) and typically manifests as erythema and/or ulceration of the oral mucosa. Acute oral infections of the mucosa (e.g. bacterial, viral and fungal), dentition/periapices and periodontium may occur due to exacerbation of latent or prior chronic infection, changes in flora that occur secondary to cancer treatment or indirect damage to oral structures and tissues, all of which may contribute to oral pain. Patients who have received allogeneic or matched unrelated haematopoietic stem cell transplants are at risk for acute and/or chronic graft-versus-host disease (GVHD), which is the result of donor cells that react with and destroy recipient tissue. Common oral findings include atrophy, erythema and lichenoid lesions and fibrosis of oral tissues, as well as persistent reduced salivary function.

Following treatment for HNC, permanent changes to tissues may result in chronic orofacial pains. RT in the head and neck causes hypovascular, hypocellular and hypoxic changes to tissues, resulting in permanent alterations of the involved tissues, also known as late effects of RT. Radiation-induced hyposalivation is a common and significant complication of cancer treatment which may cause painful dentofacial sequelae. RT changes may also result in chronic mucosal sensitivity secondary to neuropathic sensitization and/or epithelial atrophy, which may predispose oral tissues to ulceration following trauma or injury. Post-radiation osteonecrosis is another well recognized late effect of head and neck RT in which loss of bone vitality occurs secondary to cellular injury and reduction in vascular supply. These changes can lead to a reduced capacity of bone to recover from injury, predisposing to osteonecrosis, secondary infection, severe pain and pathological fracture. Additionally, fibrosis of connective tissue and masticatory muscles may develop secondary to scar formation following surgery, and RT may also contribute to the fibrosis and atrophy in the masticatory, pharyngeal and neck muscles and/or TMJ as a late radiation effect. These changes may result in reduced tongue mobility, dysphagia, limitation of neck movement and decreased range of mandibular opening. The limitation in opening which develops often interferes with oral hygiene, nutritional intake and dental treatment.

Neuropathic pain may also develop following HNC treatment. Surgical procedures may cause tissue injury at the site of tumour resection or neck dissection, leading to post-traumatic neuropathic pain. In addition, neurotoxicities due to chemotherapeutic agents or RT often initiate painful peripheral neuropathies. Following CT, the neuropathic pain often resolves with time; however, with RT, permanent neural damage may evolve into a chronically painful condition. Taste may also be altered with curative RT regimens and is often transient, though taste change present at one year following treatment is considered permanent. The loss of taste is a result of the damage to the neural component of taste and is related to the reduction in salivary flow rate. Dentists should be aware of these orofacial pain presentations which may be unique to patients who have undergone head and neck cancer treatment

General concepts in pain management for the older patient

Pain management in the older adult is a challenge due to differing responses to treatments, multiple factors that contribute to generating pain and many concomitant medical factors that alter the selection of pain therapeutic modalities. The experience of pain involves physical symptoms as well as psychosocial and affective components; therefore, a multifactorial treatment approach is recommended.

Age-associated physiological changes affect the way older adults respond to drugs. Changes in drug absorption, alterations in the duration of action, reduced activity of hepatic enzyme systems and decreased renal function may increase the risk of drug interactions and slow the elimination of medications. Medications used to manage other medical disorders may increase the possibility of adverse events or toxicity through drug interactions (see also Chapter 12 on pharmacology).

Non-steroidal anti-inflammatory drugs are the analgesics most widely used by the geriatric population. Long-term use of these drugs may produce complications such as dyspepsia and peptic ulcer disease. Interactions with anticoagulant or antiplatelet agents must also be considered. Acetaminophen (paracetamol) may be safer from haematological and gastrointestinal perspectives, but also carries risks for renal and hepatic dysfunction. TCAs, which have been widely used in the management of chronic neuropathic conditions, should be used with caution in older adult patients since anticholinergic side effects may precipitate acute confusion or cardiac arrhythmias. TCAs with less marked anticholinergic effects, such as imipramine or desipramine, may be considered, although each medication should be titrated slowly and patients should be monitored closely for side effects. Finally, opioids should also be used with caution due to a slower elimination of these drugs in older adults as well as unwanted side effects such as sedation, confusion, ataxia, respiratory depression and constipation.

In older adults, a multimodal approach to pain management is suggested, using pharmacological therapy, non-pharmacological modalities (education, exercise, weight loss, physical therapy, occlusal appliances) and psychosocial support to maximize the older adult's function and quality of life. Pain control is necessary for relief of suffering, as well as the possibility of developing pain-associated adverse health events. Poor pain control can significantly increase morbidity and mortality and has also been linked to sleep disturbance, functional disability and depression, especially in elderly individuals.

Further reading

Bigal, M.E., Liberman, J.N. & Lipton, R.B. (2006) Age-dependent prevalence and clinical features of migraine. *Neurology*, **67**(2), 246–251.

Burton, A.W., Fanciullo, G.J., Beasley, R.D. & Fisch, M.J. (2007) Chronic pain in the cancer survivor: a new frontier. *Pain Medicine*, **8**(2), 189–198.

Caraceni, A. & Portenoy, R.K. (1999) An international survey of cancer pain characteristics and syndromes. IASP Task Force on Cancer Pain. International Association for the Study of Pain. *Pain*, **82**(3), 263–274.

Dasgupta, B. & Hassan, N. (2007) Giant cell arteritis: recent advances and guidelines for management. *Clinical and Experimental Rheumatology*, **25**(1 Suppl 44), S62–65.

Eberhardt, R.T. & Dhadly, M. (2007) Giant cell arteritis: diagnosis, management, and cardiovascular implications. *Cardiology in Review*, **15**(2), 55–61.

Frampton, M. (2003) Experience assessment and management of pain in people with dementia. *Age and Ageing*, **32**(3), 248–251.

Gibson, S.J. & Farrell, M. (2004) A review of age differences in the neurophysiology of nociception and the perceptual experience of pain. *Clinical Journal of Pain*, **20**(4), 227–239.

Helme, R.D. & Gibson, S.J. (2001) The epidemiology of pain in elderly people. *Clinics in Geriatric Medicine*, **17**(3), 417–431, v.

Hsu, K.T., Shuman, S.K., Hamamoto, D.T., Hodges, J.S. & Feldt, K.S. (2007) The application of facial expressions to the assessment of orofacial pain in cognitively impaired older adults. *Journal of the American Dental Association*, **138**(7), 963–969.

Huffman, J.C. & Kunik, M.E. (2000) Assessment and understanding of pain in patients with dementia. *Gerontologist*, **40**(5), 574–581.

Jung, B.F., Johnson, R.W., Griffin, D.R. & Dworkin, R.H. (2004) Risk factors for postherpetic neuralgia in patients with herpes zoster. *Neurology*, **62**(9), 1545–1551.

Licata, A.A. (2005) Discovery, clinical development, and therapeutic uses of bisphosphonates. *Annals of Pharmacotherapy*, **39**(4), 668–677.

Lipton, J.A., Ship, J.A. & Larach-Robinson, D. (1993) Estimated prevalence and distribution of reported orofacial pain in the United States. *Journal of the American Dental Association*, **124**(10), 115–121.

Marbach, J.J. (1993) Is phantom tooth pain a deafferentation (neuropathic) syndrome? Part I: Evidence derived from pathophysiology and treatment. *Oral Surgery, Oral Medicine, Oral Pathology*, **75**(1), 95–105.

Melis, M., Lobo, S.L., Ceneviz, C., Zawawi, K., Al-Badawi, E., Maloney, G. *et al.* (2003) Atypical odontalgia: a review of the literature. *Headache*, **43**(10), 1060–1074.

Merskey, H. & Bogduk, N. (1994) *Classification of chronic pain: descriptions of chronic pain syndromes and definitions of pain terms*, 2nd edn, IASP Press, Seattle, WA.

Meyer, J.S., Terayama, Y., Konno, S., Margishvili, G.M., Akiyama, H., Rauch, R.A. *et al.* (1998) Age-related cerebrovascular disease alters the symptomatic course of migraine. *Cephalalgia*, **18**(4), 202–208, discussion 171.

Migliorati, C.A., Schubert, M.M., Peterson, D.E. & Seneda, L.M. (2005) Bisphosphonate-associated osteonecrosis of mandibular and maxillary bone: an emerging oral complication of supportive cancer therapy. *Cancer*, **104**(1), 83–93.

Oxman, M.N., Levin, M.J., Johnson, G.R., Schmader, K.E., Straus, S.E., Gelb, L.D. *et al.* (2005) A vaccine to prevent herpes zoster and postherpetic neuralgia in older adults. *New England Journal of Medicine*, **352**(22), 2271–2284.

Patton, L.L., Siegel, M.A., Benoliel, R. & De Laat, A. (2007) Management of burning mouth syndrome: systematic review and management recommendations. *Oral Surgery, Oral Medicine, Oral Pathology, Oral Radiology and Endodontology*, **103**(Suppl:S39), e1–13.

Riley, J.L., 3rd,, Gilbert. G.H. & Heft, M.W. (1998) Orofacial pain symptom prevalence: selective sex differences in the elderly? *Pain*, **76**(1–2), 97–104.

Scrivani, S.J., Mathews, E.S. & Maciewicz, R.J. (2005) Trigeminal neuralgia. *Oral Surgery, Oral Medicine, Oral Pathology, Oral Radiology and Endodontology*, **100**(5), 527–538.

Vissink, A., Jansma, J., Spijkervet, F.K., Burlage, F.R. & Coppes, R.P. (2003) Oral sequelae of head and neck radiotherapy. *Critical Reviews in Oral Biology & Medicine*, **14**(3), 199–212.

Woo, S.B., Hellstein, J.W. & Kalmar, J.R. (2006) Narrative [corrected] review: bisphosphonates and osteonecrosis of the jaws. *Annals of Internal Medicine*, **144**(10), 753–761.

Zakrzewska, J.M., Forssell, H. & Glenny, A.M. (2005) Interventions for the treatment of burning mouth syndrome. *Cochrane Database of Systematic Reviews*, **2005**(1):CD002779.

CHAPTER 22

Concepts and techniques for oral rehabilitation measures in elderly patients

Niklaus P. Lang[1]**, Frauke Müller**[2] **and J. Mark Thomason**[3]

[1]School of Dental Medicine, University of Berne, Berne, Switzerland
[2]School of Dental Medicine, University of Geneva, Geneva, Switzerland
[3]School of Dental Sciences, Newcastle University, Newcastle upon Tyne, UK

The concept of opportunistic infections

Caries and periodontal diseases represent opportunistic infections associated with biofilm formation on all hard non-shedding surfaces in a fluid system, such as teeth, prostheses or implants. Factors such as bacterial specificity and pathogenicity as well as local and general susceptibility may influence the onset, the rate of progression and clinical characteristics of the plaque-associated dental infections. Findings from animal experiments and longitudinal studies in humans, however, have demonstrated that treatment, including the elimination or the control of the biofilm infection and the introduction of careful plaque control measures, in most – if not all – cases results in dental and periodontal health. Even if health cannot always be achieved and maintained, the arrest of disease progression following treatment must be the goal of modern dental care.

While in the past the practice of reconstructive therapy was dominated by mechanical concepts, more biologically oriented treatment principles, including those of secondary prevention, have to replace the older mechanically oriented concepts. This paradigm shift has led to profound changes in oral rehabilitation. Patients with advanced oral diseases and partial or total tooth loss jeopardizing individually optimal function have to be treated primarily as patients affected by opportunistic infections and hence the elimination and control of such infections must receive first priority irrespective of the patients age.

Screening for dental caries and periodontal disease

Screening for dental caries: clinical exploration and bitewing radiographs

A patient seeking dental care is usually screened for the presence of carious lesions by means of clinical exploration and radiographic interpretation. A minimum of two bitewing radiographs is required for appropriate screening and diagnosis.

In the elderly, it may be necessary to specifically look for root surface caries and distinguish between 'soft', caries-active and arrested lesions.

Screening for periodontal disease: the basic periodontal examination

Likewise, it is imperative that such a patient is screened for the presence of periodontitis as well using a procedure termed the basic periodontal examination (BPE) (or periodontal screening record; PSR).

The goal of the BPE is to screen the periodontal conditions of a new patient irrespective of his or her age and to facilitate treatment planning. BPE scoring will allow the dentist to identify:

- a patient with reasonably healthy periodontal conditions, but in need of long-term preventive measures.
- a patient with periodontitis and in need of periodontal therapy.

In the BPE the screening of each tooth or implant is evaluated. For this purpose, the use of a thin (diameter: 0.4–0.5 mm), graduated, ball-ended periodontal probe is

Textbook of Geriatric Dentistry, Third Edition. Edited by Poul Holm-Pedersen, Angus W. G. Walls and Jonathan A. Ship.

recommended. At least two sites per tooth/implant (i.e. mesio-buccal and disto-buccal) should be probed using a light force (i.e. 0.2 N). Each dentate sextant within the dentition is given a BPE code or score, whereby the *highest* individual site score is used.

BPE system code

Code 0 = probing pocket depth (PPD) ≤ 3 mm, bleeding on probing (BoP) negative, no calculus or overhanging fillings [Figure 22.1(a)].

Code 1 = PPD ≤ 3 mm, BoP positive, no calculus or overhanging fillings [Figure 22.1(b)].

Code 2 = PPD ≤ 3 mm, BoP positive, presence of supra and/or subgingival calculus and/or overhanging fillings [Figure 22.1(c)].

Code 3 = PPD > 3 mm but ≤ 5 mm, BoP positive [Figure 22.1(d)].

Code 4 = PPD > 5 mm [Figure 22.1(e)].

If an examiner identifies one single site with a PPD > 5 mm within a sextant, the sextant will receive a code of 4 and no

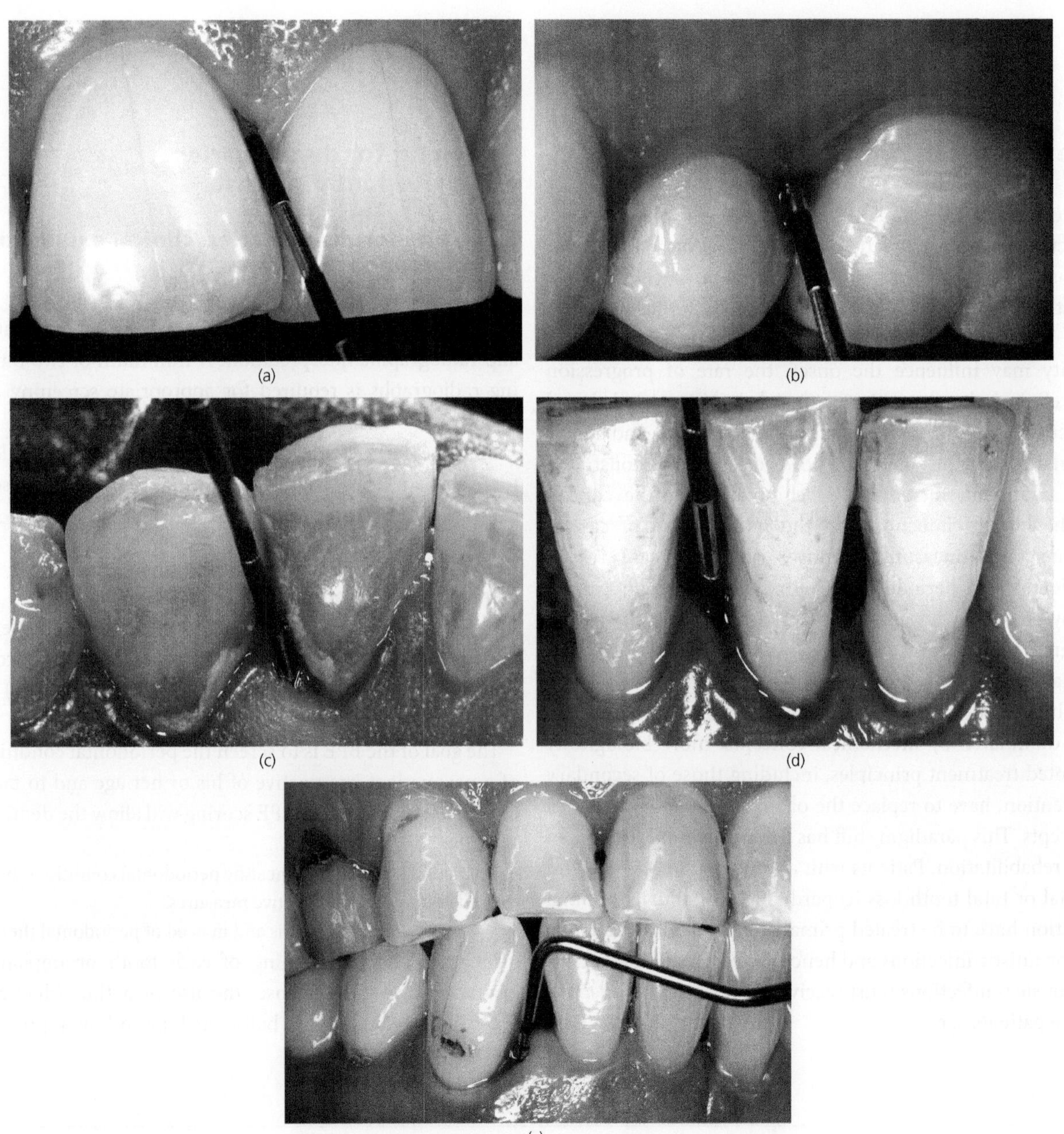

Figure 22.1 BPE system code **a)** Code 0; **b)** Code 1; **c)** Code 2; **d)** Code 3; **e)** Code 4.

further assessments are needed in this particular sextant. Patients with sextants given codes of 0, 1 or 2 belong to the relatively periodontally healthy category. A patient exhibiting a sextant with codes of 3 or 4 must undergo a more comprehensive periodontal examination. An asterix (*) may be added to any sextant displaying recession, furcation involvement or substanially increased mobility (M: 2 or 3).

Pretherapeutic single tooth prognosis

Based on the results of the comprehensive examination, including assessments of periodontitis, caries, tooth sensitivity and the resulting diagnosis, as well as considering the patient's needs regarding aesthetics and function, a pretherapeutic prognosis for each individual tooth (root) is made.

Three major questions are addressed:

1 Which tooth/root has a *'good' (safe)* prognosis?
2 Which tooth/root is *'irrational-to-treat'*?
3 Which tooth/root has a *'doubtful' (unsecure)* prognosis?

Teeth with a *good* prognosis will require relatively simple therapy and may be regarded as secure abutments for function.

Teeth that are considered *irrational-to-treat* should be extracted during initial, cause-related therapy. Such teeth may be identified on the basis of the following criteria:

Periodontal

- Recurrent periodontal abscesses.
- Combined periodontal-endodontic lesions (specifically if the lesion is primarily of periodontal origin).
- Attachment loss to the apex.

Endodontal

- Root perforation in the apical half of the root.

Dental

- Vertical fracture of the root.
- Oblique fracture in the middle third of the root.
- Caries lesions that extend into the root canal walls (soft dentine).
- Inadequate remaining coronal tooth tissue for restoration

Functional

- Third molars without antagonists and with periodontitis/caries.

Teeth with a *doubtful* prognosis are usually in need of comprehensive therapy and must be brought into the category of teeth with a *good* prognosis by means of additional therapy. Such teeth may be identified on the basis of the following criteria:

Periodontal

- Furcation involvement.
- Angular (i.e. vertical) bony defects.
- 'Horizontal' bone loss involving >2/3 of the root.

Endodontal

- Incomplete root canal therapy.
- Periapical pathology.
- Presence of voluminous posts/screws.

Dental

- Extensive root caries.

Treatment goals

Patients diagnosed with periodontitis require a treatment strategy that includes the elimination of the opportunistic infection. This strategy should also define the clinical outcomes to be reached through therapy. Such clinical parameters include:

- Reduction or resolution of gingivitis (BoP). A patient full mouth mean BoP $\leq 25\%$ should be reached.
- Reduction in PPD. No residual pockets with PPD > 5 mm should be present.
- Elimination of (through-and-through) open furcations in multirooted teeth. Beginning furcation involvement should not exceed 3 mm.
- Absence of pain.
- Individually satisfactory aesthetics and function.

Consequently, the treatment of elderly patients affected by caries, periodontal disease and tooth loss, including symptoms of associated pathological conditions such as pulpitis, periapical periodontitis, marginal abscesses, tooth migration, and so on, should follow four logical treatment phases:

1 **Systemic phase of therapy** (including smoking-cessation advice)

   The goal of this phase is to eliminate or decrease the influence of systemic conditions on the outcomes of therapy and to protect the patient and the dental care providers against infectious hazards. Since the elderly patient may take multiple medications for the control of various systemic conditions, the risk of routine dental therapy, including the risk assessment for surgical interventions, has to be assessed. If necessary, the patient's physician is consulted and appropriate measures are taken in modifying the administration of medications [1]. Moreover, in heavy smokers, efforts must be undertaken to stimulate a smoker to enrol in a smoking cessation programme.

2 **Cause-related therapy**

   The goal of this treatment phase is the establishment of optimal oral hygiene and the cleaning-up of the oral cavity. This is performed by motivating the patient for preventive measures and instructing in individually optimal plaque control protocols. Furthermore, the dentition is systematically scaled and root planed where indicated, most likely under local anaesthesia. Carious lesions are excavated, since open carious lesions also represent plaque-retaining areas. Likewise, teeth deemed to be 'irrational to treat' are extracted in this initial phase of therapy.

Cause-related therapy is concluded by a re-evaluation, 4–8 weeks after the last intervention, and planning of both additional and supportive therapies is performed.

3 **Corrective phase of therapy:**

This phase addresses the sequelae of the opportunistic infections and includes therapeutic measures such as periodontal and implant surgery, endodontic therapy, restorative and/or prosthetic treatment. The volume of corrective therapy required and the selection of means for the restorative and prosthetic therapy can be determined only when the level of success of the cause-related therapy can be properly evaluated. The patient's willingness and ability to cooperate in the overall therapy must determine the content of the corrective treatment. If this cooperation is unsatisfactory, it may not be worth initiating complex treatment procedures.

4 **Maintenance phase (supportive periodontal therapy; SPT)**

The aim of this continuous treatment is the secondary prevention of reinfection and disease recurrence. For each individual patient a recall system must be designed that includes (i) assessment of deepened sites with BoP, (ii) instrumentation of such sites and (iii) fluoride application for the prevention of dental caries. In addition, this treatment involves the regular maintenance of prosthetic restorations incorporated during the corrective phase of therapy. Routine assessment of the vitality of abutment teeth or those with crowns should be undertaken where possible as loss of vitality represents a common complication [2–4]. Based upon the individual caries activity, bitewing radiographs should be incorporated in SPT at regular (2 year-) intervals. It is suggested that elderly patients should be seen at between 3 and 6 month frequency for supportive therapy depending on their general health status and care need.

Subjective chewing comfort

The need for a complete dentition with 14 antagonistic occlusal units to maintain adequate function of the masticatory system has been a generally accepted dogma in restorative dentistry [5, 6]. Claims that a shortened dental arch may act as an etiological factor for functional disturbances in the masticatory system have been made without supporting evidence [5, 6].

This dogma has been challenged in more recent times resulting in the widespread acceptance of the functionally acceptable shortened dental arch [7–10].

In the cross-sectional study by Käyser [7, 9], the validity of two working hypotheses was substantiated (Figure 22.2):

- The masticatory function decreased slowly in the presence of a functional adaptation to the status of premolar occlusion (i.e. four remaining occlusal units), following which a rapid deterioration of the chewing function was noted (Figure 22.3).
- The masticatory function decreased linearly without a sudden deterioration. However, the level to which functional adaptation could sufficiently compensate for the loss of posterior tooth units, and thus still allow individual optimum function, was difficult to define.

From these studies it may be concluded that the functional adaptation of the masticatory system in a shortened dental arch with at least four, preferably symmetrically located, antagonistic occlusal units (premolar-occlusion) is consistent

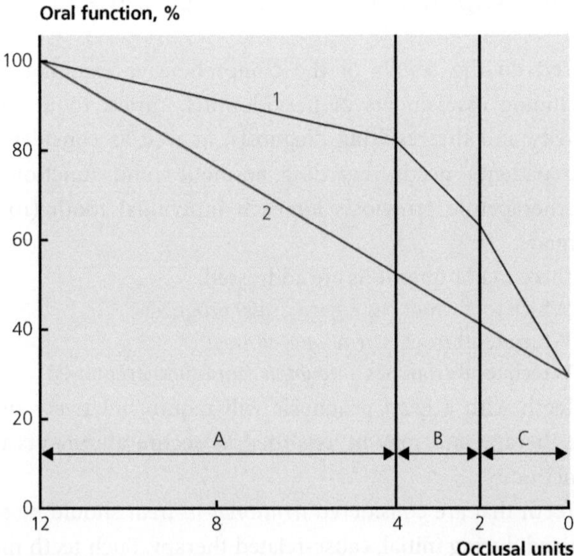

Figure 22.2 The two possibilities of the adaptive capacity of the masticatory system following the loss of teeth 25. A = zone of subjective optimal masticatory function, B = zone of adaptation, C = zone of subjective inadequate chewing function. The occlusal units are expressed as premolar equivalents (1 molar = 2 premolar equivalents).

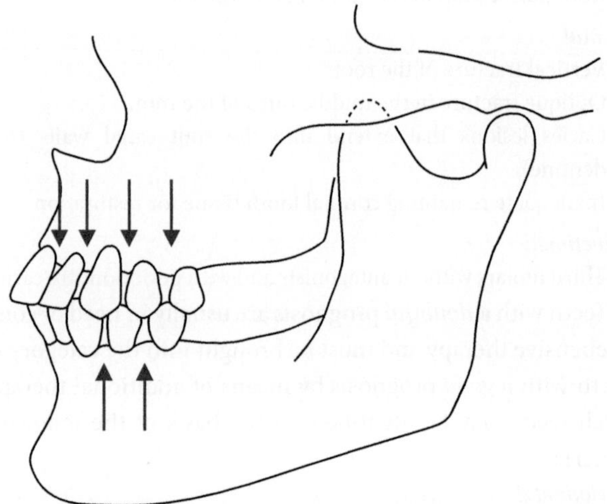

Figure 22.3 Optimal chewing function can be assured with a dentition of four premolar units bilaterally present. Functional adaptation of the masticatory system appears likely [7].

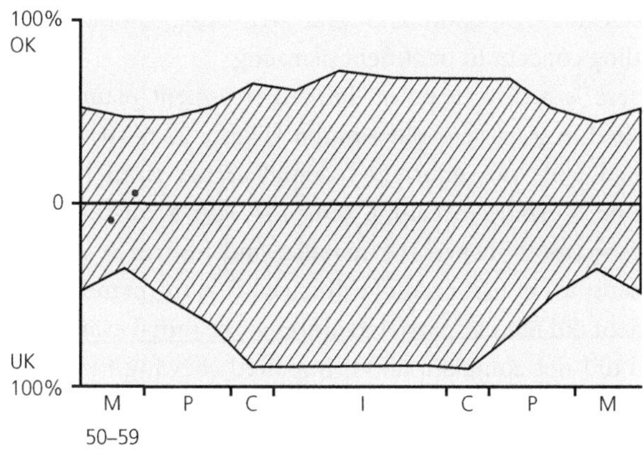

Figure 22.4 Topographical distribution of the percentage of teeth present in randomly selected subjects aged 50–59 years. M = molars, P = premolars (bicuspids), C = canines (cuspids), I = incisors, MAX = maxilla, MAND = mandible. Sixty per cent of the subjects had a shortened dental arch. However, only a quarter of these used a partial denture to replace the missing teeth [12].

with a reduced, yet adequate, function [11]. Occasionally, minor tooth migrations may be seen in dentitions with premolar occlusion. The results were confirmed by another cross-sectional study [12]. In this survey, 300 randomly selected subjects were examined and interviewed for subjective chewing comfort. In the group 50–59 years of age (Figure 22.4), approximately 10% were without teeth in the mandible and 30% had a complete dentition. The remaining 60% of the subjects demonstrated a shortened dental arch, with the incisor teeth and the canines present in all subjects. None of the 300 individuals complained about disturbances of the masticatory system or impaired chewing comfort. Only about 50% of the individuals with shortened dental arches (30% of all subjects) had partial dentures, of whom half used their dentures. The fact that, in this cohort, 45% of the individuals functioned well having a shortened dental arch demonstrated the central role of subjective chewing comfort in deciding whether to replace lost molars or premolars [11].

From an aesthetic point of view, most individuals tolerate a premolar occlusion well [11].

A more recent study [13] has investigated the objective chewing capacity of patient cohorts with various conditions. While young or elderly patients with a complete dentition use approximately 20 chewing strokes to fragment the particle size of a test food from approximately 5.5 mm to 2 mm, the patients with shortened dental arches had to apply 40 strokes to reach the same fragmentation of the test food (Figure 22.5.) Hence, it is evident that a reduced dentition will induce the need for more chewing strokes to compensate for the reduced masticatory capacity.

The shortened dental arch appeared to display a similar function as that of edentulous patients wearing full dentures with a high alveolar ridge and patients with overdentures on natural roots. The limited chewing efficiency of the patients with shortened dental arches has to be explained by the reduced occlusal surface constraining the quantity of food particles that can be trapped between the teeth.

Especially in the elderly, the individual optimum function, the person's subjective need for additional occlusal units and the person's satisfaction with the present situation should be considered in treatment planning. The replacement of lost molars has to be judged individually and the advantages and

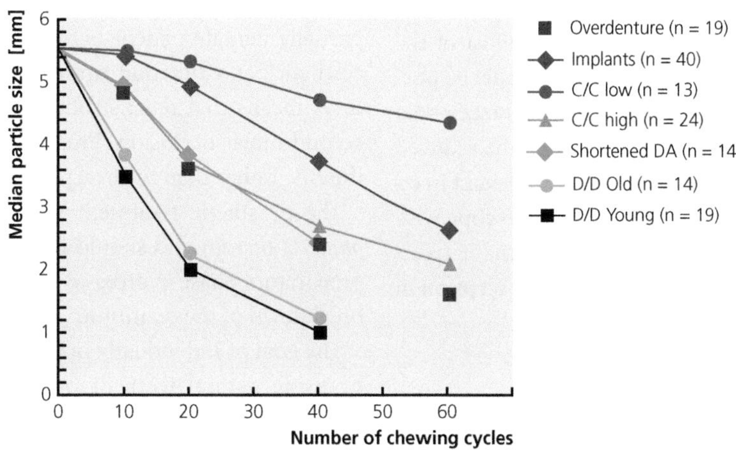

Figure 22.5 Mean median particle sizes plotted as a function of chewing strokes. black = complete dentition (young), green = complete dentition (elderly), light blue = shortened dental arch, orange = complete dentures with high alveolar ridge, red = complete dentures with low alveolar ridge, dark blue = implant-retained overdenture on low alveolar ridge, purple = tooth supported over denture. Adapted from Fontijn-Tekamp *et al.* 2000 [13].

disadvantages carefully weighed in the best interests of the patient [14, 15].

Treatment planning

Levels of treatment planning

The treatment plan usually consists of a number of treatment goals that satisfy an *ideal level* of function and aesthetics under healthy conditions. Patient's desires and chief complaints should be brought into an equilibrium with the clinical situation to meet these goals. Quite often such a treatment plan will result in complex treatment phases that may require the cooperation of various dental specialties. While it is mostly possible to fulfil optimal demands on aesthetics and function with the treatments available today, such an *ideal* treatment goal may not be entirely relevant for individual patients.

Based on their profile, financial means and physical and mental status, a cost-benefit analysis will often simplify the treatment plan to a *reasonable level* that considers all the limiting factors mentioned.

In the elderly patient, the desires of the patient may often be overshadowed by those of the family. Moreover, financial aspects may severely dominate the treatment options and reduce the reasonable treatment plan to a *feasible level.* Nevertheless, such a reduced and feasible treatment plan still requires time-consuming preparatory therapy before reconstructions can be incorporated. This pre-treatment phase should be understood as a diagnostic element to be considered in later re-evaluations. Occasionally, treatment plans have to be adapted during execution and modified to adapt to unexpected changes in health situation of the patients.

In this context, it should be realized that for most of the elderly patients the *ideal* treatment plan cannot really be pursued and hence a *reasonable* treatment plan is forseen as a rule. Quite often the treatment plan will have to be reduced further to the *pragmatic* level. This is especially relevant in elderly frail patients where the ability of a patient to cope with care can vary substantially from day to day. Pragmatic treatment planning may represent the rule rather the exception in geriatric dentistry.

Pragmatic treatment planning

Since a variety of clinical studies have established that replacing lost teeth beyond the second premolar often is not required, pragmatic and individual treatment planning should be given preference over supposedly 'ideal' professional concepts of optimum function. The subjective masticatory function and oral well-being should be the leading concept in treatment planning.

Here is a case in point: limited treatment planning was applied in a 64-year-old woman [Figure 22.6(a)] who presented with two shortened dental arches from maxillary canine (cuspid) to canine (cuspid) with a missing lateral incisor (tooth 12) in the maxilla, and from first premolar (biscuspid) to first premolar (bicuspid) in the mandible. The patient did not use partial dentures at the initial examination and did not complain about impaired chewing function or masticatory disturbances. Her grandson was to be confirmed in church and she worried about her appearance at this important family reunion. One central incisor (tooth 11) had been nonvital for many years and was discoloured; the other central incisor had already been crowned temporarily several years ago. Therefore, the treatment plan for this patient was limited to the replacement of the maxillary right lateral incisor by a cantilever bridge using one maxillary central incisors as abutment. The reconstruction was preceded by a hygiene phase to control gingivitis. Also, endodontic revision and a gold core-and-post build-up were performed on the right central incisor. Six years following this limited treatment approach, the patient showed no signs of functional disturbances or impaired chewing ability [Figure 22.6(b)]. Her main concern, the aesthetic problem, was eliminated by a simple treatment. (Twenty years later, the patient is still completely satisfied [Figure 22.6(c)], although gingival recession has occurred.)

Reconstruction of partially dentate patients

As indicated above, the goal of the reconstruction of the partially dentate patient is to satisfy the patient's needs for aesthetics and function under healthy conditions. This, in turn, means that reconstructions usually do not extend to second molar occlusion. Pragmatic treatment goals may be the rule rather than the exception.

The prosthetic treatment plan belongs in *the corrective phase of therapy* and should follow a successfully completed preparatory phase in order to prevent reinfection and further breakdown of the dentition.

The goal of individually optimal function may be realized by using natural teeth or oral implants as abutments for reconstructions or with a removable prosthesis. Whenever possible, preference is given to the preservation of natural tooth substance or existing reconstruction with satisfactory function. Using single implants as abutments may render reconstructions to be less extensive and

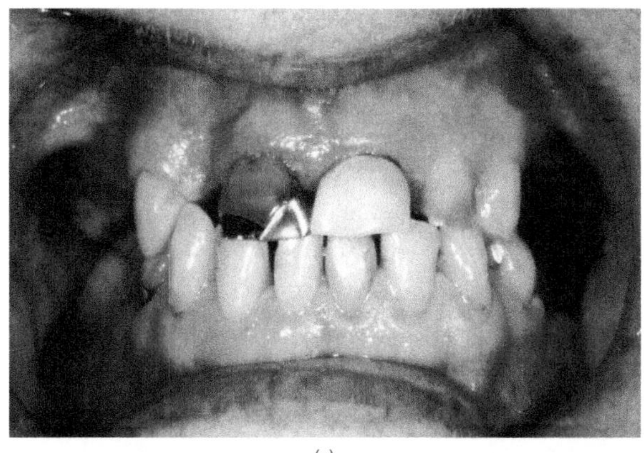

(a)

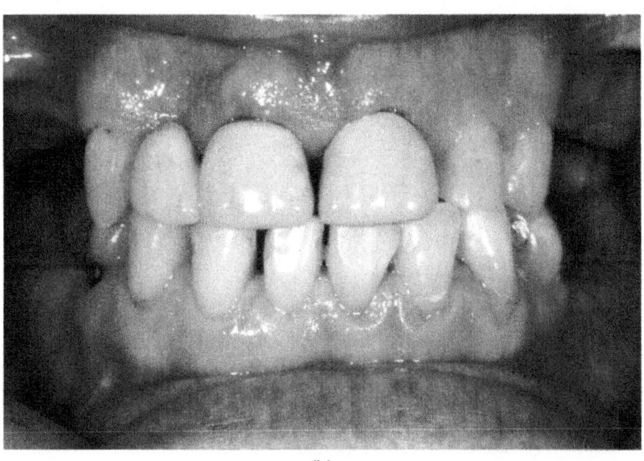

(b)

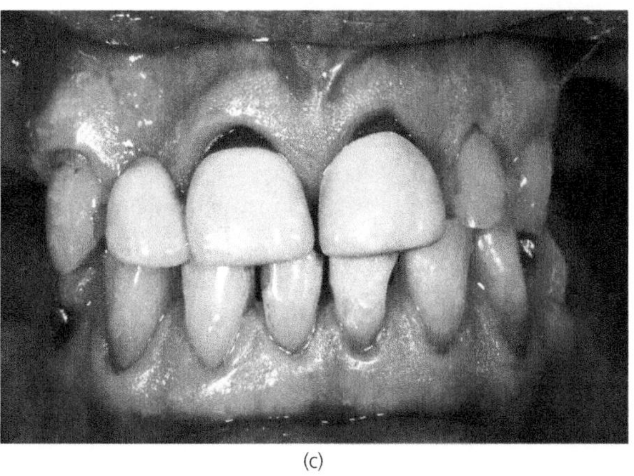

(c)

Figure 22.6 Limited treatment planning **a)** 64-year-old woman with aesthetic problems. Missing tooth 12, nonvital and carious tooth 11, temporary crown on tooth 21, shortened dental arch 13/43 to 23/33. **b)** Same patient, 6 years following the provision of a cantilever bridge from 11 replacing 12 **c)** Same patient, after 20 years follow-up. Gingival recession resulted from overzealous toothbrushing.

hence less susceptible to technical complications. Shorter spans for fixed bridgework are to be preferred over the longer spans, irrespective of the nature of the abutments chosen.

The following cases in point demonstrate the sequential planning and implementation of a treatment plan that is oriented towards individually optimal function under healthy conditions. Despite the existence of multiple problems prior to therapy, infection was successfully treated to control the infection prior to reconstructing the dentition.

Conventional and implant born reconstructions

This 61-year-old female patient came to the clinic for a second opinion after her dentist had proposed the provision of a removable partial dental prosthesis. She had read about the possibilities of implant therapy on the Internet.

The lower anterior and right posterior mandible were painful and chewing was difficult on the right side. Moreover, she was dissatisfied with the appearance of her maxillary anterior reconstruction.

Her oral hygiene practices were less than optimal with interdental cleansing being non-existent. Her general health condition was very good. Ten years earlier she had been operated on for cataracts. Otherwise, no pathological findings were known both for herself as well as for her family. She was a life-long non-smoker.

There were no significant findings on extra-oral examination and the examination of the oral soft tissues did not reveal any pathological changes.

The dental examination showed numerous teeth responding negatively to a thermal vitality assessment (teeth 17, 14, 13, 12, 11, 31, 32). Radiographic assessment revealed that 17 had an incomplete root canal filling and 31 and 32 presented with periapical radiolucencies. 18, 27, 28, 36, 38, 41, 46, 47, 48 were missing.

There were numerous splinted crowns (17, 16, 15, 14 and 13, 12, 11, 21, 22, 23 as well as 24, 25, 26 and 44, 45, 46, 47) with over-contoured margins and caries around their margins (17, 16 and 13, 12). Severe wear and chipping was seen on most of the acrylic veneers used with these cast restorations [Figure 22.7(a),(b),(c)].

Functionally, a prematurity in centric relation (CR) was diagnosed between 23 and 33 with a horizontal, vertical and lateral slide between centric relation and centric occlusion (CR-CO) of 1.0 mm. Both the right and the left lateral movements were canine guided. No non-working side interferences were present. Wear facets were visible on the functional surfaces of 45 to 33.

The inter-incisal distance in maximal mouth opening was 53 mm. The overbite was 4 mm and the overjet 6 mm. There was a Class II skeletal base.

The BPE revealed a score of 4 in the molar sextants, a score of 3 in the anterior sextants, with stars due to furcation involvement and because of aesthetic recession problems:

4*	3	4*
4	3*	4*

This justified the detailed periodontal chat presented in Figure 22.7(d),(e),(f).

It is evident that 17, 16 and 36 presented with periodontal Probing Pocket Depths (PPD) of up to 12 mm and attachment loss to close to the apex at some aspects.

The dental panoramic tomogram [Figure 22.7(e)] confirmed severe bone loss at 17, over-contoured crowns, caries at 13, periapical pathology at 32 and 31 and showed a clearly

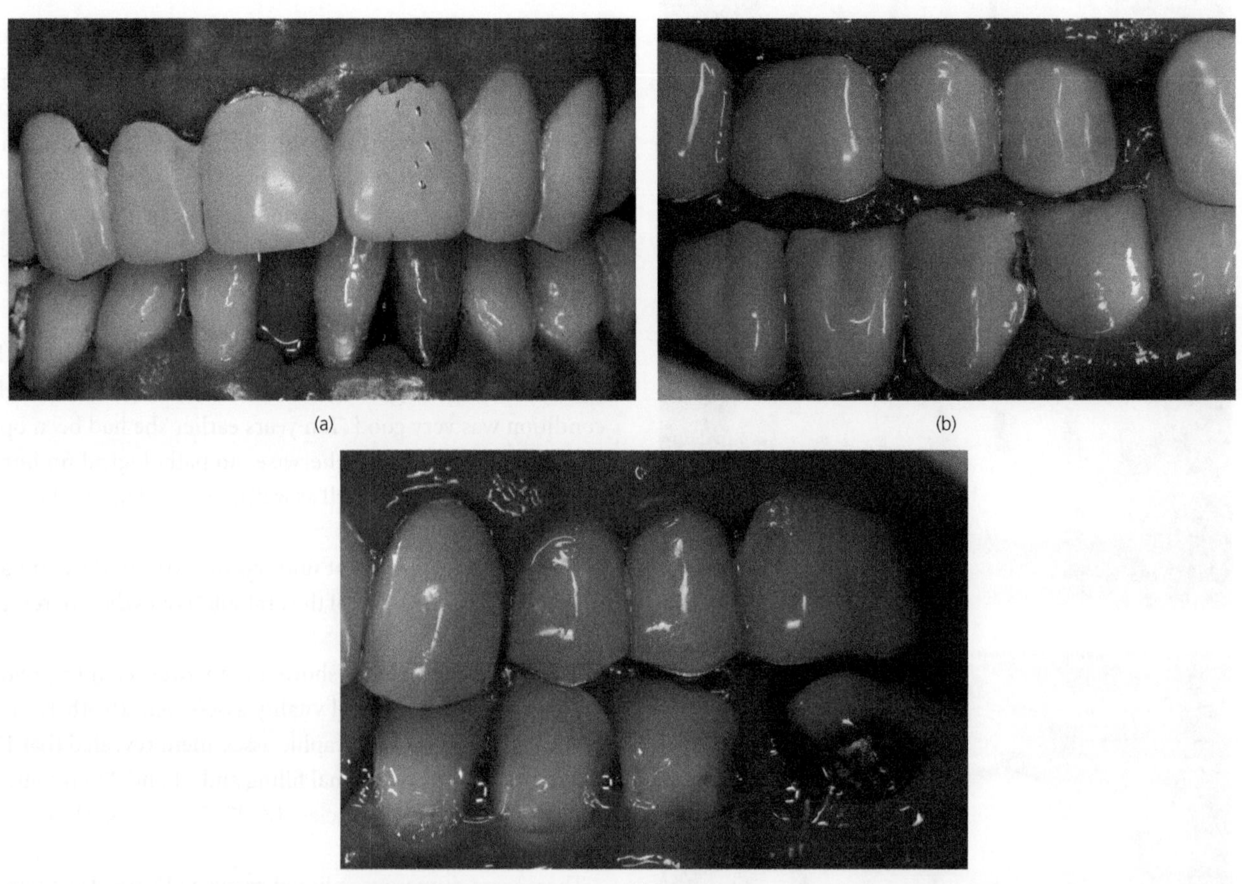

(a) (b) (c)

Figure 22.7 Case presentation: 61-year-old female. **a)** Anterior view shows inflamed gingiva in the region of 13. Please note also the gingival recession on 13, 12 and quite healthy looking gingiva in the 2nd quadrant. Front bridge shows traces of damage to the acrylic veneer. In the mandible, tooth 41 is missing and teeth 31 and 32 are severely discoloured. **b/c)** Lateral views with space between bridge in 1st quadrant and front area, front bridge moved towards the front, inflammation, edematous gingivae, chipping of acrylic; in the 4th quadrant, extension bridge following a root fracture of 47 (removed) lesions in the maxillary right and mandibular left molar region. Likewise, tooth 31 yields substantial attachment loss. **d)** Periodontal chart revealing advanced periodontal lesions in the maxillary right and mandibular left molar region. Likewise, tooth 31 yields substantial attachment loss. **e)** Orthopantomogram confirming the findings of the periodontal chart. Moreover, periapical radiolucencies around the apices of 17, 13, 32, 31 are visible. Tooth 45 shows signs of trauma from occlusion due to inadequate bridge reconstruction in the 4th quadrant. Root canal fillings of teeth 14, 12, 11 are adequate without periapical pathology. **f)** Scheme for the classification of teeth into 'secure prognosis', 'doubtful prognosis' and 'irrational to treat' as a pretherapeutic risk assessment on the tooth level. **g)** Provisional composite splint 42 × 31 & 32. **h)** Periodontal chart at the re-evaluation following the successful completion of the hygiene phase therapy. Only one residual pocket of 5 mm is diagnosed at 45. All teeth irrational to treat have been extracted during hygiene phase. However, 31 and 32 were still maintained. **i)** Treatment planning for the corrective phase (crosses demarcate the teeth judged 'irrational to treat' and extracted). **j)** Same patient as in (i) after completed treatment. In the anterior mandible, a mixed tooth-implant supported bridge with screw retention is provided. A harmonious gingival margin is visible, resulting from the surgical lengthening of the clinical crown. **k/l)** Lateral views; some plaque is still visible in the 4th quadrant but much better hygiene is performed compared with the beginning of the treatment. 3rd quadrant cervical fillings were performed at the same time as the pictures were taken. Teeth 33, 34, 35, 43 have not been crowned. **m)** X-ray. **n)** Panoramic overview; implant placement on the regions of 13, 36 and 32, FDP with one cantilever in the 4th quadrant. Please observe that the periodontal ligament of 45 is no longer widened, indicating that the trauma from occlusion has been eliminated with a correct occlusal scheme of the FDP. **o)** No pockets >4 mm, 5 years after the completion of the corrective phase.

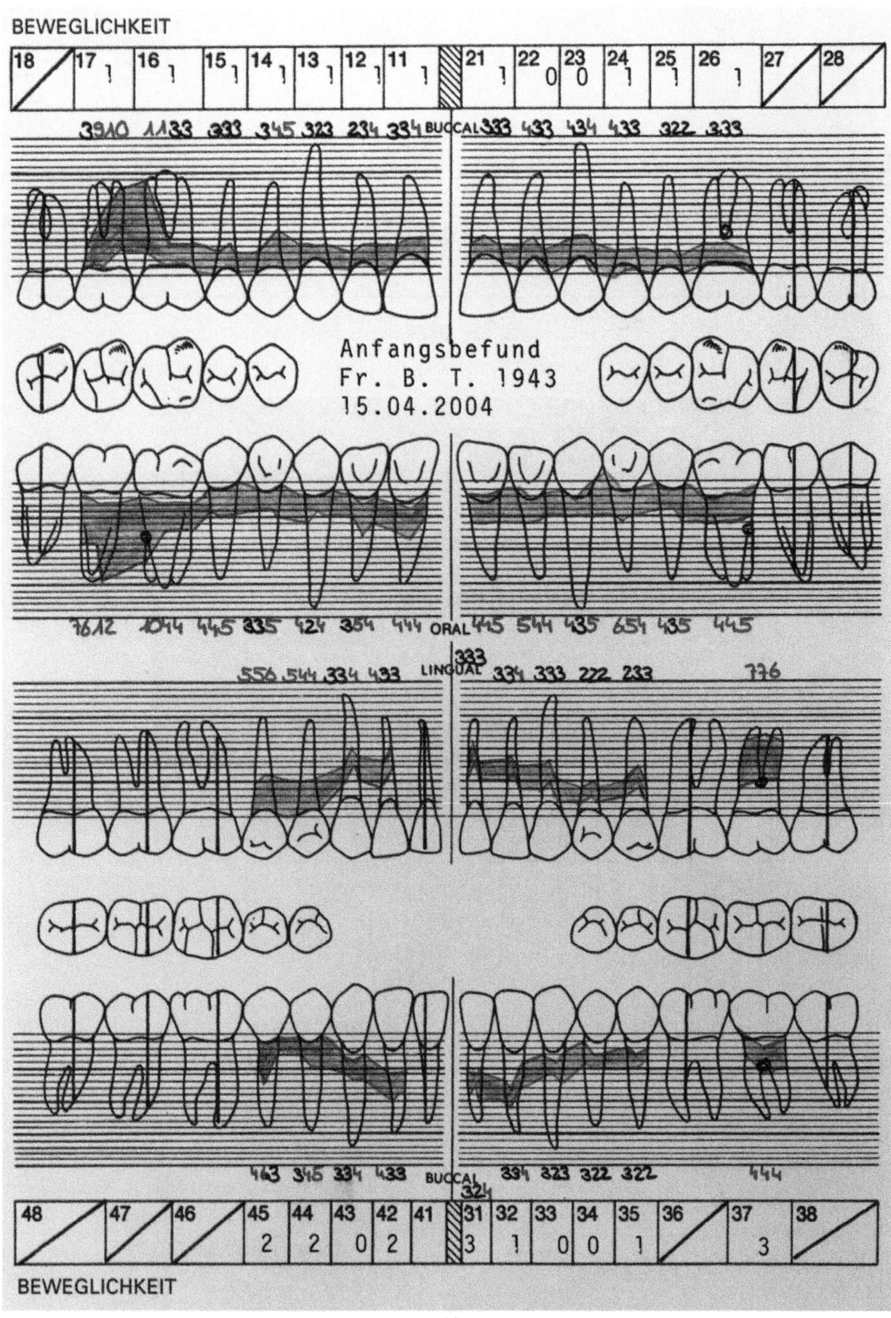

(d)

Figure 22.7 (*Continued*)

widened periodontal ligament space at 45 in association with a cantilever bridge that does not appear to have been designed as such. 37 presented with a deep mesial angular defect (Figure 22.7).

The Plaque Index was 79% and the BoP was 90%.

Since the patient wanted improved aesthetics, chewing function and oral health, a comprehensive treatment plan was presented with the goal of incorporating a fixed reconstruction.

The pretherapeutic risk assessment for each tooth is depicted in Figure 22.7(f):

17, 13, 37, 32 and 31 were judged to be 'irrational to treat'.

16, 12, 11 and 45 had a doubtful prognosis. The remainder of the teeth presented with a good prognosis.

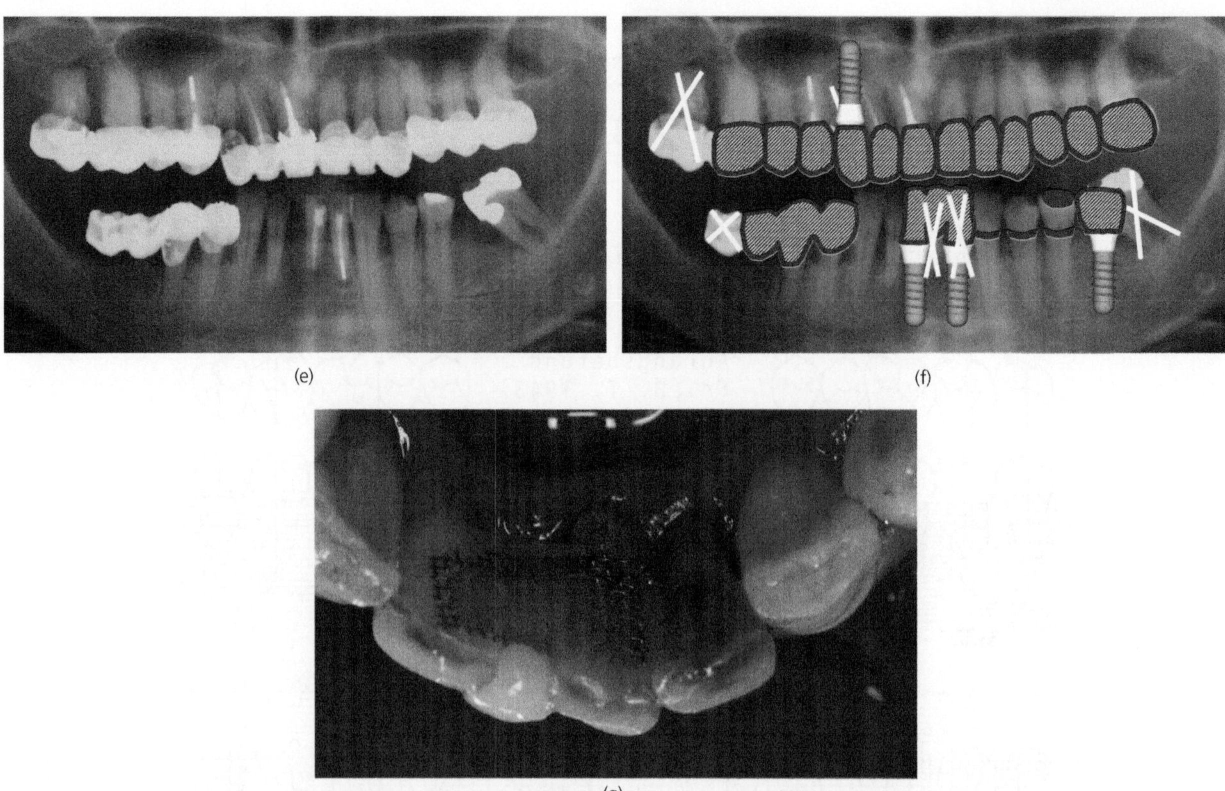

(e) (f) (g)

Figure 22.7 (*Continued*)

The treatment plan was followed meticulously for the first two phases:

1 *Systemic phase*
  - No further examination required.
2 *Hygiene phase*
  - Motivation.
  - Oral hygiene instructions; bass technique and interdental brushes.
  - Removal of cantilever units 46, 47.
  - Scaling and root planing of all teeth.
  - Extraction of 17, 13, 37, 32 & 31.
  - Caries management 16, 12 & 11.
  - Provisional restorations 16, 15, *14* × *12*, 11, 21, 22, 23, 24, 25, 26, 44 & 45.
  - Provisional composite splint 42 × 31 & 32 [Figure 22.7(g)].
  - Re-evaluation after 6 weeks following the last instrumentation.

After re-evaluation [Figure 22.7(h)], the *Corrective phase* was planned in detail [Figure 22.7(i)]. Restoration of the edentulous spaces could have been achieved with a removable partial denture (RPD), a tooth-supported fixed reconstruction, an implant-supported fixed reconstruction or a combination of the above. The patient requested a fixed rather than a removable prosthetic appliance.

3 *Corrective phase*
  - *Surgical phase*
    - Surgical lengthening of the clinical crowns in the 1st quadrant.
    - Implant installation in region 13, 36 and 32, if possible also 41. However, due to lack of bone volume the implant in region 42 could not be placed which led to a change in the reconstructive treatment plan. Now a combined tooth-implant supported bridge was to be incorporated from tooth 42 to implant 32.
  - *Reconstructive phase*
    - A composite post and core build-up was placed on tooth 12.
    - Further composite build-ups were placed on teeth 16, 14 & 11.
    - Fixed reconstructions (FDPs) were provided: a cantilever bridge ×45 44 replaced the missing 46.
    - The missing anterior mandibular incisors were replaced with a combined tooth–implant-borne FDP Tooth 42 × Implant 32.
    - The reconstructions of teeth 16, 15, 14, implant 13, teeth 12, 11, 21, 22, 23, 24, 25, 26 and implant 36 were single porcelain fused to metal crowns.
    - Finally, cervical composite fillings on teeth 33, 34 and 35 were placed.

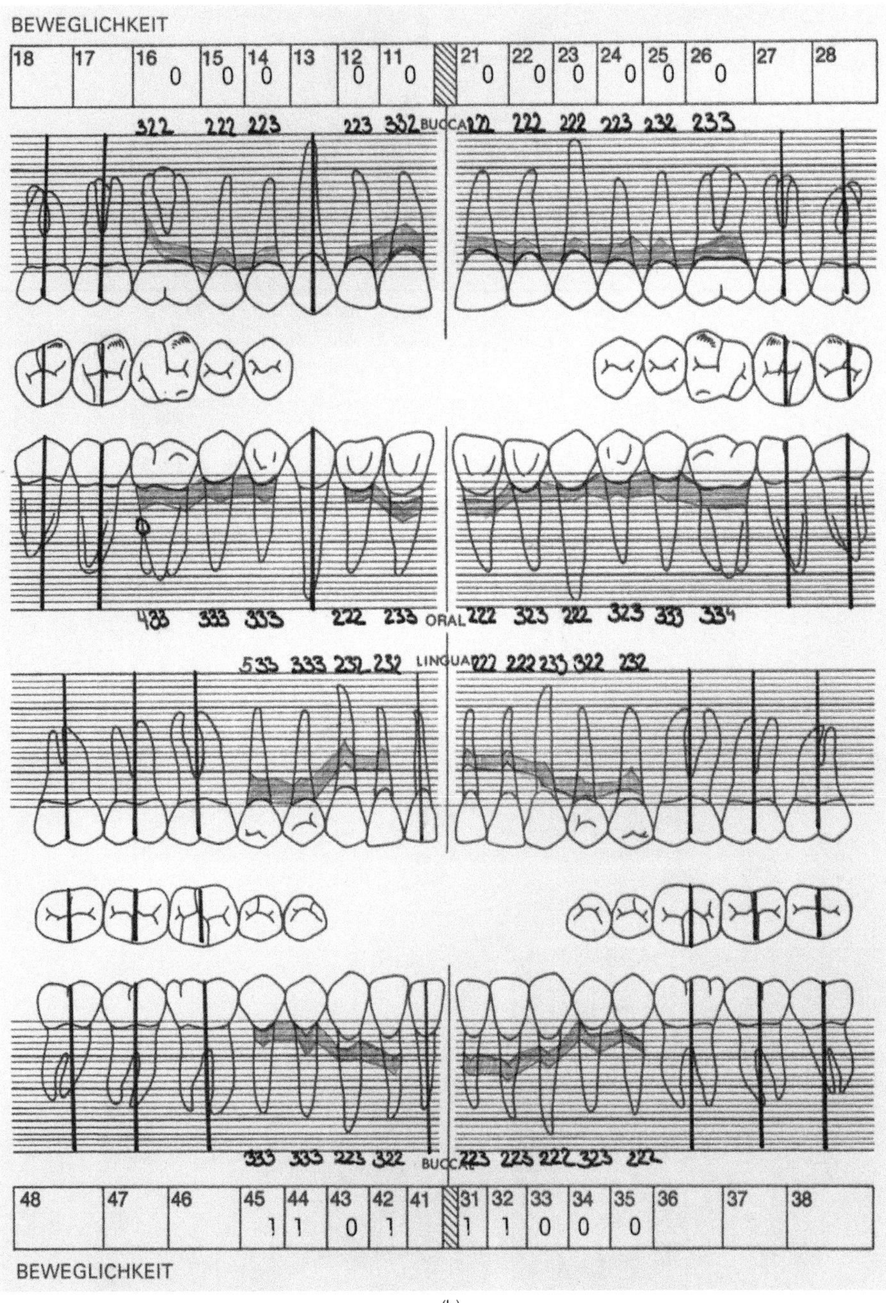

(h)

Figure 22.7 (*Continued*)

◦ Eventually, a re-evaluation completed the case [Figure 22.7(j),(k),(l),(m)].

4 *Maintenance phase*

- Initially, recall visits were scheduled at 4 month intervals. Depending on an adequate performance in home care, the recall interval could be prolonged to 6 and then 8 months. After five years, the excellent condition of the dentition and the reconstructions were evident [Figure 22.7(o)].
- At each recall visit, BoP and PPD were registered. Subsequently, bleeding sites were instrumented and calculus was removed. If necessary, instruction in oral hygiene practices was repeated. The dentition was meticulously cleaned and polished and topical fluorides were applied. All reconstructions were checked. The alveolar bone around the implants has been maintained [Figure 22.7(n)].

Removable dental prosthesis (RDP)

Older independent and systemically healthy patients should be treated like any others with the principles governing

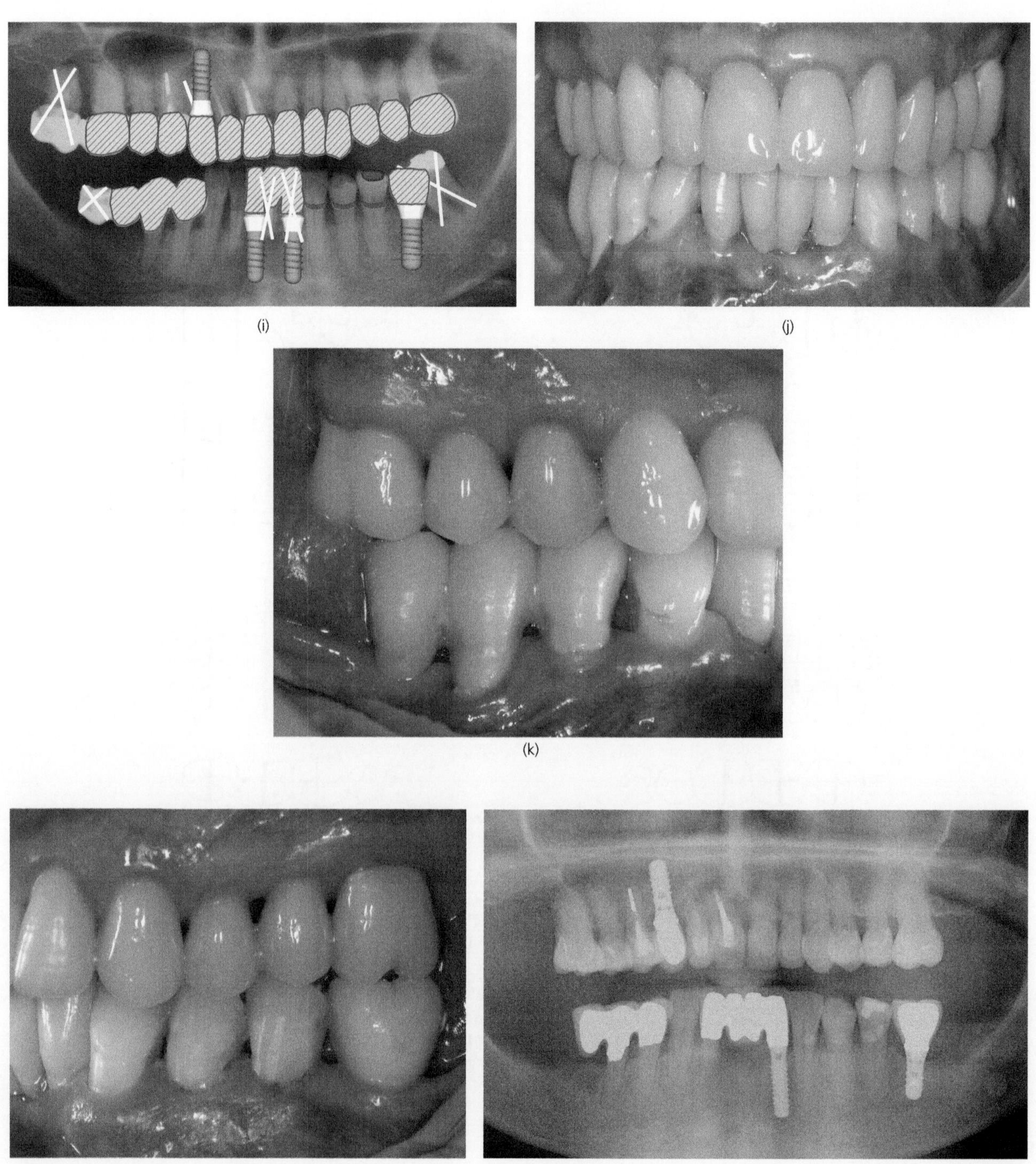

Figure 22.7 (*Continued*)

treatment planning applying independently of the patient's age. However, in elderly and frail geriatric patients, the reconstruction of a mutilated dentition may follow principles of a reasonable or even pragmatic care, rather than an ideal treatment plan [16]. This, in turn, means that prosthetic replacement of missing teeth may have to be simplified. Likewise, limited budgets of elderly patients may require more simple and cost-effective prosthetic treatment.

In this context, the use of a removable prosthesis may satisfy the functional needs and aesthetic demands of the patient.

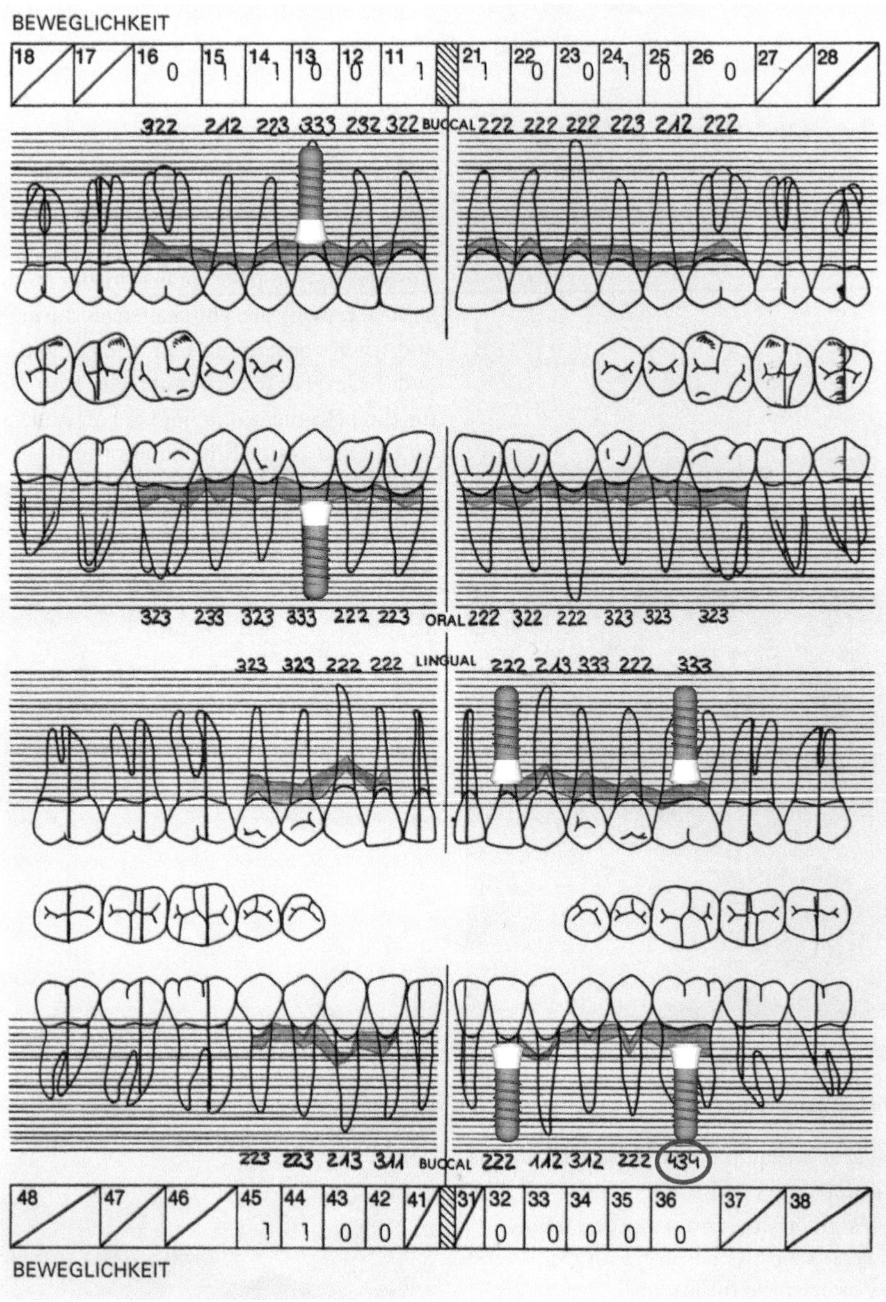

(n)

Figure 22.7 *(Continued)*

It has to be realised that elaborate prosthetic treatment requires not only major efforts during the fabrication and insertion of reconstructions, but also life-long regular maintenance. If dexterity and physical ability to manage prosthesis are no longer guaranteed, adaptation of the plan of care becomes a requirement (Figure 22.8). Basically, the same principles of RPD design apply to younger and elderly frail patients [17]. In addition, the design of RPDs for frail elderly adults should maximize the potential for cleaning and minimize complexity. Equally, the resin surfaces need to be smoothly polished, refraining from complex imitations of natural tissue texture. Likewise, retentive elements and major connectors should be designed to favour periodontal health (Figure 22.9). Proximal surfaces of the abutment teeth should leave an appropriate space for saliva access and for the application of interdental brushes. Where possible,

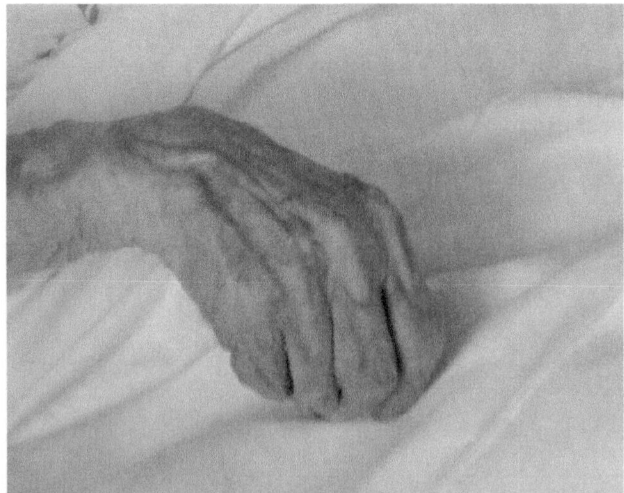

Figure 22.8 The manual dexterity of a patient can often be judged by looking at his hands.

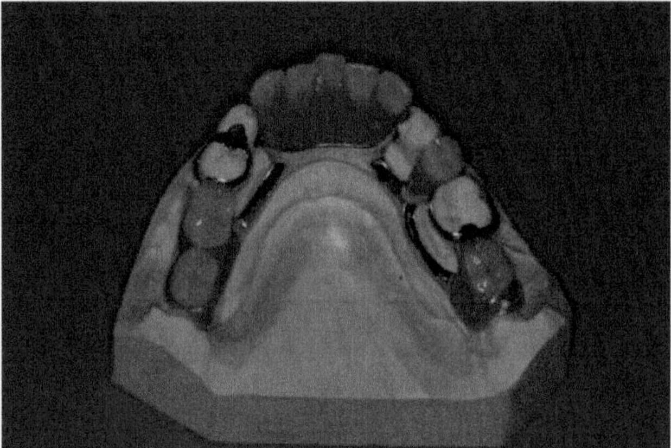

Figure 22.9 The design of a removable partial denture for elderly patients should be simple and rigid. The major connectors should stay clear from the gingival margins to foster periodontal health.

a 3 × 3 × 3 mm space is required but, especially in the aesthetic zone, this is not always realistic (Figure 22.10). The guidelines for RPD design may be summarized as follows:

1 The design should be as simple as possible, with saddles and connectors avoiding proximity to the marginal gingiva.
2 Saddles should be supported by adjacent abutments where possible. In distal extension RPDs, occlusal rests should be placed to avoid tilting of abutment teeth.
3 The metal framework of RPDs should be sufficiently rigid to withstand and distribute occlusal forces as well as ensure stability in case of occasional clumsy handling by the patient.
4 The RPD should be designed with appropriate retention by at least two retentive elements placed on diagonally opposing abutment teeth. In distal extension RDPs, retention is improved by adding indirect retention with occlusal rests on the opposite side of the axis of rotation of the RPD when possible.
5 Occlusal contacts should be bilateral and simultaneous in CR at an appropriate vertical dimension. When muscular control of mandibular movements is no longer indicated in frail and multi-morbid patients, the occlusal pattern may have to be established in a more anterior, comfortable, muscle-determined position.

A particular, but common, clinical challenge arises from gingival recession and/or over-eruption, leading to abutment teeth with a high clinical crown. The unfavourable ratio of the latter and the clinical root requires particular attention when considering the load applied to the tooth. Teeth with high clinical crowns present challenges during impression taking and when considering both the aesthetics of the prosthesis and the level of the occlusal table. They may leave little space for the placement of a lingual bar. A 'dental bar', which sits on cingular rests of the anterior teeth but stays clear of the gingival margin, may help to solve this problem and provide flexibility in case of further tooth loss (Figure 22.11).

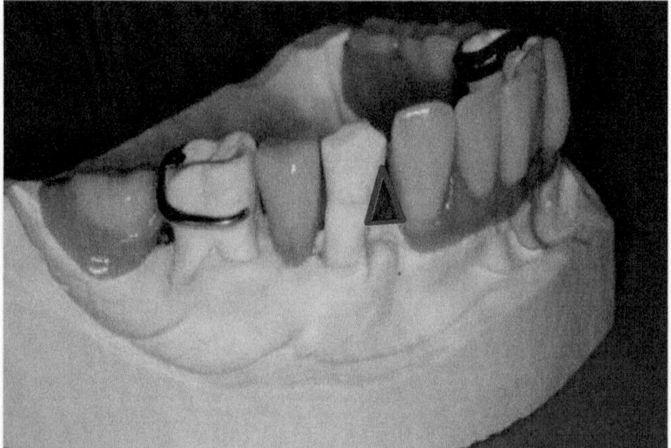

Figure 22.10 Interdental spaces of 3 × 3 × 3mm size allow the saliva to access the dental and periodontal tissues and thus protect the abutment teeth. However, when space and aesthetics are an issue, they are not always possible.

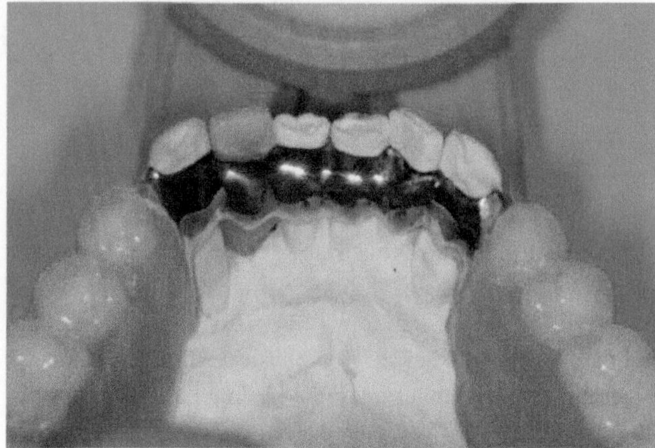

Figure 22.11 'Long teeth' often preclude a lingual bar. In these cases the major connector can be placed lingually on the lower teeth with cingulum rests.

Alternatives to removable dental prostheses

If, after careful evaluation of the patient's needs for aesthetics and masticatory function, it is decided to replace lost occlusal units, several prosthodontic alternatives other than removable partial dentures are available. They include osseointegrated dental implants and cantilever bridges, which are especially useful if the dental arch is to be lengthened unilaterally or by one occlusal unit only. This concept is beneficial in the elderly patient since such reconstructions are more comfortable and easier to maintain than removable partial dentures. Oral hygiene is facilitated and the restored occlusal plane remains stable. This may play a central role when cantilever bridges are constructed as antagonistic occlusal units to a complete maxillary denture, providing bilateral and protrusive stability for the denture during function.

Despite recent developments where implants have become a predictable treatment, cantilever bridges may remain a treatment choice in elderly patients. Especially with compromised health precluding surgical interventions or where there is the need for extensive augmentation procedures prior to implantation, cantilever bridges may be an option. However, technical aspects have to be considered.

Recent systematic reviews on the 10-year survival rate of cantilever bridges [18, 19] and conventional bridges [20] revealed that cantilever bridges presented with 81.8% survival in comparison with 89.1% for the conventional reconstructions.

Biological complications, such as recurrent periodontitis or the development of pulpal infections, do not appear to be linked to the type of fixed bridgework [21]. Also, the rate of technical failures may only be slightly higher in cantilever bridges than in conventional reconstructions with distal abutments [22, 21].

By far the most common technical complication is the failure of the luting cement. This has been reported to occur over an approximate observation period of 5 years between 3.3% [21] and 15% [22]. To avoid this, an optimal retention form of every abutment tooth [23] with optimal height and minimal taper should be achieved. Also, total bridge retention may be enhanced by paralleling the surfaces with the same topographical position (mesial, distal) in the dental arch and tipping the prepared abutment in the direction opposite the load of the cantilevered pontic (Figures 22.12 and 22.13). This means that, in cases replacing a lost molar or premolar with a distal cantilever bridge, the abutment teeth (premolar and/or canine) should be prepared with a slightly mesial angulation.

Root fractures have been reported to occur in 2.4% of cases over approximately 5 years [21]. The incidence of these fractures seems to increase when loosening of the bridge remains undiagnosed for a prolonged period of time [22]. Root fractures were three times as frequent in non-vital than in vital teeth, especially when the root canals were weakened by short and thick posts [21]. Therefore, tooth vitality should be maintained as long as possible.

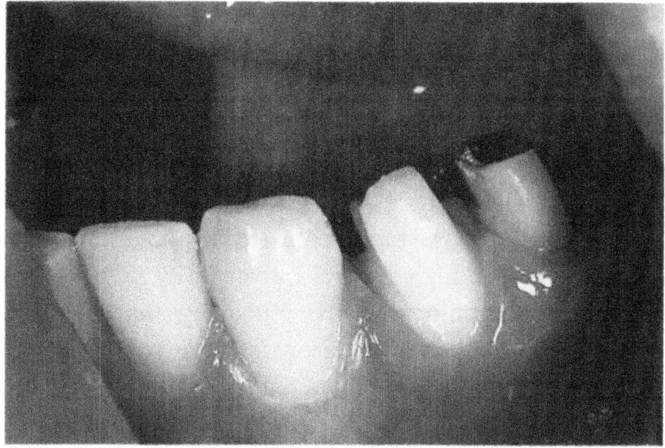

Figure 22.12 Preparation of abutment teeth for a cantilever bridge. The mesial surfaces of the abutments compensate for the load on the cantilevered pontic. The abutments are prepared slightly to the mesial aspect to assure locking-in of the bridge 34, 35 ×.

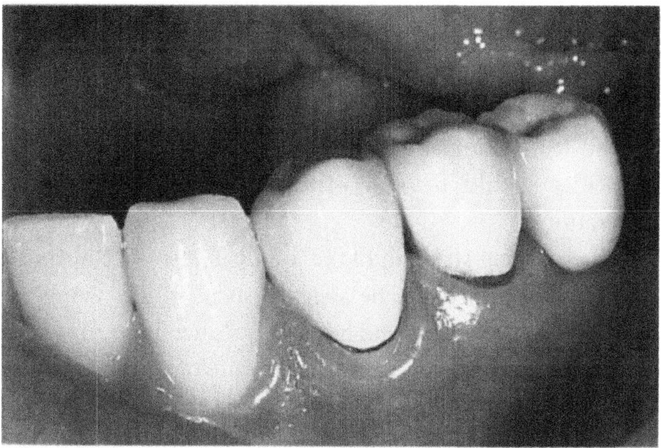

Figure 22.13 Cantilever bridge 34, 35 × on a 64-year-old female to avoid a removable partial denture (same patient as in Figure 22.12).

In summary, cantilever bridges provide a suitable and often welcome alternative to removable partial dentures in the elderly, especially when a treatment plan with limited goals for replacing lost teeth is preferred. However, great caution should be exercised in fabricating these restorations.

Replacing teeth with resin-bonded bridges

The development of electrolytic etching of cast alloy frameworks provided the basis for improved bonding strength of resin-bonded bridges (RBB). This technique also led to thinner, but stronger, frameworks allowing bonding to the enamel surface without additional mechanical retention.

Further developments of adhesive luting agents have led to more predictable clinical outcomes without the need for the complicated surface etching process and have contributed to more widespread use of this type of restorative dentistry in older adults. A recent systematic review on the scientific evidence from longitudinal studies on RBBs has indicated that the 5-year survival rates amount to approximately 87.7% [24]. Despite this high survival rate of RBBs after 5 years, technical complications, such as debonding, were frequent. Hence, indications for such reconstructions have to be selected carefully keeping in mind that these bridges may not withstand occlusal forces on a long-term basis and should probably be chosen to predominantly satisfy aesthetic needs in the elderly patient. In many ways they should be considered as viable alternatives to removable partial dentures [25] or the incorporation of a complex fixed reconstruction. Owing to the physical conditions of many older patients it has to be realized that less invasive treatment options are to be favoured over stressful and invasive procedures.

This is particularly true for frail individuals who present with age-dependent muscle atrophy, so that occlusal load for the RBB would be reduced. The ideal abutment teeth for RBBs should be caries-free and devoid of previous restorations.

If the bonding strength of the joint between the abutment and the framework can be assured, such bridges would be the treatment of choice and have been shown to be preferred by patients and markedly reduce the rate of development of caries in the mouths of patients compared with RPDs [26].

Management of the substantially reduced dentition

The substantially reduced dentition often triggers a debate over whether or not to retain the remaining teeth, since such teeth are often in a compromised status. Logically, the extraction of these teeth may be the easiest, fastest and least expensive treatment. However, the extraction of the remaining dentition may also challenge the patient's ability to cope with change and in maintaining adequate function, even if complete dentures are provided.

From the patient's perspective, the following reasons may justify the preservation of individual teeth at least on a medium-term basis:

1 Emotional attachment of the patient to his/her 'last' tooth.
2 Maintenance of retention and denture stability.
3 Maintenance of chewing efficiency.
4 Facilitating denture adaptation or the transition to a complete denture.
5 Providing psychosocial 'security'.

The residual teeth may be root-treated, domed to a level slightly above the gingival level and retained as abutment teeth for an overdenture. Vital teeth may also be used within the context of a so-called transitional denture. Simple wrought wire clasps provide retention and some stability to the denture. Even a continuous Roach clasp, which is supposed to provide lateral guidance, may help the patient to adapt to the prosthesis and to integrate the foreign body into the oral environment. Thus, the transition to the complete denture may be facilitated.

Rehabilitation with overdentures

In addition to the mentioned advantages from the patient's perspective there are some clinical advantages from retaining some tooth roots to support an overdenture, especially in the mandible.

These would include:

1 Load transmitted to the denture is shared between the denture bearing mucosa and the teeth, resulting in a reduced load on the oral mucosa which is a tissue not 'designed' for load taking.
2 The periodontal ligament can fulfil its normal purpose of taking occlusal load and dissipating this load to the supporting alveolar bone, which reduces future bone loss beneath the prosthesis and helps to retain bone around the root.
3 Equally, retaining the periodontal ligament also retains its ability to provide some proprioception which may give the patient more intraoral discrimination than would occur without the presence of the natural teeth/roots.
4 Retention can be gained by adding attachments to the tooth/root structure.
5 An increase in denture stability can be gained as the vertical extension of the tooth/root into the fitting surface of the prosthesis can resist lateral forces placed on the prosthesis.
6 Reduction of the height of the tooth, by definition, improves the crown/root ratio, which helps to reduce the tooth mobility and hence may allow a tooth that would otherwise be too mobile for consideration as an abutment for a partial denture to be retained.

There are really no serious disadvantages in using overdentures over natural teeth (compared with loosing the teeth) in any patient, particularly the older patients, even if the teeth will need endodontics. However, there will be an ongoing need for caries control and prevention of periodontal disease in a patient who has had difficulties in these areas in the past. One small disadvantage that may need to be managed is the slightly larger bulk of the completed prosthesis which needs to envelop the retained tooth roots. When anterior teeth are minimally reduced to provide overdenture abutments this may adversely impact on facial aesthetics, and there may be some compromise to the strength of the prosthesis as the bulk of acrylic resin is significantly reduced

Whilst an overdenture may be advantageous to almost all patients compared with the alternative of a conventional

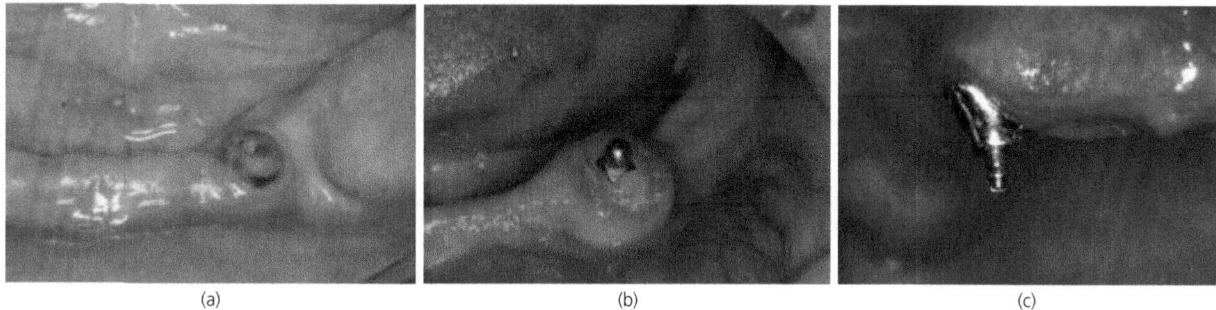

Figure 22.14 A simple filling of an overdenture abutment root is often sufficient **(a)**, but when retention is required various attachment systems exist without **(b)** or with **(c)** the use of cold copings.

complete denture, they have specific advantages in the following situations.

In patients with:

- a bruxist habit, as the additional support and stability may make denture wearing tolerable, and in cases where there has been widespread attrition an overdenture may be the most feasible way of re-establishing the appearance of teeth.
- a need for a removable prosthesis where there is insufficient freeway space to insert a prosthesis without an increase in occlusal face height. Toleration of this increase in vertical dimension is usually better accomplished if the removable prosthesis is supported in part by teeth/roots
- difficulties in adapting to complete dentures in patients where a reduced neuroplasticity or poor motor control is anticipated, for example in patients with dementia or Parkinson's disease. Adaptation problems may also arise from a variety of personality traits or psychological conditions such as depression or neuroticism.

As with all treatment, provision must begin with a clinical examination that will give sufficient information to facilitate the selection of the most appropriate teeth to overlay.

Ideally, a tooth that will be overlaid will:

- have at least half of its original periodontal attachment and be surrounded by attached gingiva;
- exhibit no anatomical features that would be incompatible with good quality endodontic treatment;
- have sufficient coronal structure for a residual supragingival height of 2–3 mm, which will allow a dome-shaped contour. If decay means that this is not possible in sound tooth structure, the deficiency can be made good with a suitable plastic filling material or by using a cast coping made to an ideal contour and cemented into place.

Canines are frequently used as overdenture abutments as they are often the longest remaining teeth and are ideally located to provide support and have easily accessible single root canals.

The least invasive and least costly treatment would be a simple sealing of the root canal with an appropriate material, which could be glass ionomer cement, composite resin or amalgam [Figure 22.14(a)]. This should be appropriately contoured and polished to provide a dome shaped coronal support with a surface contour that is easy to clean. Copings can usually be reserved for the restoration of the remaining tooth structure where caries results in a remaining root shape that cannot be restored with a conventional restoration, or if it is felt to be appropriate to incorporate some form of precision attachment. For this indication, various attachment systems are available for the construction of overdentures on such single teeth [Figure 22.14(b,c)]. Smooth contours are advantageous if the patient chooses to stop wearing the denture, which may occur during palliative care when chemotherapy renders the oral mucosa very sensitive and hence denture wearing uncomfortable. In this case, cutting a disturbing or sharp attachment may be indicated.

The importance of plaque control needs to be stressed as the microenvironment under an overdenture is particularly favourable to the development of a largely undisturbed plaque biofilm. Development of the appropriate brushing technique is essential to control plaque on and around the abutment teeth supporting overdentures [27]. An aggressive prevention regime would also be recommended for such cases.

Reconstruction of the edentulous patient

Immediate complete dentures are dental prostheses constructed to replace the teeth immediately after the removal of the last tooth/teeth.

Complete dentures

Immediate complete dentures

Immediate dentures may ease the patient's psychological distress of becoming edentulous, as they restore the appearance and facilitate speech and function, allowing the patient to continue a normal social and work life. Furthermore the dentures will initially act as a bandage for the healing tissues and stabilize the position of the mandible in relation to the cranial base, maintaining the occlusal vertical dimension.

Although there are no definite contraindications for immediate dentures when treating elderly patients who are otherwise fit, a transitional denture using a progressive series of extractions and immediate replacement plan may be preferred, especially in the mandible where denture retention is more difficult to achieve. The only group where immediate dentures may not be sensible would be patients where healing of the extraction sockets could be compromised, for example in patients taking bisphosphonates (see Chapter 12).

For immediate complete dentures the following treatment sequence is suggested:

1 Removal of posterior teeth 3–4 weeks prior to impression taking (right and left side consecutively to avoid bilateral block anaesthesia. Where possible occlusal stops should be maintained in the premolar region to maintain the occlusal vertical dimension).
2 Preliminary impression taking.
3 Functional secondary impression taking in a customized tray.
4 Recording of the jaw relationship in centric relation and at a reasonable vertical dimension (if not otherwise prescribed by the remaining teeth).
5 Mounting of posterior teeth and trial of the set-up to ensure patient satisfaction with the appearance of those elements of the prosthesis that are visible at that stage.
6 Replacement of the natural anterior teeth on the plaster cast by denture teeth, usually one by one in the same position as the natural teeth to support neuromuscular and psychological adaptation to the dentures.
7 After extraction the dentures are inserted and the patient instructed to keep the dentures in place until the following morning.
8 Denture use and care instructions are provided and postoperative care is provided as needed. Occlusal adjustments are performed once the denture has settled into the denture bearing tissues.
9 Gross tissue changes are usually completed 3–6 months after extraction. At this time a permanent denture can be constructed or the immediate denture can be relined or rebased.

Complete dentures

In a stage of life when the context of oral health care is dominantly influenced by multiple comorbidities, loss of autonomy as well as functional (and sensorial) impairment, treatment options are often limited to removable prostheses without tooth or implant support. These have to be designed to meet the individual's requirements in terms of comfort, aesthetics, cleaning ability, handling and chewing stability.

Requirements for dentures for the oldest old include:

- well polished surfaces which facilitate cleaning;
- absence of crevices which exacerbate food and plaque retention;
- rigid denture body which can withstand occasional clumsy handling;
- moderate cusp inclination and some 'freedom' in centric occlusion to meet the age-related function of the TMJ (flattened condylar inclination, loosened ligaments);
- mutually acceptable tooth colour and dental appearance (this may include darker shade selection, simulation of incisal wear, increased visibility of the lower anterior teeth and reduced visibility of the upper anterior teeth);
- labelling of the dentures (label with the patient's name and identify corresponding upper and lower dentures), especially when the patient lives in a long-term care facility (Figure 22.15)

The patient's adaptation to complete dentures is a complex process which may be influenced by:

- the dimensions of the supporting tissues, particularly in the mandible;
- the physical retention of the prosthesis which is enhanced by localized tissue compression during functional impression taken in combination with a film of saliva;
- a balanced articulation which stabilizes both dentures on the denture bearing tissues during function;
- motor skills of the cheeks, lips and tongue to manage the denture during chewing and speech;
- neuroplasticity which enables adjusting neuromuscular pattern to the altered oral environment.

Physical retention is greatest when a well made new denture has settled into the tissues, but during the life-span of the prosthesis this reduces as the quality of adaptation of the denture base to the underlying supporting tissues deteriorates as a result of continued alveolar bone resorption. As the physical aspects of retention decrease, the wearer has to rely

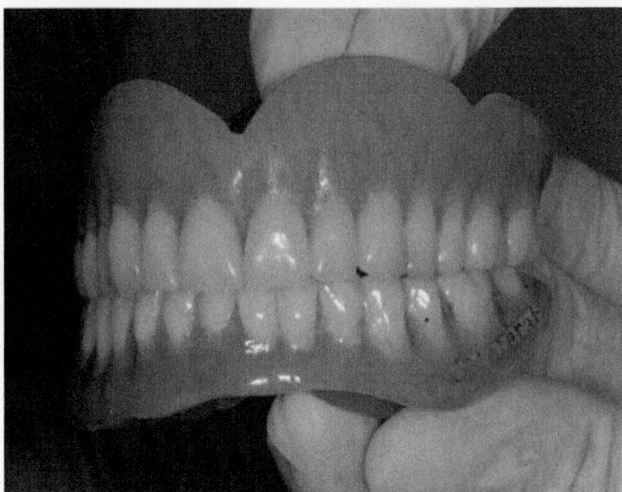

Figure 22.15 Especially in institutionalized patients, it is wise to label sets of dentures with the patient's name or initials.

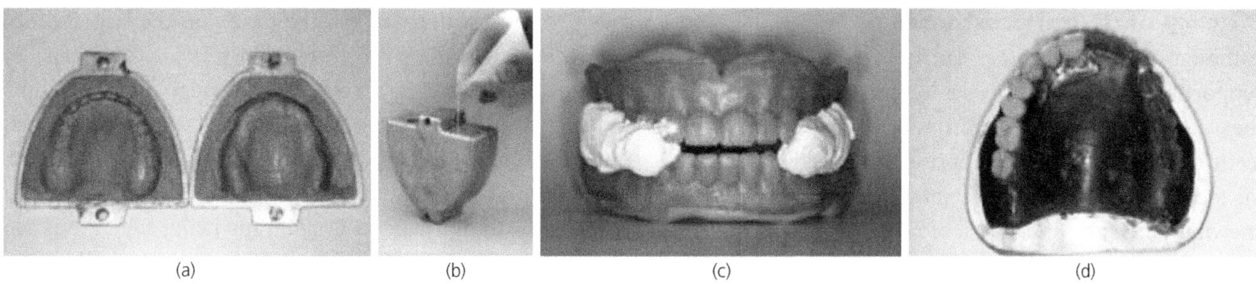

Figure 22.16 For renewing an existing complete denture by means of duplication techiques, the old denture is first flasked in alginate **(a)**, poured in cold-cure acrylic **(b)**, relined and, after registration of the RC **(c)**, mounted in the articulator. Before flasking, the 'pink' teeth are replaced one by one with white denture teeth **(d)**. This allows replication of selected features of an existing denture in the new prosthesis.

increasingly on learned muscular skills [28]. Patients become 'oral acrobats' to a degree, which allows them to manage a denture which has little or no physical retention or may even be fractured into several pieces.

Complete dentures for the oldest old

The aging process may render wearing complete dentures particularly difficult, because the anatomical conditions become less favourable with advanced alveolar ridge resorption. Xerostomia will reduce the amount of available saliva and tends to increase its viscosity altering the delicate balance required for physical denture retention. Furthermore, the protective effects of saliva are reduced, increasing the fragility of the oral mucosa which may also lose its elastic properties and mechanical resistance with age. Further problems may arise from poor motor control and slow reflex modification, in particular when the physiological aging is compounded by age-related neuromuscular degeneration in conditions such as Parkinson's disease or mandibular dyskinesia. Finally, depression, cognitive impairment and dementia may lead to serious complete denture adaptation problems. When aging and disease impair the muscular skills, care should be taken to avoid aspiration or swallowing of the dental prostheses which can become a significant choking risk [29]. When the conditions are unfavourable to gain denture stability, it is of particular importance to place the artificial teeth in the muscular equilibrium between lips, tongue and cheeks. 'Neutral zone' impression techniques can be helpful to determine the ideal placement of the artificial dental arch.

Treatment modalities should be considered which take the old patient's reduced adaptation capacity into account and aim to limit the change of the intraoral environment. Hence, modifications of existing dentures should be performed step-wise and preferably by means of reversible measures in case the change exceeds the patient's neuroplasticity. It is wise to leave an existing successful restoration 'untouched'. Duplication techniques allow selected successful features of an existing denture to be imported into the new one [Figure 22.16(a)–(d)]. Features which can be copied from the old prostheses comprise:

1 the fitting surface/adaptation to the denture bearing tissues (if a spare, identical denture is manufactured);
2 occlusal surfaces, including cusp inclination;
3 polished surface morphology of the denture body;
4 location and shape of the dental arch;
5 vertical dimension of occlusion;
6 static and dynamic occlusal relationships;
7 colour and shape of the front teeth.

Whereas the fitting surface and the occlusal surface are usually changed during the duplication of a complete denture to improve retention and food comminution, most other features are kept during manufacturing the new prostheses to minimize the need for adaptation to a new prosthesis. Obviously improving the denture retention by replacing the fitting surface with one that is better adapted to the denture bearing area also has the benefit of reducing the dependence on learned muscular skills to achieve denture function. This is also a valuable treatment approach for all patients with reduced motor control or cognitive impairment. Worn occlusal surfaces are also replaced in most duplicated dentures, as they help with cutting the food.

Denture adhesives are a valuable, cost-effective and non-invasive part of our armamentarium to help with achieving denture retention and improving chewing stability. They are not a substitute for a well-fitting prosthesis and their use as a palliative when poor denture design or with age of the prosthesis should be discouraged. However, many patients will find them of benefit, even with well-fitting prostheses, and we need to educate our patients about denture hygiene and the challenges of removal of fixative from the denture base. They are of limited benefit to patients with xerostomia as they depend on adequacy of saliva for hydration and function.

Efficacy of dental prostheses

Although dental prostheses can replace lost tissue volume supporting the lips and cheeks to provide aesthetic benefit, they can only partly restore orofacial functions. Denture teeth do not provide the proprioceptive feedback of natural teeth. Complete dentures show a considerably inferior chewing efficiency and bite force compared with a natural dentition. Consequently most patients gradually adapt their diet towards softer and more easy to chew foods. Improving chewing function by restorative means does not automatically improve a patient's nutritional intake [30]. Careful nutritional intervention is recommended to translate the benefit of an improved chewing efficiency into a balanced and healthy nutritional intake [31] (see Chapter 11). Nevertheless, the majority of complete wearers are subjectively satisfied with their tooth replacement. The older the patient, the less pronounced is the demand for improvement [32], yet efficient chewing might be beneficial in fighting malnutrition and morbidity in certain systemic conditions [33].

Recall, maintenance and repair

The insertion of a denture must not be regarded as the end of the treatment for any patient as resorption of the alveolar bone continues with age and is potentially increased if the oral mucosa becomes inflamed. Regular recall visits are required to assure the continuous adaptation of the denture base to the edentulous ridges and to verify denture retention and stability. It is also important to ensure oral mucosal health during these visits for both the denture bearing area and elsewhere in the mouth. Irregular bone resorption and a lack of saliva may lead to sore-spots on the denture bearing tissues which usually heal within a few days following denture base adjustment. More advanced bone resorption might require compensation through relining of the denture. Prolonged low-grade trauma at the periphery of an ill-fitting denture base can result in the development of a 'denture granuloma' that will then further complicate denture placement. An upper denture that becomes loose within a few weeks might not only require a reline but also a general health examination as it might be a first indicator of a neurodegenerative decline [34].

Implant-supported overdentures

Once the last tooth roots have been removed, options for treatment have been significantly reduced. In the past this meant that the patient could realistically only be offered, and some would now say condemned to, conventional complete dentures. Whilst there are many patients who are content with conventional complete dentures resting on the oral mucosa, the dental literature is littered with examples of patients who struggle with these prostheses. By far the largest problem is associated with the lower denture, which has a smaller support area, often on a relatively flat ridge, surrounded by the active muscles of the tongue and the lips. To see this in context it should be noted that simply being edentulous fulfils the World Health Organisation's (WHO) definition of a physical impairment. In addition, being edentulous can be recognized as a disability, as it impacts on eating and speaking. This often leads to individuals modifying their interactions with others. Thus, for example, when they avoid eating in the company of others because of problems with chewing, this fulfils the WHO definition of a handicap.

Before the advent of reliable osseointegrated implants to help to support dental prostheses for edentulous subjects there was little that could be done other than trying to minimize these problems by fabricating removable prostheses of a high quality. With the above observations in mind, it is hardly surprising that the initial clinical work using osseointegration was targeted at edentulous people, but rather than removable prostheses it was the fixed restorations that were regarded as the 'gold standard' of treatment at that time. This is understandable as it represents the opportunity to mimic the state that existed before the ravages of disease caused the patient to be rendered edentulous. It also reflected the country of origin where modern implants were pioneered where the first choice option for missing teeth would be a fixed rather than removable prosthesis. On an individual basis it is quite easy to make a case for the fixed options being preferable, but if we want to make a difference to the whole population of edentulous patients it is unlikely that this would be a realistic option either professionally or financially in the next few decades at least. This then was the premise that underlined the meetings that developed the McGill and York Consensus Statements [35, 36]. These statements proposed that edentulous patients should be offered mandibular overdentures supported by two osseointegrated dental implants, rather than conventional complete dentures, as the minimum standard of care.

The premise is not that an implant-supported overdenture is the best available treatment for edentulous patients, but rather that it is better than the alternative of a conventional complete denture. This gives the prosthodontist a greater opportunity to achieve a *reasonable level* of function and aesthetics and so help to fulfil a patient's wishes or to offer a *reasonable* or a *feasible level* of treatment planning. For edentulous patients, the implant-supported overdenture is perhaps the lowest standard of care that an affluent developed society should offer these disabled people.

Surprisingly little work has been done looking at long- or short-term cost effectiveness of prosthetic treatment as opposed to the cost of the prosthesis. Cost means different things to patients, dentists, and to research economists. Takanashi *et al.* (2004) for instance have shown that the time taken to construct a removable overdenture by a prosthodontist is exactly the same as for a conventional complete denture [37]. Nevertheless, although the 'cost' in terms of the prosthodontist will be the same, the charge the prosthodontist makes to the patient for this care is usually quite different (much greater for the implant-supported overdenture). There will be some modest extra expense for an implant-supported prosthesis in terms of any 'implant hardware' that needs to be used at the prosthodontic stage. However the discrepancy between costs for conventional and implant-supported prostheses is greater than the sum of the two. Studies have attempted to look at the actual cost for the construction and maintenance of conventional complete dentures and two implant-supported overdentures [38]. Although limited data are available, it is clear that the additional cost of implant overdenture treatment over the life expectancy of the patient is relatively small compared with the cost in the first year. Little or no work has been undertaken to compare the cost effectiveness of removable and fixed implant-supported prostheses. Indeed there has been a specific call for 'additional meta-analyses on well conducted randomized-controlled trials that include relevant economic assessments' [39].

Despite this lack of relevant cost effectiveness data, the clear advantage of overdentures supported by two implants in the mandible is that they directly address the most serious problems encountered by complete denture wearers. These are of stability and support for the mandibular denture which has a much smaller denture bearing area to dissipate the occlusal load and a less favourable contour than the maxilla to provide stability. As such, resources are targeted at the area where they can be most effective and potentially give the greatest single benefit for patients. Data from the Montreal Group have consistently shown substantial improvements in general satisfaction, comfort, stability and chewing ability in the order of 30% or more compared with conventional dentures [40–42], with similar levels of impact on oral health-related quality of life [43] (see Chapter 23). The limited published qualitative data relating to prosthetic rehabilitation has highlighted the social restrictions that conventional complete denture wearing can lead to [44–47]. Patients are often concerned about being embarrassed when eating with strangers, friends or even family, although they often do not disclose this information unless specifically questioned. Indeed, those with extensive problems may even avoid social situations completely. Hyland *et al.* showed that patients provided with implant-supported overdentures were much more likely to report improvements both in what they could eat and in how they felt eating with others than those provided with conventional dentures [45].

Masticatory function/chewing ability

In addition to patient perceived improvements in chewing ability with implant-supported overdentures, a recent systematic review [48] assessed studies objectively measuring masticatory performance published between 1996 and 2007. The trials included in this review compared masticatory performance of implant-supported dentures with conventional dentures using standardized masticatory tests. They concluded that implant-supported overdentures provide significant improvements in masticatory performance compared with conventional dentures for both the mandible and maxilla of those having persistent functional problems.

There is an increasing number of both randomized and non-randomized studies that support the view that implant-supported mandibular overdentures are perceived by patients to be preferable to conventional dentures and that these data are supported by objective measures of denture function. This tends not to be the case for maxillary implant overdentures where there have been specific and very marked problems.

Implant placement

Traditionally, two implants have been placed in the region between the mental foramina in the anterior mandible as part of a two-stage procedure, but more recently, the usual practice is to use a one-stage rather than a two-stage approach. Some work is also being undertaken with 'mini implant' fixtures that are smaller in diameter and shorter than conventional implants. Early data for these systems are encouraging but currently are insufficient to warrant widespread advocacy. Attachments are added to the implant to provide both support and retention for the overdenture. Different attachment systems have resulted in different overall outcomes with the greatest benefit seeming to be offered by a bar joining the 2 implants, followed by separate ball attachments and then individual magnetic attachments (for a review see reference [49]).

It is important that the implant is positioned so that the attachment can be contained within the planned 'envelope' of the final denture and so it is advisable to start the procedure with an optimized denture so that the final contour of the definitive denture is known and the implant placement can be managed accordingly. The procedure for denture construction is the same as for conventional mandibular overdentures over dental roots, though it is critical that the position of the implant abutments is recorded with

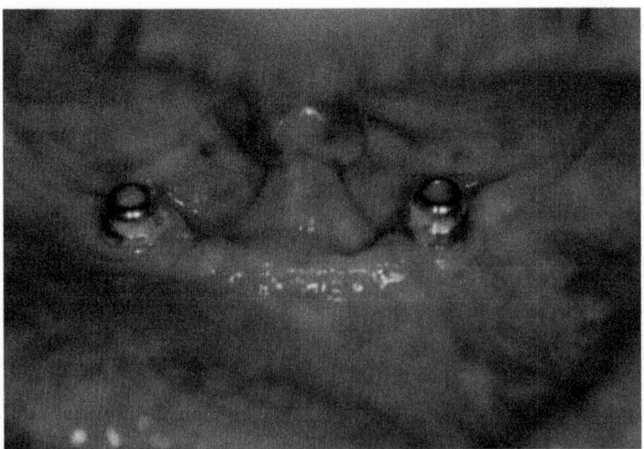

Figure 22.17 Implants to retain and support overdentures provide functional, structural and psychosocial benefits to edentate patients, whereby the number of implants and the chosen attachment system seem to have little impact on the patient's satisfaction.

precision. This is usually managed with a transfer impression which allows abutment-analogues to be located in the stone models on which the dentures will be made. It has generally been thought that implant-supported prostheses 'must' be more difficult or complicated than conventional therapies. However, whilst the processes will have more stages these are not necessarily more complicated or difficult. Indeed clinical stages such as registration are easier to undertake as the record blocks are held consistently in place by the implants. The little work that has been undertaken asking clinicians about the level of difficulty suggests that it is perhaps actually easier to construct an implant-supported overdenture, rather than a conventional denture [50].

Implants are not however the solution for all patients as they may not be accepted by fragile and dependent patients who fear the time and surgical intervention, even if cost does not play a role [51] (Figure 22.17). Further contraindications may arise from general health conditions.

Plaque control and denture hygiene

Plaque control is enhanced by proper motivation and instruction of the patient and monitored and maintained by using an individual recall system for professional oral hygiene. Most elderly denture-wearers respond favourably to motivation and instruction in oral hygiene. The frequency of recall and review should be based on the level of disease risk an individual patient presents with. Recall intervals should be reduced for those with increased risk of decay or periodontal disease based on past levels of disease and change associated with both oral rehabilitation and general health. Thus a recall interval should be short for someone being provided with a removable prosthesis for the first time to ensure that the changes in oral hygiene practices required by this change in their oral health status are being achieved. The recall interval can then be extended once an appropriate pattern of personal oral heath care has been established. It should be realized, however, that the person's ability or willingness to deliver personal oral health care may suddenly change due to debilitating diseases, change of living conditions or loss of relatives. These situations may result in neglect of oral hygiene followed by a rapid deterioration of teeth and more widespread mucosal infections. In such situations patients need professional care more often, such as monthly.

Professionals should be reluctant to introduce new brushing techniques to elderly people, as they may have difficulty in conforming with them. However, special brushing techniques are essential to control plaque on teeth adjacent to denture saddles and on the abutment teeth supporting overdentures. In overdenture wearers, removal of the dentures at night is very important to prevent caries and periodontal breakdown of the abutments [52, 27].

Removal of all prostheses at night should be recommended to reduce the risk of inflammatory change of the oral mucosa beneath the prosthesis. There is an increasing awareness that mucosal inflammation may result in both accelerated bone resorption and in the presence of circulating markers of inflammatory disease with potential implications for systemic health

Chemical agents may be important adjuncts in oral hygiene care of elderly people who are physically unable to maintain sufficient oral and denture hygiene. Thus, daily mouth-rinsing with chlorhexidine solutions or the application of chlorhexidine gels, as well as the immersion of dentures in chlorhexidine, are effective means in chemical plaque control but may profoundly change the environmental conditions of the oral cavity. This treatment may also stain teeth and dentures. Daily mouth-rinsing and denture immersion in chlorhexidine should only take place in association with monthly recalls for professional oral hygiene care.

Topical treatment with fluoride is an important means of reducing caries activity, especially on the root surfaces particularly exposed to caries. Thus, caries has been dramatically reduced in the abutment teeth for overlay dentures by topical fluoride therapy in caries-active patients.

A wide range of commercial chemical denture cleansers is available to the general public, but their effectiveness has not been proven conclusively, and they are no substitute for mechanical cleansing [53]. Thus, peroxide cleansers have only limited effect on denture plaque; hypochlorite cleansers are effective, but may cause tarnish to metal components and have a bad taste; acid cleansers that are based on hydrochloric acid are hazardous to use and should not be recommended. Bleaching of acrylic components of dentures is associated with the temperature of the solution into which the denture is placed for cleaning rather than any specific cleansing agent. It is essential that patients understand that denture cleaning solutions should be cold not hot.

Not wearing the dentures at night and keeping them dry is the most efficient way to control biofilms on dentures. However, some elderly patients may feel uncomfortable leaving their teeth 'on the dry'.

References

1 Lang, N.P., Ramseier, C.A. & Baur, H.R. (2013). Systemic phase of periodontal therapy. In: N.P. Lang & J. Lindhe (eds), *Periodontology and Implant Dentistry,* 6th edn, Ch. 35, Wiley Blackwell, Oxford, UK.

2 Bergenholtz, G. & Nyman, S. (1984) Endodontic complications following periodontal and prosthetic treatment of patients with advanced periodontal disease. *Journal of Periodontology,* **55,** 63–68.

3 Lang, N.P., Pjetursson, B.E., Tan, K., Brägger, U., Egger, M. & Zwahlen, M. (2004) A systematic review of the survival and complication rates of fixed partial dentures (FPDs) after an observation period of at least 5 years. II. Combined tooth--implant-supported FPDs. *Clinical Oral Implants Research,* **15,** 643–653.

4 Lulic, M., Brägger, U., Lang, N.P., Zwahlen, M. & Salvi, G.E. (2008) Ante's (1926) law revisited. A systematic review on survival rates and complications of fixed dentalprostheses (FDPs) on severely reduced periodontal tissue support. *Clinical Oral Implants Research,* **18**(Suppl. 3), 63–72.

5 Franks, A.S.T. (1967) The dental health of patients presenting with temporomandibular joint dysfunction. *British Journal of Oral Surgery,* **5,** 157–166.

6 Gerber, A. (1971) Kiefergelenk und Zahnokklusion. *Deutsche Zahnärztliche Zeitschrift,* **26,** 119–141.

7 Käyser, A.F. (1976). *De gebitsfuncties bij verkorte tandbogen. Tandheelkundige Monografieën 20.* University of Nijmegen, Stafflen & Tholen, Leiden.

8 Käyser, A.F. & van der Hoeven, J.S. (1977) Colorimetric determination of the masticatory performance. *Journal of Oral Rehabilitation,* **4,** 145–148.

9 Käyser, A.F. (1981). Shortened dental arches and oral function. *Journal of Oral Rehabilitation,* **8,** 457–462.

10 Witter, D.J., van Elteren, P. & Käyser, A.F. (1988) Signs and symptoms of mandibular dysfunction in shortened dental arches. *Journal of Oral Rehabilitation,* **15,** 413–420.

11 Battistuzzi, P.G.F.C.M. (1982) *Het gemutileerde gebit. Een beschrijvend epidemiologisch onderzoek.* Universiteit te Nijmegen, Klijsen b.v., Tilburg.

12 Imperiali, D., Grunder, U. & Lang, N.P. (1984) Oral hygiene habits, dental care and subjective chewing capacity in socioeconomically different population classes in Switzerland. *Schweizer Monatsschrift für Zahnmedizin,* **94,** 612–624.

13 Fontijn-Tekamp, F.A., Slagter, A.P., van der Bilt, A., van t'Hof, M.A., Witter, D.J. et al. (2000) Biting and chewing in overdentures, full dentures, and natural dentitions. *Journal of Dental Research,* **79,** 1519–1524.

14 Pilot T. (1978) Pleidooi tegen het verlengen van de verkorte tandboog. *Nederlandse Tijdschrift voor Tandheelkunde,* **85,** 477–480.

15 Pilot, T. (1980). Moet de verkorte tandboog verlengd worden met een partiële prothese? *Nederlandse Tandartsenblad,* **35,** 258–270.

16 Riesen, M., Chung, J.-P., Pazos, E. & Budtz-Jorgensen, E. (2002) Interventions bucco-dentaires chez les personnes âgées. *Médecine & Hygiène,* **2414,** 2178–2188.

17 Budtz-Jorgensen, E. (1999) *Prosthodontics for the elderly: diagnosis and treatment.* Quintessence, Chicago, IL.

18 Pjetursson, B.E., Tan, K., Lang, N.P., Brägger, U., Egger, M. & Zwahlen, M. (2004) A systematic review of the survival and complication rates of fixed partial dentures (FPDs) after an observation period of at least 5 years. *Clinical Oral Implants Research,* **15,** 625–642.

19 Pjetursson, B.E., Tan, K., Lang, N.P., Brägger, U., Egger, M. & Zwahlen, M. (2004) A systematic review of the survival and complication rates of fixed partial dentures (FPDs) after an observation period of at least 5 years. *Clinical Oral Implants Research,* **15,** 667–676.

20 Tan, K., Pjetursson, B.E., Lang, N.P. & Chan, E.S. (2004) A systematic review of the survival and complication rates of fixed partial dentures (FPDs) after an observation period of at least 5 years. *Clinical Oral Implants Research,* **15,** 654–666.

21 Nyman, S. & Lindhe, J. (1979) A longitudinal study of combined periodontal and prosthetic treatment of patients with advanced periodontal disease. *Journal of Periodontology,* **50,** 163–169.

22 Landolt, A. & Lang, N.P. (1986). Technical failures in extension bridge restorations. Results after four to eight years. *Journal of Oral Rehabilitation,* **14.**

23 Hegdahl, T. & Silness, J. (1977) Preparation areas resisting displacement of artificial crowns. *Journal of Oral Rehabilitation,* **4,** 201–207.

24 Pjetursson, B.E., Tan, W.C., Tan, K., Brägger, U., Zwahlen, M. & Lang, N.P. (2008) A systematic review of the survival and complication rates of resin-bonded bridges after an observation period of at least 5 years. *Clinical Oral Implants Research,* **19,** 131–141.

25 Thomason, J.M., Moynihan, P., Steen, I. & Jepson, N. (2007) Time to Survival for the Restoration of the Shortened Lower Dental Arch. *Journal of Dental Research,* **86,** 646–650.

26 Jepson, N.J.A., Allen, P.F., Moynihan, P.J., Kelly, P.J. & Thomason, J.M. (2003) Patient Satisfaction following the Restoration of Shortened Lower Dental Arches. *International Journal of Prosthodontics,* **16,** 409–414.

27 Budtz-Jørgensen, E. (1994) Effects of denture-wearing habits on periodontal health of abutment teeth in patients with overdentures. *Journal of Clinical Periodontology,* **21,** 265–269.

28 Müller, F., Heath, M.R., Ferman, A.M. & Davis, G.R. (2002) Modulation of mastication during experimental loosening of complete dentures. *International Journal of Prosthodontics*, **15**, 553–558.

29 Arora, A., Arora, M. & Roffe, C. (2005) Mystery of the missing denture: an unusual cause of respiratory arrest in a nonagenarian. *Age and Ageing*, **34**, 519–520.

30 Moynihan, P., Bradbury, J. & Müller, F. (2011) Dietary consequences of oral health in frail elders. In: M.I. MacEntee, F. Müller & C.C. Wyatt (eds), *Oral Healthcare and The Frail Elder*, pp. 73–94, Wiley-Blackwell, Ames, IA.

31 Bradbury, J., Thomason, J.M., Jepson, N.J., Walls, A.W.G., Allen, P.F. & Moynihan, P.J. (2006) Nutrition counseling increases fruit and vegetable intake in the edentulous. *Journal of Dental Research*, **85**, 463–468.

32 Müller, F. & Hasse-Sander, I. (1993) Experimental studies of adaptation to complete dentures related to ageing. *Gerodontology*, **10**, 23–27.

33 Faxen-Irving, G., Basun, H., & Cederholm, T. (2005) Nutritional and cognitive relationships and long-term mortality in patients with various dementia disorders. *Age and Ageing*, **34**, 136–141.

34 Magri, F., Borza, A., del Vecchio, S., Chytiris, S., Cuzzoni, G., Busconi, L., Rebesco, A. & Ferrari, E. (2003) Nutritional assessment of demented patients: a descriptive study. *Aging Clinical and Experimental Research*, **15**, 148–153.

35 Feine, J.S., Carlsson, G.E., Awad, M.A., Chehade, A., Duncan, W.J., Gizani, S. *et al.* (2002) The McGill consensus statement on overdentures. Mandibular two-implant overdentures as first choice standard of care for edentulous patients. *Journal of Prosthetic Dentistry*, **88**, 123–124.

36 Thomason, J.M., Feine, J., Exley, C., Moynihan, P., Müller, F., Naert, I. *et al.* (2009) Mandibular two implant-supported overdentures as the first choice standard of care for edentulous patients - the York Consensus Statement. *British Dental Journal*, **207**, 185–186.

37 Takanashi, Y., Penrod, J.R., Lund, J.P. & Feine, J.S. (2004) Cost Analysis of Mandibular 2-implant Overdenture Treatment from a Randomized Clinical Trial. *International Journal of Prosthodontics*, **17**, 181–186.

38 Heydecke, G., Takanashi, Y., Lund, J.P., Penrod, J.R., Feine, J.S. & Thomason, J.M. (2005) Cost-Effectiveness of Mandibular Conventional and Two-Implant Overdentures. *Journal of Dental Research*, **84**, 794–799.

39 Emami, E., Heydecke, G., Rompré, P.H., de Grandmont, P. & Feine, J.S. (2009) Impact of implant support for mandibular dentures on satisfaction, oral and general health-related quality of life: a meta-analysis of randomized-controlled trials. *Clinical Oral Implants Research*, **20**, 533–544.

40 Awad, M.A., Lund, J.P., Shapiro, S.H., Locker, D., Klemetti, E., Chehade, A. *et al.* (2003) Oral health status and treatment satisfaction with mandibular implant overdentures and conventional dentures. A randomized trial in a senior population. *International Journal of Prosthodontics*, **16**, 390–396.

41 Pan, S., Awad, M., Thomason, J.M., Dufresne, E., Kobayashi, T., & Kimoto, S. (2008) Sex differences in denture satisfaction. *Journal of Dentistry*, **36**, 301–308.

42 Thomason, J.M., Lund, J.P., Chehade, A. & Feine, J.S. (2003) Patient Satisfaction with Mandibular Implant Overdentures and Conventional Dentures Six months after Delivery. *International Journal of Prosthodontics*, **16**, 467–473.

43 Heydecke, G., Locker, D., Awad, M.A., Lund, J.P. & Feine, J.S. (2003) Oral and general health related quality of life with conventional and implant dentures. *Community Dentistry and Oral Epidemiology*, **31**, 161–168.

44 Fiske, J., Davis, D.M., Frances, C. & Gelbier, S. (1998) The emotional effects of tooth loss in edentulous people. *British Dental Journal*, **184**, 90–93.

45 Hyland, R.M., Ellis, J., Thomason, M., El-Feky, A. & Moynihan, P.J. (2009) A qualitative study on patient perspectives of how conventional and implant-supported dentures affect eating. *Journal of Dentistry*, **17**, 718–723.

46 MacEntee, M.I., Hole, R. & Stolar, E. (1997) The significance of the mouth in old age. *Social Science & Medicine*, **45**, 1449–1458.

47 Trulsson, U., Engstrand, P., Berggren, U., Nannmark, U. & Branemark, P.-I. (2002) Edentulousness and oral rehabilitation: experiences from the patients' perspective. *European Journal of Oral Sciences*, **110**, 417–424.

48 Fueki, K., Kimoto, K., Ogawa, T. & Garrett, N.R. (2007) Effect of implant-supported or retained dentures on masticatory performance: a systematic review. *Journal of Prosthetic Dentistry*, **98**, 470–477.

49 Thomason, J.M., Heydecke, G., Feine, J.S. & Ellis, J.S. (2007) How do patients perceive the benefit of reconstructive dentistry with regard to oral health related quality of life and patient satisfaction? *Clinical Oral Implants Research*, **18**, 168–188.

50 Esfandiari, S., Lund, J.P., Thomason, J.M., Dufresne, E., Kobayashi, T., Dubois, M. *et al.* (2006) Can general dentists produce successful implant overdentures with minimal training? *Journal of Dentistry*, **34**, 796–801.

51 Walton, J.N. & MacEntee, M.I. (2005) Choosing or refusing oral implants: a prospective study of edentulous volunteers for a clinical trial. *International Journal of Prosthodontics*, **18**, 483–488.

52 Budtz-Jørgensen, E. (1992) Prognosis of overdenture abutments in the aged: effect of denture wearing habits. *Community Dentistry and Oral Epidemiolology*, **20**, 302–306.

53 Budtz-Jørgensen, E. (1979) Material and methods for cleaning dentures. *Journal of Prosthetic Dentistry*, **42**, 619–623.

CHAPTER 23

Oral health-related quality of life

Finbarr Allen[1] and Jimmy Steele[2]

[1]Department of Restorative Dentistry, University College Cork, Cork, Ireland
[2]School of Dental Sciences, Newcastle University, Newcastle upon Tyne, UK

What is 'quality of life?'

In recent medical and dental literature, 'quality of life' has become a ubiquitous term. However, it is clear that it means different things to different authors. In an effort to focus on the assessment of health and quality of life issues, the term 'health-related quality of life' is now widely used. Other terms used include 'subjective health status' and 'functional status' [1].

There is a complex relationship between health, disease and quality of life and the nature of the inter-relationships are not clearly defined. Locker [2] proposed a model to explain the interaction between oral health, disease and quality of life which will be described later in the chapter. In this model, while health problems may affect quality of life, such a consequence is not inevitable. Examples of this relationship are found in studies of quality of life issues in both medical and dental literature. For example, Decker and Schultz [3] found that satisfaction with quality of life of middle aged and spinal cord injury patients was reported as only slightly worse than controls. Evans [4] has reported that a group of patients receiving haemodialysis had levels of quality of life satisfaction which exceeded that of a healthy population.

The implication of such studies is that people with chronic disabling disorders often perceive their quality of life as better than healthy individuals; that is, poor health or presence of disease does not inevitably mean poor quality of life. Indeed these findings suggest that the way people rate their quality of life is capable of adjustment according to circumstances. Allison *et al.* [5] attempted to further explain this phenomenon by suggesting that quality of life was a 'dynamic construct'. Individuals' attitudes are not constant: they vary with time and experience and are modified by phenomena such as coping, expectancy and adaptation. They give as an example an individual who had eating problems due to pain and discomfort, who would have rated this problem as extremely important at one point in time. However, when this problem is diagnosed as oral cancer and treated with radiotherapy and surgery, the same individual may report the original problem as relatively unimportant.

Models of health and disease

The traditional biomedical model has focused on measurement of stages in diseases processes. In dentistry this might be the decayed, missing, filled teeth index (DMFT), community periodontal index of treatment needs (CPITN) or any of a range of similar measures of disease. However, important as these measures are, they only reflect the disease processes. They give no indication of the impact of the disease on function or psychosocial well-being. Increasingly, it is recognized that disease impacts upon people differently and this, in turn, may influence attitudes to health care and response to treatment intervention.

The limitations of the 'biomedical' paradigm of health have been recognized. However, health and disease are themselves, in sociological terms, independent dimensions of human experience and not part of a continuum [2]. This was recognized by WHO as early as 1948, when health was defined as 'a complete state of physical, mental and social well-being, and not merely the absence of illness'. More recently, distinctions have been made between disease ('abnormalities in anatomical structures, physiological or biochemical processes') and illness ('subjective perception of changes in his/her physical, mental and social well-being') [6]. Consequently,

Textbook of Geriatric Dentistry, Third Edition. Edited by Poul Holm-Pedersen, Angus W. G. Walls and Jonathan A. Ship.

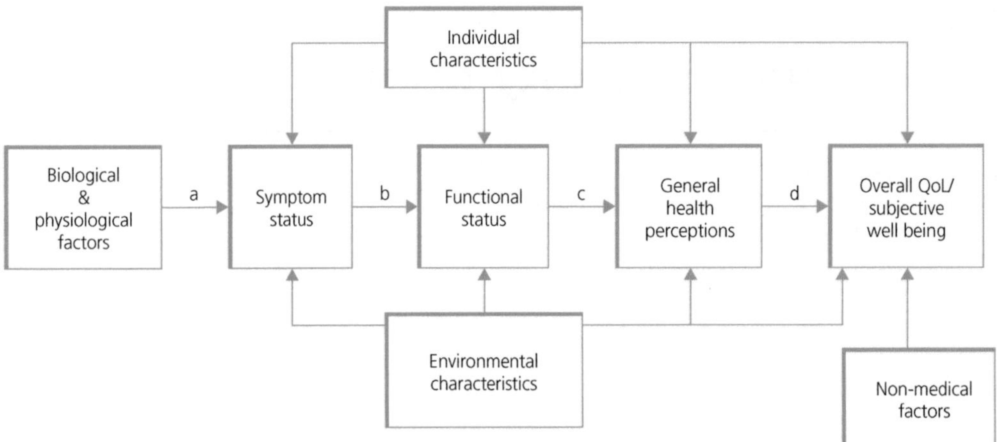

Figure 23.1 Links between clinical variables and quality of life. Model proposed by Wilson and Cleary, 1995 [7].

any measure of health needs to assess social and emotional aspects of health as well as assessing the presence or absence of disease.

In the socio-environmental model of health, each of these separate conceptual domains is recognized; the complex multi-dimensional nature of health is encompassed, including cultural, environmental and psycho-social influences. Various conceptual frameworks for measuring health have been described, an example of which is shown in Figure 23.1 [7].

When interpreting a model such as this, it is important to recognize that the component variables may operate independently of one another, or be of varying importance at certain points in time.

Oral health-related quality of life and older people

One of the implicit purposes of managing disease in the young is to intercept its progression, reducing any impairment through tooth loss or damage at an early stage, with lifetime benefits. In this environment the traditional importance attached to early detection and management of oral disease as the focus of oral health care is understandable, despite the obvious limitations. When we start to consider the aims of individual dental treatments or how we can evaluate the success of our oral health services, the conceptual models such as those described above can help us to look beyond disease and to understand the impact of dentistry and oral health services on 'oral health-related quality of life'. Thinking about and understanding the impact of clinical interventions at this level is a fundamental step in understanding what it is that dentists and dental services do. This approach focuses on the patient rather than the disease.

In older people the management of all disease may be neither feasible, nor desirable, nor cost effective. When thinking about the aims of dental care in older people, intercepting disease, whilst still relevant, is not always the predominant aim of treatment. The restoration of function, with a view to nutrition, would be one important aim. A focus on maintaining or improving quality of life may be the other. The result may be a different way of thinking about treatment planning.

The dynamic construct described by Allison *et al.* [5] is particularly important in this context. On one hand, the cumulative nature of dental disease and its 'cradle to grave' impact mean that the level of physical impairment can be high by old age. At its worst the impairment may be a complete loss of teeth and alveolar bone, rendering function and comfort severely impaired. On the other hand, competing health demands might be expected to ameliorate the impact of declining oral health. The way that these two considerations play out at an individual level might be a useful, all be it imprecise, way to think about how treatment need can be defined in older people.

Theoretical framework for measuring oral health

The concept of quality of life may be useful to inform decision making, including clinical decisions, but to do that you have to be able to measure it. Measuring quality of life would allow populations to be understood, informing everything from health policy to the effectiveness of individual interventions. The detailed uses will be discussed in the next section but it is important to first grasp the concepts of measurement.

Measuring quality of life is a conceptual challenge, not least because of the highly individualized nature of the human experience. However, a number of health status measures have

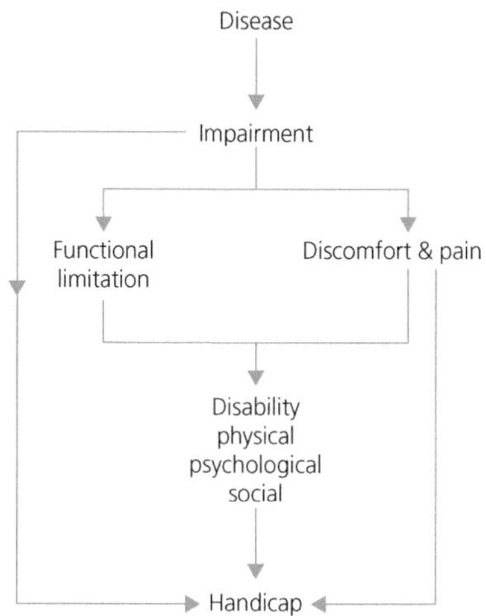

Figure 23.2 Conceptual model for measuring oral health. Reproduced from Locker, 1988 [2].

been derived, based on the impact of oral health on the individual. These measures are now fairly widely used and serve as the best proxy available for measures of oral health-related quality of life. Some of these count the negative impacts of problems related to the mouth and order them according to a structure, others attempt to capture both positive and negative influences. All are questionnaire-based instruments, but rather than being a selection of questions plucked out of the atmosphere, they are generally based on a conceptual framework which gives them their structure. The same conceptual frameworks we discussed earlier in this chapter.

The basis for several of these measures is the conceptual framework for measuring oral health status described by Locker [2] shown in Figure 23.2. This is based on the WHO [8] classification of impairment, disability and handicap, and attempts to capture all possible functional and psycho-social outcomes of oral disorders (see Chapter 10).

The publication of this conceptual framework has been pivotal to the development of this research theme in dentistry. Until relatively recently, the psycho-social consequences of oral conditions had received little attention, as they are rarely life threatening. Furthermore, the oral cavity has historically been dissociated from the rest of the body when considering general health status. However, research has highlighted that oral disorders have emotional and psycho-social consequences as serious as other disorders.

Subjective appraisal of oral health – qualitative methodology

Qualitative research is commonly used to explore, interpret or obtain a 'deeper understanding' of certain aspects of human beliefs, attitudes or behaviour, such as personal experiences and perspectives [9]. It is not quantitative and seeks to ascribe meaning rather than measuring a specific outcome. Qualitative methods are used to study individual responses to specific contexts and to attempt to ascribe meaning to these phenomena. Accordingly, this type of research is not guided by the rules used in quantitative research such as representative sampling, power calculations and probability testing.

Qualitative methodology follows either an 'inductive' process whereby a hypothesis is developed by gathering data from patients (e.g. 'Grounded Theory') or a 'deductive' process whereby data are gathered to confirm a predetermined theory or hypothesis. Sampling for this type of research is purposive; that is, subjects are selected in order to broadly represent a particular condition. For example, if one were interested in assessing the partially dentate state, the researcher would select subjects based on age, gender, missing tooth spaces restored and unrestored and denture wearing experience. This is an iterative process aimed at obtaining a study group broadly representative of the condition of interest. Data can be collected using a variety of approaches. These include:

1 Focus groups
2 Interviews (structured, semi-structured, unstructured)
3 Observation

In dentistry there are a number of reports published which have used qualitative methodology. Friedman *et al.* [10] have described three classes of maladaptive responses to complete dentures:

1 maladaptive class 1: patients who can adapt physically but not emotionally,
2 maladaptive class 2: patients who cannot adapt physically or emotionally,
3 maladaptive class 3: patients who cannot and do not wear dentures, who are chronically depressed and who isolate themselves from society.

Using a qualitative approach, they also describe three influences they believe influence the maladaptive response. *Parental influence* may affect how an individual may perceive themselves and their teeth. Teeth may also have a *symbolic significance*, and loss of teeth may be reflect impending loss of virility, facial attractiveness and body degeneration. Finally, *current life circumstances* may strongly influence the adaptive response to tooth loss. If there are strong extraneous influences (e.g. recent bereavement, unemployment, diagnosis of life threatening illness etc.), the ability of the individual to accept complete loss of natural teeth may be seriously compromised.

Another example of the use of a qualitative approach to assess the emotional effects of tooth loss has been reported by Fiske *et al.* [11]. Using an unstructured interview technique, 50 edentulous individuals were invited to discuss their feelings about tooth loss, from the time of being rendered edentulous. The study sample was recruited from patients attending for conventional prosthodontic treatment at an undergraduate student clinic. There was no suggestion in the paper that any of the study subjects demonstrated maladaptive tendencies. Common themes which emerged from these interviews were: feelings of bereavement, lowered self-confidence, altered self-image, dislike of appearance, an inability to discuss this taboo subject, a concern about their dignity, behaving in a way that keeps tooth loss secret, altered behaviour in socializing and forming close relationships and premature aging. The conclusion of this study was that tooth loss can profoundly affect the psycho-social well-being of patients, even those apparently coping well with dentures.

These findings were similar to those reported by MacEntee *et al.* [12], who advocated the use of qualitative methodology to explore fully the significance of the mouth in old age. The findings reported in these studies should be interpreted with some caution, as subjects were recruited from specialist treatment centres. Many of these patients will have been referred from general practice for specialist advice and care and as such may not be truly representative of the whole population.

In terms of partially dentate older adults, the impact of tooth loss and its treatment has been assessed in Irish [13] and British [14] adults. In the Irish context, key themes to emerge were the rising importance older adults ascribe to teeth, particularly conservation of teeth, and the relationship between dentists and patients. It was interesting to note that patients under the age of 65 years had higher expectations of what dentists can provide for them and expected to have significant input into decision making about their oral health. Patients over the age of 65 years appear to have lower expectations and are more likely to accept without question the recommendations of dentists. Graham *et al.* [14] were investigating the possible reasons for non-compliance with partial denture (RPD) wearing by partially dentate adults. They conducted two sets of semi-structured interviews, one with dentists and a second with patients. For dentists, RPD provision was indicated by patient demand and physical function of the remaining teeth but was mediated by NHS fee structures and professional satisfaction. For patients, RPD use was influenced by the trade-off between improved appearance and the unpalatable presence of an RPD in their mouth. The location of the gap(s) was important, but other issues were relevant such as ability to 'manage' without the RPD. They concluded that this divergence in priorities may partly explain why some patients provided with partial dentures fail to wear them. In view of the considerable waste of public resource that this represents, further research on the relationship between denture use and social identity was suggested.

When interpreting qualitative research, it is important to remember that the findings are context specific. For example, the responses can be influenced by the nature of the health care system in the country in which the sample resides. Accordingly, it cannot be assumed that results from a particular study are generalizable. Nonetheless, qualitative research improves our understanding of particular conditions and their impact on daily living. Additionally, qualitative research using grounded theory can be used to develop health status measures for quantitative research.

Uses of health status measures

Quantitative methods can be used to overcome the aforementioned limitation of context specificity in qualitative research. At the outset, it is important to acknowledge the role of qualitative methods to aid the development of quantitative tools such as health status measures. On a population level, the importance of assessing both patients' perceptions of health and presence or absence of disease lies in the need to have accurate data to promote health, to evaluate disease prevention programmes [15] and to allow sensible allocation of health resources [1]. Furthermore, as patients' assessment of their health-related quality of life is often markedly different to the opinion of health care professionals [16], patients' assessment of health care interventions are warranted. Uses of health-related quality of life measures have been described by Fitzpatrick *et al.* [1], and are shown in Box 23.1.

Box 23.1 Uses of measures of health-related quality of life.

- Screening and monitoring for psychosocial problems in individual patient care.
- Population surveys of perceived health problems.
- Medical audit.
- Outcome measures in health services or evaluation research.
- Clinical trials.
- Cost-utility analysis.

Slade and Spencer [17] have also suggested that such measures may also be used to advocate oral health, especially when attempting to secure public funds for oral health care. The information provided by these measures facilitates an increasing understanding of how individuals perceive oral health needs and what oral health outcomes drive them to seek health care.

The appropriate terminology for such measures when applied to oral health is slightly problematic. All of those which are widely used in oral health and described as 'oral health-related quality of life' measures might be more accurately described as measures of subjective oral health status, and this is the term we will use from now on.

Methodological requirements in health status measurement

Before going further with oral health status measurement, we should first cover some more generic methodological issues. As research into health-related quality of life has grown, so has the use of health status measures. Patient-based assessments of the impact of a wide variety of chronic conditions have been reported. The sophistication of measures currently available varies widely, and a number of theoretical issues need to be considered when selecting a health status measure.

The main requirements of a health status measure have been summarized by Fitzpatrick *et al.* [1]. These are: (1) multidimensional construct; (2) reliability; (3) validity; (4) sensitivity to change; (5) appropriateness and 6) practical utility.

Multidimensional construct. In keeping with the socio-environmental model of health, a measure must assess many dimensions. The dimensions of 'quality of life' incorporated in available health status measures are summarized in Box 23.2:

Box 23.2 Dimensions of quality of life.

- Physical function - e.g. mobility, self-care.
- Emotional function - e.g. depression, anxiety.
- Social function - e.g. intimacy, social contact.
- Role performance - e.g. work.
- Pain.
- Other symptoms - e.g. fatigue, nausea.

Reliability of a measure refers to its ability to produce the same results with repeated use under the same conditions.

Validity is a broad term which has a number of different components, the most important of which are construct and discriminant validity. Validity relates to how well we actually measure what we are trying to measure. *Construct* validity is concerned with the pattern of relations of the instrument with other more established measures. *Discriminant* validity is the ability of the instrument to detect differences in specific conditions between different populations. Once validity properties have been demonstrated for assessment of specific conditions or populations, it cannot be assumed to be valid for all circumstances [18]. For example, a measure which demonstrates good validity properties in the assessment of rheumatoid arthritis in elderly adults may not be valid in the assessment of juvenile rheumatoid arthritis.

Sensitivity to change is an essential requirement of a health status measure in clinical trials and longitudinal studies [18]. This property is also referred to as the 'responsiveness' of the measure. Ideally, a measure should be capable of detecting small changes over time. Fitzpatrick *et al.* [1] identified four factors which may affect the responsiveness of a measure. Firstly, the use of a generic measure with a large number of statements may include several items not relevant to the group in question. Secondly, the measure may contain too few quality of life domains and may not therefore be sensitive to subtle changes. Thirdly, the instrument may contain items not readily affected by a clinical intervention, such as the pattern of social relationships. Finally, the measure may be subject to ceiling or floor effects; that is, unable to register further improvement or deterioration in subjects (if a narrow range of responses is available).

Appropriateness refers to how relevant the measure is to the group being assessed. It is not appropriate, for example, to use a measure developed for psychiatric patients in a non-psychiatric population. It is essential to think carefully about what is being assessed prior to using a health status measure. A 'scatter gun' approach, where a battery of instruments is used to uncover unexpected problems, may result in significant findings by chance because of the large number of variables tested.

Practical utility involves using an instrument which only contains sufficient items to answer the research question. This is particularly relevant in clinical settings, as using a large generic questionnaire may not be feasible. Care is required with this approach, however, as shorter instruments may omit items which may be relevant to the population in question.

When interpreting data using an oral health status measure, the considerations above are important. However no one tool will be perfect in terms of these requirements, and certain attributes may be more desirable in certain circumstances. So for example, excellent sensitivity to change would be essential for a tool to be used as an outcome measure in a trial, but may be less important when comparing populations. Most of the widely used oral health status measures have been through a process of validation, often in a variety of circumstances and groups. Matching the measure to the purpose is clearly an important step.

Oral health status measurement

Indices such as CPITN and DMFT have been used frequently to assess prevalence of dental diseases and to inform policy on provision of oral health care. These measures indicate disease extent and reflect measurement of the progress of the biological disease process. They provide no information on how disease affects daily living for individuals or of patients' judgement of their health status. The literature in the medical field illustrates that a dichotomy often exists between patient-based and professionally assessed treatment need. Frequently, preconceived notions that disease status adversely affects quality of life have been proved incorrect.

Such information is important when planning health care and monitoring the effect of clinical interventions, and nowhere more so than in older people.

The need for patient-based assessment of oral health was first recognized in the mid-1970s by Cohen and Jago [19]. The next landmark was the publication of a report by Reisine [20] in 1984 which indicated that working days lost in the USA due to dental problems numbered in the millions. Locker [2] suggested that whilst such information was important on a societal level it provided no information at an individual level. Some workers had used generic measures such as the Sickness Impact Profile to assess the impacts of oral disorders on quality of life, but Locker suggested that these measures were not sensitive to oral disorders. Since then, a plethora of measures has been developed, as shown in Table 23.1. These range from a three item measure to a 49 item profile.

During a consensus conference in 1996 [30], a variety of these measures of oral health-related quality of life were reviewed. Since then, many have been used in cross-sectional surveys of oral health. The data from these studies have consistently demonstrated the value of good oral health to older adults.

Uses to date and remaining problems

The literature in this area has grown steadily over the past 10 years. Much of the effort has consisted of testing and retesting measures in large population studies, usually of older adults. The research indicates that patients with poorer self-rated oral health have fewer teeth, more problem-based dental visits and come from poorer socio-economic backgrounds.

Table 23.1 Oral specific measures of health currently available

Authors	Name of measure
Cushing *et al.*, 1986 [21]	Social Impacts of Dental Disease
Atchison and Dolan, 1990 [22]	Geriatric Oral Health Assessment Index
Strauss and Hunt, 1993 [23]	Dental Impact Profile
Slade and Spencer, 1994 [17]	Oral Health Impact Profile
Locker and Miller, 1994 [24]	Subjective Oral Health Status Indicators
Leao and Sheiham, 1996 [25]	Dental Impact on Daily Living
Kressin, 1996 [26]	Oral Health Related Quality of Life Measure
Cornell *et al.*, 1996 [27]	Oral Health Quality of Life Inventory
Adulyanon and Sheiham, 1997 [28]	Oral Impacts on Daily Performances
McGrath and Bedi, 2001 [29]	OHQoL UK

No measure has emerged as the 'measure of measures', and this area is now becoming the focus of research activity.

Whilst most of the measures currently available have good reliability and validity properties, a number of methodological issues still remain. These include the length of the measures (ease of use has to be balanced against psychometric properties), whether items are weighted to give a score (some do this), questions about cross-cultural relevance (within diverse populations or when comparing between different populations), versatility (fitness for different purposes) and whether disease or condition specific measures are even relevant at all. There is no perfect measure but there are several which are fit for purpose and the field is improving all the time.

Most of the research to date has been in two areas: descriptive population studies and clinical intervention trials.

Descriptive population studies

These studies have been almost exclusively cross-sectional and a number of predictors of poor oral health-related quality of life have been identified. In addition to the clinical condition of teeth and supporting tissues, socio-economic and cultural status, dental anxiety, problem motivated dental visits have been shown to be associated with a higher prevalence of self-reported negative oral health impacts [31, 32]. A number of national population studies of oral health have used the short version of the Oral Health Impact Profile (OHIP-14) to collect patient rated health status data. One such study [33] used data from two national population studies to assess the impact of age and toothloss on oral health-related quality of life. Using data from the UK and Australia, the authors showed that age and tooth loss had independent effects on oral health-related quality of life. Intriguingly, the older cohorts in both countries reported the fewest negative impacts, i.e. had the best oral health-related quality of life, after correcting for the effect of tooth loss. This was unexpected, and it was suggested that the oldest cohorts may have had the lowest expectations of oral health once the effect of physical impairment was taken into account.

A further important outcome in this study related to the effect of the number of retained teeth on oral health-related quality of life. Figure 23.3 illustrates this and shows that, having controlled for age and gender, people with 25 or more teeth had significantly better scores than all other groups in both countries. Functionally oriented treatment planning is underpinned by the shortened dental arch concept which, in turn, is reliant upon the retention of twenty natural teeth with 3–5 occluding pairs of teeth. However, the data seem to suggest that the relationship between number of retained teeth and quality of life is complex. There was a difference between the Australian and UK populations, which suggests that such 'thresholds' are influenced by cultural background.

Using a 'lifecourse' epidemiological approach, Mason *et al.* [34] reported that factors from both early and adult lifespan contributed to oral health-related quality of life. However, an apparent gender difference emerged; the number of remaining teeth in adulthood had a more prominent impact on oral health-related quality of life of females in the study. The relevance of this may be that health promotion activities aimed at improving tooth retention rates may have a more positive impact on women than on men.

Clinical intervention studies

The literature in relation to clinical intervention studies is much more sparse and dominated by assessment of the impact of implant retained prostheses on quality of life of edentulous patients.

The use of osseointegrated implants provides an obvious opportunity to use oral health status measures for the evaluation of outcome; they have an immediate and substantial impact on various aspects of mechanical and social functioning. Prior to the mid-1990s, a variety of approaches were used to assess the impact of implant retained prostheses, but these studies were hampered by the failure to include control groups and use of health status measures unsuited to oral health measurement.

A more sophisticated approach was used by a team of researchers in Montreal. In a within subject, crossover clinical trial, de Grandmont *et al.* [35] compared fixed and removable mandibular implant-supported prostheses. Fifteen edentulous subjects were involved and all subjectively evaluated their existing dentures and oral health status prior to active treatment using Visual Analogue Scales (VAS) and a categorical functional questionnaire (CAT). Variables assessed were general satisfaction, fit and retention, chewing ability, appearance, ability to speak and social interaction. Each subject received 4–5 Brånemark implants in the anterior mandible, and following a quasi-randomization process, eight subjects received a fixed bridge and seven were provided with a removable overdenture supported by a long bar. Following implant prosthesis insertion, all subjects completed VAS and CAT as before. The prostheses were then changed (fixed prostheses exchanged for removable and vice versa) and the

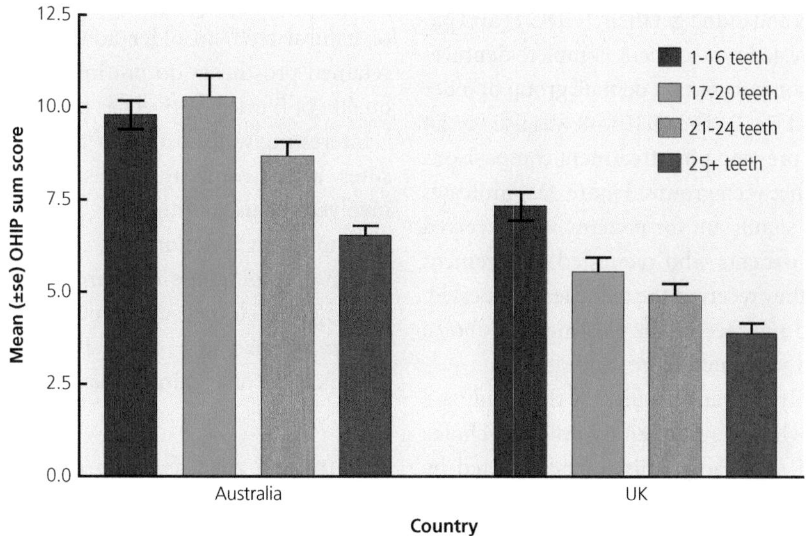

Figure 23.3 Mean and SE for OHIP-14 scores in UK and Australia according to number of teeth. Reproduced from Steele *et al.*, 2004 [33].

procedures repeated. At the end of the trial, subjects were asked to choose the prosthesis they wished to keep as their definitive prosthesis. They concluded that subjects rated both types of implant supported prosthesis significantly higher than their original conventional dentures. The only significant differences between scores for different types of implant supported design were that subjects rated their ability to chew hard foods higher with a fixed prosthesis. At the end of the trial, eight subjects elected to keep a fixed prosthesis and seven chose a removable implant-supported overdenture.

In a further study conducted by this group, Tang *et al.* [36] used the same method to compare attitudes to both implant-supported mandibular overdentures with bar retention (primarily implant-supported) and overdentures retained using ball attachments (support shared between implants and oral mucosa). They tested the hypothesis that the influence of prosthesis support on patient satisfaction would be greater than the mechanism of prosthesis attachment to the implants. They concluded that satisfaction with both forms of prosthesis was higher than with the original conventional dentures. However, subjects rated satisfaction with bar retained overdentures on four implants higher than ball attachment retained overdentures on two implants, thus supporting their hypothesis. When offered the prosthesis of choice at the end of the trial, all 16 subjects chose the overdenture supported completely by implants. The authors conceded that a requirement to 'bury' two implants if the ball attachment option were chosen may have influenced this choice.

In a non-randomized longitudinal trial, Allen and McMillan [37] assessed the impact of implant retained prostheses (either fixed or removable) and conventional dentures across three groups of edentulous patients, namely: patients who requested implants and got them (IG), patients who requested implants and didn't get them (CDG 1) and patients who simply requested replacement complete dentures (CDG 2). For comparison purposes, a dentate group of older adults was also included (DG). The OHIP-49 was used as an outcome measure, and pre- and post-treatment comparisons were made within and between groups. Figure 23.4 indicates that improvement was significant for patients who received implants (IG) and for patients who requested replacement dentures (CDG 2), i.e. they received the treatment requested. For the group who did not receive the treatment of choice (CDG 1), improvement was much more modest.

A number of clinically relevant features of this study are worth noting. Patients who received their treatment of choice were likely to respond favourably. This was also noted by Feine and co-workers [38] who discussed the possible influence of treatment preference bias on randomized study designs. Secondly, the post-treatment OHIP scores for patients

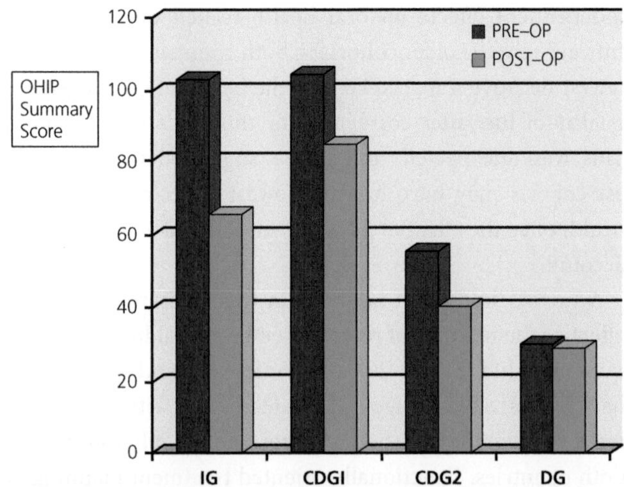

Figure 23.4 Comparison of mean pre- and post-treatment summary OHIP-49 scores for edentulous patients (IG, CDG 1 and CDG 2) and dentate older adults (DG). Reproduced from Allen and McMillian, 2003 [37].

who received implants were higher than the pre-treatment scores of patients who requested dentures; that is, they still had poorer oral health-related quality of life after implant treatment. From a funding perspective, this might on the surface suggest that implant retained prostheses may not be worth the costs involved. However, a more positive view is that the magnitude of difference between the levels of improvement achieved was substantially greater for the implant group. The authors used 'effect sizes' for the OHIP summary score change to give an indication of the clinical relevance of the pre/post-treatment difference, and reported that the IG group effect size was 1.2 (a very large change), whereas that for CDG 2 was 0.5 (a moderate change). Finally, the best oral health-related quality of life was reported by the dentate patients. This gives further indication of the importance of natural teeth to older adults and suggests that implant retained prostheses do not impact upon oral health-related quality of life as positively as healthy pain-free natural teeth.

Interestingly, almost all of the uses of health status measures as outcome measures in intervention trials have involved the use of implants. The use of implants make such an impact on function that even measures not specifically designed as outcome measures can fulfil this purpose. The efficacy of such measures around other interventions where the impact is more subtle is not clear and may require modification of existing tools.

Summary and future directions

It would seem that use of subjective health status measures is increasing, and the data from national population surveys are becoming more and more substantial. Our understanding of the impact of oral disease on quality of life has improved, and public health policy has a more robust database to tap into than ever before. Further work is required to assess the relative impact of treatment to restore missing teeth and to evaluate new treatment strategies such as dental implants. Measurement of subjective oral health status will indicate the value of good oral health to older adults, and this is also vital as the population ages and clinical decision making becomes more diverse and complex.

References

1 Fitzpatrick, R., Fletcher, A., Gore, D., Spiegelhalter, D. & Cox, D. (1992) Quality of life measures in health care. I: Application and issues in assessment. *British Medical Journal*, **305**, 1074–1077.

2 Locker, D. (1988). Measuring oral health: A conceptual framework. *Community Dental Health*, **5**, 3–18.

3 Decker, S.D. & Schultz, R. (1985) Correlates of life satisfaction and depression in middle-aged and elderly spinal cord injured patient. *American Journal of Occupational Therapy*, **39**, 740–745.

4 Evans, R.W. (1991) Quality of life. *The Lancet*, **338**, 636–639.

5 Allison, P.J., Locker, D. & Feine, J.S. (1997) Quality of life: a dynamic construct. *Social Science and Medicine*, **45**, 221–230.

6 Culyer, A.J. (1983) *Health Indicators*. Martin Robertson, Oxford.

7 Wilson, I. & Cleary, P. (1995) Linking clinical variables with health-related quality of life: a conceptual model of patient outcomes. *Journal of the American Medical Association*, **273**, 59–65.

8 WHO. (1980) *International classification of impairments, disabilities and handicaps*. World Health Organisation, Geneva.

9 Silverman, D. (ed) (2000) *Doing Qualitative Research: A Practical Handbook*. Sage Press, London.

10 Friedman, N., Landesman, H.M. & Wexler, M. (1988) The influences of fear, anxiety, and depression on patient's adaptive responses to complete dentures. Part II. *Journal of Prosthetic Dentistry*, **59**, 45–48.

11 Fiske, J., Davis, D. M., Frances, C. & Gelbier, S. (1998) The emotional effects of tooth loss in edentulous people. *British Dental Journal*, **184**, 90–93.

12 MacEntee, M.I., Hole, R. & Stolar, E. (1997) The significance of the mouth in old age. *Social Science & Medicine*, **45**, 1449–1458.

13 Cronin, M., Meaney, S., Jepson, N.J. & Allen, P.F. (2009) A qualitative study of trends in patient preferences for the management of partial dentition. *Gerodontology*, **26**, 137–142.

14 Graham, R. S., Mihaylov, S., Jepson, N.J., Allen, P.F. & Bond, S. (2006) Determining need for a Removable Partial Denture: a qualitative study of factors that influence dentist provision and patient use. *British Dental Journal*, **200**, 155–158.

15 Locker, D. (1995) Social and psychological consequences of oral disorders. In: E.J. Kay (ed) *Turning strategy into action*. Eden Bianchi Press, Manchester.

16 Slevin, M.L., Plant, H., Lynch, D., Drinkwater, J. & Gregory, W. M. (1988) Who should measure quality of life, the doctor or the patient? *British Journal of Cancer*, **57**, 109–112.

17 Slade, G.D. & Spencer, A.J. (1994) Development and evaluation of the Oral Health Impact Profile. *Community Dental Health*, **11**, 3–11.

18 Guyatt, G.H., Kirshner, B. & Jaeschke, R. (1992) Measuring health status: what are the necessary measurement properties? *Journal of Clinical Epidemiology*, **45**, 1341–1345.

19 Cohen, L.K. & Jago, J.D. (1976) Toward formulation of socio-dental indicators. *International Journal of Health Services*, **6**, 681–698.

20 Reisine, S. (1984) Dental disease and work loss. *Journal of Dental Research*, **63**, 1158–1161.

21 Cushing, A., Sheiham, A. & Maisels, J. (1986) Developing socio-dental indicators-the social impact of dental disease. *Community Dental Health*, **3**, 3–17.

22 Atchison, K.A. & Dolan, T.A. (1990) Development of the Geriatric Oral Health Assessment Index. *Journal of Dental Education*, **54**, 680–687.

23 Strauss, R. & Hunt, R. (1993) Understanding the value of teeth to older adults: influences on the quality of life. *Journal of the American Dental Association*, **124**, 105–110.

24 Locker, D. & Miller, Y. (1994) Evaluation of subjective oral health status indicators. *Journal of Public Health Dentistry*, **54**, 167–176.

25 Leao, A. & Sheiham, A. (1996) The development of a socio-dental measure of Dental Impacts on Daily Living. *Community Dental Health*, **13**, 22–26.

26 Kressin, N.R. (1996) Associations among different assessments of oral health outcomes. *Journal of Dental Education*, **60**, 501–507.

27 Cornell, J.E., Saunders, M.J., Paunovich, E.D. & Frisch, M.B. (1997) Oral Health Quality of Life Inventory. In: G. Slade (ed) *Measuring Oral Health and Quality of Life*. Dental Ecology, University of North Carolina, Chapel Hill, NC.

28 Adulyanon, S. & Sheiham, A. (1997) Oral Impacts on Daily Performances. In: G. Slade (ed) *Measuring Oral Health and Quality of Life*. Dental Ecology, University of North Carolina, Chapel Hill, NC.

29 Mc Grath, C. & Bedi, R. (2001) An evaluation of a new measure of oral health related quality of life--OHQoL-UK(W). *Community Dental Health*, **18**, 138–143.

30 Slade, G.D., Strauss, R., Atchison, K., Kressin, N., Locker, D. & Reisine, S. (1998) Conference summary: assessing oral health outcomes--measuring health status and quality of life, *Community Dental Health*, **15**, 3–7.

31 Slade, G.D., Spencer, A.J., Locker, D., Hunt, R.J., Strauss, R.P. & Beck, J.D. (1996) Variations in the social impact of oral conditions among older adults in South Australia, Ontario, and North Carolina. *Journal of Dental Research*, **75**, 1439–1450.

32 McGrath, C. & Bedi, R. (2004) The association between dental anxiety and oral health-related quality of life in Britain. *Community Dentistry & Oral Epidemiology*, **32**, 67–72

33 Steele, J.G., Sanders, A.E., Slade, G.D., Allen, P.F., Lahti, S., Nuttall, N. *et al.* (2004) How do age and tooth loss affect oral health impacts and quality of life? A study comparing two national samples. *Community Dentistry & Oral Epidemiology*, **32**, 107–114.

34 Mason, J., Pearce, M.S., Walls, A.W.G., Parker, L. & Steele, J.G. (2006) How do factors at different stages of the lifecourse contribute to oral-health-related quality of life in middle age for men and women? *Journal of Dental Research*, **85**, 257–261

35 De Grandmont, P., Feine, J.S., Tache, R., Boudrias, P., Donohue, W.B., Tanguay, R. *et al.* (1994) Within-subject comparisons of implant-supported mandibular prostheses: psychometric evaluation. *Journal of Dental Research*, **73**, 1096–1104.

36 Tang, L., Lund, J.P., Tache, R., Clokie, C.M. & Feine, J.S. (1997) A within-subject comparison of mandibular long-bar and hybrid implant-supported prostheses: psychometric evaluation and patient preferences. *Journal of Dental Research*, **76**, 1675–1683.

37 Allen, P.F. & McMillan, A.S. (2003) A longitudinal study of quality of life outcomes in older adults requesting implant prostheses and complete removable dentures. *Clinical Oral Implants Research*, **14**, 173–179.

38 Feine, J.S., Awad, M.A. & Lund, J.P. (1998) The impact of patient preference on the design and interpretation of clinical trials. *Community Dentistry and Oral Epidemiology*, **26**, 70–74.

CHAPTER 24

Influences on older adults' use of dental services

H. Asuman Kiyak†
School of Dentistry, Institute on Aging, University of Washington, Seattle, WA, USA

Introduction and some definitions

Access to health care is defined by the Institute of Medicine as 'the timely use of personal health services to achieve the best possible health outcomes' [1]. This includes the process of obtaining needed services from the health care system and seeking preventive care even when the individual has no symptoms or emergency needs. Both the US Public Health Service and the American Cancer Society recommend annual oral assessments for all adults age 40 and older. It is widely recognized that good oral health is a basic right and an important component of general health and quality of life. Preventive dental care is particularly important for older adults who have multiple chronic diseases and who often use medications with oral side effects such as xerostomia [2].

Despite this widespread recognition of the need for regular preventive care and access to restorative treatments, many older adults do not use dental services except for emergencies. The current cohort of elders varies widely in its use of dental services, from regular preventive users to non-users who report that they have not been to a dentist in more than 20 years. In 2002, according to the National Health Interview Survey (NHIS), 55.4% of older adults reported that they had visited a dentist, the lowest rate of any age group beyond 18 [3]. The NHIS revealed wide disparities across subgroups of the population age 65 and older. For example, they found that 65% of the non-poor had used dental services in the past year, compared with 35% of poor elders. Among white respondents to the NHIS, 58% had sought dental care in the past year, compared with 34% of African Americans. Likewise, differences exist across regions and between urban and rural elders. Nevertheless, there is some hope for future cohorts of elders; the NHIS found the greatest increase in utilization rates among the population age 65+, rising from 16.2% who reported at least one dental visit in the 1957–1959 survey to 55.4% in the 2002 survey. These rates were approaching one of the objectives of *Healthy People 2010*: to increase utilization among the older population to 56% by 2010 [4].

The purpose of this chapter is to explore some of the determinants of older persons' dental service utilization, those that help or hinder access to dental care, as a means of understanding why some people continue seeking preventive dental care throughout their lives while others are lifelong irregular users and still others discontinue regular use after retirement or relocation to a new community or long-term care facility. Based on the epidemiological and psychosocial literature available on this topic, barriers to be discussed include cohort and age, race and ethnicity, income and education, availability of dental and medical insurance, urban versus rural residence, physical access to a dental office and systemic and functional health. Some of these same variables are valuable in enabling elders to access dental care. Attitudes towards oral health and dental care, as well as perceived need, can also influence older adults' decision to seek services. Dental providers can be potent enablers of, or barriers to, older adults' access to dental care as well. Each of these factors will be examined in turn, focusing on situations where they help or hinder elders' use of dental services. It is noteworthy that most studies have not conducted multivariate analyses to compare the relative power of each barrier or enabler. A few studies that have simultaneously examined multiple predictors will be described later in this review.

Demographic variables

Cohort and age

Perhaps the most obvious demographic factor affecting dental utilization is age and cohort. Let us examine cohort

† Author is deceased.

Textbook of Geriatric Dentistry, Third Edition. Edited by Poul Holm-Pedersen, Angus W. G. Walls and Jonathan A. Ship.

first, because it shapes our socioeconomic and psychosocial lives. Historical events as well as social and health policies of a given era influence our view of the world. An interesting approach to the role of cohort differences on oral health was first introduced by Ettinger [5]. By comparing socioeconomic and dental events of each decade, one can track the impact of these developments on each generation's oral health behaviours. For example, the 1930s was a time of significant social and health policies in the USA, with the passage of the Social Security Act in 1935 and the first health insurance plans through Blue Cross in 1933. Dental researchers were developing new anaesthetics to make dentistry a less painful experience. The cohort born during this decade was more likely than previous decades to benefit from such developments. Those born in the 1950s would be more likely to have access to fluoridated water and to be influenced by toothpaste commercials with the advent of television. However, those age 65+ in that era would be more likely to avoid dental services because of their earlier experiences with painful extractions and restorative procedures. This may be why utilization rates were so low among the older cohort in the 1957–1959 NHIS (16.2%) [3]. In recent decades, the concept of preventive and aesthetic dentistry has reached a wider public as orthodontics, dental implants, commercial tooth bleaching and new dental materials have become more common. Thus, cohorts born in the 1930s, 1950s and 1980s have widely varying views of the purpose of teeth, as well as the maintenance and appearance of teeth. Socio-historical and dental influences on each cohort during the past century are shown in Table 24.1.

Perhaps one should not expect current cohorts of older adults – born before 1943 – to value oral health and dental

Table 24.1 A history of socioeconomic events and dentistry (1900–2003)

Decade	Socioeconomic events	Dental events
1900		1890 – Benzocaine (ester) 1905 – Procain: Einhorn & Braun (ester)
1910	1913 – Personal Income Tax 1914–1918 – WWI	1910 – Hunter Theory of Focal Infection
1920	1922 – Model T 1925 – Radio 1929–1939 – Depression	1921 – Dental Act (License of Dentists)
1930	1933 – Blue Cross 1935 – Social Security Act	1930 – Tetracaine: Fussanger (ester)
1940	1940–1945 – WWII 1942 – Women in the Work Force 1945 – Income Tax as a Fiscal Instrument 1946 – Television – Post-WWII Baby Boom	1943 – Lidocaine: Lofgren (amide) 1945 – First public fluoridation of H_2O
1950	1950 – National Conference on Aging 1950–53 – Korean War	1955 – Buncore, sealants 1955 – Borden: air turbine handpiece 1957 – Carbocaine: Ekenstram (amide)
1960	1961 – First White House Conference on Aging 1965 – Medicare & Medicaid 1965 – Older Americans Act	1960's – Dental Insurance Plans 1960 – Citanest: Lofgren (amide) 1962 – Astra: Cartridge local anaesthetic fissure sealants 1968 – Plaque control programmes
1970	1971 – Second White House Conference on Aging 1973 – National Institute on Aging 1974 – Supplemental Security Income 1978 – Area Agency on Aging	1971 – Acid-etch technique
1980	1981 – Third White House Conference on Aging 1986 – Elimination of Mandatory Retirement 1987 – Nursing Home Reform Act 1989–1990 – Medicare Catastrophic Health Care passed, then repealed	1980 – Osseointegrated dental implants in USA 1989 – The first commercial home tooth bleaching product is marketed.
1990	1995 – Fourth White House Conference on Aging 1996 – Family and Medical Leave Act 1999 – United Nations: International Year of Older Persons	1990s – New tooth – coloured restorative materials, increased usage of bleaching, veneers and implants inaugurate an era of aesthetic dentistry. 1997 – FDA approves the erbium YAG laser, the first for use on dentine, to treat tooth decay.
2000	2000 – National Family Caregiver Support Program 2003 – Medicare Prescription Drug Bill	

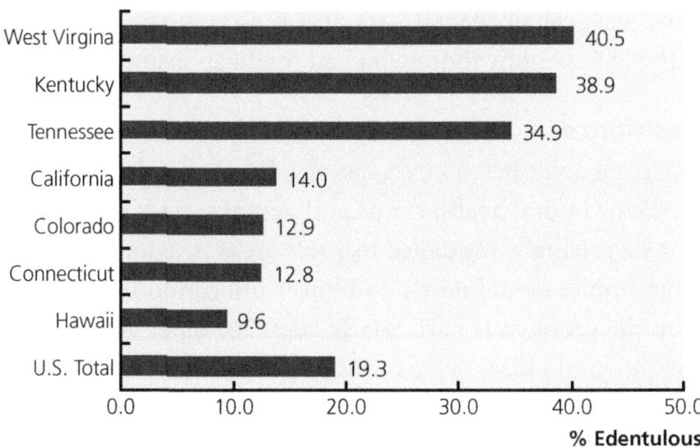

Figure 24.1 Variations in edentulism rates across the USA. Reproduced from CDC, 2006 [18].

aesthetics in the same way younger generations do. Nevertheless, as we learn more about the link between oral and systemic health, and as more people keep their natural teeth into old age, it is critical to help older adults learn and practise preventive oral health care.

This discussion of cohort effects suggests that it may not be age per se, but cohort differences that affect oral health practises and values. Several researchers have reported significant differences between younger and older adults in oral health status and utilization patterns. These include epidemiological studies comparing different countries such as the International Collaborative Studies I and II [6], surveys in Australia [7, 8], Great Britain [9], Denmark [10] and the USA [11–16]. In studies where age groups are compared, significant differences generally emerge, with older adults more likely to report not seeking dental care within the most recent five or more years. Utilization appears to peak in middle age, and declines dramatically by age 65; 2002 NHIS data revealed that only 55.4% of adults 65+ had seen a dentist in the past year, compared with 63% of 45–64 year-olds [3]. Dental care was far less frequent than blood pressure and cholesterol screenings in the 1999 NHIS, reported by at least 95% and 72% of older adults respectively [17]. Utilization rates vary from state to state, from 41% of older adults in Kentucky to 75% in Hawaii reporting a dental visit in the past year. This may be related to the rates of edentulism across states; West Virginia and Kentucky have the highest rates and Hawaii the lowest (40.5%, 38.9% and 9.6% respectively) [18]. The impact of dentition status on utilization patterns will be discussed later in this chapter.

Racial and ethnic differences

The oral health status of ethnic minority elders is worse than that of white elders and younger cohorts in the same ethnic groups. Findings of the ICS II [6] revealed greater differences between white and disadvantaged minorities in the USA than between whites in the USA and their counterparts in other countries (Germany, Poland and Japan). For example, adults who participated in this study from the Navajo and Lakota tribes, as well as African American adults in Baltimore and Latinos in San Antonio had worse oral health status and poorer utilization patterns than whites in the same communities. Differences were particularly dramatic between older adults in these ethnic and racial groups.

The 1996 MEPS revealed sharp differences in dental visits between non-Hispanic white, Latino and African American elders, with adjusted odds ratios of 0.58 and 0.38, respectively, for the two minority groups compared to whites [16]. The more recent 2002 NHIS data suggest that differences may not be as great as those found in the 1996 MEPS; African American elders used dental services at 0.59 the rate of whites [3]. Other national studies have revealed higher rates of untreated dental caries and periodontal diseases in African American and Latino elders and more edentulism among the former, which results in higher DMFT scores for these ethnic and racial minorities. Data from the 1988–1991 NHANES revealed that African Americans had on average 4.3 decayed coronal and 4.1 root surfaces, compared with 3.5 and 1.7 for Latinos, 1.5 and 1.4 for white elders respectively. Despite having worse oral health status and utilization than whites, Latino elders appear to be better off than their African American counterparts.

There is some association between poor oral health status and perceived oral health among disadvantaged ethnic minorities but generally they do not report difficulty chewing or discomfort with the appearance of their teeth [11, 19] Such complacence with one's oral health status represents a barrier to seeking care even when symptoms of oral diseases are present.

Education and income

Educational achievement and income (both real and perceived) are significant predictors of utilization among older adults. A national survey in Australia among the population age 15 and older found that age at leaving school was most significantly associated with utilization among the oldest groups [8]. Those who had continued their education beyond age 18 were 1.85 times more likely to have visited a dentist in the past year than those who had never attended school or had quit at age 15. Occupational status, closely related to education, was also significant, with blue collar workers only half as likely as higher occupational levels to have made dental visits in the past year. Blue collar workers were 2.5 times more likely to have had an extraction at their last visit than those in managerial or professional occupations. The role of education has been supported in US surveys as well but it may be confounded with occupational level, income and access to dental insurance.

A survey of black and white adults in Florida reported that both poverty and race were related to utilization, such that the lowest rates were found among the poorest African Americans, and that non-poor African Americans used dental services at about the same rate as the poorest whites in this sample [14]. This same study revealed that *perceived* ability to pay for dental care predicted utilization as well as did actual income level. The 2002 NHIS revealed that older adults classified as poor had an adjusted odds ratio of 0.54 for utilization, compared to those classified as non-poor [3].

Dental and medical insurance

Unlike medical care, dental services are not covered by Medicare, and only a minority of states in the US provides adequate benefits for adult dental services. This discrepancy is illustrated by the fact that oral health care represented only 5.3% of all health expenditures in 2002. This compares with 36% each for physician and hospital services and 12% for prescription drug costs, all of which are covered in whole or in part by Medicare for older adults and by Medicaid for low income populations [20]. Among the population age 65+, one would expect even greater discrepancies between health expenditures for medical versus dental services.

The availability of dental insurance has been found to be a significant predictor of utilization. Estimates of coverage range from 14.5% among all those 65 and older [21] to 28.4% of 65–74-year-olds and 16.5% of those aged 75+ [22]. When only private dental insurance is considered, adults aged 65+ are *least* likely to be covered, with rates as low as 10% [23]. The importance of third party coverage is highlighted by the fact that older adults with dental insurance are 2.53 times more likely to make regular dental visits [16], significantly more likely to be dentate, with more natural teeth remaining, and to hold more favourable oral health beliefs [24]. In the 2000 MEPS, 77% of all dental expenditures for older adults was paid out of pocket, and only 15% by private dental insurance [22]. These findings suggest that offering affordable dental insurance to older adults may serve as an enabler of dental service utilization. This will become even more important as more and more people keep their natural teeth into advanced old age.

Even the availability of supplemental medical insurance (*Medigap*) increases one's chances of using dental services, presumably because the older person can divert some of the savings from their medical care to their out-of-pocket dental expenses. The 1993 Medicare Current Beneficiary Survey (MCBS) revealed that older adults covered by Medicare spent $310 per year on dental care and prescriptions, compared with $585 spent by those who had Medigap insurance [25].

Residence

Where an older person lives has also been considered to be a predictor of oral health status and dental service utilization. Not surprisingly, residence in rural areas is associated with more unmet dental needs and lower utilization rates. However, the problem is particularly acute for older adults, with 46% of rural elders versus 58% of urban dwellers reporting a dental visit in the past year, 51% versus 42% reporting unmet dental needs and 37% versus 28% who are edentulous, respectively [3]. The availability of private dental insurance, reflecting lower income status among rural populations, is lower among this group of elders. Similar findings are reported by Chalmers [7] in Australia, where rural elders had significantly more missing and decayed teeth than their urban counterparts and fewer filled coronal and root surfaces. One must ask if these differences could be alleviated by increasing the number of dental practitioners in rural communities, thereby increasing access. However, inadequate financial resources and unfavourable oral health attitudes among rural elders most likely would preclude their use of dental services even if they became more available.

Another residential variable is whether the individual lives alone or in a long-term care facility (LTC). Oral health is generally poor among older adults living in LTC. This problem can be attributed to a combination of access issues such as the difficulty of making visits to dental providers and the unavailability of dentists who provide dental care in LTC settings. But it may also be linked to poor functional health and a focus on systemic conditions that overrides oral health concerns. In an epidemiological study of older adults in Australia who were living independently in the community or in nursing homes, and chronically mentally ill elders in boarding homes, dramatic differences were found across the three groups, with independent elders having 2.5 times more filled coronal surfaces than the institutionalized groups. The former group had, on average 0.3 decayed coronal surfaces, compared with 1.7 among nursing home dwellers and 5.4 among institutionalized chronically ill elders [7], as shown in Figure 24.2. These findings highlight the impact of limited access to professional care and the availability of daily oral hygiene.

Impact of dentition status and health status

One might hypothesize that dental service utilization is related to the individual's dentition status. Certainly the studies

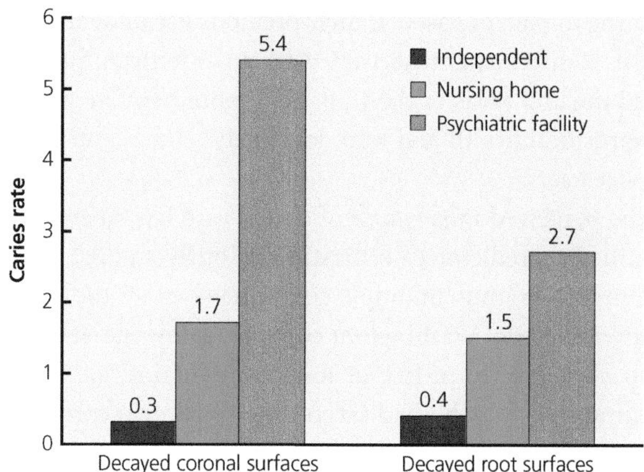

Figure 24.2 Impact of residential setting on caries rates. Reproduced from Chalmers, 2001 [7].

comparing edentulous and dentate elders support this hypothesis; one national survey revealed that dentate elders are 6.5 times more likely to seek dental care than their edentulous counterparts [16]. Those with more teeth make more visits than their counterparts with fewer teeth. The likelihood of seeking dental care increases fourfold if the older person is edentulous in one arch only or has at least one tooth in each arch, compared with those who have no natural teeth [13]. To date there have been no reports of dental service utilization among older adults who wear an implant-supported bridge; this would be an interesting group to compare with elders wearing complete dentures because of the additional care needed for implants.

These findings suggest that future cohorts, who will retain more natural teeth, will be more likely than their predecessors to seek dental care. Evidence for this emerges from the dramatic increase in utilization rates between 1957 and 2002, rising from 16.2% to 55.4% who reported any visits in the past year [3]. However, the presence of large numbers of decayed root and coronal surfaces and deep periodontal pockets does not necessarily mean the individual will seek dental care, as illustrated by the barriers described above. Poor systemic health and multiple chronic diseases can also deter the older person from obtaining needed dental care. Indeed, those who make frequent medical visits and who spend more on medications and medical visits are *less* likely to use dental services. This is most probably due to their focus on the chronic conditions that impair their activities of daily living (ADL), and the time and energy required to deal with medical problems [26]. In fact, even among educated elders who have had a history of regular dental service use, the more ADL limitations an older person reports, the less likely s/he is to seek dental care [12].

Physical access and mobility

There is a widespread belief among community health providers and elders themselves that they would be more likely to use dental services if the clinics were located nearby, or delivered directly via mobile units, or were less costly. Indeed, surveys of community-dwelling older adults in the 1980s reported that respondents wanted dental treatment but had difficulty climbing stairs and could not find dentists with ground floor offices [27] or that mobility problems prevented up to 30% of elders from obtaining dental services [28]. Even in more recent surveys, such as one conducted in a community north of London, 52% of housebound older adults who responded said that they had difficulty leaving their homes to receive dental care, and complained of inadequate transportation options to dental providers. The overwhelming number of these frail elders (93%) said they only made a dental visit when they had dental problems, but 86% perceived no need! [9]

However, in our own experience and in reports of other programmes that have attempted to provide such services, there is little support for the concept, 'If you build it, they will come'. In one survey of dentists and residential care supervisors in northern Scotland, no more than 25% of elderly residents in these facilities had had contact with a dentist in the past year, despite the fact that 86% of dentists were willing to do home visits and 93% of facilities provided transportation to dental providers. These low rates of dental utilization by elders in domiciliary care did not vary by frailty [29]. A recent assessment of users of a university-sponsored mobile dental clinic that provided services to elders at adult day health sites found that only about 25% elected to use this clinic. Those who did and did not seek care in this on-site programme did not differ in the number and severity of their systemic diseases, but users were less likely to have a private dentist or to be able to pay out-of-pocket for dental care [30].

Psychosocial variables as barriers and enablers

Perceived versus normative needs

The primary reason why people seek health services is their belief that they *need* health care and that the situation will get worse without professional help. Furthermore, individuals must believe that their health status will get better by obtaining clinical services. However, researchers have demonstrated that many older adults accept chronic disease as an inevitable and even normal part of the aging process. Low income and less educated elders have been found to have lower expectations of good health in their old age [5, 31]. Such acceptance of poor health is particularly striking in the area of oral health. Whether this means living without natural teeth or with poorly fitting dentures, or with pain and halitosis due to caries, some older persons attribute their condition to aging and do not seek dental care. Numerous studies have reported a consistent finding; older people who are irregular or non-users of dental care do so not because of cost or fear but because they believe that they do not need any treatment [14, 32, 33]. In a comparison of adults under age 55 with those who were 55 and older, Abrams and colleagues found that almost twice as many of the younger group cited cost and fear as reasons, while 'no need' was cited by 38.5% of the former and 72.5% of the latter [32]. In other studies, as many as 90% of older adults give 'no need' as a reason. A comparison of these reasons in two studies is shown in Figure 24.3.

Dental attitudes

A related barrier to seeking dental care is the *attitude* of the individual towards oral health and towards dental providers. The Florida Dental Care Study interviewed dentate African American and white adults ages 45+ to determine the impact of dental attitudes and demographic characteristics on dental service utilization [14]. As noted above, race and poverty (both objective income levels and perceived ability to pay for dental care) had independent effects on utilization patterns. However, six attitudinal constructs significantly discriminated between regular users of dental services and irregular users and non-users. These included questions regarding respondents' beliefs about the importance of dental visits in preventing future problems, perceived quality and effectiveness of dental care received in the past, cynicism toward dentists and dental care, eventuality of dental decline

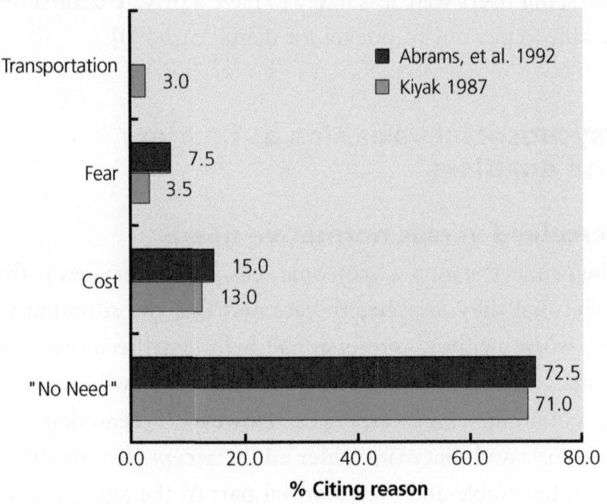

Figure 24.3 Low income elders' reasons for not using dental services.

and the impact of costs on their previous use of dental treatment. Respondents who were African American, poor and lived in rural areas of the state held more negative attitudes towards oral health and were less likely to be regular dental service users.

The perceived *importance* of dental care has emerged as a significant predictor of utilization in other studies. One of the first to examine multiple components of attitudes was a study in Seattle, Washington, comparing low income elders who had enrolled in free or low cost dental services in the community and who had (according to clinic records) used the service regularly (preventive users) or only for emergency purposes, or not at all since enrolling two or more years prior to being interviewed [33]. As in other communities where dental services have been developed for those who cannot pay, these clinics have experienced high levels of utilization initially but, once emergency needs are attended to, return visits become irregular. Attitudes were measured as a multidimensional concept, including beliefs regarding oral health and the importance attributed to each belief. The importance component of attitudes could discriminate among the three groups better than beliefs or the multiplicative attitude score.

Using Andersen and Newman's [34] model of predisposing, enabling and need variables, several demographic and health characteristics were also included in the design. Even with this expanded model, the importance attributed to oral health remained the best predictor of preventive versus emergency or non-utilization, together with perceived need and the number of natural teeth. For example, one barrier cited by older adults in other studies has been transportation or physical access. In this study, none of these indicators of access could discriminate between users and non-users and did not emerge among the list of significant predictors.

A subsequent study by Gilbert and colleagues [13] also tested Andersen and Newman's model of health behaviour to predict older adults' reported interval since their last dental visit. As with the study described above, perceived importance attributed to oral health and perceived value of dental care were significantly associated with utilization. Other significant predictors were educational status, income and being dentate versus edentulous. In both of these studies, attitudes served as both a barrier to, and an enabler of, utilization. Older people who placed more importance on oral health, who viewed it as valuable and who perceived a need for dental care (a key predictor described above) were more likely to seek dental services on a regular basis.

Social support

Another psychosocial variable that is gaining more attention as a predictor of health status and health service utilization is social support and 'social connectedness'. The MacArthur Studies of Successful Aging have found this variable, together with income adequacy and functional health, to be a significant predictor of successful aging [35]. In the area of dental care and utilization, there is growing evidence that older adults with strong interpersonal ties maintain their oral health better than their peers who are isolated. When 'social connectedness' is measured in terms of marital status and living arrangement, elders who are married or living with others have better periodontal health, more filled and fewer decayed coronal and root surfaces than those who are unmarried or are living alone [36]. Similarly, a study of dentate community-dwelling adults aged 80+ in Denmark found that those who had lived alone or became alone during the preceding 7 years had 2.4 times greater likelihood of coronal caries. Those who were dissatisfied with their level of social contacts were 2.9 times more likely to develop root caries during this interval [10]. Another Scandinavian study examined predictors of utilization among older men. Functional ability and general health status were less predictive of time since last dental visit than were social relations and lifestyle factors [37].

Thus, it behooves dental practitioners to encourage regular dental visits by their older patients who experience increased social isolation through widowhood or loss of close friends and family, or who have recently relocated to a new community and are lacking a social network.

Other psychosocial barriers and enablers

Self-efficacy, self-concept, and the desire to look attractive may also play a role in older adults' willingness to seek dental care. The first of these concepts (the belief that one has control over and can perform specific behaviours) has been widely tested in the health behaviour area. Across diverse ages, people who have high levels of self-efficacy relevant to a particular aspect of health (e.g. weight loss, smoking cessation) are more likely to improve their habits in that area. In our own research we have found an association between low self-efficacy, gingivitis and caries incidence over 1–2 years [38]. Self-concept also has been found to be an important predictor of various behaviours across the lifespan. Adolescents who have high levels of self-concept in multiple domains perform better in school and are less likely to experiment with drugs and alcohol. Young adults with high self-concept are more likely to adhere to orthodontic regimens. In the same manner, a high self-concept may help older adults maintain their oral health and dental appearance. Finally, although there is no research testing this observation, the desire to look attractive has become more important for baby boomers than for their predecessors, as evidenced by the increasing numbers seeking plastic surgery and botox treatments, as well as the growing numbers of 50- and 60-year-olds turning to orthodontics after a lifetime of experiencing malocclusion and the trend towards cosmetic dentistry and tooth whiteners among middle-aged adults. To the extent that such an aesthetic focus can motivate people to maintain their oral health in the later years, dental service utilization will improve for future cohorts of older adults.

A summary of the best predictors of utilization

This review supports the conclusion that multiple variables influence dental service use by older persons. In one of the few multivariate analyses available, Kiyak and colleagues found the best predictor of dental utilization by elders to be perceived importance of dental care [33]. Additionally, this study demonstrated that perceived importance best predicted the use of preventive or emergency services or non-utilization. In addition to perceived importance, perceived need and number of teeth remaining also influence older adults' utilization patterns. Gilbert and colleagues confirmed these findings [13, 14]. They showed that the importance attributed to oral health and perceived value of dental care are the major predictors of elders' utilization patterns. Educational status, income, race and ethnicity and number of teeth remaining also influenced these patterns. However, it is important to recognize the interactions among many of these variables; in the USA today, racial and ethnic minority elders have lower incomes, less education and fewer teeth than their white, non-Hispanic counterparts. This seemingly inconsistent pattern of lowest utilization rates among elders who have the greatest normative need but with low perceived need has been described as the 'paradox of dental need' [39]. That is, older adults who self-report oral problems and pain are more likely to seek dental care than those with multiple clinically determined needs and chewing difficulties. One might conclude from this that many elders are 'satisfied' with poor oral health, but such findings should challenge dental providers to educate their older patients to help them recognize symptoms of caries and periodontal disease and to make regular preventive visits in order to avoid these conditions.

Health services researchers have attempted to determine the best predictors of elders' medical care utilization. Shah and colleagues used logistic regression to identify symptom onset within four hours of seeking care. They found that older age, deficiencies in activities of daily living, worse physical and social functioning, less education, living alone and higher comorbidity scores predicted higher use of emergency medical services [40, 41]. Most of these variables are also linked to dental service utilization, although the number of chronic diseases has the opposite effect on elders' use of dental services, as described above. Similarly, McCusker and colleagues used regression analyses to determine the best predictors of emergency room visits by older adults [42, 43]. The researchers found that number of functional problems, hospitalization in the last six months, feeling depressed, cognitive impairment, a lack of social support, some medical diagnoses, a history of heart disease and diabetes, marital status, recent emergency visits and previous functional problems best predicted repeated ER visits. Parallel data for emergency dental visits are not available.

Predictors of elders' and family caregivers' use of home health services were evaluated by Houde [44]. Residence in older housing, recent hospitalization, gender, limitations in daily living, being a recipient of Medicaid, age, quality of informal care and number of household members were the best predictors of an older person's use of home services. In comparing the findings of studies on dental versus medical and home services utilization, it is apparent that subjective health and patient perceptions are more likely to predict dental service utilization, whereas objective health status is a better predictor of ER and home services utilization.

Dental provider characteristics that help or hinder utilization

Dentists' beliefs, stereotypes and comfort level with older patients can encourage or discourage the use of dental services by this population. Dentists who believe that older adults are unable or unwilling to maintain their teeth, or that they cannot afford dental care, may drive away potential patients. In contrast, dentists who assume that retirees have more time and money may expect them to be available for extensive and costly dental visits. In fact, one study that examined expectations of dentists and middle-aged and older patients regarding dental treatment found that dentists significantly overestimated their older patients' reluctance to receive dental treatment [45].

It is difficult to gauge from dentists' favourable responses to a survey whether they would actually provide care to a frail or institutionalized elder if asked to do so. The interpretation becomes more problematic when response rates to surveys are low; does a non-response convey more negative attitudes or a lack of interest in the issue? In a survey of Vancouver, BC, dentists, 55% who received the survey responded. Despite having dental practices near long-term care facilities, only 19% had ever provided dental care (mostly emergency services) in these settings, although 37% indicated a willingness to provide services if asked. Even among these dentists who reported favourable intentions towards treating institutionalized elders, they perceived barriers such as low demand (56%) and inadequate equipment and space for dental care (91%) in these facilities. Almost one-fourth of the respondents also felt unprepared to treat frail older patients [46, 47]. Data from this same survey revealed that interest in treating patients in long-term care settings was associated with lack of concern for time lost in one's private practice, training in managing medically compromised patients and positive attitudes towards older persons [48]. It is difficult to generalize these findings since 45% of dentists contacted did not respond; it is unclear if the self-reported level of interest in treating frail elders would be even lower.

Hope for the future

The patterns of utilization found among current cohorts of older adults may change in the future with the improving oral health of younger Americans. More people are retaining their natural teeth into advanced old age, and the evidence from multiple studies described above, both in the USA and in other countries, is that dentate elders are far more likely than their edentulous peers to use dental services. Although private dental insurance plans are becoming less available through employers, many baby boomers who grew up with dental insurance elect to continue this benefit by paying the premiums themselves and will be more likely than earlier cohorts to continue doing so into their retirement. This can only help increase utilization, as demonstrated by the significant association between insurance and access to dental care.

Other factors that enhance utilization rates are higher income and educational levels. Both are increasing for newer cohorts of elders, with poverty rates among those 65+ declining to their lowest levels in recent years, and with the majority of young-old having completed 12 or more years of education. Among all adults age 65+ today, over 72% have a high school diploma, an increase from 53% in 1990. During this same period the proportion with a college degree has increased from 11% to 17%. More-educated, middle-class elders are most likely to seek regular dental care from private practitioners. In fact, a 1998 survey of 237 dentists in five states found that older persons composed almost 20% of their patient load, up from 16.4% in a similar survey conducted 10 years earlier [49]. These older adults accounted for 17.5% of services and 22% of patient expenditures in the private practices that responded, both at higher levels than 10 years previously (see Figure 24.4). Although these private practitioners reported a decline in fees per visit for all age groups, adults age 65–69 paid the highest mean fees, as shown in Figure 24.5. To the extent that more baby boomers

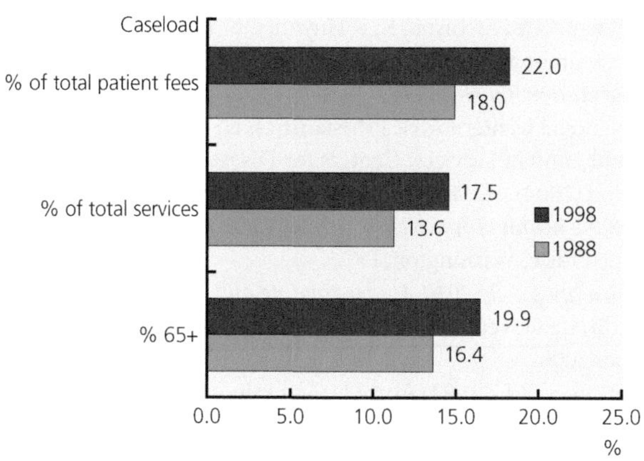

Figure 24.4 Private practitioner reports of older patients in practice. Reproduced from Meskin and Berg, 2000 [49].

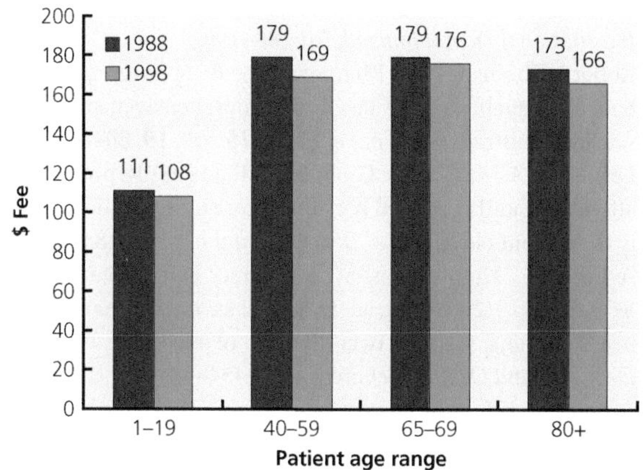

Figure 24.5 Average fees for dental services. Reproduced from Meskin and Berg, 2000 [49].

can pay for their dental care through private insurance or out-of-pocket, they will be an important segment of the private practice patient load in their later years.

Research to improve dental service utilization by diverse older adults

Despite the improving socioeconomic status of future cohorts of older adults, it is unrealistic to expect all baby boomers to enter old age with high levels of education, income and private Medigap and dental insurance. It is also unreasonable to assume that a lifetime of poor utilization patterns and low priority attributed to oral health can be modified in old age. What are some interventions that might enhance utilization among this latter group, particularly among disadvantaged ethnic minorities and immigrant populations who have had low access to dental care during adulthood? Community-based health promotion efforts are one method of addressing this problem. In our own research, we have tested alternative preventive oral health regimens such as intensive educational interventions, fluoride varnish applications and long-term rinsing with chlorhexidine [50, 51]. These interventions, aimed at low income ethnic minority and immigrant elders who have been irregular users of dental services, have yielded mixed results in terms of improving oral health parameters measured in each study. However, they have had an indirect effect of enhancing participants' interest in and desire to seek dental care. Follow-ups with these elders up to 3 years after completing the 5-year clinical trial have found many of them with a regular dental provider, often through a public health or community dental clinic. Their greater awareness of the importance of oral health in the later years has led most of these older persons to become preventive dental users. In a study testing the impact of an intergenerational oral health promotion programme on older adults' retention and practise of new oral health and nutrition knowledge, ethnically, culturally and linguistically diverse elders demonstrated higher rates of seeking dental care in their local communities [51].

Health promotion has become an important means of improving older adults' behaviours in a variety of areas, including exercise, weight loss, management of diabetes and hypertension. Unfortunately it has received less attention in dentistry except for some early efforts more than 20 years ago. With the rapid advances in materials and methods for home-based oral hygiene and materials and techniques in dental practice, it is important to educate the general population on an ongoing basis. Even those who make semiannual dental visits generally do not receive much systematic oral health education. Many patients would welcome such efforts, as illustrated by the findings of Abrams and colleagues [32] that 73% of adults younger than 55 and 62% of those 55 and older indicated a desire for educational programmes in their dentist's office. For those who do not seek regular dental care, this information is even more critical and should be provided in alternative settings such as primary care providers' offices (which older adults utilize at higher rates than any other age group), senior centres, assisted living facilities and adult day health centres, as well as non-traditional settings such as churches and malls. Advocates of oral health care for current and future cohorts of elders can adopt many of the techniques used by the medical community to assist patients with chronic systemic diseases. The dental care community must find creative ways to reach out to underserved segments of older adults.

Medicaid is the second largest expenditure in most states' budgets. Not surprisingly, it is the largest insurer in the country and is the primary third-party payer for long-term care services. Ongoing cuts to adult Medicaid dental services in many states and cuts by the federal government in bloc grants to states will reduce money available for elder dental care. For this reason, other ways to increase opportunities for intervention are needed.

Currently, licenced dentists must complete a certain number of hours in continuing education courses. One way to increase elders' access to elder oral health care is by requiring dentists and hygienists to promote oral health care in underserved areas (e.g. nursing homes, community clinics) as part of a continuing education requirement. The communities in need could also be accessed through mobile dental units. This could make oral health care accessible to more elders and give back to the community. Dental residency programmes represent another avenue for increasing access. Increasing numbers of Advanced Education in General Dentistry residency programmes train recently graduated dental students. The curriculum of these programmes could focus on providing care to underserved populations, one of which would be low-income older adults.

In some states, dental hygienists can be licenced to perform expanded dental functions. One way to increase oral health promotion is by allowing hygienists to work with underserved older populations by completing simple restorations, as well as cleanings and fluoride treatments, under this expanded function law without direct supervision by a dentist. Dentists can then be called in for more complex procedures. Under this law more elders could receive basic dental services.

Another way to increase oral health care to older adults is through interdisciplinary training. Providing oral health training to physicians, nurse practitioners, nutritionists and pharmacists in addition to dentists and hygienists would increase the frequency and amount of oral health information provided to elders and their caregivers. Finally, it would be beneficial to introduce the practise of good oral hygiene skills to the general public at an earlier age and provide better oral hygiene training to all age groups. Such awareness in the younger years can help instil lifelong preventive oral health habits, including making regular dental visits. These patterns should help reduce oral health problems among future cohorts of elders.

Acknowledgements

Portions of this work originally appeared in a different form in the *Journal of Dental Education*, Volume 69(9), September 2005. Used by permission of the American Dental Education Association, www.jdentaled.org.

References

1 Institute of Medicine. (1993) *Access to health care in America*. National Academy Press, Washington, DC.

2 Dolan, T.A., Atchison, K. & Huynh, T.N. (2005) Access to dental care among older adults in the United States. *Journal of Dental Education*, **69**, 961–974.

3 National Center for Health Statistics, US Department of Health and Human Services, Centers for Disease Control and Prevention (2004). *Health, United States, 2004, with chartbook on trends in the health of Americans*. pp. 265–266, US Government Printing Office, Washington, DC.

4 *Healthy people 2010: Understanding and Improving Health*, 2nd edn, US Government Printing Office, Washington, DC, November 2000.

5 Ettinger, R.L. (1992) Attitudes and values concerning oral health and utilisation of services among the elderly. *International Dental Journal*, **42**, 373–384.

6 Davidson, P.L. & Andersen, R.M. (1997) Determinants of dental care utilization for diverse ethnic and age groups. *Advances in Dental Research*, **11**, 254–262.

7 Chalmers, J.M. (2001) Geriatric oral health issues in Australia. *International Dental Journal*, **51**, 188–199.

8 Roberts-Thomson, K., Brennan, D.S. & Spencer, A.J. (1995) Social inequality in the use and comprehensiveness of dental services. *Australian Journal of Public Health*, **19**, 80–85.

9 Lester, V., Ashley, F.P. & Gibbons, D.E. (1998) Reported dental attendance and perceived barriers to care in frail and functionally dependent older adults. *British Dental Journal*, **184**, 285–289.

10 Avlund, K., Holm-Pedersen, P., Morse, D.E., Viitanen, M. & Winblad, B. (2003) Social relations as determinants of oral health among persons over the age of 80 years. *Community Dentistry and Oral Epidemiology*, **31**, 454–462.

11 Ahluwalia, K.P. & Sadowsky, D. (2003) Oral disease burden and dental services utilization by Latino and African-American seniors in Northern Manhattan. *Journal of Community Health*, **28**, 267–280.

12 Dolan, T.A., Peek, C.W., Stuck, A.E. & Beck, J.C. (1998) Functional health and dental service use among older adults. *Journals of Gerontology, Series A: Biological Sciences and Medical Sciences*, **53**, M413–M418.

13 Gilbert, G.H., Duncan, R.P., Crandall, L.A. & Heft, M.W. (1994) Older Floridians' attitudes toward and use of dental care. *Journal of Aging and Health*, **6**, 89–110.

14 Gilbert, G.H., Duncan, R.P., Heft, M.W. & Coward, R.T. (1997) Dental health attitudes among dentate black and white adults. *Medical Care*, **35**, 255–271.

15 Jones, J.A., Fedele, D.J., Bolden, A.J. & Bloom, B. (1994) Gains in dental care use not shared by minority elders. *Journal of Public Health Dentistry*, **54**, 39–46.

16 Manski, R.J., Goodman, H.S., Reid, B.C. & Macek, M.D. (2004) Dental insurance visits and expenditures among older adults. *American Journal of Public Health*, **94**, 759–764.

17 Janes, G.R., Blackman, D.K., Bolen, J.C., Kamimoto, L.A., Rhodes, L., Caplan, L.S. *et al.* (1999) Surveillance for use of preventive health-care services by older adults, 1995-1997. *MMWR CDC Surveillance Summaries*, **48**, 51–88.

18 Centers for Disease Control and Prevention. *Prevalence data: Oral health 2006*. http:apps.nccd.cdc.gov/brfss/list.asp?cat=OH&yr=2006&qkey=6606&state=all. [Accessed February 2008].

19 Kiyak, H.A., Kamoh, A., Persson, R.E. & Persson GR. (2002) Ethnicity and oral health in community-dwelling older adults. *General Dentistry*, **50**, 513–518.

20 Centers for Medicaid and Medicare Services. *National health, personal and other personal expenditures aggregate and per capita amounts, percent distribution, and average annual percent growth, by source of funds, and type of expenditure, selected years 1980-2002*. Vol. 2004. Tables 1, 4, 8, and 9. CMS, Washington, DC.

21 Wall, T.P. & Brown, L.J. (2003) Recent trends in dental visits and private dental insurance, 1989 and 1999. *Journal of the American Dental Association*, **134**, 621–627.

22 Brown E, Manski R. *Dental services: use, expenses, and sources of payment, 1996-2000. MEPS Research Findings No. 20. AHRQ Pub. No. 04-0018*. Rockville, MD: Agency for Healthcare Research and Quality, 2004.

23 Dolan, T.A. & Atchison, K.A. (1993) Implications of access, utilization and need for oral health care by the non-institutionalized and institutionalized elderly on the dental delivery system. *Journal of Dental Education*, **57**, 876–887.

24 Adegbembo, A.O., Leake, J.L., Main, P.A., Lawrence, H.L. & Chipman, M.L. (2002) The effect of dental insurance on the ranking of dental treatment needs in older residents of Durham Region's homes for the aged. *Journal of the Canadian Dental Association*, **68**, 412.

25 Gross, D.J., Alecxih, L., Gibson, M.J., Corea, J., Caplan, C. & Brangan, N. (1999) Out-of-pocket health spending by poor and near-poor elderly Medicare beneficiaries. *Health Services Research*, **34**, 241–254.

26 Kuthy, R.A., Strayer, M.S. & Caswell, R.J. (1996) Determinants of dental user groups among an elderly, low-income population. *Health Services Research*, **30**, 809–825.

27 Smith, J.M. & Sheiham, A. (1980) Dental treatment needs and demands of an elderly population in England. *Community Dentistry and Oral Epidemiology*, **8**, 360–364.

28 Hoad-Reddick, G., Grant, A.A. & Griffiths, C.S. (1987) Knowledge of dental services provided: investigations in an elderly population. *Community Dentistry and Oral Epidemiology*, **15**, 137–140.

29 Hally, J., Clarkson, J.E. & Newton, J.P. (2003) Continuing dental care for Highlands elderly: current practice and attitudes of dental practitioners and home supervisors. *Gerodontology*, **20**, 88–94.

30 Walker, R.J. & Kiyak, H.A. (2007) The impact of providing dental services to frail older adults: Perceptions of elders in adult day health centers. *Special Care in Dentistry*, **27**, 139–143.

31 Stoller, E.P. (1982) Patterns of physician utilization by the elderly: a multivariate analysis. *Medical Care*, **20**, 1080–1089.

32 Abrams, R.A., Ayers, C.S. & Lloyd, P.M. (1992) Attitudes of older versus younger adults toward dentistry and dentists. *Special Care in Dentistry*, **12**, 67–70.

33 Kiyak, H.A. (1987) An explanatory model of older persons' use of dental services. Implications for health policy. *Medical Care*, **25**, 936–952.

34 Andersen, R. & Newman, J.F. (1973) Societal and individual determinants of medical care utilization in the United States. *Milbank Memorial Fund Quarterly: Health and Society*, **51**, 95–124.

35 Rowe, J.W. & Kahn, R.L. (1999) The future of aging. *Contemporary Longterm Care*, **22**, 36–8, 40, 42–4.

36 Persson, G.R., Persson, R.E., Hollender, L.G. & Kiyak, H.A. (2004) The impact of ethnicity, gender, and marital status on periodontal and systemic health of older subjects in the Trials to Enhance Elders' Teeth and Oral Health (TEETH). *Journal of Periodontology*, **75**, 817–823.

37 Osterberg, T., Lundberg, M., Emilson, C.-G., Sundh, V., Birkhed, D. & Steen, B. (1998) Utilization of dental services in relation to socioeconomic and health factors in the middle-aged and elderly Swedish population. *Acta Odontologica Scandinavica*, **56**, 41–47.

38 Persson, R.E., Persson, G.R., Kiyak, H.A. & Powell, L.V. (1998) Periodontal effects of a behavioral prevention program. *Journal of Clinical Periodontology*, **25**, 322–329.

39 Gilbert, G.H., Shelton, B.J., Chavers, L.S. & Bradford, E.H. Jr., (2003) The paradox of dental need in a population-based study of dentate adults. *Medical Care*, **41**, 119–134.

40 Shah, M.N., Glushak, C., Karrison, T.G., Mulliken, R., Walter, J., Friedmann, P.D. *et al.* (2003) Predictors of emergency medical services utilization by elders. *Academic Emergency Medicine*, **10**, 52–58.

41 Shah, M.N., Rathouz, P.J. & Chin, M.H. (2003) Emergency department utilization by noninstitutionalized elders. *Academic Emergency Medicine*, **8**, 267–273.

42 McCusker, J., Healey, E., Bellavance, F. & Connolly, B. (1997) Predictors of repeat emergency department visits by elders. *Academic Emergency Medicine*, **4**, 581–588.

43 McCusker, J., Cardin, S., Bellavance, F. & Belzile, E. (2000) Return to the emergency department among elders: patterns and predictors. *Academic Emergency Medicine*, **7**, 249–259.

44 Houde, S.C. (1998) Predictors of elders' and family caregivers' use of formal home services. *Research in Nursing & Health*, **21**, 533–543.

45 Wilson, M.C., Holloway, P.J. & Sarll, D.W. (1994) Barriers to the provision of complex dental treatment for dentate older people: A comparison of dentists' and patients' views. *British Dental Journal*, **177**, 130–134.

46 MacEntee, M.I., Weiss, R., Waxler-Morrison, N.E. & Morrison, B.J. (1987) Factors influencing oral health in long term care facilities. *Community Dentistry and Oral Epidemiology*, **15**, 314–316.

47 MacEntee, M.I., Weiss, R.T., Waxler-Morrison, N.E. & Morrison, B.J. (1992) Opinions of dentists on the treatment of elderly patients in long-term care facilities. *Journal of Public Health Dentistry*, **52**, 239–244.

48 Weiss, R.T., Morrison, B.J., MacEntee, M.I. & Waxler-Morrison, N.E. (1993) The influence of social, economic, and professional considerations on services offered by dentists to long-term care residents. *Journal of Public Health Dentistry*, **53**, 70–75.

49 Meskin, L. & Berg, R. (2000) Impact of older adults on private dental practices, 1988-1998. *Journal of the American Dental Association*, **131**, 1188–1195.

50 Kiyak, H.A. *et al.* (2007) *Trials to enhance elders' teeth and oral health (TEETH)*. NIDCR grant RO1 DE12215. Final report October 2007.

51 Kiyak, H.A. (2005) *Community-wide strategies to promote oral health*. CDC grant U48 CCU 009654. Final report December 2005.

CHAPTER 25

Oral health care programmes for homebound people, nursing home residents and elderly inpatients

Ronald L. Ettinger[1] **and Jane M. Chalmers**[†2]
[1]Department of Prosthodontics and Dows Institute of Dental Research, College of Dentistry, University of Iowa, Iowa City, IA, USA
[2]Department of Preventive and Community Dentistry, The University of Iowa, College of Dentistry, Iowa City, IA, USA

Introduction

In modern medical education and practice there is an increasing emphasis on treating the whole patient and on the interaction among the physical, mental, social and economic aspects of health and disease. There are increasing attempts to normalize and rehabilitate people within institutions and to change from custodial care to optimum independence. Dentistry plays a role in such a total care programme because it can influence people's quality of life by allowing them to be free of pain and infection and to maintain their dentition at an adequate level so that they may enjoy mastication and communication.

Definition of the population

In all societies the majority of elderly people live in the community, while a small minority is homebound or institutionalized. This minority can be defined as very frail or functionally dependent elderly individuals whose capacities are so impaired by chronic debilitating physical, medical and/or emotional problems that they are unable to maintain independence [1].

The homebound comprise a specific group of people whose mental handicaps, chronic illness or frailty confine them to their homes. It is difficult to define exactly when a person is homebound, but such a person has been described as being unable to leave the house or garden without some mechanical assistance such as a stretcher or a wheelchair. In fact, with the exception of mental illness, especially dementia, the frail older adults living outside nursing homes may not be very different from those in nursing homes.

Epidemiology

The world's population is aging. Population growth has been slowing down, primarily as a result of the reduction in fertility in the majority of countries, both in the industrialized and in the industrializing world. The number of children born per woman was 5 in 1950 and 2.5 in 2011. Between 1970–1975 there were just 19 countries with below-replacement fertility, but by 2000–2005 there were 65. Over the same time period, the number of countries having very low fertility – that is, a total fertility lower than 1.3 children per woman – passed from zero to 17. Today about 40 per cent of the world's population live in countries with below-replacement fertility and 13 per cent live in countries with very low fertility. In parallel to the decline of fertility, mortality has declined considerably in most countries over recent years. In some industrialized countries, life expectancy at birth for females has already exceeded or is now approaching 80 years and is not slowing down [2].

Because of these rapid transformations, population age distributions are changing markedly as the number of older persons increases and there is a relative decrease in the number of younger persons. Thus, the 21st century is projected to be the century of population aging, and even the size of the

[†] Author is deceased.

Textbook of Geriatric Dentistry, Third Edition. Edited by Poul Holm-Pedersen, Angus W. G. Walls and Jonathan A. Ship.

population is expected to decrease considerably in a number of countries over the coming decades [2, 3].

In 2005 Japan became the country with the oldest population in the world with a mean age of 43.5 years. Other countries with high rates of elderly are in Western Europe, which includes Italy, Greece, Spain, Belgium, France, Germany, Monaco, the Netherlands and Switzerland, followed by northern Europe, which includes Denmark, Finland, Iceland, Norway, Sweden and the United Kingdom. In 2002, although only a quarter of the world's population lived in the more industrialized countries, 45% of the people aged over 65 years resided in them. Among people aged 80 years or older, 60% live in the more industrially developed regions. The five countries with the highest numbers of elderly are: China with 16.8% of the world's total, USA 13.1%, India 8.7%, Japan 6.6% and Russia 4.2%. The current figures for the proportion of elderly people as a proportion of the total population in six of the most populous countries are shown in Table 25.1. Some of these countries, owing to their size, like China and India, have large numbers of older people but do not have an aging problem, as these older people do not make up a large proportion of their population; others have both large numbers and proportions such as the USA and Japan. In 1997 the characteristics of people over 80 years of age in the USA were reviewed. They found that women made up 69% of the group; only 21% were married, 70% were widowed, 24% were institutionalized and 48% were disabled. This group increased in number by 141% between 1960 and 1980 and is projected to triple from 5.7 million in 2011 to 14.1 million in 2040 [4]. It is estimated that between 2000 and 2025 women over age 80 will increase from 9.5% of the population to 13.3% [5]. Those over age 80 are the fastest growing age group in any of the more industrially developed countries.

The proportion of older women in the general population is increasing in both the industrialized countries and industrializing countries. Currently older women in the more industrialized countries make up 10% of the total population, but are projected to exceed 15% by 2025. In Japan and Italy older women will account for 18% of the total population. This is due to the gap in the life expectancy between men and women which is currently about 7 years. In some countries (e.g. Russia, Romania and Belarus) life expectancy differences have risen to 10 years due to the high levels of male mortality. In the less industrialized countries the difference is only about 3 years, probably due to maternal mortality [5].

The fastest growing age groups are persons aged 80 years and older. In the more industrialized countries women aged 80 years and older make up 19% of all older women and by 2025 that number will have increased to 25%. In the less industrialized countries this age group currently makes up 9% of all older women but it will triple in numbers by 2025. The implications of this growth of the oldest old are that several of these persons are more likely to be in poorer health and require more services and are more likely to be dependent on others [6].

Table 25.1 The elderly population of the world[a]

Country	% over age 65	Country	No. in millions over age 80
1 Monaco	22.4	1 China	11.8
2 Italy	19.3	2 USA	9.2
3 Japan	18.8	3 India	6.2
4 Greece	18.6	4 Japan	4.6
5 Germany	17.9	5 Russia	3.0
6 Spain	17.5	6 Germany	2.9
7 Sweden	17.5	7 United Kingdom	2.4
8 Belgium	17.4	8 Italy	2.3
9 Bulgaria	17.1	9 France	2.2
10 San Marino	16.7	10 Spain	1.5

[a]Data sourced from references [60] and [61].

Homebound people

There is still very little information on the distribution and characteristics of older adults who are confined to their homes or homebound. In a review of the characteristics of the homebound, Ganguli *et al.* [7] state that the 'scientific literature on the topic, while somewhat sparse, falls into two groups'. They found that the biggest group of reports was on the demographics and burden of illness in the population but all of the studies had selection bias and targeted the homebound who were receiving services. The second group of studies tried to examine representative samples and compared them to the general population but the samples were usually very small.

In the USA in 1996 it was estimated that 1.75 million elderly people aged 65 years and older were using home health care services [8]. These consumers were predominantly women (70%) aged 75–84 years (47%), white (69%), widowed (47%), living in private residences (92%) and living with at least one family member (50%). The most frequent help they received was with bathing (53%), dressing (46%), transferring from their bed to a chair (3%) and toileting (23%). Although no official national data are available on homebound elderly due to a difficulty in defining who they are, in 2005 the American Academy of Home Care Physicians stated that at least 2 million persons aged 65 and older were permanently homebound; this number will increase over the next decade [9].

These frail individuals tend not to seek elective services and are not inclined to volunteer for household studies. In a recent study [10] in New York, 131 out of 334 homebound elderly receiving home-based primary care services agreed to participate in an oral health survey. The authors found that 92% needed some type of dental treatment beyond oral hygiene needs. Also, 96% had not seen a dentist since they became housebound. The percentage of people in the community who are frail can be estimated from data reporting limitation of activity due to disability. A good indicator for the number of people who are homebound might be how many people require a home visit by a physician. National Health Interview Survey data in 2005 in the USA indicated that 24% of the population over age 65 years had a limitation in a major activity. The highest rate of home visits was in people aged 65 years and older: 46 per 1000, which is similar to the often quoted figure that 5% of elderly people are homebound [11].

The only dental data come from a US pilot study which, by means of a dental chart audit, evaluated the differences between homebound and institutionalized people. The only difference they found was that nearly 80% of the homebound had to pay privately for dental care compared with 33% of those in nursing homes. The homebound had slightly fewer teeth and less need for care but were essentially similar to nursing home residents.

In Japan it was estimated that 2.8 million would require long-term care [12]. In 2000 the Japanese government expanded the public long-term care insurance system to cover the cost and promote health care services for functionally dependent elderly people. This now includes oral health care services.

It is estimated that of the 9 ½ million persons in Britain who are aged 65 and older, 10% are functionally dependent or institutionalized. In Britain general dental practitioners have provided domiciliary visits to patients who could not attend a private dental office. In 1999–2000 there were 330 000 visits; of these, 76% were to people aged 75 or older. In 2000 the Dental Practice Board restricted the travel claims for domiciliary visits by general dentists to two per day. The care of the homebound and the institutionalized has been delegated to salaried dentists working within the Community Dental Service (CDS). The CDS however is constrained in the amount of domiciliary care it can provide because it is a small service and has limited resources [13].

A similar domiciliary dental care system exists for older adults who are eligible for public-funded dental care in Australia – this is a constrained system with many challenges to providing care for homebound and institutionalized older adults [14].

Hospice

The hospice movement was begun in Britain by Dame Cicely Saunders at St. Christopher's hospice in London in 1967. The first hospice in the USA was the Connecticut Hospice which opened in 1974. There are currently more than 3200 hospices across the USA, some part of hospital systems, some independent, many are non-profit agencies [15].

A hospice is a programme and/or a hospital-type facility that is designed to care for the dying and treat their special needs, which include adequate pain control, psychosocial support for the patient and the family, medical services; and an interdisciplinary team approach which includes dentistry to care for the integrated needs of the dying patient.

The oral and dental needs of many of these patients have been neglected. Gordon *et al.* [16] reported that over 50% of the patients complained of dry mouth (62%), problems talking (59%), bad bite (59%), general oral discomfort (55%), poor chewing ability (52%) and poor dental appearance (52%). The dental administrators did not believe that the patients had a lot of problems but they did suggest that the patients' problems were food under dentures (86%), dentures that did not stay in place (72%) and discomfort with dentures (57%). None of the administrators felt that 'maintaining or improving the dental and oral condition of the mouth' was very important to their patients whereas 45% of the patients rated it high. Other studies have also reported a high level of oral symptoms in this population [17–19] (Table 25.2).

The care for these patients has been called palliative care and is the management of patients with active, progressive, far advanced disease for whom the prognosis is limited and the focus of care is on the quality of their life. The principles of palliative care state that a palliative care dentist, in collaboration with the patient, must first assess his/her difficulties. Then one should try to help the patient to eliminate or at least alleviate the pain and discomfort and provide relief if comfort is not possible for the patient. This may include emotional comfort such as replacing lost anterior maxillary teeth with

Table 25.2 Prevalence of oral problems in terminally ill patients

Symptoms	Gordon *et al.*, 1985 [16] (%)	Jobbins *et al.*, 1992 [62] (%)	Aldred *et al.*, 1991 [63] (%)
Xerostomia	62	58	97
Oral soreness	55	42	31
Oral candidiasis	10	70	NA
Dysphasia	NA	37	51
Difficulty talking	59	NA	66
Denture problems	59[a]	71[a]	40[a]

[a] % in patients wearing dentures.

a denture to help with dignity and self-esteem for the *patient and the family*.

Institutionalized people

In the last two decades several large representative studies have evaluated the oral and dental problems of people who have been institutionalized. These were in the USA, the Department of Veterans Affairs Nursing Home study in 1987 [20], and in the UK, the National Diet and Nutritional Survey in 1998 [21], which compared two representative groups of older adults, one free-living, the other institutionalized. Other more numerous studies have focused on states (in the USA) or regions and cities. Thus, information on these populations is more reliable. In 1977, about 1.28 million elderly people resided in 16 200 nursing homes in the USA. By 2011, there were 1.50 million in 15 683 homes. They make up about 3.6% of the population over age 65, but it has been projected that 20% of the people over age 65 years will spend at least part of their life in a nursing home [22]. In recent years, there has been an increase in alternatives to nursing homes, such as assisted living or community housing. The number of persons needing short-term, post-acute care has also increased. Thus, the nursing home population has decreased in size but has become older and sicker when they enter this kind of long-term care institution. Residents of nursing homes in the USA are said to have a number of common characteristics [23].

- They are old (the average age is 83 years, 70% are over 75 years and 45.2% are over age 85).
- They are mainly women (71.2%).
- They are widowed (62%).
- They are disabled (99% due to poor physical health and 54% are mentally impaired).
- Less than 40% are ambulatory.
- They are confused: 42% have dementia, 12% have schizophrenia or other mood disorders.
- They need help: over 75% need assistance with three or more activities of daily living (ADL) and 51.1% need help with all five ADLs.
- They take multiple drugs (an average of 4.9 drugs each day per person).
- They are alone (more than 40% have no close relatives or relations).
- Few will leave before they die.

Similar data have been published for other industrialized countries. In addition, many countries are developing innovative home-based care delivery systems for people who are assessed as being high level care nursing home patients.

Elderly inpatients

National dental data for elderly inpatients are virtually nonexistent in most countries. However, increasing numbers of hospital inpatient beds are occupied by older adults, especially those aged 85+ years, and these older patients have much longer hospital stays. These patients complain of problems associated with loose dentures and dry mouth and a bad taste, also problems swallowing and bad breath, and so on. Many have dental problems that could be helped by palliative care, and many need help with daily oral hygiene [24].

Oral health status and needs

Among functionally dependent elderly people around the world, 55–80% are edentulous and 60–80% have immediate dental needs. Their last dental visit was approximately 8–10 years ago and the average age of their dentures is at least 15–20 years.

The oral health of the elderly is poor, with the most neglected group being the persons who are homebound, hospitalized or institutionalized. Elderly persons enter long-term care with high levels of oral diseases, and disease continues to be ongoing during their nursing home stay [25]. Many community-living older adults with dementia have the onset of high levels of oral disease in the early moderate stages of cognitive impairment. In the past, most of the elderly in institutions were edentulous, so oral health care services have not always been urgently needed, as the staff could always remove the dentures and place the person with problems on a soft diet. However, evidence shows that this is changing. In many areas, elderly people in institutions have many more natural teeth than in the past. This increases the need for oral health care services, and the provision of oral health care will be much more complex than the past emphasis on 'dentures for the old folks' [26].

Nevertheless, elderly people in long-term care facilities are among the most dentally neglected members of their communities. It has been suggested that this neglect has a multifactorial etiology. Some of the factors identified are elderly people's ignorance of treatable oral and dental conditions and their fear of treatment. As a group, the old old have had a stereotypical view of the dentist as a mechanically oriented individual who 'pulled teeth and made plates' [26]. They also believed that dentures should last for a lifetime. Thus, they sought care only when previous unmet dental needs could no longer be ignored. In the USA, residents in long-term care facilities have to pay for extra services within an institution; many do not have the resources to purchase dental care. The majority of long-term care residents are single, divorced or widowed elderly women, who also have the highest rate of poverty [27]. Most health workers, especially physicians, have not been sensitized to the oral health care needs of their elderly clients or patients. It has also been suggested that, since a physician coordinates the health care of elderly people and since dentistry falls outside the sphere of their direct influence and control, the dentist usually has not been part of the coordinated health care team. Therefore, if the physician does not suggest dental care, none is likely to be carried out. However, more importantly, the evidence indicates the physicians may either lack interest and avoid nursing home residents or, if interested, find that they have less control, back-up or support in the nursing home than in the acute-care hospital and that their recommendations are not translated into action by an overworked and often unskilled staff. Furthermore, as many older persons had dental experiences prior to the universal use of good local anaesthesia and high-speed turbine handpieces, they associate dentistry with pain [26]. Therefore, it is not surprising that they seek care only if they are in discomfort or pain. A further complication has been the dental profession itself. In the past, few dentists have had the opportunity to treat medically compromised, institutionalized and bedridden patients during their training. Most dental curricula did not prepare dentists either philosophically or technically to treat patients outside the dental offices [28]. Thus, such a dentist with little or no experience with mobile equipment or out-of-office procedures may either refuse or be reluctant to treat elderly patients in long-term care facilities or geriatric hospitals. Studies [29, 30] have shown that, for elderly people living in the community, there is a strong relationship between education, income, place of residence and utilization of dental services. Studies [25, 31, 32] carried out in long-term care facilities have shown that over 80% need treatment, of which only 65–75% are mentally or physically healthy enough to benefit from treatment. The amount of treatment required depended on the socioeconomic level of the residents in the facility and on the degree of severity of their mental or physical disabilities. In a study evaluating the perceived need of institutionalized elderly people, it was found that those who were edentulous and not wearing dentures were least likely to seek care [23]. The ability to get to a dentist or mobility status was also found to correlate highly with seeking care. Those most likely to seek care were persons with natural teeth who had painful lesions, growths and bleeding gums. In fact, 57% of the institutionalized elderly perceived specific clinical needs. If free treatment was offered to residents of long-term care facilities, then persons under 75 years were more likely to accept treatment than those over 75 years and men more frequently than women. Also, the persons who practised personal grooming more frequently were more likely to accept dental treatment. By knowing whether a resident was dentate combined with data from the resident's medical chart, it was possible to predict who would need oral health care without a clinical examination. However, this information could not be used to accurately predict who would accept dental treatment. The best predictor of acceptance was the availability of third-party payment, especially public funding.

Several international studies have investigated the perceptions of Directors of Nursing (DONs) and dentists about nursing home dentistry. Overall, these studies have highlighted significant barriers to dental care for nursing home residents, and differing perceptions between DONs and dentists. Most of the dental care for residents is provided at dentists' offices and not on-site at nursing homes. Dentists and DONs held several common and many varying perceptions of the problems associated with dental care provision in nursing homes [33]. Both identified a group of nursing home environmental constraints and a lack of portable dental equipment. DONs further identified a group of resident-related problems such as families and residents disinterest about dental care, problems obtaining consent for dental care, residents' behaviour and cognitive problems, while dentists discussed some dental practice-related problems such as increased time needed for dentistry at nursing homes, low priority of dental care by nursing home staff and staff's dislike of providing regular oral care. Overall, dentists' interest in providing dental care on-site at nursing homes was very low, and DONs also perceived this to be true.

Oral health programmes

The majority of oral health care services for elderly people in the USA are provided in community-based offices by private practitioners. For well and ambulatory elderly, a few modifications in office design to allow for normal aging changes will allow private practitioners to treat this population [34]. For non-ambulatory nursing home residents and for homebound people, different delivery systems are needed. This section discusses six methods of dental care delivery for homebound and institutionalized elderly people and evaluates their advantages and disadvantages: transfer to a dental office; on-site dental programmes; teledentistry; mobile dental vans; portable dentistry interventions; and hospital-based mobile programmes.

1. Transfer to a dental office/practice

This method is best for dentists, as they can treat patients in their own offices with all their auxiliary personnel and equipment. It is the most cost-effective means for a dentist, as no travelling or set-up time is required. However, this is rather expensive and time-consuming for a nursing home if a staff member must accompany their resident to the dentist. Nursing homes are often reluctant to contract such an arrangement and thus little care under these circumstances is voluntarily offered to nursing home residents [35]. A study of a representative sample of the institutionalized population of the city of Edinburgh [36] evaluated the residents' ability to attend the office of a general practitioner. They found 30% physically capable of using public transport. If accompanied, an additional 46% could be transported in a private vehicle providing that the dentist's office was accessible (either on a ground floor and having ramps and/or elevators). Another 20% would require an ambulance and the remaining 4% were bedfast. This study did not evaluate the ability of these residents to withstand the documented emotional trauma of being transported. Data from a statewide study in Vermont [37] indicated that more than 50% could be cared for in dentists' offices. A survey in California [38] reported that 66.1% of residents in the homes studied could be transported, but they excluded patients with dementia and severely ill and uncooperative patients. Table 25.3 summarizes some of the studies that have reported on the ability to transport residents to private dentists' offices; the rates vary from a low of 34% to a high of 90%.

Several factors need to be taken into account before an institutionalized person can be transported to a dentist's office such as: the person's activity level, continence, transferability appointment times, communication and legal and ethical considerations.

The person's activity level

Many residents who are underweight or need special padding to sit cannot tolerate procedures in which they have to sit for more than two hours. These two hours must include loading the person into a vehicle, travel time and the actual time in the dental office as well as the return trip.

Continence

Even when a resident is ambulatory or using a walker, many older residents need to use bathroom facilities on a regular schedule because of weakness of the bladder sphincter. Dentists must therefore evaluate bathroom facilities in the office for access and safety and know the patient's schedule. The dentist's staff also needs to know how to help a patient (especially if the patient is wheelchair-bound) to use bathroom facilities.

Transferability

The ability to transport an institutionalized person depends on the home having a vehicle available that can safely and easily carry the resident to a dental office. If the resident is in a wheelchair, then a van with a wheelchair lift is ideal. Such vans could belong to the nursing home or an agency or be part of a government programme. The accessibility of the office is also important, including adequate and safe parking, ramps, doors and elevators, and so on. [34]. Many people in wheelchairs can be treated in a wheelchair with appropriate headrests if there is adequate office space or they may have to be transferred into the dental chair. The dentist needs to train the staff in the skills of safe wheelchair transfers but it is preferable if family or the accompanying staff person transfer the patient as they do it regularly.

The ability to bring residents to a dental office can be affected by the weather. Frail, older people are susceptible to hypothermia and hyperthermia. It is difficult to manoeuvre a wheelchair in ice and snow. If walks and parking lots are not cleared after a snowstorm, it is difficult to bring someone for care. Thus, winter weather is a major factor affecting transportability.

Appointment times

A patient's disability affects the time of day he or she should be appointed. Mid-morning appointments are good for many patients, such as those with heart disease, because

Table 25.3 The transportability of long-term care residents

Authors/year/reference	Location	No. of residents	% who can betransported	Sample type[a]
Martinello & Leake, 1971 [64]	Ontario	517	90	C
Manderson & Ettinger, 1975 [36]	Edinburgh	442	76	B
Terrili & Elliott, 1979 [65]	Montana	3780	83	A
American Dental Association, 1980 [66]	Vermont	375	71	B
Ekelund, 1984 [67]	Finland	480	71	B
Shareff & Strauss, 1985 [68]	North Carolina	161	34	C
California Dental Association, 1986 [69]	California	286	66	B
McIntyre et al. 1986 [70]	Ontario	345	77	B
Ettinger et al. 1988 [71]	Iowa	853	53	C

[a] A = total sample; B = stratified random; C = convenience.

they are strongest after a night's rest. Also, there is a diurnal variation in the stickiness of platelets, thus the patient should not be seen between 6 am and 9 am to avoid a cardiovascular event [39]. Mid-morning or early-afternoon appointments are preferable for other elderly patients, especially when interviewing the patient, to avoid any changes in mental status that may occur due to the oversedation from night time hypnotics. In addition, patients with osteoarthritis, a major disability of nursing home residents, need time to loosen up after a night's sleep, so they also need later morning appointments. Mildly demented patients, because of decreased auditory and visual stimuli, exhibit increased confusion as evening approaches, which is called 'sundowning'.

Many nursing homes have staff changes at 7 am and 3 pm. If personnel from nursing homes need to accompany residents, early-morning appointments and mid-afternoon appointments need to be avoided or the nursing home will have to pay the accompanying staff member overtime.

Communications

Most nursing homes in the USA require permission from a resident's physician when they take that resident to the dentist. The nursing home staff requires dental progress notes from the dentist after each appointment as well as written instructions so that the staff can cooperate and accurately carry out any care prescribed for the resident and monitor the resident's ability to follow instructions. The dentist who performs procedures in a nursing home should be aware that it operates differently from an acute-care hospital. The ratio of either registered nurses (RN) or licensed practical nurses (LPN) is significantly lower in nursing homes and the majority of care in most homes is carried out by nurses' aides who, at best, have had only minimal training. For post-surgery patients requiring close monitoring, the dentist may have to keep in close telephone contact with the nursing staff to assure that instructions are carried out.

Legal and ethical considerations

Developing dental care programmes for homebound or institutionalized elderly people pose ethical and legal problems not often encountered in caring for ambulatory, healthy adults. The legal system in most countries has established that adults must freely consent to care. The consent must be: (1) voluntary; that is, given without coercion or excessive influence on the person's exercise of choice; (2) competent; that is, given by a person legally capable of giving consent; and (3) informed; that is, given by a person who has been provided sufficient information to make an intelligent decision. The homebound or institutionalized elderly person may not be capable of providing informed voluntary consent. It has been suggested that dentists must consider four major principles of biomedical ethics when caring for compromised patients:

- to do no harm,
- to do good,
- to respect patient autonomy,
- to treat patients fairly and justly.

It is estimated that more than half of the institutionalized elderly have either primary degenerative or secondary dementia. Data for homebound elderly people are not available, but for non-institutionalized elderly, the prevalence of primary degenerative and secondary dementia is estimated to be 5–6% for the elderly population over age 65 years [40]. It has been reported that dementia affects about 2.8% of those aged 65–74 years in the USA; in the age group 75–84 years this increases to 9% but by age 85 increases to 28% [41]. For these cognitively impaired people, the dental practitioner or nursing home consultant will need to assess the need for legal intervention to protect the rights of the patient and reduce liability before proceeding with care. A number of cognitively impaired people have court-appointed conservators or guardians. For these patients, the dentist needs to obtain informed consent from that appointed person. For the patient with questionable cognitive functioning and no appointed conservator or guardian, the dentist needs to determine competence before proceeding with care. The decision should be based on an evaluation of cognitive function using one of the many mental status tests [42] and consultations with the patient's physician, family and nursing staff. If it is determined that the patient is not capable of giving voluntary informed consent, then the courts must appoint a guardian or conservator before dental care is rendered. Nevertheless, emergency care should be rendered using similar guidelines as for a dependent child.

2. On-site dental programmes

These programmes have established dental units in hospitals and nursing home facilities. Depending on the size of the hospital or home, its ownership and the mechanism of financing available, the equipment belongs either to the government or to the institution. The institution needs at least 150–200 residents to make such a dental facility financially feasible. The advantage is that residents can be treated within their own environment, for it has been shown that frail elderly people do not withstand well the disruption of being transported. Residents who are incontinent or catheterized are best treated at their place of residence. It is also less disruptive to the functioning of a nursing home to have residents treated within the facilities, as the institution must either arrange for the family to transport the resident or they must send a staff member and have a vehicle available. The problems of transport; that is, having a suitable vehicle and using volunteer drivers or subsidized transport or ambulances creates problems of coordination, organization and financing. A further advantage of on-site facilities is that it can become a regional outpatient health centre for eligible, ambulatory, elderly people living nearby, and on-site dental facilities were utilized significantly more than off-site dental facilities. The number of routine dental visits per person per year was twice as great when services were available on-site [43]. The disadvantages of such on-site facilities are that they cannot be easily moved to treat residents in nearby smaller facilities and they cannot be moved to the bedside of a bedridden patient. Thus, such a programme is somewhat inflexible and not cost-effective unless the home is very large and mobile equipment is also available.

3. Teledentistry

Teledentistry provides the opportunity for patients in remote locations being treated by their local general dentist to have their problems and their treatment reviewed by dental specialists. Teledentistry is the provision of real time dental care such as diagnosis, treatment planning, consulting and follow-up, via electronic transmission from a different site [44]. The first group to put teledentistry into practice was the US Army in 1994 [45].

This technology has been used by the University of Southern California's Mobile Dental Clinic with children living in a rural area [46]. It has also been used for the diagnosis and treatment of orofacial pain. In Japan, teledentistry has been used as a means of preventive patient education for homebound patients. We believe that it has a very real potential for dentists working in long-term care or with isolated populations in that it allows consultation with specialists without having to transport the patient. This is firstly cost-effective and less traumatic on the more confined, fragile residents of nursing homes.

4. Mobile dental vans

Portable equipment has been developed substantially in the recent past. This equipment ranges from simple units carried on mopeds and golf carts, to mobile vans of various sizes and to the military dental units that can be parachuted into a combat zone.

Mobile dental vans can be of two types. In one type, the van carries all the supplies and equipment to the treatment location, and the equipment is unloaded and carried into the home or facility and set up inside. Laboratory and film-processing equipment may remain in the van. In the second type, the van is equipped as a dental operatory so that dental care can be delivered within the vehicle itself (Figure 25.1). Such a self-contained mobile van may also have a laboratory incorporated for polishing and repairing dentures. Several companies have developed a variety of vans. However, as Mulligan [47] points out, conversion of a bus or motor home creates some functional problems. The electrical capacity of the motor home needs to be upgraded to support dental equipment as well as air conditioning and heating units. If the unit is a trailer, then a connection to a suitable power outlet at the side where treatment is to be carried out is required. The second major problem is in transferring the person from the home to the van. This requires a wheelchair lift or a ramp, which often means enlarging an existing door in the motor home or trailer. Many elderly people who are homebound or institutionalized are physically disabled and are stressed by being moved from the controlled environment of a facility through inclement weather into the van. A particular problem is

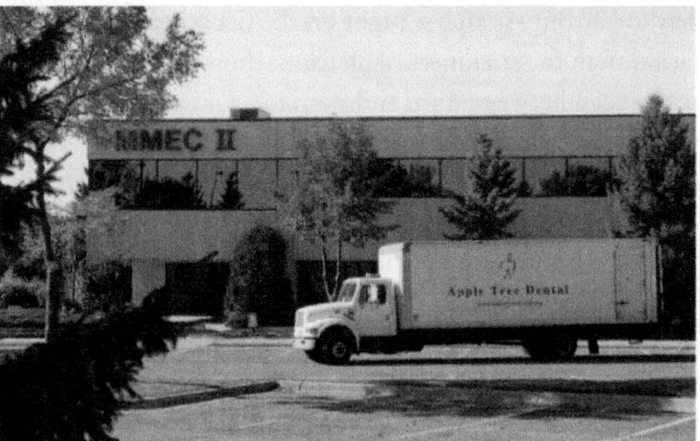
MMEC II
Apple Tree Dental
Apple Tree's Multi-Site Delivery Vehicle
Transports (3) Apple Tree Mobile Dental Offices
(a)

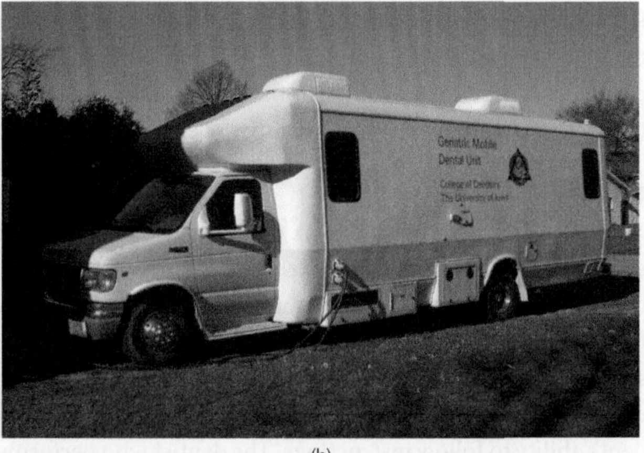

(b)

Figure 25.1 a) The Appletree Dental truck, which transports a portable dental office to nursing homes (courtesy Dr M. Helgeson). b) Mobile dental office, University of Iowa.

the possibility of hypothermia in cold weather, especially if the van cannot be parked right next to the nursing home. Another disadvantage associated with a van is the freezing of water lines. The only solution for this problem is to have storage tanks within the van, but these take up a lot of space. The main advantage of the self-contained mobile dental units is the ability to have modem standard equipment available, such as fibre-optic handpieces and good suction. The primary disadvantages are the initial capital costs and the maintenance required for the equipment and the van. Other problems complicating the use of mobile vans are issues that may vary from city to city and state to state such as:

- the need for a local business license;
- regulations for radiographic equipment, including safety checks;
- special regulations from some dental boards;
- special registration of the vehicle;
- security of the van, with the ability to lock up syringes and needles, and so on;
- insurance for protection from damage due to vandalism; and
- support services to repair dental equipment or the van.

5. Portable dentistry interventions

This equipment varies depending on its purpose. The simplest is the 'little black bag' concept, which includes enough equipment to carry out only emergency care such as extraction of teeth and adjustment of dentures. The next level of *portable equipment* consists of a variety of dental units constructed by individuals as well as companies to include high- and low-speed handpieces (Figure 25.2). These units are small, compact and lightweight. The advantages of these portable systems are that: (1) they can be easily loaded into almost any car; (2) they are compact and light enough in weight to be transported virtually anywhere; and (3) they are self-contained to run off a small air compressor or a pressurized carbon dioxide tank.

The disadvantages of the small portable systems are that they were designed for limited work and thus cannot be used continuously. For this kind of care, larger mobile units are required [43]. *Mobile dental units* are complete units constructed so that they can be transported by vehicle. These units are either modified standard units that need a separate compressor or come with a built-in compressor. Many of

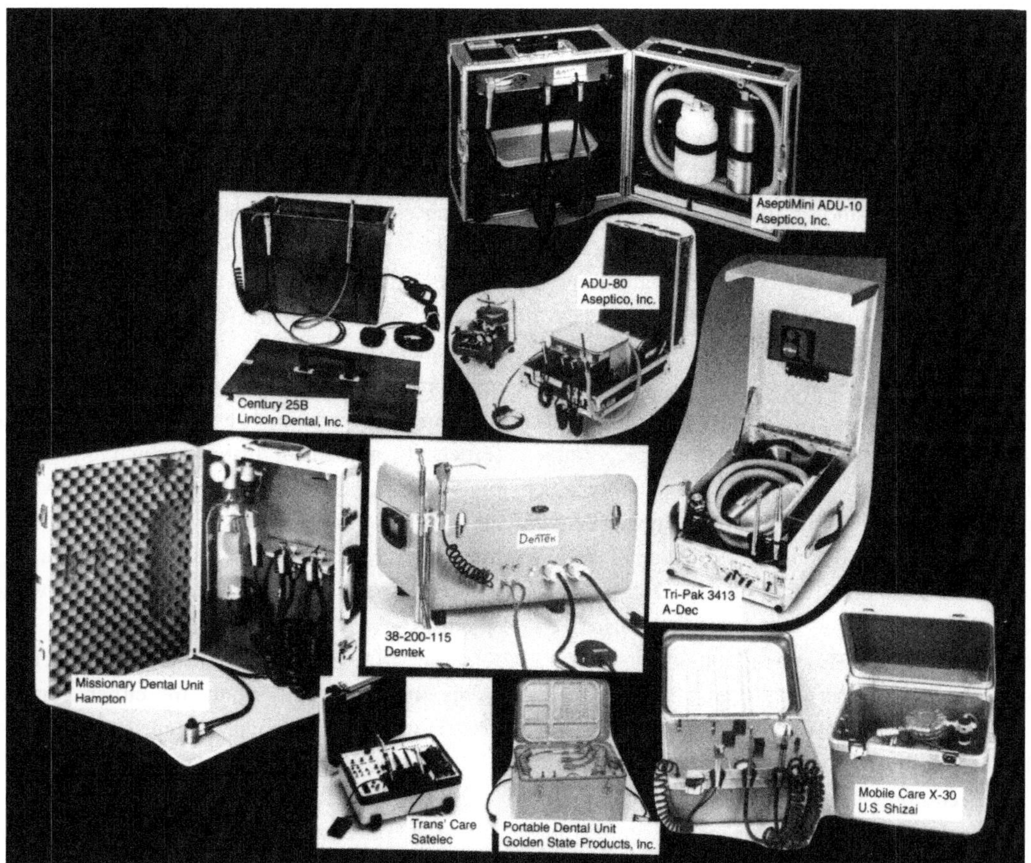

Figure 25.2 A variety of commercially produced portable units.

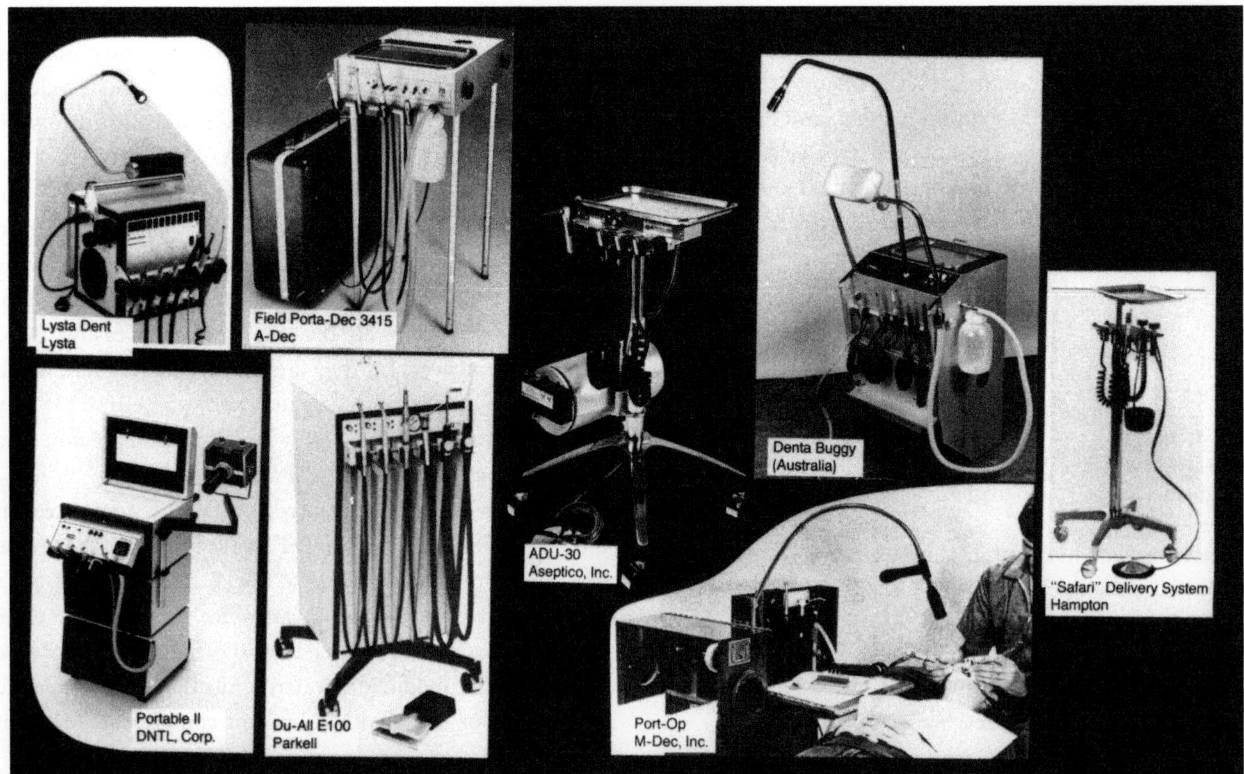

Figure 25.3 A variety of commercially produced mobile dental units (picture of Dentabuggy, bottom left, courtesy of Dr D. Crack, Melbourne, Australia).

the earlier models tended to overheat with continuous use but most of these design problems have been eliminated (Figure 25.3). The advantages of mobile units are that they can be transported to a site and set up to carry out comprehensive care. These systems are best used by bringing them to a central site such as a nursing home or small hospital and bringing patients to the unit. Once all the patients have been seen, the unit can be packed up and transported to another site.

Carrying out effective dental care for isolated elderly populations, especially if they are to receive a complete range of dental services, requires not only a dental unit but portable dental chairs, headrests and X-ray units. A variety of dental units with high- and low-speed handpieces including suction are shown in Figures 25.2 and 25.3. Headrests (Figure 25.4), portable chairs (Figure 25.5) and X-ray units have also been developed to use with these systems to allow delivery of a complete range of restorative services (Figure 25.6).

The advantages of these mobile dental systems are: (1) They can be brought to the patient virtually anywhere (Figure 25.7). A compressor run by electricity or a carbon dioxide tank can provide pressure for the air-turbine hand-pieces. (2) These systems are flexible and can potentially provide much more cost-effective care (Figure 25.8). (3) The systems can also be used for homebound people (Figure 25.9). Cost-effective dental care can be delivered to nursing home residents and hospital patients but delivering care to the individual homebound person is very difficult. There is inefficiency due to travelling time, setting up the equipment, treatment for only one person and then dismantling and storing the equipment. This allows no more than three patients per half day, even when they are geographically close. Other possible problems are related to communication, such as obtaining an adequate history (especially a medical history which often means calling the patient's physician). Communication with the patient and getting informed consent may be difficult. The most difficult problem is funding. Who will pay for the care? Who will reimburse the dentist at an adequate level to cover the expenses?

In the USA, these programmes have taken a number of forms, but essentially they are either community-based programmes or individual entrepreneur ventures designed for the needs of various social groups.

A good example of a community programme is the Dental Treatment of Homebound Persons in Louisville, Kentucky. It is a cooperative effort among three Louisville organizations: the Rotary Club of Louisville, Inc., the Louisville Dental

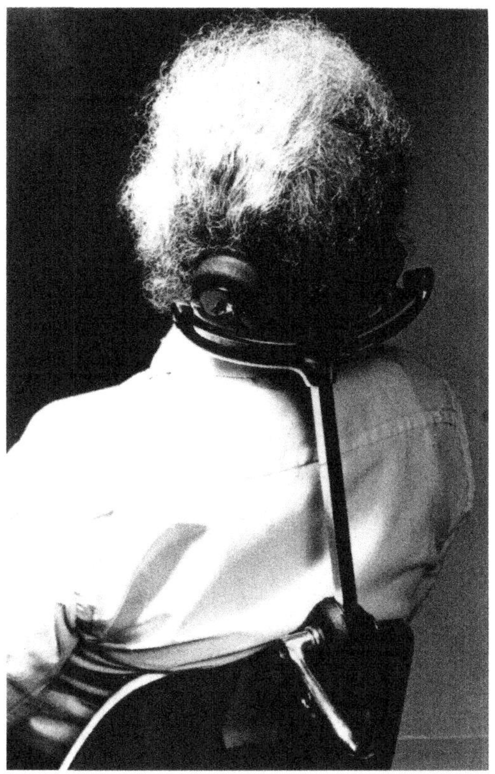

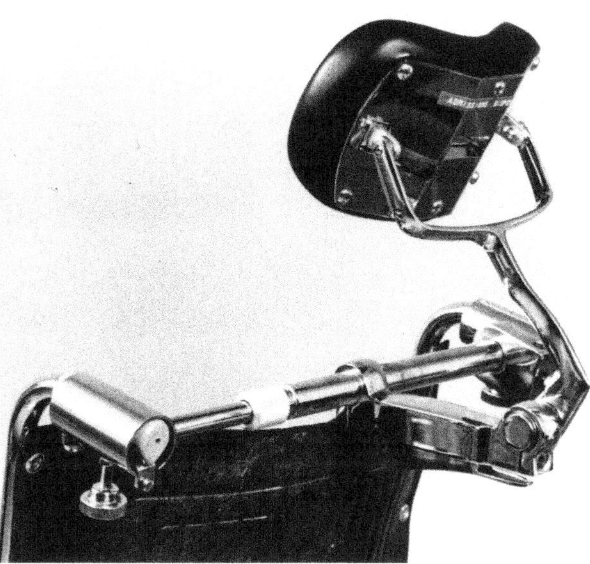

Figure 25.4 On the left is a headrest that can be attached to a straight-backed chair, to the right a unit that attaches to a wheelchair.

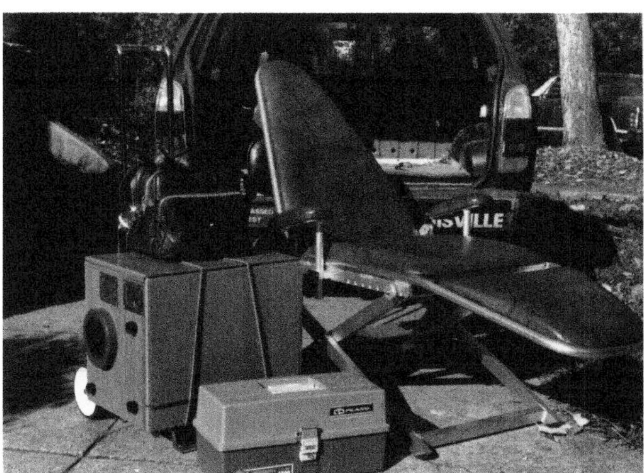

Figure 25.5 A portable chair (courtesy of Dr B.W. Ceridan, Louisville, Kentucky, USA).

Society and the Visiting Nurse Association of Louisville, Inc. They address the dental care needs of homebound people in their community, estimated to be 20 000 people. Basically, the Rotary Club supplied the funds for the purchase of equipment. The Visiting Nurse Association supplied the administrative support. The Dental Society trained the dental personnel in the use and care of the equipment and its members supplied the dental services as volunteers.

The multiple objectives included:

- screening for oral cancer and dental needs;
- providing dental treatment and oral health education;
- providing lectures on geriatric dentistry to dentists, nurses and dental hygienists;
- coordination with physicians and other treatment centres for holistic care;
- coordination with social agencies providing care;
- informing the public about the programme; and
- training dentists in homebound techniques.

In effect, such programmes are designed to deliver oral health care to elderly people in a home setting on a long-term basis (Figure 25.10).

6. Hospital-based/dental school-based mobile programmes

Hospital-based programmes have only recently begun to appear. The programme is usually based in a hospital or teaching institution that provides dental care for long-term care facilities within a nominated radius of the institution. The dental school in Iowa has developed such a programme that has been in operation since 1981. The programme uses portable and mobile equipment. Under the supervision of members of the faculty, six senior students spend a continuous four-week rotation on the mobile unit or in a special care clinic set-up in the dental school. The rest of the staff

NOMAD® PRO 2

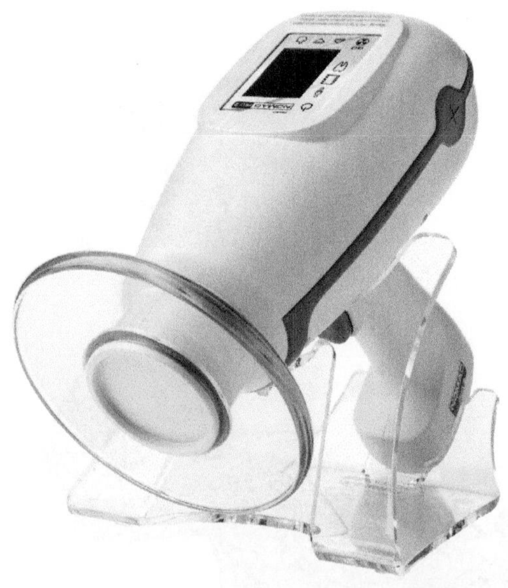

Figure 25.6 Aribex NOMAD Pro 2 handheld dental X-ray unit. *Source:* Aribex, Inc. Reproduced with permission of Aribex, Inc.

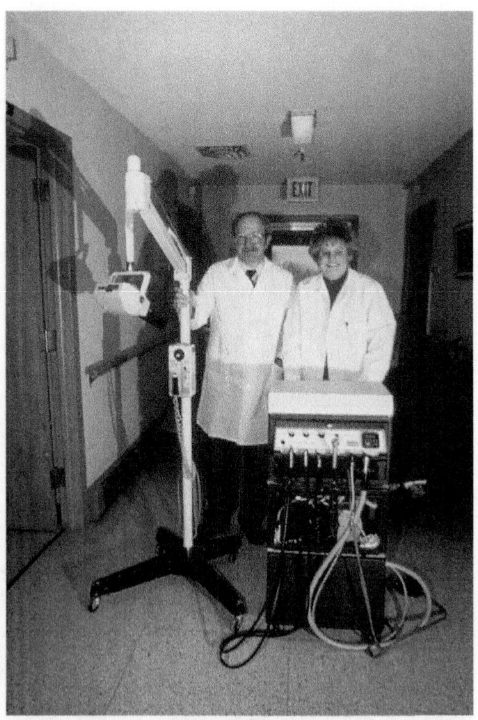

Figure 25.8 A mobile unit (DNLT) and a portable X-ray unit being moved down the hall of a nursing home to care for a bedridden patient.

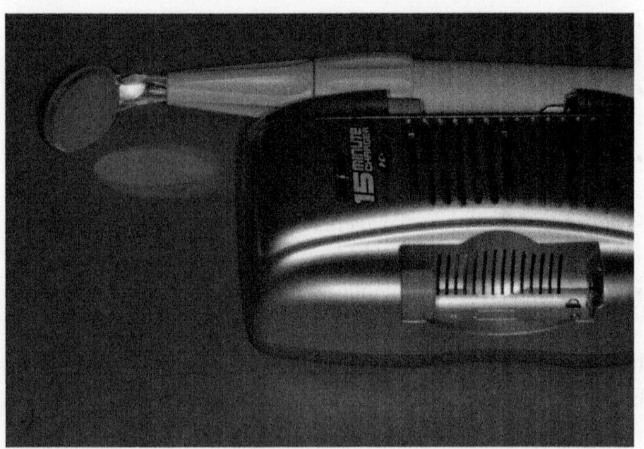

Figure 25.7 Denlite cordless portable dental light with battery charger.

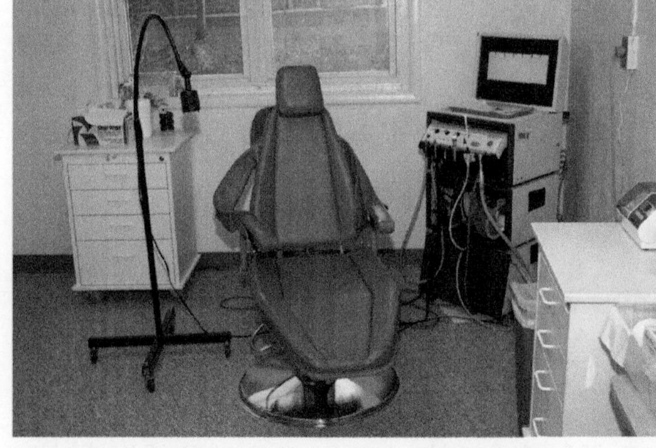

Figure 25.9 Complete unit set-up with portable dental equipment.

consists of three dental assistants and a hygienist. This team services a series of nursing homes in a radius of 100 km from the dental school. The mobile unit contracts with nursing homes to carry out comprehensive oral health care on a fee-for-service basis for its residents. All residents wishing to be treated and requiring oral health care are treated, and the unit moves to another facility when all their treatment is complete. Follow-up care is carried out at the nursing home, or the person is brought to the special care clinic within the dental school [48]. Other hospitals and dental schools in the USA and in other countries are developing similar programmes (e.g. University of British Columbia, Canada; University of Melbourne, Australia; Ohio State University, USA; and University of Maryland, USA). The advantage of such a system is that it provides both a service component for older people in need of care and superimposes a teaching component on this service. There is some evidence that the

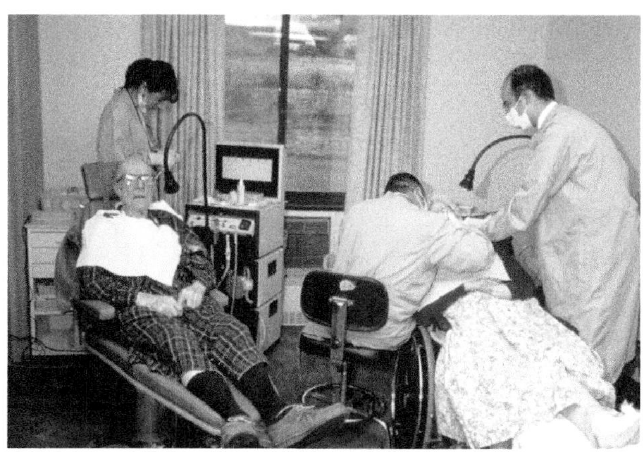

Figure 25.10 University of Iowa Geriatric Mobile Unit and portable dental office set up in a nursing home.

dentists of the future, after having had these experiences as students, will feel more competent and willing to treat homebound and institutionalized people [49].

Preventive programmes

There are abundant international data to evidence that homebound and institutionalized older adults have the poorest oral health of nearly any group in society. The preservation of the natural dentition of these older adults requires three key components be addressed: (1) regular oral assessment; (2) regular oral hygiene care; and (3) provision of dental treatment [43].

The personal care of dependent homebound older adults is usually provided by family or visiting caregivers, while that of residents in nursing homes is provided by nurse aides/personal care attendants (NAs). Incorporating lifelong practices and preferences into care routines provides a sense of familiarity to the older person. Oral care has received the highest importance ratings among activities such as bathing, toileting and mouth care among older adults. Registered and trained nurses do not provide this hands-on oral hygiene care unless a prescribed dental product requires their presence for its administration. Many home caregivers have little experience in providing oral hygiene care for other people, and it appears from research in nursing homes that NAs also have little training in this personal care activity. NAs often have a relatively low level of education, come from a lower socioeconomic background and receive only limited training for their work. NAs are paid minimum wage and their job turnover is over 400% annually – many stay working in a nursing home for less than a year, although there is often a small core of NAs that have worked for 5–10 years. Many aides have poor oral health themselves and may have experienced poor access to dental care. A significant body of research has tried to understand why oral hygiene care is so neglected in nursing homes. Disturbing US observational research has indicated that the oral hygiene care reported by NAs in previous studies was overstated, and that many basic standards of care such as the wearing of gloves, mouth rinsing and the use of toothpaste are being neglected [47]. The main reasons identified in these studies [50–54] were: (1) lack of time dedicated for oral hygiene care provision; (2) lack of priority of oral hygiene care by nursing home nursing managers and administrators; (3) disruptive behaviours of residents; (4) NAs fear of being bitten or physically hurt (hit/kicked); (5) communication problems with cognitively impaired residents; (6) low prioritization of oral hygiene care among all other personal care activities; and (7) the results of oral hygiene care are less observable by supervisors than are other activities of daily living. A model detailing these issues is presented in Figure 25.11 [52, 53]. Four main cycles contribute to poor oral hygiene care in nursing homes: residents' medical and medication issues cycle into residents' dental problems and disruptive behaviours. These then cycle into barriers to accessing dental care and also a nursing home organizational and carer cycle. These cycles are ongoing and constantly build upon each other to escalate the poor oral hygiene care for residents.

Many excellent in-service training programmes for NAs and family caregivers have been implemented successfully in the UK, Scandinavia, Australia, Canada and the US – many have evaluated the short and long-term effectiveness of the programme on residents' oral health [54]. A single 'annual dental in-service' has not been evidenced as successfully improving residents' oral health. A key component of the more recent successful programmes is the 'hands-on' training in small groups, with a dentist or dental hygienist participating on a regular weekly/monthly basis. Other newer training programmes for NAs educational curricula have been developed with a story-based focus rather than the traditional 'show and tell of bad mouths' that has often been used. NAs require very basic skills in organization, preparation and execution of activities rather than intensive knowledge of oral diseases and conditions to provide adequate oral hygiene care. Key skills are likewise needed in communication and behaviour management strategies for dementia. MacEntee *et al.* [50] have also highlighted the importance of a 'dental champion' in the nursing home for the provision of successful dental treatment and oral hygiene care. Also key is the regular implementation of interdisciplinary screening oral assessments by non-dental nursing home staff and/or physicians. Several of these have been validated and researched and provide a basis for individualization to suit the policies and procedures of each country/region [55]. It is essential

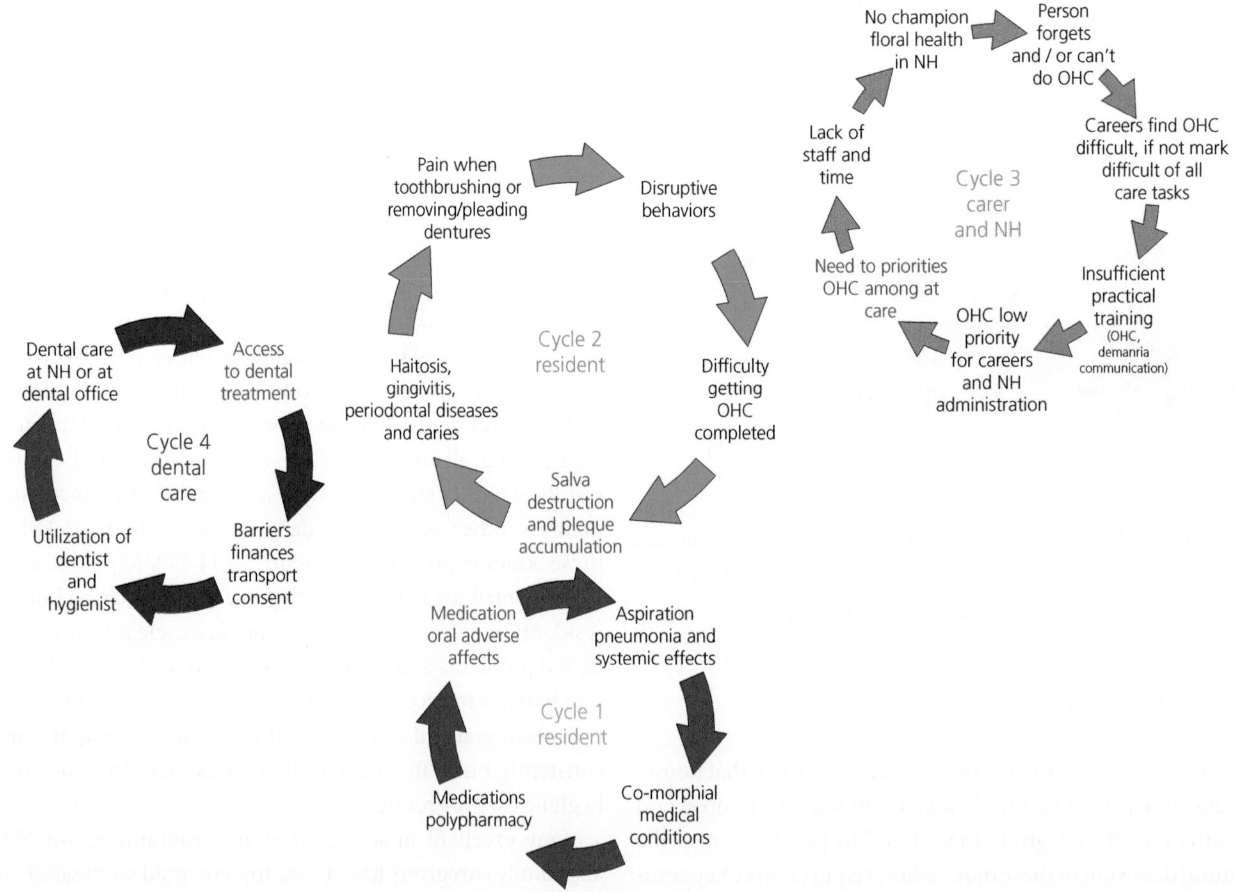

Figure 25.11 Model of cycles of poor oral hygiene care in nursing homes. Reproduced from Pyfferoen *et al.*, 2007 [52] and Cody *et al.*, 2007 [53].

for each screening assessment tool to have an accompanying training programme.

Reviews of oral hygiene care provision for older adults and studies of dental products have evidenced the standard of care for frail and dependent older adults to incorporate the use of: (1) chlorhexidine gluconate mouthrinse/spray/gel/varnish (or another chemoprophylactic agent) for the management of dental plaque and dental caries; (2) fluoride products such as 1000 ppm/5000 ppm toothpaste and 22 600 ppm fluoride varnish; and (3) saliva substitutes and stimulants [56]. Clinical research has evidenced that chlorhexidine (CHX) gel is more efficacious than mouthrinse, and that CHX products without alcohol are as efficacious as those with alcohol [56]. Application of CHX mouthrinse in a small spray bottle is clearly a good option for dependent older adults that need assistance from carers [56]. The use of a mouth prop or a backward-bent toothbrush is helpful to break perioral muscle spasms to gain better access to the mouth. Frequency of CHX mouthrinse application has traditionally been twice daily, however it is clear that once daily is adequate. Fluoride toothpastes and other products containing sodium lauryl sulfate (SLS) need to be used carefully together with CHX otherwise they may ionically negate each other – generally use them at least 2 hours apart. Table 25.4 provides some examples of the use of product combinations. The use of fluoride mouthrinses (generally 0.05% and 0.2%) has decreased in recent years with the increasing use of 5000 ppm toothpastes and 22 600 ppm fluoride varnishes. Neutral sodium fluoride or amine fluoride products are used in older patients in preference to acidulated and stannous fluorides, mainly due to the adverse effects that the two latter products have on dental materials such as composite and porcelain. Professional fluoride varnish application in these high caries risk older adults is recommended several times yearly – whenever access to dental professionals is possible!

It is essential to evaluate all older patients for saliva dysfunction and xerostomia. The term xerostomia is a person's subjective self-perception that they have a dry mouth (assessment of xerostomia can be undertaken using a short

Table 25.4 Examples of oral hygiene care protocols for older adult patients[a]

Older adult patient dental issues	Chlorhexidine gluconate 0.12% mouthrinse (rinse or use spray bottle) (no alcohol preferred)	Toothpaste	Recaldent product (MI Paste Plus and/or Trident White Gum) or Novamin product (Sensodine repair and protect)	Fluoride varnish 22 600 ppm
Low caries risk and hypersensitivity related to exposed root surfaces	Not needed	1000 ppm 2 times daily (morning and night)	Use gum and/or MI Paste Plus (either after brushing or in tray) several times daily; for severe hypersensitivity also rub MI Paste Plus directly onto hypersensitive tooth surface several times initially	0–1 times annually
Moderate to high caries risk and/or saliva dysfunction	Once daily after lunch for 4 weeks and then review oral bacteria and caries rate to gradually reduce frequency	1000 ppm 2 times daily (morning and night)	Use gum and/or MI Paste Plus (either after brushing or in tray) several times daily for saliva dysfunction and caries	Several times annually
Very high caries risk, prevention of demineralization and treatment of saliva dysfunction (e.g. for patients before, during and after head and neck radiotherapy/ chemotherapy; GERD etc)	Once daily after lunch for 4 weeks and then review oral bacteria and caries rate to gradually reduce frequency	1000 ppm 2 times daily (morning and night)	Use gum and/or MI Paste Plus (either after brushing or in tray) multiple times daily for saliva dysfunction (up to 10 or more times is OK; especially apply MI Paste Plus before sleeping) and caries	Monthly initially, and then reduced to several times annually

[a]Reproduced from references [72, 73] and [74].

self-completion questionnaire like the xerostomia inventory [57] (Table 25.5). However, xerostomia is also often incorrectly and 'globally' used to describe a reduction in saliva flow. When a person has a change in the quality and/or quantity of saliva, they have salivary dysfunction or Salivary Gland Hypofunction (SGH), in which the minor and/or major salivary glands are affected. Thus, xerostomia can only be assessed by directly questioning patients, while SGH can be determined using clinical assessment of secretions, viscosity and pH and using sialometry (collecting unstimulated and stimulated saliva).

To further complicate our understanding of 'dry mouth', epidemiological studies have evidenced that *not all patients with xerostomia have SGH and not all patients with SGH perceive dry mouth*! In a review of geriatric oral epidemiological studies of non-institutionalized older adults [58], it was estimated that xerostomia prevalence was approximately 21% and SGH prevalence was slightly higher than this in the range of 22–40%. However, it has been reported that as low as 5.7% of study cohorts of such older adults had both xerostomia and SGH (see Chapter 19).

Assessment of xerostomia can be easily undertaken before or at the dental appointment by the use of a short questionnaire, such as the Xerostomia Inventory (1999) [57] (Table 25.5).

Assessment of SGH can be broken down into two main steps: (1) a clinical screening step for all patients and (2) more comprehensive testing using 'kits' (e.g. GC Saliva Check or Vivadent CRT Buffer) for patients with a probably higher risk of salivary dysfunction. A clinical visual screening assessment is useful to review:

- salivary consistency (watery, bubbly, frothy, ropey),
- salivary pooling,
- minor salivary gland function:
  - sit the patient upright,
  - roll out the lower lip and dry with a gauze square,
  - measure the time taken for droplets of saliva to appear at the orifices of the minor gland ducts,
  - apply a single ply of tissue to make it easier to see the droplets of saliva [59].

The testing 'kits' that are available provide a simple and efficient way to further assess the pH of unstimulated and stimulated saliva, and the buffering capacity of the saliva to neutralize acids. Mean whole-saliva flow rates reported are 0.3 mL/min for unstimulated saliva and 1.7 mL/min for stimulated saliva. A flow rate of less than 0.1 mL/min for unstimulated saliva and 0.7 mL/min for stimulated saliva is considered pathological for SGH [59]. This is a clinical task that a dental auxiliary can easily perform, especially with systems such as

Table 25.5 The Xerostomia Inventory (XI) (After answering the XI, the response option scores are summed to compute the single XI scale score. Higher XI scores are equated with a greater severity of xerostomia symptoms)[a]

This is a short questionnaire about any signs of dry mouth that you may or may not have experienced **in the last 4 weeks**. Please complete this questionnaire and add any additional comments or questions at the bottom.

Please circle the answer which BEST applies to you during the last 4 weeks.

	Never	Hardly ever	Occasionally	Fairly often	Very often
1. I sip liquids to aid in swallowing food	1	2	3	4	5
2. My mouth feels dry when eating a meal	1	2	3	4	5
3. I get up at night to drink.	1	2	3	4	5
4. My mouth feels dry.	1	2	3	4	5
5. I have difficulty in eating dry foods	1	2	3	4	5
6. I suck candy or cough drops to relieve dry mouth	1	2	3	4	5
7. I have difficulties swallowing certain foods	1	2	3	4	5
8. The skin of my face feels dry	1	2	3	4	5
9. My eyes feel dry	1	2	3	4	5
10. My lips feel dry	1	2	3	4	5
11. The inside of my nose feels dry	1	2	3	4	5

[a]Reproduced from reference [75].

the GC Saliva Check kit which comes with a user-friendly 'mat' to facilitate the 'steps' in the testing process.

Saliva substitutes/buffers are buffering, rehydrating or mucosal protective products to help 'replace' the functions and feeling of the missing saliva [59]. A range of substitutes are available as gels, liquids and sprays from a variety of distributors. The Laclede Oral Balance products have wide international clinical acceptance from dental professionals and patients and include a gel and liquid which contain bio-active enzymes with essential amino acids. These substitutes can be gently rubbed all over the oral soft tissues and teeth, as well as on the internal and external surfaces of dentures (Biotene Oral Balance or Denture-Grip). A bicarbonate mouthrinse can also be helpful to neutralize acids in thick dental plaque and make the mouth feel more comfortable: mix 1/2 tsp baking soda with 1 cup warm water, rinse gently for 30 seconds several times per day [59]. *Saliva stimulants* are either non-prescription or prescription. Over-the-counter gums and candies are well-accepted by many patients – ensure they are sugar-free and if possible contain xylitol (e.g. Biotene gum, Trident White with Recaldent gum, Spry gum, Theragum, Theramints). Another product to stimulate saliva is the SalivaSure tablet which contains fruit acids and a phosphate buffer; a tablet is placed at one of the major salivary gland duct openings (parotid or submandibular) and sucked until dissolved. While a variety of prescription-only cholinergic mediations can increase salivary flow (pilocarpine and cevimeline), all have significant side effects (particularly on the cardiovascular system) and it is advisable to consult a patient's medical practitioner before prescribing such medications.

Other newer investigations are highlighting the need for additional use of calcium and phosphate products for caries management such as the Recaldent CPP-ACP mouth crème and chewing gum, or the Novamin product range. When using calcium/phosphate products it is important not to directly combine them with the use of higher level fluorides such as 5000 ppm toothpaste or 22 600 ppm varnish – brush with 1000 ppm toothpaste and then apply a product such as MI Paste (Tooth Mousse) straight after to the teeth and soft tissues.

Role of the interdisciplinary team

An interdisciplinary health care team is where a group of diverse health professionals develop a joint treatment plan for each patient and makes the decision together. This is different from multidisciplinary input to a physician who makes all the decisions.

There is very little literature on the role of dentists or dental hygienists in interdisciplinary health teams. However, now that the association between oral health and overall systemic health has been established, it is easier to argue for dentists to be part of geriatric assessment teams. These teams usually function as an outpatient service in a health care centre, in hospitals or long-term care centres, usually associated with a university training health care professional. The most common members of a geriatric assessment team are:

- the patient and his/her family;
- the primary care physician/geriatrician;
- nursing staff – registered nurse practitioner;

- pharmacist;
- dietician;
- social worker.

On call would be a psychologist or psychiatrist, speech pathologist, occupational therapist and other medical specialists, but rarely a dentist or hygienist.

The patient

The patient's autonomy and desires are important in setting the treatment goals. If the patient is incompetent there can be problems determining informed consent unless the patient has given durable power of attorney to a significant other. The patient and/or the health care guardian will have final approval of the treatment plan.

The physician

The primary care physician or geriatrician makes the medical diagnoses and usually prescribes the medication to treat these diseases. If the dentist is not a team member, then the physician needs to be consulted with regard to the severity of the patient's diseases and their ability to withstand the planned oral/dental treatment.

The pharmacist

The clinical pharmacist advises the physician on appropriate pharmacotherapeutic choices. He/she helps to reduce potential adverse effects or monitor and treat side effects when polypharmacy is required to treat the patient. If the dentist is not part of the team, then the pharmacist needs to be consulted when potent drugs such as local anaesthetics or antibiotics, and so on, are being prescribed by the dentist.

The dietician

Many older patients live alone and as a result of low income or isolation have poor or inadequate diets. Many older patients have a dry mouth due to the medications they have been prescribed. Oral lesions may result in the patient avoiding certain foods. The dentist can help the dietitian recommend an appropriate diet by informing the dietitian that the patient has painful oral ulcers, inadequate chewing pairs of teeth or malfunctioning dentures. Also, the dentist can help the dietician assess if the patient needs a mechanically altered diet to prevent choking or aspiration, which could lead to aspiration pneumonia which can be life threatening.

The social worker

Many older adults, especially women, live alone and some of them are living at or below the poverty level. The social worker can help these people find transport, meal services and/or alternate sources of funding so that they afford to pay for their care. The social worker knows the community resources and understands the limits of eligibility and so can counsel the patient and their family with regard to making important health care decisions.

Role of the dental hygienist

The dental hygienist is a key participant in the delivery of oral health care not only to homebound, frail and dependent persons utilizing private dental offices but also for long-term care or institutionalized patients.

The hygienist's role as part of the clinical team is to perform any clinical hygiene procedure necessary (as is permitted by national or regional dental board regulations) and to develop and maintain oral hygiene care plans for each resident. The hygienist also provides 'hands-on' regular in-service training and support for the nursing home staff, assists the staff to incorporate oral hygiene care into residents' personal care plans and assists in the administration of dental policies and procedures. Hygienists can also contribute to caregiver training programmes in local groups such as Alzheimer's Association and other caregiver support groups.

Whether the hygienist is working in the nursing home itself or seeing patients only at a private practice location, their role is key to monitor and coordinate the nursing home dental programme with the identified 'dental champion' of the nursing home. The hygienist can work in an interdisciplinary fashion with medical, nursing, dietary and other nursing home staff to ensure residents are regularly screened. They are also essential for the efficient coordination of an 'on-site' dental treatment programme at the nursing home, including coordination of care so that sufficient patients are scheduled to make it financially worthwhile for the dentist/hygienist to take portable equipment and work in the nursing home. Positive financial incentives can thus be created for private practice-based dentists and hygienists to treat this population. Gradually, more regions in the USA and other countries are introducing independent practice for dental hygienists in nursing homes, and regional regulations concerning this need to be obtained from administrative regional dental boards. If hygienists are to perform this role in nursing homes there needs to be sufficient hygiene curricula and continuing education available to ensure adequate training in geriatric dentistry. In some countries dental therapists combine the skills of a hygienist with training and ability to provide plastic restorations to restore carious lesions. These additional skills can be of great benefit when teamworking to provide care for clients in long-stay care.

Role of the consulting dentist

Every nursing home or institution should have a consulting dentist who has a contractual agreement with them to carry out regular comprehensive dental examinations and treatment for all of its consenting residents. The consultant dentist needs to work with the administrator, the director of nursing and the medical director/consultant to develop a dental programme that suits the policy and procedural needs of the nursing home. A dental programme contractual policy agreement needs to incorporate the following points while also incorporating regional regulations (e.g. Minimum Data Set or similar guidelines/standards):

- the institution should have a consulting dentist on staff;
- participation by competent residents in a dental programme must be voluntary, but the institution should have a short dental screening of all residents at or about the time of admission, which is documented in the resident's record and can be carried out by a medical practitioner, a registered nurse, a hygienist or a dentist
- the initial short dental screening should be followed by a thorough dental examination by a dentist within six weeks of admission;
- both dentate and edentulous residents should have a dental examination at least once yearly;
- if dental treatment is required, the rational/realistic treatment plan should have the following priorities:
  - all patient modifying factors should be reviewed and incorporated;
  - pain should be relieved and acute infections treated;
  - if a person's life expectancy is very short, dental treatment should be limited to emergency and maintenance procedures;
  - in some instances restoring aesthetics may be a valuable contribution to the psychological welfare of patients and their families, however short their life expectancy.
- a written policy for oral hygiene care for its residents which could include concepts such as:
  - a 'dental champion' or liaison person should be identified for each nursing home that can work with the dental team and who can be an advocate for implementation of the oral hygiene care policy;
  - natural teeth and dentures should be regularly cleaned (preferably on a daily basis) by the resident with support as is required from personal care staff;
  - where required, toothbrushes should be soft for natural teeth and hard for dentures and they can be adapted to the patients' specific needs
  - all dentures should be removed at night, as the tissue needs 6–8 hours of rest per day to remain healthy, and all denture containers should be either able to be sterilized or disposable and regularly replaced
  - all dentures should be cleaned before being stored overnight using a firm brush and liquid soap to remove soft debris and/or a commercial soaking tablet regime. Subjects who suffer from Candida infections will benefit from their dentures being soaked for a half hour in 2% sodium hypochlorite solution, readily available as the disinfectant 'Milton'. All soaking and disinfecting solutions should be cold when the dentures are placed in them to avoid the risk of bleaching of denture color.
  - preventive oral hygiene care products should be available for all residents as is required, including but not limited to chlorhexidine, fluorides, saliva substitutes and stimulants, amorphous calcium phosphates, xylitol and other mouthrinses;
  - all personal care staff should wear clean gloves while assisting residents with oral hygiene care;
  - persons who are semicomatose need special care to prevent the oral tissues from drying; the teeth, tongue and gums should be wiped 2–3 times each day with a piece of gauze moistened with water and/or a 10% solution of sodium bicarbonate (baking soda) to remove the coating that forms on the tissues, and lips and intraoral soft tissues should be lightly lubricated with a saliva substitute (e.g. Lansinoh, MI Paste/Tooth Mousse, Oral Balance Gel, KY Jelly, but not Vaseline).
  - to maintain the oral health of the residents, regular 'hands-on' in-service training and support of nurses and personal care staff is required (incorporating concepts of systemic health and dementia care); this will help to alert the dentist/hygienist of any changes in the resident's ability to masticate or to maintain oral hygiene and of the presence of any potentially dangerous oral lesions;
  - if possible, ultrasonic cleaners should be used for regular denture care;
  - dentures should be marked with an identifying name or number for each resident (an economical and effective way is to use a marking pencil on the buccal flange of a denture – the area is first prepared by removing the high polish with an abrasive material, such as sandpaper. After the name or number is written, it is then covered with two layers of clear nail enamel. A commercial system for marking dentures is the Identure System (3M Co., St. Paul, MN, USA).

Summary

The homebound and institutionalized people in a community can be defined as being very frail or functionally dependent and thus unable to maintain independent living without reliance on others. The oral health status and needs of this population have been described. Many of these people are edentulous and are reluctant to seek care. However, this status is changing and many are now dentate and therefore require more frequent and complex oral health care. Five essential types of dental care delivery systems are available for these persons. For the individuals who can be transported, transfer to a dental office is a possibility providing that such factors as appointment times, adequate vehicles and office safety are taken into account. On-site dental programmes are useful, but there are disadvantages if the equipment is not portable. Mobile dental vans are useful but have limited use in inclement weather. Mobile dental programmes are most useful, and the range of equipment varies from portable equipment for palliative care to mobile equipment for comprehensive care. Hospital-based mobile programmes have the advantage of having a hospital and a full medical staff available to which high-risk patients can be referred. These latter programmes often incorporate a teaching and training component. Preventive programmes and oral health programmes in institutions and the role of hygienists and dentists within them are described and discussed. Finally, a model policy for an oral health care programme in an institution is presented.

References

1 Ettinger, R.L. & Beck, J.D. (1984) Geriatric dental curriculum and the needs of the elderly. *Special Care in Dentistry*, **4**, 207–213.

2 Lutz, W., Sanderson, W. & Scherbov, S. (2004) *The end of the world population growth in the 21st century: new challenges for human capital formation and sustainable development*, Earthscan London and Sterling, VA.

3 United Nations. *World population prospects: the 2012 revision population database*, Department of economic and social affairs, Population division New York, NY. http://esa.un.org/wpp [Accessed 12/15/14]

4 Administration on Aging (2012). *A profile of older Americans: 2012.* US Department of Health and Human Services. http://www.aoa.gov?Aging_Statistics/Profile/Index.aspx [Accessed 3/26/14]

5 Gist, Y.J. & Velkoff, V.A. (1997) *International brief gender and aging, demographic dimensions.* Bureau of the Census 1B/97-3, Washington, DC.

6 United Nations. *World population ageing 1950-2050. Population division DESA.* http://www.un.org/esa/population/publications/worldageing19502050/ [Accessed 12/15/14].

7 Ganguli, M., Fox, A., Gilby, J. & Belle, S. (1996) Characteristics of rural homebound older adults: A community-based study. *Journal of the American Geriatrics Society*, **44**(4), 363–370.

8 Munson, M.L. (1999) Characteristics of elderly home health care users: data from the 1966 National Home & Hospice Care Survey. *National Center for Health Statistics, Advance Data*, No. **309**, pp. 1–12.

9 American Academy of Home Care Physicians. Public policy statement. http://www.aahcm.org/?Pub_Policy_Statement [Accessed 3/26/14]

10 Gluzman, R., Meeker, H., Agarwal, P., Patel, S., Gluck, G., Espinoza, L. *et al.* (2013) Oral health status and needs of homebound elderly in an urban home-based primary care service. *Special Care in Dentistry*, **33**, 218–226.

11 Schiller, J.S., Lucas, J.W. & Peregoy, J.A. (2012) Summary health statistics for U.S. adults: National Health Interview Survey, 2011. *Vital and Health Statistics*, Series 10, No. **256**, pp. 1–153.

12 Morishita, M., Takaesu, Y., Miyatake, K., Shinsho, F. & Fujioka, M. (2001) Oral health care status of homebound in Japan. *Journal of Oral Rehabilitation*, **28**, 717–720.

13 Simons, D. (2003) Who will provide dental care for housebound people with oral problems? *British Dental Journal*, **194**, 137–138.

14 Chalmers, J.M. (2001) Geriatric oral health issues in Australia. *International Dental Journal*, **51**, 188–199.

15 A brief history of the Hospice movement. http://www.hospiceworld.org/history.htm (accessed 3/26/14).

16 Gordon, S.R., Berkey, D.B. & Call, R.I. (1985) Dental needs among hospice patients in Colorado. *A pilot study. Gerodontics*, **1**, 125–129.

17 Berkey, D.B., Ofstehage, J.C., Crane, C.A. & Malley, K.J. (1987) Is there a role for dental professionals within hospice programs? *Journal of Palliative Care*, **3**, 35–37.

18 Wyche, C.J. & Kerschbaum, W.E. (1994) Michigan hospice oral healthcare needs survey. *Journal of Dental Hygiene*, **68**, 35–41.

19 Wilwert, M. (2003) Should dentists be included as members of the hospice care team? *Special Care in Dentistry*, **23**, 84–85.

20 Weyant, R.J., Jones, J.A., Hobbins, M., Niessen, L.C., Adelson, R. & Rhyner, R.R. (1993) Oral health status of a long-term-care, veteran population. *Community Dentistry and Oral Epidemiology*, **21**, 227–233.

21 Sheiham, J., Steele, J.G., Marcenes, W., Finch, S. & Walls, A.W.G. (1999) The impact of oral health on stated ability to eat certain foods; findings from the National Diet and Nutrition Survey of older people in Great Britain. *Gerodontology*, **16**, 11–20.

22 Centers for Medicare and Medicaid services. (2013) *Nursing home data compendium 2012 edition.* Centers for Medicare and Medicaid services, Baltimore, MD.

23 Jones, A. (2009) The National Nursing Home Survey: 2004 Overview National Center for Health Statistics, *DHHS Publication No (PHS) 2009-1738*, Hyattesville, MD.

24 Wyatt, C.C.L. (2002) Elderly Canadians residing in long-term care hospitals. Part I. Medical and dental status. *Journal of the Canadian Dental Association*, **68**, 353–358.

25 Chalmers, J.M., Carter, K.D., Fuss, J.M., Spencer, A.J. & Hodge, C.P. (2002) Caries experience in existing and new nursing home residents in Adelaide, Australia. *Gerodontology*, **19**, 30–40.

26 Ettinger, R.L. (1993) Cohort differences among aging populations: a challenge for the dental profession. *Special Care in Dentistry*, **13**, 19–26.

27 Minkler, M., Fuller-Thomson, E. & Guralnik, J.M. (2006) Gradient of disability across the socioeconomic spectrum in the United States. *New England Journal of Medicine*, **355**, 695–703.

28 Mohamad, A.R., Preshaw, P.A. & Ettinger, R.L. (2003) Current status of predoctoral geriatric education in U. S. dental Schools. *Journal of Dental Education*, **67**, 509–514.

29 Kiyak, H.A. & Reichmuth, M. (2005) Barriers to and enablers of older adults' use of dental services. *Journal of Dental Education*, **69**, 975–986.

30 Robbertz, A.A., Lauf, R.C., Rupp, R.L. & Alexander, D.C. (2006) A qualitative assessment of dental care access and utilization among the older adult population in the United States. *General Dentistry*, **54**, 361–365.

31 Ettinger, R.L., Beck, J.D. & Jakobsen, J. (1988) Prediction of need and acceptance of dental services for institutionalized patients. *Gerodontics*, **4**, 109–113.

32 Frenkel, H., Harvey, I. & Newcombe, R.G. (1993) Oral health care among nursing home residents in Avon. *Gerodontology*, **10**, 90–97.
33 Chalmers, J.M., Hodge, C., Fuss, J.M., Spencer, A.J., Carter, K.D. & Mathew, R. (2001) Opinions of dentists and directors of nursing concerning dental care provision for Adelaide nursing homes. *Australian Dental Journal*, **46**(4), 277–283.
34 Bill, D.J. & Weddell, J.A. (1986) Dental office access for patients with disabling conditions. Special Care in Dentistry, **6**, 246–252.
35 Berkey, D. (1987) Improving dental access for the nursing home resident: portable dentistry interventions. *Gerodontics*, **3**, 265–268.
36 Manderson, R.D. & Ettinger, R.L. (1975) Dental status of the institutionalized elderly population of Edinburgh. *Community Dentistry and Oral Epidemiology*, **3**, 100–107.
37 Council on Dental Health and Health Planning Bureau of Economic and Behavioral Research (1982) Oral health status of Vermont nursing home residents: results of a pilot study. *Journal of the American Dental Association*, **104**, 68–69.
38 California Dental Association. (1986) *California skilled nursing facilities' residents: a survey of dental needs*. California Dental Association Sacramento, CA.
39 Panza, J.A., Epstein, S.E. & Quyyumi, A.A. (1991) Circadian variation in vascular tone and its relation to alpha-sympathetic vasoconstrictor activity. *New England Journal of Medicine*, **325**, 986–990.
40 Prince, M., Bryce, R., Albanese, E., Wimo, A., Ribeiro, W. & Ferri, C.P. (2013) The global prevalence of dementia: A systematic review and metaanalysis. *Alzheimer's & Dementia*, **9**, 63–75.
41 Plassman, B.L., Langa, K.M., Fisher, G.G., Heeringa, S.G., Weir, D.R., Ofstedal, M.B. *et al.* (2007) Prevalence of dementia in the United States: The aging, demographics, and memory study. *Neuroepidemiology*, **29**, 125–132.
42 Pfeiffer, E. (1975) A short portable mental status questionnaire for the assessment of organic brain deficit in elderly patients. *Journal of the American Geriatrics Society*, **23**, 433–441.
43 Berkey, D. (1987) Improving dental access for the nursing home resident: portable dentistry interventions. *Gerodontics*, **3**, 265–268.
44 Fricton, J. & Chen, H. (2009) Using teledentistry to improve access to dental care for the underserved. *Dental Clinics of North America*, **53**, 537–548.
45 Rocca, M.A., Kudryk, V.L., Pajak, J.C. & Morris, T. (1999) The evolution of a teledentistry system within the Department of Defense. *Proceedings of the AMIA Symposium*, **1**, 921–924.
46 Chang, S.W., Plotkin, D.R., Mulligan, R., Polido, J.C., Mah, J.K. & Meara, J.G. (2003) Teledentistry in rural California: a USC initiative. *Journal of the California Dental Association*, **31**, 601–608.
47 Mulligan, R. (1987) Considerations for using mobile dental vans to deliver dental care to the elderly. *Gerodontics*, **3**, 260–264.
48 Ettinger, R.L. (2012) A 30-year review of a geriatric dentistry teaching programme. *Gerodontology*, **29**, 1252–1260.
49 Ettinger, R.L., McLeran, H. & Jakobsen, J. (1990) Effect of a geriatric educational experience on graduate activities and attitudes. *Journal of Dental Education*, **54**, 273–278.
50 MacEntee, M.I., Thorne, S. & Kazanjian, A. (1999) Conflicting priorities: oral health in long-term care. *Special Care in Dentistry*, **19**, 164–172.
51 Coleman, P. & Watson, N.M. (2006) Oral care provided by certified nursing assistants in nursing homes. *Journal of the American Geriatric Society*, **54**, 138–143.
52 Pyfferoen, M., Cody, K., Chalmers, J. & Coleman, P. (2007) Observation of mealtime and oral hygiene cares for dementia residents. *Journal of Dental Research*, **86**(Special issue A), 0955.
53 Cody, K., Pyfferoen, M., Chalmers, J. & Coleman, P. (2007) Morning and evening oral hygiene care for residents with dementia. *Journal of Dental Research*, **86**(Special issue A), 0957.
54 Frenkel, H.F. (1999) Behind the screens: care staff observations on delivery of oral health care in nursing homes. *Gerodontology*, **16**, 75–80.
55 Chalmers, J.M. & Pearson, A. (2005) The assessment of oral health in residential aged care facilities – a systematic review. *Special Care in Dentistry*, **25**, 227–233.
56 Pearson, A. & Chalmers, J.M. (2004) Oral hygiene care for adults with dementia in residential aged care facilities: a systematic review. *JBI Reports*, **2**, 65–113.
57 Thomson, W.M., Chalmers, J.M., Spencer, A.H. & Williams, S.M. (1999) The Xerostomia Inventory: a multi-item approach to measuring dry mouth. *Community Dental Health*, **16**, 12–17.
58 Orellana, M.F., Lagavere, M.O., Boychuk, D.G.J., Major, P.W. & Flores-MIR, C. (2006) Prevalence of xerostomia in population-based samples: a systematic review. *Journal of Public Health Dentistry*, **66**, 152–158.
59 Walsh, L.J. (2005) Lifestyle Impacts on Oral Health. In: G.J. Mount & W.R. Hume (eds), *Preservation and Restoration of Tooth Structure*. Ch. 7, Knowledge Books and Software, Brisbane, Australia.
60 US Census Bureau, International Program Center Population Division. (2004) *Global Population Profile 2002, Appendix B, Population Projections and Availability of Data*. International Population Reports WP/02, US Government Printing Office, Washington, DC.
61 McDevitt, T.M. & Rowe, P.M. (2002) *The United States in international context: 2000*. US Census Bureau, Washington, DC, 20233.
62 Jobbins, J., Bagg, J., Finlay, I.G., Addy, M. & Newcombe, R.G. (1992) Oral and dental disease in terminally ill cancer patients. *British Medical Journal*, **304**(6842), 1612.
63 Aldred, M.J., Addy, M., Bagg, J. & Finlay, I. (1991) Oral health in the terminally ill: a cross-sectional pilot survey. *Special Care in Dentistry*, **11**, 59–62.
64 Martinello, B.P. & Leake, J.L. (1971) Oral health status in the three London, Ontario, homes for the aged. *Journal of the Canadian Dental Association*, **37**, 429–432.
65 Terrill, A.J. & Elliott, J. (1979) The Montana Advisory Dentist Program. *Journal of the American Dental Association*, **98**, 402–406.
66 Council on Dental Health and Health Planning. Bureau of Economic and Behavioral Research (1982) Oral health status of Vermont nursing home residents: results of a pilot study. *Journal of the American Dental Association*, **104**, 68–69.
67 Ekelund, R. (1984) The dental and oral condition and the need for treatment among the residents of municipal old people's homes in Finland. *Proceedings of the Finnish Dental Society*, **80**, 43–52.

68 Shareff, H.L. & Strauss, R.P. (1985) Behavioral influences on the feasibility of outpatient dental care for nursing home residents, *Special Care in Dentistry*, **5**, 270–273.
69 California Dental Association. (1986) *California skilled nursing facilities' residents: a survey of dental needs*. California Dental Association, Sacramento, CA.
70 McIntyre, R.T., Jackson, M. & Shosenberg, J.W. (1986) Dental health status and treatment needs of institutionalized seniors. *Ontario Dentist*, **63**, 12–14, 18–23.
71 Ettinger, R.L., Beck, J.D., Miller, J.A. & Jakobsen, J. (1988) Dental service use by older people living in long-term care facilities. *Special Care in Dentistry*, **8**, 178–183.
72 Chalmers, J.M. (2006) Minimal Intervention Dentistry: strategies for the new caries challenge in our older patients. *Journal of the Canadian Dental Association*, **72**, 325–331.
73 Hay, K.D. & Thomson, W.M. (2002) A clinical trial of the anticaries efficacy of casein derivatives complexed with calcium phosphate. *Oral Surgery, Oral Medicine, Oral Pathology, Oral Radiology and Endodontology*, **93**, 271–275.
74 Reynolds, E.C. and Walsh, L.J. (2005) Additional aids to the remineralisation of tooth structure. In: G.J. Mount & W.R. Hume (eds), *Preservation and Restoration of Tooth Structure*, Knowledge Books and Software, Varsity Lakes, Australia.
75 Thomson, W.M., Chalmers, J.M., Spencer, A.H. & Williams, S.M. (1999) The Xerostomia Inventory: a multi-item approach to measuring dry mouth. *Community Dental Health*, **16**, 12–17.

CHAPTER 26

Clinical management of the cognitively impaired older adult and the terminally ill older patient

Jane M. Chalmers†[1], Ronald L. Ettinger[2] and Michael Wiseman[3]

[1]Department of Preventive and Community Dentistry, The University of Iowa, College of Dentistry, Iowa City, IA, USA
[2]Department of Prosthodontics and Dows Institute of Dental Research, College of Dentistry, University of Iowa, Iowa City, IA, USA
[3]Faculty of Dentistry, McGill University, Montreal, Quebec, Canada

Clinical dental care provision for older patients with dementia or a terminal illness holds many challenges for the dental team. High levels of oral diseases and conditions have been evidenced in these older patients. An understanding of dementia, how it is treated, and how behavioural and communication problems can be managed is essential for successful dental care provision. Rational dental treatment planning reviews all patient modifying factors, together with oral environmental factors such as saliva, and helps to provide realistic dental care for both the dementia and terminally ill patient.

Clinical management of the cognitively impaired older adult

What is dementia?

Some of the most challenging but yet rewarding patients to care for are those with dementia. An understanding of dementia and cognitive impairment is essential to adequately care for these patients. Neuropsychological and medical research in recent years has enhanced our knowledge concerning the diversity of dementia in older adults. Dementia is not a specific diagnosis, but is a group of signs and symptoms that can be caused by a variety of systemic or primary central nervous system diseases. Dementia, as formally described in the *Diagnostic and Statistical Manual of Mental Disorders Fourth Edition (DSM-IV)*, is characterized by the development of multiple cognitive deficits (including memory impairment and at least one of the following cognitive disturbances: aphasia, apraxia, agnosia or a disturbance of executive functioning) that are due to the direct physiological effects of a general medical condition, the persisting effects of a substance or to multiple aetiologies. The cognitive deficits must be sufficiently severe to cause impairment in occupational or social functioning and must represent a decline from a previously higher level of functioning [1]. DSM-IV defines aphasia as a disturbance of language, apraxia as impaired ability to carry out motor activities despite intact function, and agnosia as failure to recognize or identify objects despite intact sensory function. Executive functions include planning, organizing, sequencing and abstracting [1]. Dementing disorders share a common symptom presentation but are differentiated based on aetiology [1]. Although DSM-V uses the concept of neurocognitive disorders instead of dementia, it has been stated that 'the term dementia is retained in DSM-V for continuity and may be used in settings where health care professionals and patients are accustomed to this term' [2]. In this chapter the term dementia will not be replaced by neurocognitive disorders.

More than 70 different causes of brain dysfunction can be associated with dementia, and differential reversible diagnoses for dementia must always be considered, including thyroid hormone and vitamin B_{12} deficiencies, substance abuse, surgical brain lesions, depressive disorders, delirium and iatrogenic medication effects (Table 26.1). Table 26.1 also summarizes the irreversible types of dementia [3]. The dementias associated with cortical brain degeneration show little or no major motor abnormalities early on; these include Alzheimer's disease (AD), Creutzfeldt–Jakob disease, frontotemporal dementias, and Korsakoff's psychosis. Subcortical structures are involved and there are more prominent

† Author is deceased.

Textbook of Geriatric Dentistry, Third Edition. Edited by Poul Holm-Pedersen, Angus W. G. Walls and Jonathan A. Ship.

Table 26.1 Types of dementia[a]

Reversible dementias	Irreversible dementias		
	Cortical (no early motor abnormalities)	*Sub-cortical (early motor abnormalities)*	*Infectious*
Thyroid disorders	Dementia of Alzheimer's type	Dementia with Lewy bodies	Acute encephalitis
Vitamin (B_{12}) deficiencies	Creutzfeldt–Jakob disease	Vascular dementia	Subacute CNS infections
Depression	Frontotemporal dementia (Pick's)	Dementia of Parkinson's disease	Neurosyphilis
Substance abuse	Korsakoff's psychosis	Progressive supranuclear palsy	HIV and AIDS opportunistic diseases
Surgical brain lesions		Huntington's disease	Prion diseases (e.g. Creutzfeldt–Jakob)
Delirium		Normal pressure hydrocephalus	
Polypharmacy adverse effects		Cortico-basal ganglionic degeneration	

[a]Data taken from references [44] and [3].

motor abnormalities in dementia with Lewy bodies (DLB), vascular dementia (VasD), dementia of Parkinson's disease, Huntington's disease, and progressive supranuclear palsy [3]. AD, DLB and VasD are the most common age-associated causes of dementia and also the most frequent diagnoses for people comprehensively assessed for memory problems; AD has been estimated to account for between 50 and 80% of dementia cases [4].

Alzheimer's disease has characteristic neuropathological and neurochemical features according to the WHO *ICD-10 Classification of Behavioural and Mental Disorders*, with a marked reduction in the population of neurons, particularly in the hippocampus, temperoparietal cortex and frontal cortex; appearance of neurofibrillary tangles made of paired helical filaments; progressive neuritic plaques of amyloid; granulovacular bodies; a marked reduction in the enzyme choline acetyltranferase in acetylcholine; and a reduction in other neurotransmitters [5]. AD is insidious in onset and develops steadily over a period of several years. A more rapid course of deterioration is seen in adults with AD onset before age 65 years. The most important risk factor for AD is old age, in addition to a family history of Alzheimer's disease [6]. In a small percentage of AD cases, especially the earlier-onset type, several causative genes have been identified, which are mutations of the beta-amyloid precursor gene on chromosome 21 and the presenilin genes on chromosomes 1 and 14. In the more common late-onset AD, specific combinations of three alleles of the apolipoprotein E gene (APoE) on chromosome 19 have been identified [7]. The other group of individuals at risk for AD are those with Down's syndrome, who have the beta-amyloid precursor gene on chromosome 21 [8].

Previously, VasD was ranked as the second most common dementia after AD. However, research during the last decade has identified DLB to be more prevalent, thus VasD is now ranked third. DLB appears to now account for 17–36% of dementias. DLB is described as a clinical syndrome characterized by cognitive deficits similar to those in AD, together with prominent visual hallucinations, Parkinsonian motor symptoms and fluctuations in levels of consciousness resulting from autonomic instability, with cortical Lewy bodies present. The survival time for people with DLB is shorter than for AD. Risk factors and protective factors for DLB have not been adequately studied at the present time. DLB needs to be correctly recognized by clinicians as: (1) some DLB patients respond positively to treatment with cholinesterase inhibitors, while others have an increased sensitivity to them and (2) typical antipsychotic medications can induce life-threatening extrapyramidal reactions in patients with DLB [9].

Vascular dementia is estimated to account for approximately 10% of dementias, with additional cases of mixed diagnosis [3]. VasD results when acute or cumulative, single or multiple, strokes destroy areas of the brain that subserve memory and intelligence, as a result of vascular disease. Onset is often abrupt, but can be gradual. The main feature of VasD is that cognitive deficits are not evenly distributed; for example, memory may be severely affected, but thinking, reasoning and information processing may be only mildly affected. The e4 allele of the APoE gene has also been identified as a risk factor for VasD [10].

It must be noted that 20–30% of dementias are of mixed VasD/AD/DLB diagnosis [3]. Infectious causes of dementia include acute encephalitis, subacute central nervous system infections, neurosyphilis, HIV and AIDS opportunistic infections and prion diseases (e.g. Creutzfeldt–Jakob disease) [11]. It is important to emphasize the variability in the cognitive impairments associated with the different causes of dementia; sub-cortical dementias reveal early motor abnormalities, while cortical dementias do not. For example, the subcortical brain structures are affected in Huntington's disease and so there is little or no aphasia, unlike in AD. Dementia of Parkinson's disease is a result of subcortical degeneration with bradyphenia (a general slowing of mental processes), inattention, apathy and inability to sustain effort at tasks [5]. Up to one-third of people with Parkinson's disease also have additional AD-like cognitive impairments [3]. Frontotemporal dementia is typified by a slowly progressive dementia dominated at first by personality and behavioural changes with disinhibition, apathy and lack of insight. There are also language abnormalities present [3]. These dementias result from cerebral frontotemporal atrophy and are called Pick's disease when Pick's bodies are present. The AIDS dementia complex begins in the later stages of the disease and progresses much more rapidly and severely than other dementias, in just a few weeks or months, to death. Also, multiple causes of dementia (for example, AD and VasD) and/or a co-existent depression may be present, which may complicate the assessment and diagnosis of dementia.

Recent research [12] has revealed that there is a variable and often prolonged period between the occurrence of the first cognitive symptoms and the development of the full clinical syndrome of dementia. This predementia period has been termed either amnestic mild cognitive impairment (aMCI) or cognitive impairment no dementia (CIND). Neuropsychological definitions limit the use of the term aMCI to being a precursor of Alzheimer's disease, whereas CIND is more generally used with respect to all dementias. The prevalence of aMCI has been reported in the range of 3–10% compared with CIND with a reported range of 10–20% in adults aged 65+ years. Vascular disease and related risk factors, including diabetes, stroke, myocardial infarction and hypertension, have been related to aMCI and CIND [13].

Dementia diagnosis

The diagnosis of dementia is one of exclusion, with often a specific diagnosis only able to be confirmed by brain autopsy after death. All reversible causes of dementia are first excluded, then neuroimaging (computerized axial tomography) and magnetic resonance imaging and other testing is completed to exclude other dementia causes. Neuropsychological testing is also used to investigate specific cognitive impairments and their effect on social and daily activities. These tests include The Mini-Mental State Exam (MMSE) [14], The Clock Drawing Test [15] and the Global Deterioration Scale (GDS) [16]. These are just several of the many commonly used screening tests for dementia. Other important assessment tools are used to evaluate changes over time in the person's ability to function in daily life (Instrumental Activities of Daily Living (IADL) [17]; Activities of Daily Living (ADL) [18].

Dementia severity has been categorized as mild, moderate or severe, as is illustrated in the GDS [16]. In the mild stage of dementia, initial short-term memory loss, personality changes, emotional instability and decision-making problems become evident. Continued progression of memory loss can advance within months or years to the moderate stage, with additional problems with slowing of movement, speech and communication, loss of ability to care for themselves independently, wandering, aggression and a range of other behavioural difficulties. As they progress into the severe stage, they become more and more dependent upon others. By the severe stage, people have difficulty with understanding instructions, speaking and communicating; many also have incontinence of urine and faeces.

Who has dementia?

Meta-analyses have provided prevalence and incidence estimates for dementia in many industrialized and developing countries. In general, every 5 years, the age-specific prevalence of dementia almost doubles, from a low of 1.5% in adults aged 60–69 to a high of 40% in older adults 90+ years [19]. In 2005, a global prevalence estimate of dementia in adults aged 60+ years was 3.9%. Regionally, there are estimates of 1.6% in Africa, 3.9% in Eastern Europe, 4.0% in China, 4.6% in Latin America, 5.4% in Western Europe and 6.4% in North America. The 2001 global estimate of numbers of people with dementia was 24 million and will double every 20 years. However, although the prevalence is higher in industrialized countries, the greatest number of people with dementia is in developing countries. The prevalence of dementia subtypes such as AD, DLB and VasD are similar internationally. Although the majority of people with dementia live in the community, increasing levels of cognitive impairment are evident in older adults living in residential care – for example, over 50% of low dependency (hostel/assisted living) and over 80% of high dependency residents (nursing home) have dementia in Australia, with similar percentages reported in other industrialized countries. This is reflected in the annual informal caregiving costs attributable to dementia which are over $18.5 billion in the USA; these informal caregivers provide most of the care for community-living adults with dementia. The global estimate of annual incidence of dementia is around 7.5 per 1000 population. There appears to be little difference in this incidence across countries with the exception of lower incidence in Africa. There is a clear exponential increase in incidence of dementia after the age of 65 years [6].

Treatment of dementia

Changes in the conceptualization of cognitive impairment and its related emotional, psychological and behavioural problems have resulted in the recognition of quality of life as a major goal of dementia treatment and management.

Recent advances are improving quality of life by pharmacological and non-pharmacological treatment of specific dementias and of the accompanying delusions, hallucinations, depression, wandering, fearfulness, aggression and other psychological and behavioural problems.

At present, there are no definitive pharmacological or other dementia 'cures' available. Pharmacological research has evidenced that cholinergic deficits are the underlying cause of cognitive impairments, and the acetylcholinesterase inhibitors (AChEI) appear to either stabilize or slightly ameliorate the cognitive deficits [3]. The most commonly used AChEI is still donepezil (Aricept), with other newer drugs such as rivastigmine (Exelon), and galantamine (Reminyl) also increasing in use. Not all people with AD will improve with donepezil and up to one-third may become worse. For donezepil there appear to be few general adverse effects and no specific adverse oral effects [3]. However, some of the other AChEIs have increased adverse effects. Memantine (Ebixa), a newer drug, is a low affinity antagonist drug to N-methyl-D-aspartate (NMDA) type receptors and may prevent excitatory amino acid neurotoxicity without interfering with the physiological actions of glutamate required for memory and learning. It appears that memantine is well tolerated and has a low incidence of adverse effects.

A host of controversial pharmacological agents are used in up to 90% of people with dementia for the management of the accompanying delusions, hallucinations, depression, wandering, fearfulness, aggression and other psychological and behavioural problems. These problems often become distressing, exhausting and difficult for carers to manage, contributing to carer stress and burden. Current best-practice advocates that the behavioural and psychological problems of dementia should be managed first by non-pharmacological approaches and those pharmacological therapies are not particularly effective for management of neuropsychiatric symptoms of dementia. However, a host of medications have been widely used to manage these problems, the most common group being the oral and intramuscular antipsychotics (neuroleptics) [3]. The potentially responsive behaviours and symptoms may include agitation, psychosis, resistiveness and nocturnal awakening. The traditional antipsychotics include: haloperidol, thioridazine, fluphenazine, pericyazine, pimozide, trifluoperazine, chlorpromazine and lithium carbonate. Their mode of action is via blockade of D2 dopamine receptors [3]. Traditional antipsychotics have many adverse effects including: extrapyramidal disturbances, tardive dyskinesia, neuroleptic malignant syndrome, anticholinergic effects such as xerostomia, peripheral oedema, weight gain, incontinence, arrhythmias, orthostatic hypotension, haematological disturbances, hepatic and ocular changes, in addition to other CNS disturbances such as impaired alertness and drowsiness [3].

Newer atypical antipsychotics are clozapine, olanzapine and risperidone. They have fewer of the traditional adverse effects but may still have other serious adverse effects and act additionally at the 5HT2 serotonin receptors, in a different pharmacodynamic manner to the traditional antipsychotics [3]. An adverse effect often observed by dentists is tardive dyskinesia (TD). TD is a syndrome of choreoid and athetoid involuntary movements that commence during sustained treatment with neuroleptics and continue after withdrawal of these medications. These involuntary movements include oculogyric crises (staring and rotation of the eyes), grimacing, sucking of the lips, tongue protrusion, chewing and grinding of teeth and jaw trismus, laryngeal/pharyngeal constriction, torticollos (twisting and extension of the neck) and abnormal posturing of the trunk and limbs. Nearly every person who takes neuroleptic medications has one or more identifiable risk factors for tardive dyskinesia and risk increases with increasing interruptions to neuroleptic doses and with age.

Another group of drugs commonly used in people with dementia are the antidepressants. Depressive features and syndromes are common and seen in at least 50% of people at some stage during the dementia [3]. It is generally advocated that depressive symptoms be treated with antidepressant medication: in early to moderate dementia, when insight is retained and symptoms of tearfulness, indecision and helplessness are prominent; where classical endogenous depressive symptoms are present; or in severe dementia when there is marked anguish or apathy [3]. The dry mouth (xerostomia) perceived by people taking antidepressants has been well documented in the dental literature, as has their associated increased risk for developing dental caries.

Many people with dementia are also prescribed sedative hypnotic medications for the management of mild anxiety, insomnia and disruptive behaviours. These medications will have prominent sedative effects which can cause increased urinary incontinence, falls, depression and confusion. The use of benzodiazepines in people with dementia has been found to be less effective than antipsychotics and 'can cause paradoxical worsening of symptoms'. If at all used in older adults, the shorter acting benzodiazepines should only be used, such as oxazepam or temazepam. There is no conclusive evidence of benzodiazepine efficacy in dementia and they should only be used for short periods [3].

Behavioural approaches to dementia care

The varying, and often limited, success of the above-described pharmacological approaches in people with dementia has resulted in individualized non-pharmacological approaches. Behavioural and psychological problems cause the most stress for carers and frequently precipitate the move to residential care. Philosophies of dementia care are centred on the individual person and advocate non-pharmacological approaches to care. The need for preparation and organization is essential as creative planning can avoid many difficulties [20]. This requires the involvement of a multidisciplinary team, including physicians, other medical professionals, physiotherapists, occupational therapists, dental professionals, other allied health professionals and social workers. Care that is poorly adapted to patients' resources, loss of abilities and needs, leads to the emergence of disruptive behaviour. Behaviours may be related to the type and/or stage of dementia but there is a wide spectrum of variability [21]. Some behaviours are consistent and follow a regular pattern, some are triggered by specific events and others are more variable. These behavioural problems are an attempt by the person with dementia to cope and are an adaptive response to internal or external stressors or to an unfulfilled need or feeling [21]. Feelings of fear and confusion usually precede behavioural problems. The most common causes of behavioural problems are medical and physical, environmental, task-related and communication-related; all of these are apparent in the dental office setting [20] (Table 26.2).

As yet, researchers and clinicians do not have a good understanding of dementia's impact on pain sensation. Research has indicated that pain responses will vary depending upon the areas of the brain affected by the varying types of dementia. The diversity of behavioural responses to pain include vocalizations, crying out, grimacing, wincing, wrinkling of forehead, restlessness, rocking, rubbing or guarding of a body part, irritability, aggression and resistance to personal care. Most behavioural problems can be prevented by focusing on four main non-pharmacological interventions related to the person with dementia's personal and environmental systems (Box 26.1): decreasing environmental stressors, meeting primary self-needs, increasing quality and quantity of social interactions and balancing inner-retreat time with active time [20].

Box 26.1 Interventions for the prevention of behavioural problems.[a]

Intervention

Decreasing environmental stressors

- simplify environment and limit choices
- decrease multiple stressors
- remove person from stressful situations
- allow time for responses
- offer activities person is capable of managing
- use task breakdown
- maintain consistency of carers
- observe patterns during activities
- keep a consistent routine and daily rituals
- schedule activities around stressful times
- create privacy for self care activities
- use clocks to orient time
- minimize shadows, glare and mirrors
- introduce new ideas/activities slowly
- avoid background conversations/noises
- turn off auditory stressors
- ensure room temperature is comfortable
- keep background colours soft and muted
- use contrasting colours to differentiate items

Meeting primary self needs

- ensure person is comfortable
- ensure positioning is comfortable
- provide rummage boxes, busy aprons/boards/cushions
- use massage and gentle touch
- look to person's lifestyle and preferences to ensure person is not bored or frustrated
- respond to their emotions
- do not force person to do activities

Increasing quality and quantity of social interactions

- use both verbal and non-verbal communication
- use quiet conversation time to convey a message of safety, caring and connection
- encourage interactions with others at meal-times, prayers etc.
- visits from children, family and friends

Balance inner retreat and active times

- physical removal from others when wanted
- respect and recognize person's need to display null/somnolent behaviour or perseverating/rhythmic behaviour
- inactivity and rest when needed
- maintain safe environment, especially for wanderers
- encourage outings and outdoor activities

[a]Data taken from references [20] and [45].

Table 26.2 Causes of behavioural problems in adults with dementia[a]

Medical and physical causes	Environmental causes	Task-related causes	Communication causes
Medication adverse effects	Environment too large	Tasks too complicated	Not understanding others
Impaired vision or hearing	Environment too cluttered	Too many steps combined	Not able to make themselves understood
Acute illness and infections	Excessive stimulation	Task not modified for increasing impairment	
Chronic illness and pain	No orientation information or cues	Task unfamiliar	
Dehydration and constipation	Poor sensory environment		
Depression and fatigue	Environment unstructured		
Physical needs not met	Environment unfamiliar		

[a]Data taken from references [20] and [45].

Table 26.3 Specific communication techniques for use during a dental examination for cognitively impaired adults[a]

Technique		Dental examination example
Task breakdown	The activity or task is broken down into all component steps, which are individually and slowly presented	*The examiner breaks down the steps involved to move a resident back to their room for the dental examination*
Rescuing	A second carer enters a situation and tells the first carer to leave so that the second carer can 'help' their friend, the resident	*The examiner is not able to remove the resident's dentures, so a carer enters, takes over and removes the dentures*
Distraction	The use of singing, holding items, gentle touch and talking to distract the resident from a distressing situation	*A rummage box, busy apron or busy board (with a familiar theme) is used to occupy the active hands of a resident during the examination*
Bridging	To improve sensory connection and task focus the resident holds the same object while the carer carries out an activity	*The resident holds a toothbrush while the examiner uses a backward-bent toothbrush to access the resident's oral cavity*
Hand-over-hand	The carer's hand is placed over the resident's hand to guide the resident through the activity	*The examiner places their hand over the resident's hand to guide them to a chair*
Chaining	The person/carer starts the activity and the resident completes it	*The examiner places the upper denture back in the resident's mouth and the resident then places the lower denture back in their mouth*

[a]Data taken from reference [20].

Both quantitative and qualitative dementia research have improved our understanding of the communication bridge between people with dementia and their carers. 'People with dementia know intuitively whether they are being accepted by a carer – caring touch, gentleness, speed of movement, tenderness of voice and body posture do not escape their sensitive awareness' [20]. Table 26.3 presents newer communication strategies that highlight how people with dementia communicate via inconsistencies that do not necessarily conform to the symptom-based descriptions of dementia stages, with adaption of these concepts into the dental setting (e.g. with examinations, radiographs, oral hygiene care) [20].

The extent and severity of oral diseases and conditions in adults with dementia

Research conducted during the last decades of the 20th century has validated clinicians' observations of poor oral hygiene and increased dental caries experience and more dental problems in older adults with dementia [22–25] (Figure 26.1). People with dementia have been reported to have poor oral health as a result of poor oral hygiene and impaired salivary output, and oral hygiene deteriorated with dementia severity [22, 26–29]. However, the importance of oral health in older adults with cognitive impairment is often neglected and misunderstood. The dental literature concerning dementia has mainly focused on:

1 descriptions of dementia and dementia care;
2 clinical approaches for the dental management of people with dementia;
3 cross-sectional investigations of the oral health status and normative dental needs of institutionalized older adults and people with dementia (case reports/groups) and carer's oral hygiene care provision; and
4 four longitudinal investigations of oral disease incidence in people with dementia.

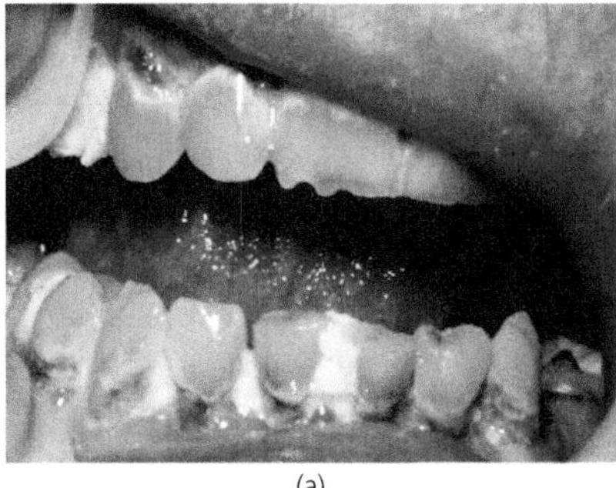
(a)

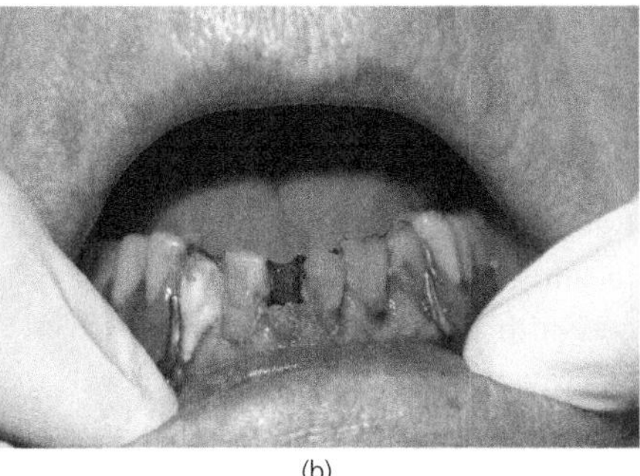
(b)

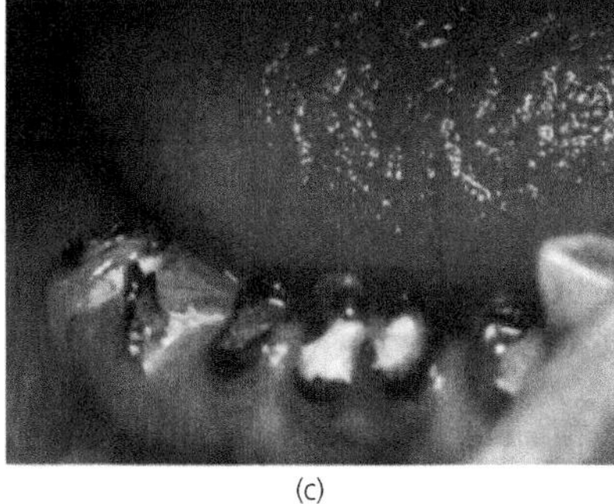
(c)

Figure 26.1 Oral diseases in older adults with dementia. (a) Plaque and caries; (b) Root caries and retained root; (c) Decayed retained roots.

The majority of the dementia research investigations were conducted in the USA, Europe, and Australia [30]. Some of these geriatric dental research studies focused on people with dementia in general, while others were specifically focused towards people with Alzheimer's disease. A few studies, such as those by Jones *et al.* (1993), Akiyama *et al.* (1993), Ship and Puckett (1994), Warren *et al.* (1997), Chalmers *et al.*, (2002) and Adam and Preston, (2006) have used comparison or control groups of older adults without dementia, with only those by Jones *et al.* (1993), Ship and Puckett (1994), Chalmers *et al.* (2002) and Ellefsen *et al.* (2009) being longitudinal in design [23, 27–29, 31–33]. Study subjects varied greatly and ranged from institutionalized older adults, some in Veterans' Affairs facilities, to different groups of community-dwelling older adults. A review of studies of people with dementia studies completed in 2006 highlighted the limited scientific data published and concluded that, from the studies conducted, people with dementia have more oral health problems than people without dementia [30]. Data from the four longitudinal studies Jones *et al.* (1993), Ship and Puckett (1994), Chalmers *et al.* (2002) and Ellefsen *et al.* (2009) highlighted the following findings:

1 Ship and Pucketts's research reported that: participants with Alzheimer's disease had a significantly reduced output of unstimulated and stimulated submandibular/sublingual saliva, but did not have lower output of parotid saliva; significant negative correlations were found between MMSE score and number of teeth with coronal caries and root caries; participants with Alzheimer's disease had significantly more sites with gingival plaque, bleeding and calculus; no significant differences were seen for any of the periodontal parameters. These authors suggested that older adults with Alzheimer's disease may have a different pattern of dental caries to that seen in generally healthy older adults without dementia.
2 Jones *et al.*'s research reported: annualized mean coronal caries increments per 100 available surfaces was 2.3 for participants with dementia and 0.9 for comparison participants; annualized mean root caries increments per 100 available surfaces was 2.4 for dementia and 0.3 for comparison participants.
3 Chalmers *et al.*'s research reported significant differences at one-year follow-up for: higher coronal and root caries experience, incidence and increments in participants with dementia; coronal and root caries increments [adjusted caries increment (ACI)] from baseline to 1 year were higher for participants with dementia (dementia = 3.6 decayed coronal and 1.9 decayed root surfaces; non-dementia = 1.4 decayed coronal and 0.9 decayed root surfaces); caries experience and increments were evident in the great majority of participants with dementia but only in a subgroup of those without dementia; coronal caries incidence occurred in 71.8% of dementia and 48.7% of non-dementia participants; root caries incidence occurred in 62.1% of participants with dementia and 44.2% of non-dementia participants; higher number of root surfaces covered in plaque (dementia = 9.0 surfaces; non-dementia = 2.1 surfaces); and a higher number of decayed retained roots (dementia = 0.3; non-dementia = 0.06). Caries experience, incidence and increments were related to dementia severity and not to specific dementia diagnoses. Caries experience and increments were higher in dementia participants with moderate-severe dementia, government cardholders, those with no private health insurance, the more functionally dependent, those taking neuroleptic medications with high anticholinergic adverse effects, those with eating and swallowing problems, those not attending the dentist regularly, people who needed assistance with oral hygiene care, those who were behaviourally difficult during oral hygiene care and whose carers had a higher burden.
4 Ellefsen *et al.*, in a study of old people referred to two memory clinics, reported a significantly higher mean number of decayed tooth surfaces (coronal and root) at 1 year follow-up than at baseline for all participants. The 1-year adjusted caries and filling increments were high for participants with and without dementia, but were highest for participants with a diagnosis of Alzheimer's disease and a dementia diagnosis other than Alzheimer's disease, indicating that older people referred to a memory clinic are of particular high risk of developing multiple carious lesions during the first year after diagnosis. Baseline risk factors for developing elevated coronal and root adjusted caries and filling increments included having caries, having many teeth and being older than 80 years. The findings

underscore the importance of addressing the oral health needs of elderly people suspected of having experienced cognitive decline.

The cross-sectional research mainly conducted in the 1990s has reported similar findings. Warren *et al.*, 1997 reported that patients without dementia had significantly more filled root surfaces and a lower gingival index score compared with the Alzheimer's group; patients with severe dementia had higher gingival index scores and higher debris scores than patients with normal cognition [28]. Recent cross-sectional geriatric dental studies conducted in Japanese nursing homes with dementia residents reported that residents with dementia had more non-functioning teeth, more teeth that were not restorable, fewer sound teeth and fewer filled teeth [31].

Restraint, consent, legal guardians and ethical issues with dementia patients

Perhaps the most challenging aspect of dental treatment for adults with dementia is obtaining adequate consent for care, and the ethical issues that surround this challenge. Yellowitz (2005) described the ethical dilemmas when providing oral health care for such patients, based on the ADA's Principles of Ethics and Code of Professional Conduct [34]. The two main principles guiding treatment decision-making are beneficence and autonomy. Beneficence means that professionals have a duty to act for the benefit of others with due consideration being given to the needs, desires and values of the patient; autonomy means that professionals have a duty to treat the patient according to the patient's desires, within the bounds of accepted treatment and to protect the patient's confidentiality [34]. Specific requirements for consent vary regionally and by country and all practitioners should consult their local dental associations and other appropriate regulatory bodies for specific regulations and information. However, in general, for informed consent to be valid the patient must have been clearly informed about the dental treatment, they must have free choice and they must have the capacity to give that consent [34].

Thus, the key to ethical care provision is the identification of patients' cognitive impairments (and behavioural and communication problems) before obtaining consent and initiating dental treatment [34]. This becomes complicated, especially in the earlier stages of cognitive impairment, often when a dementia diagnosis has not been definitively given. All dental providers should consult with the dementia patient's appropriate responsible parties which may include their family, caregiver, spouse, children, nursing home director and primary care physician. In many cases, it is the primary care physician who can confirm any dementia diagnoses, describe any related medical issues that may complicate the consent process and determine the person's capacity to consent [34]. If a dementia diagnosis is confirmed, determine if the patient has a legally responsible party allocated to give consent on their behalf for: (1) medical issues (a durable power of attorney for health care) and (2) financial issues – these may often be different individuals. Patients with dementia may have previously expressed desires concerning their dental/medical care that need to be incorporated into the consent process, such as in their advanced directives. It is also helpful to gain assent for the treatment from the person with dementia and to document it – this involves communication with the dementia patient in the appropriate manner ranging from in writing to orally, or by gesture. A more difficult situation is when the person with dementia declines treatment and definitive medical consent from the person responsible must be obtained, including consent for the use of restraint. This will often occur as the person with dementia has increasing behaviour and communication problems. Guidelines for the use of restraint are presented in Box 26.2. The level of restraint to be used can vary greatly from hand-holding, to holding of arms/legs, wrapping/stabilization/holding of the head and to the use of adult papoose boards. Each dental practitioner will find their own level of comfort in using these various levels of restraint and should attempt to use other behaviour management techniques as have been previously described, such as task breakdown, distraction and bridging. Often oral

Box 26.2 Guidelines for use of restraint.[a]

Restraint is necessary for safe, effective treatment
Restraint is not for punishment of the patient or the convenience of carers/staff
The least restrictive alternative should be used
Restraint should cause no physical trauma and minimal psychological trauma
Reasonable benefits are expected as a result of the treatment
There is consent for dental treatment
There is consent for the use of restraint
The type of restraint is specifically selected based on the planned treatment
Dental staff are trained in the safe use of the restraint
Restraint is clearly documented, including type, duration and reason for use
If appropriate, the person responsible for giving consent for the patient can be present or nearby to assist with decision making during treatment
If appropriate, the caregiver most familiar with the person should be present to assist with behaviour management and communication during the dental treatment

[a]Data taken from reference [46].

sedation may also be used in conjunction with restraint in the clinical dental practice and this needs to be clearly discussed with all parties involved. The use of benzodiazepines is common for oral sedation, but be aware that such drugs are contraindicated for many patients with dementia and indeed may increase their behavioural problems. If used, benzodiazepines should be short-acting. Optimum results will often be achieved with the use of an increased dosage of an existing medication the dementia patient is taking, rather than the addition of another psychotropic medication. When the use of restraint, with or without oral sedation, is not consented to or is not able to be used, the dental practitioner needs to evaluate the use of a form of intravenous sedation or general anaesthesia [35].

Rational dental care for dementia patients

Maintaining adequate oral health is essential for older adults with dementia for their quality of life and for medical reasons. Older adults need to eat and talk comfortably, to feel happy with their appearance, to stay pain free, to maintain self-esteem and to maintain habits/standards of hygiene and care that they have had throughout their life. Behavioural problems in people with dementia such as disinterest in food and not eating, "pulling" at the face or mouth, chewing of the lip, tongue or hands, grinding of teeth or dentures, not wearing of dentures, aggression (especially during activities of daily living) and alterations in activity (such as somnolence, tiring, screaming and restlessness) can be caused by dental pain and problems. Adequate oral hygiene and dental treatment are needed for people with dementia: to prevent medical problems such as aspiration pneumonia and bacteraemias; to manage medication side effects such as dry-mouth, speech problems, swallowing problems, tardive dyskinesia and gingival overgrowth; to maintain adequate nutrition and hydration; and to manage consequences of co-morbid medical conditions such as Sjögren's syndrome, arthritis, strokes, radiation and chemotherapy. The cognitive deficits of dementia also reduce a person's ability to perform regular oral hygiene care for themselves and they gradually require more and more reminders and assistance to complete this task. Thus, it is essential to provide regular dental care and oral hygiene care maintenance as soon as possible for a patient with dementia.

Regular dental care provision for people with dementia requires the implementation of the concept of 'rational' or 'realistic' care. Rational dental care should only be provided after careful consideration of all the patient's modifying factors (Box 26.3). In the overall context of Geriatric Minimal Intervention Dentistry (GMID), consideration is also needed of a group of primary oral factors and plaque/biofilm factors [36] (Figure 26.2).

Box 26.3 Modifying factors for treatment planning a patient with dementia.

- The patient's desires and expectations
- The caregiver, family and other desires and expectations
- The patient's medical/neurological conditions and current/past medications
- The patient's financial, social, transport and residential situation
- The patient's ability to tolerate the stress of treatment
- The type and severity of the patient's dental pain and dental needs
- How the dental problems affect the patient's quality of life
- The patient's ability to maintain oral hygiene care
- The probability of positive treatment outcomes
- The availability of reasonable and less-extensive treatment alternatives
- The dental team's ability to deliver the care needed (skills and equipment available)
- Other issues (for example, the patient's lifespan, bioethical issues)

Data taken from reference [47].

GMID uses a medical model for oral disease control and comprises: (1) oral disease risk assessment with early detection and prevention; (2) external and internal remineralization therapy; (3) use of a range of restorations, dental materials and equipment; and (4) surgical intervention only after disease is controlled [36]. Thus, it is imperative to evaluate home oral hygiene care and caregiver involvement to ascertain how to optimally maintain the influential primary

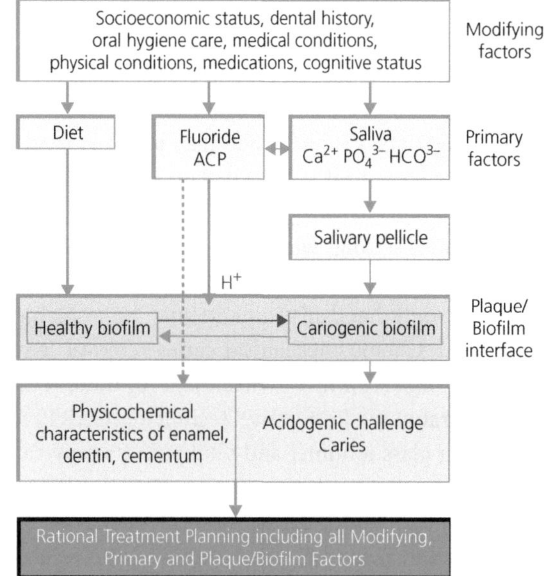

Figure 26.2 Geriatric minimal intervention dentistry for dementia patients. *Source:* Chalmers, 2006 [36]. Reproduced with permission of the Canadian Dental Association.

oral factors such as diet, fluoride, amorphous calcium phosphate and saliva. These factors are discussed in detail in other chapters in this text. Achieving good compliance with home care products is a challenge, especially when carers are involved in oral hygiene care. When deciding which preventive or therapeutic dental product to prescribe it is necessary to: (1) review the oral diseases present and identify the greatest modifying factors contributing to them; (2) try one product first; (3) add products over time; and (4) have ongoing adjustment and review of the oral hygiene protocol [36].

Geriatric MID helps dentists to address the ever-increasing restorative challenges faced with older patients with dementia, including: erosion, abrasion, demineralization, rampant coronal and root caries, retained roots, recurrent caries (crowns, repairs), subgingival caries, 'wet' oral environments, saliva dysfunction, patient disruptive behaviours, poor compliance with preventive care, high plaque levels and financial and other restrictions on care options. In Geriatric MID, the choice of the direct restorative material to be used cannot be made until: (1) caries removal is complete and (2) field control has been evaluated. Caries removal utilizes conventional hand instruments, rotary handpieces and if available may use air abrasion or lasers. The final factors to weigh into the choice of restorative material are aesthetic requirements, longevity required for the restoration, if the restoration is being repaired versus replaced, availability of a dental assistant and patient behavioural problems [37].

One of the most challenging restorative situations in older patients occurs with deep, subgingival caries, where there is excessive saliva and bleeding. If rubber dam and isolation cannot be adequately obtained to enable the use of amalgam or composite resin, then an alternative material is Fuji Triage/Fuji VII, which has a better tolerance for wet conditions and which can be carved in difficult access situations [25]. Fuji Triage/Fuji VII and other glass ionomer materials can also be used as a root surface sealant in high caries risk older patients [37].

In some clinical settings where access to rotary handpieces is limited, such as in nursing homes or in the dementia patients' homes, only hand instruments may be available for caries removal. Chemo-mechanical caries removal may also be of some benefit in this environment. In these settings, a Geriatric Atraumatic Restorative Technique (GART) technique utilizing glass ionomer and vital pulp therapy can be used [37]. The choice of glass ionomer material will be limited only by the ability of the dental professional to access a triturator and a curing light. The diversity of conventional glass ionomer materials is increasing and provides choices from: (1) hand-mix, (2) paste-pak and (3) triturated capsules. At present, resin-modified glass ionomers are available in: (1) paste-pak and (2) triturated capsules and require the use of a curing light. Both conventional and resin-modified glass ionomers require a seal and in these settings a varnish or a light-activated resin enamel bond can be applied.

Treatment planning and dental care under general anaesthesia for dementia patients

The numbers of dentate older adults with dementia are increasing, and research has documented their high levels of caries and retained tooth roots. As dementia progresses, so do their behavioural and communication problems. This has resulted in a group of older dementia patients in whom dental treatment cannot be provided in the dental office, and who seek dental treatment under intravenous sedation or general anaesthesia (GA). Some of the indications for GA include: acute pain, infection, decreased nutritional intake, increased behavioural problems, as well as for regular radiographic and clinical examination and dental treatment. Careful planning and consultation is required for any prospective GA patient with dementia – there are many risks associated with GA to be weighed by the person with dementia, dental team, physician, medical and financial persons responsible, caregivers and family. These risks include nausea, temporary delirium, hypoxia, prolonged sedation, cardiac events and death. The risks of GA (pre- and postoperative) versus the benefits of dental treatment must be carefully considered. All prospective GA dental patients must have a comprehensive medical evaluation by their physician, an anaesthetist and other relevant medical specialists – the results of these evaluations need to be conveyed to the dental team in writing, including all blood test, electrocardiograph and other medical test results. Professional national associations of anaesthetists usually provide clear guidelines for such evaluations [38]. Another consideration for a GA procedure is whether the medical and social conditions of the patient require them to have an overnight hospital stay after the GA procedure versus being a day-stay only patient. Most dementia patients will require preoperative sedation. It also is essential to determine how the patient will be premedicated, how they will be transported, who will accompany them to and from the GA procedure, who will pay for the GA procedure and hospital stay and who will coordinate the preoperative issues such as fasting and administration of medications (e.g. regular medications and additional medications such as antibiotics).

GA dental treatment for people with dementia encompasses the full range of care including radiographs, prophylaxis, restorations, extractions/surgery and in some specific situations periodontics, endodontics, and prosthodontics. GA is not appropriate for frequent recall visits involving dental prophylaxis or preventive measures [38]. GA should be a treatment option every 3–5 years, with regular dental examinations and prophylaxis attempted in the dental office in the intervening period [38]. Regular oral hygiene care and dental maintenance is a key aspect of treatment planning for GA dental treatment. Attempt a dental examination and radiographs prior to the GA to obtain as much information for treatment planning. Sometimes very little dental information is available prior to the GA, and it is essential to obtain a blanket or open consent which covers all of the treatment possibilities listed above. A detailed informed written consent must be obtained from the appropriate person responsible for the dementia patient. Patients with dementia may present with a large number of grossly carious teeth and tooth roots, and the decision concerning extraction of all remaining teeth/roots needs to be carefully weighed – dentures may or may not be able to be fabricated for these patients. All persons responsible for the dementia patient must be fully informed of this when consent is obtained for the GA.

GA dental procedures require the administration of local anaesthetics to: provide postoperative pain management; assist with haemostasis; minimize cardiac adverse events related to pain; reduce the amounts of general anaesthetics used during the procedure [38]. Adequate postoperative pain relief needs to be prescribed and clearly communicated orally and in writing to all nurses and caregivers. A 0.12% oral chlorhexidine lavage should be administered to all patients prior to administration of local anaesthetics. Other issues to be addressed in older GA patients are urinary continence, positioning and additional padding, removal of dentures and other prostheses and adequate thermoregulation [38].

After the patient has been intubated and prepared by the anaesthetist, and a throat pack is placed, radiographs need to be made (extra and intraoral as required) to assist with treatment planning. It is essential to use mouth props to keep the mouth open and to protect the tongue. Whilst radiographs are being developed, a detailed dental examination can be completed. Photographs may also be taken pre- and post-operatively. If a blanket or open consent has been obtained the dental team can complete any treatment needed, otherwise they will have to obtain further consent from the person legally responsible. A dental/nursing assistant should be present to document the treatment plan. The order of dental treatment procedures under GA will often depend upon the location of the restorations and extractions to be completed and the ensuing bleeding problems. Ghezzi *et al.* (2000) presented four general GA dental treatment planning scenarios for older adults with cognitive impairment; these are based on the restorability of the dentition and the level of cooperation of the patient [38] (Table 26.4). In cases where the clinician is not comfortable managing specific aspects of surgical care required, an oral surgeon may also participate in the GA. All dental equipment should be carefully organized, with all infection control requirements addressed. Adequate supplies of dental equipment should be available, with clear access available in the operatory to all radiographic equipment and dental handpieces. Some hospitals will provide all dental equipment, while others will require the dental team to bring their own supplies. All dentists need to be accredited by the hospital that they are using.

Clinical management of the terminally ill older patient

What is palliative oral care?

Palliative oral care has been defined as the study and management of patients with active, progressive, far-advanced disease in whom the oral cavity has been compromised either by the disease directly or by its treatment, and the guiding principle is symptom relief. The goal of palliative care is achievement of optimum quality of life for terminally ill patients and their families [39]. The palliative care team consists of physicians, nurses, social workers, psychologists, dieticians, clergy and dentists. This team of professionals targets their care to both the patient and their loved-ones. Figure 26.3 presents the five components of care for terminally ill older adults. In addition to medical and dental treatment, optimal palliative oral care encompasses humanistic, spiritual and metaphysical aspects of care. Humanistic care is that in which the patient always comes first and the care is what is best for the patient. Empathy gives us insight into the patient's concerns and feelings. When we identify with these feelings, compassion follows, in which we have sympathetic concern for the patient's suffering. We try to alleviate the cause of and problems arising from the patient's concerns and feelings. Spirituality is a person's life philosophy – it is 'why' you are here and extends beyond religious boundaries. A spiritual healer is a conduit of powers; a palliative care dentist is a communicator and facilitator of spiritual essence – trust, love, pain, fear, happiness, confusion. Metaphysical abilities are the natural form of communication of the spirit – forces of the earth, nature and cosmos; metaphysical forces include palmistry, aromatherapy, meditation and 'healing hands' (a form of healing massage). A palliative care dentist uses metaphysical abilities such as hypnotherapy, touch and desensitization while providing dental care for their terminally ill patients.

Good communication is the key to effective palliative oral care and encompasses the use of humanistic, spiritual and metaphysical abilities of the dentist and the dental team.

Table 26.4 Dental treatment planning guidelines for general anaesthesia (modified by Chalmers, 2007)[a]

Oral condition and findings	Behaviour	GA treatment plan	Ongoing treatment
Severe decay Non-restorable dentition	No cooperation	**1** Oral examination **2** Radiographs/photos **3** Chlorhexidine (CHX) lavage **4** Full-mouth extractions	Postoperative review of extraction sites Annual oral examinations
Severe decay Non-restorable dentition	Limited cooperation	**1** Oral examination **2** Radiographs/photos **3** CHX lavage **4** Full-mouth extractions **5** Possible immediate dentures	Postoperative review of extraction sites 24 h and 1 week recall for immediate dentures Annual oral examinations
Multiple dental needs Restorable dentition	No cooperation	**1** Oral examination **2** Radiographs/photos **3** CHX lavage **4** Scale, root plane, prophy **5** Restorations **6** Extraction of teeth with poor prognosis	Postoperative review of extraction sites 3–6 monthly oral examinations (prophy, fluoride varnish) with use of oral/i.v. sedation if necessary Oral hygiene care (e.g. CHX, fluoride, amorphous calcium phosphate, saliva substitutes/stimulants)
Multiple dental needs Restorable dentition	Limited cooperation	**1** Oral examination **2** Radiographs/photos **3** CHX lavage **4** Scale, root plane, prophy **5** Restorations **6** Extraction of teeth with poor prognosis **7** Extensive dental procedures (e.g. endodontics, preparation and impression for fixed and removable prostheses)	Postoperative review of extraction sites Further return visits to complete extensive treatment (e.g. fixed and removable prostheses) 3–6 monthly oral examinations (prophy, fluoride varnish) with use of oral sedation if necessary Oral hygiene care (e.g. CHX, fluoride, amorphous calcium phosphate, saliva substitutes/stimulants)

[a]Data taken from reference [38].

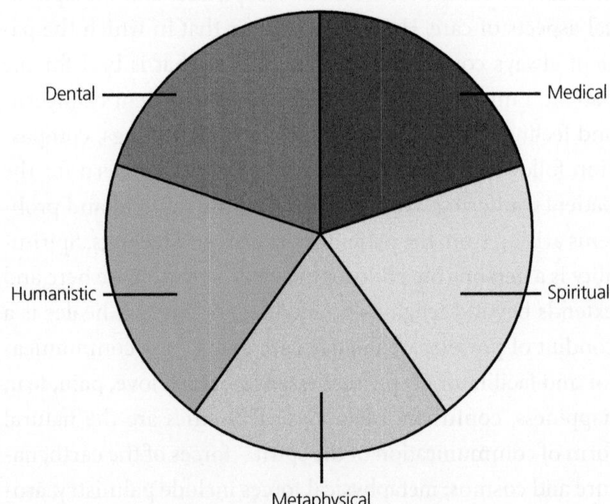

Figure 26.3 Components of care for terminally ill older dental patients. *Source:* Jolly, D.E. (2004) *Wellness, oral health and the spirit.* Lecture given at the Ohio State University College of Dentistry. Reproduced with permission of D.E. Jolly.

Palliative care supports the patient in preparing the mind to the reality of death. Dentists need to be able to openly talk about dying with patients and their families and address issues such as fear, progressive pain and discomfort, financial hardships and feelings of being a burden on others. This broadens the focus of the dentist from the oral cavity to the whole person.

Oral conditions in palliative care

The mouth is often a site of pain, loss of function and poor quality of life for a palliative care patient. The main oral conditions evident are: dry mouth (xerostomia/salivary gland hypofunction); mucositis; candidiasis; viral infections; caries; periodontal diseases; problems with dentures; dysphagia, oral pain, taste disorders, speech problems and poor aesthetics (see Figure 26.4). In addition, nausea, vomiting, poor nutrition and poor hydration also involve the oral cavity. These conditions may not always be resolved but the dentist should strive to at least alleviate symptoms, minimize pain and suffering and provide symptom control [40]. Use of the previously described concept of rational treatment planning is essential for terminally ill patients to ensure realistic dental care is provided. Also, provision of adequate

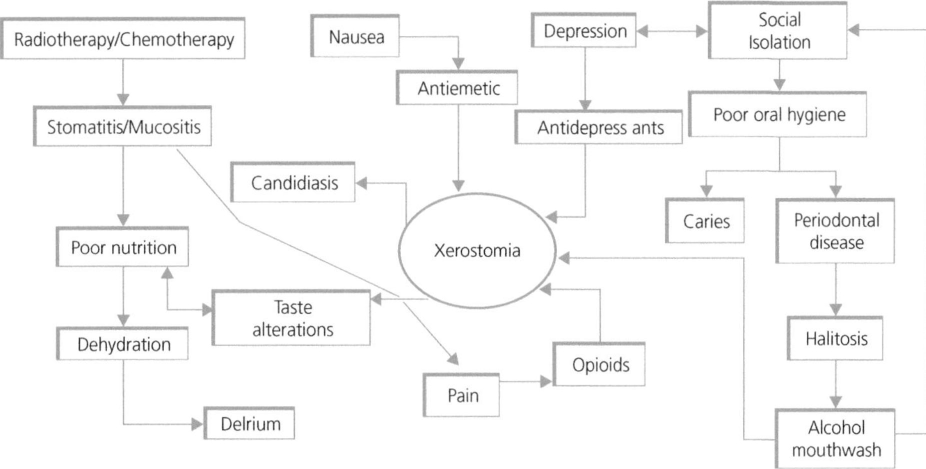

Figure 26.4 The main oral conditions evident in palliative care.

oral hygiene care is important to help prevent many oral conditions, in addition to other medical conditions such as aspiration pneumonia. Wherever possible, the dentist should be an integral member of a palliative care team and as such can help to prevent these oral conditions rather than having to treat them once they have occurred [40].

Oral mucositis (severe ulceration) occurs commonly in patients undergoing chemotherapy and head and neck radiotherapy. Chemotherapy is used in cancer patients to act on tissues with a high rate of mitosis, with the oral cavity frequently affected as coincidentally the oral mucosal tissues have a high rate of turnover. The oral mucosa undergoes atrophy leading to ulceration and sometimes microbial invasion [41]. Up to 80% of patients with head and neck cancer and up to 40% of patients undergoing chemotherapy have oral mucositis. Chemotherapeutic agents such as 5-fluorouracil and methotrexate will produce oral mucositis within 5–7 days. Radiation to the head and neck will destroy salivary gland tissue resulting in salivary dysfunction, rendering the oral mucosal tissues more susceptible to trauma and microbial invasion. Systematic reviews conducted to date have reported the following as effective (from a weak to strong degree) in preventing or reducing the severity of oral mucositis: allopurinol amifostine, antibiotic paste or pastille, benzydamine, granulocyte macrophage-colony stimulating factor, hydrolytic enzymes, ice chips and povidone. Mucositis pain is generally most successfully treated using opiates (morphine), often as a 0.2% solution used topically [41]. Many oncologists prescribe 'magic mouthwash' (antihistamine, topical anaesthetic, antibiotic and/or antifungal) but systematic reviews have concluded that it is ineffective. All mucositis patients should have any potential traumatic areas in the mouth restored and should avoid spicy foods, alcohol and smoking [41]. The use of alcohol-free chlorhexidine gluconate has not been evidenced as effective for the management of oral mucositis but may be helpful in the control of periodontal diseases and dental caries – it may be rinsed, applied as a gel or used in a spray bottle [42].

Candidiasis occurs in the majority of palliative care patients and is related to poor oral hygiene, dry mouth, immunosuppression, use of corticosteroids, use of antibiotics, poor nutritional status, diabetes and denture-wearing [41]. *Candida albicans* is the most common causative organism. Candidal infections manifest as acute pseudomembranous (thrush), erythematous (atrophic), hyperplastic (denture stomatitis) or angular cheilitis (corners of the mouth) [41]. White plaques are present in acute pseudomembranous candidiasis – these plaques rub off to reveal an erythematous area of tissue. Erythematous candidiasis occurs as red patches on the palate and dorsum of the tongue. Angular cheilitis commonly has not only a candidal but a bacterial component. If any dentures are present, they must be regularly sterilized and scrubbed – diluted sodium hypochlorite (15 mL bleach/250 ml water) is adequate for non-metal dentures. However, any metal containing dentures should be sterilized in benzalkonium chloride (1 : 750 dilution). All denture containers should be regularly sterilized or disposable. Candidiasis can be treated topically and systemically [41]. Nystatin has long been used to treat candidiasis but its success requires long contact time with the tissues, which is generally minimal with the commonly prescribed oral suspension (200 000–500 000 IU, swished and swallowed three to five times daily). Nystatin suspension also has a high sugar content because of its bad taste and should be used with caution in dentate patients. Nystatin (100 000 IU, four times per day) or clotrimazole (100 mg day for 7 days) vaginal troches can be sucked, but this can be difficult for patients with dry mouth. Clotrimazole 1% cream can be applied to the surface of dentures several times daily for 7 days. Angular cheilitis can be treated with a nystatin cream and the corners of the mouth washed regularly with an antibacterial soap, chloramphenicol eye ointments can also be used topically to manage the bacterial element of angular cheilitis. If topical agents are ineffective, systemic drugs can be used with care, as they are expensive and many have renal/hepatic toxic adverse effects –fluconazole (100–200 mg on day 1, then 50–100 mg orally daily for 7–14 days) and itraconazole (100–200mg daily for 7–14 days) are most commonly used [41].

Xerostomia (self-perceived dry mouth) and salivary gland hypofunction (reduced salivary quality and/or quantity) can be present in most terminally ill older adults. It may range from mild to extremely severe. If any salivary gland tissues are remaining then saliva stimulants can be used – these include the chewing of sugarless gum and candy, SalivaSure tablets (fruit acid in a buffered pH placed near the saliva duct outlets) and the systemic drugs pilocarpine and cevimeline [43]. Pilocarpine and cemiveline may have adverse effects that preclude their use. If there is little or no salivary gland tissue remaining, saliva substitutes can be used on the oral soft tissues and in dentures – when dry mouth is severe these may need to be applied many times daily. A large range of these are available in most countries and include: the Oral Balance Gel/Denture Grip products (Laclede Professional Products, Gardena, California); and MI Paste Plus (GC Corporation). Petroleum-based products should not be used as they will absorb water from oral tissues and should not be used near oxygen [43]. Additionally, petroleum-based products may allow for opportunistic infections as these products may create a 'protective' barrier for the pathogen from the body's own defence mechanisms. Avoid using toothpastes with sodium lauryl sulfate and also alcohol-containing mouthwashes. Carers can apply products intraorally using a small foam brush, a toothbrush or a spray bottle [41].

One of the major problems noted in palliative care patients is dehydration. This can accentuate the effect of xerostomia. The palliative care patient should be encouraged to drink as much as possible. Using additional means such as IV or SC hydration do not actually prolong life but may improve the quality of the death process. A common side effect of poor hydration is decreased drug clearance. This can lead to an accumulation of opioid metabolites and nitrogenous waste products. This could induce a state of delirium in patients. A healthy oral cavity can allow the patient to self hydrate.

Depression is very common in palliative care patients. The use of antidepressants, even the newer 'saliva saving' varieties, do induce a state of xerostomia. It is important for the dental professional to be part of the palliative care team (clergy, music therapists, art therapists, social workers) and attempt to raise the spirits of the palliative care patient and family but always trying to be honest with the prognosis.

Depression can always lead to a disconnect to their oral hygiene and their finality of life. Halitosis may prevent some family members from displaying their emotions appropriately to their loved ones. The palliative care patient should be provided alcohol-free mouth rinses to limit the extent of the xerostomia.

As many of these patients may have used bisphosphonates to retard the metastasis of their cancer (such as seen in breast and prostate cancer), prudent oral care must be provided. Figure 26.5(a) demonstrates how a 70-year-old female palliative care patient with breast metastasis to the brain, who was

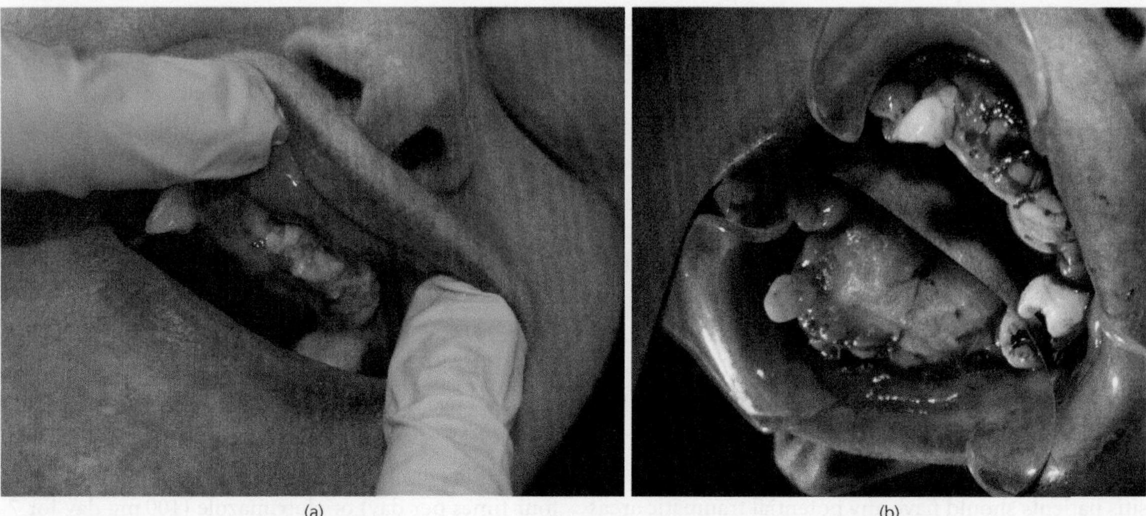

Figure 26.5 a) Bisphosphonate induced osteonecrosis of the jaw. b) Using local anaesthesia with premedication the sequestra portions of bone were removed and primary closure was achieved.

previously given pamidronate i.v. to hinder metastasis, had poor oral hygiene and began to lose teeth from periodontal disease. This led to a diagnosed bisphosphonate-induced osteonecrosis of the jaw. Under local anaesthesia, with premedication with clindamycine 300 mg qid, and chlorhexidine gluconate rinses qid, sequestra portions of bone were removed and primary closure was achieved [Figure 26.5(b)]. This patient's oral pain decreased. She died one month post-treatment without oral pain.

Essential concepts for the dental professional from this chapter

- High levels of oral diseases and conditions have been evidenced in older patients with dementia and terminal illness.
- Rational treatment planning reviews of all patient modifying factors and oral environmental factors aids the dental team to provide realistic dental care for patients with dementia and terminal illness.
- In addition to dental care provision, all treatment plans must include comprehensive oral hygiene care strategies for ongoing maintenance of oral health.
- Both pharmacological and non-pharmacological strategies are available to manage behavioural and communication problems in patients with dementia.
- General anaesthesia is an alternative for dental care provision for patients with dementia but needs to be carefully assessed and implemented by a dental and medical team.

References

1 American Psychiatric Association (1994) *Diagnostic and Statistical Manual of Mental Disorders Fourth Edition (DSM-IV)*, pp. 133–134, American Psychiatric Association, Washington, DC.

2 American Psychiatric Association (2013) *Diagnostic and Statistical Manual of Mental Disorders Fifth Edition (DSM-V)*, p. 591, American Psychiatric Publishing, Arlington, VA.

3 Ancill, R.J., Holliday, S.G., Thorpe, L. & Rabheru, K. (eds) (1999) *Treating dementia: cognition and beyond*. Canadian Academic Press, Vancouver, BC.

4 Plassman, B.L., Langa, K.M., Fisher, G.G., Heeringa, S.G., Weir, D.R., Ofstedal, M.B. *et al.* (2007) Prevalence of dementia in the United States: The aging, demographics, and memory study. *Neuroepidemiology*, **29**, 125–132.

5 WHO. (1992) *The ICD-10 Classification of Mental and Behavioural Disorders. Clinical descriptions and diagnostic guidelines*. World Health Organisation, Geneva.

6 Reitz, C. & Mayeux, R. (2014) Alzheimer disease: Epidemiology, diagnostic criteria, risk factors and biomarkers. *Biochemical Pharmacology*, **88**, 640–651.

7 Bertram, L. & Tanzi, R.E. (2012) The genetics of Alzheimer's disease. *Progress in Molecular Biology and Translational Science*, **107**, 79–100.

8 McCarron, M., McCallion, P., Reily, E. & Mulryan, N. (2014) A prospective 14-year longitudinal follow-up of dementia in persons with down syndrome. *Journal of Intellectual Disability Research*, **58**, 61–70.

9 Weisman, D. & McKeith, I. (2007) Dementia with Lewy bodies. *Seminars in Neurology*, **27**, 42–47.

10 Jellinger, K.A. (2013) Pathology and pathogenesis of vascular cognitive impairment-a critical update. *Frontiers in Aging Neuroscience*, **5**, 17, doi: 10.3389/fnagi.2013.00017.

11 Mawanda, F. & Wallace, R. (2013) Can infections cause Alzheimer's disease? *Epidemiologic Reviews*, **35**, 161–180.

12 Forlenza, O.V., Diniz, B.S. & Gattaz, W.F. (2010) Diagnosis and biomarkers of predementia in Alzheimer's disease. *BMC Medicine*, **8**, 89, doi: 10.1186/1741-7015-8-89.

13 Ward, A, Arrighi, H.M., Michels, S. & Cedarbaum, J.M. (2012) Mild cognitive impairment: Disparity of incidence and prevalence estimates. *Alzheimer's & Dementia*, **8**, 14–21.

14 Folstein, M.F., Folstein, S.E. & McHugh, P.R. (1975) Mini-mental state: a practical method for grading the cognitive state of patients for the clinician. *Journal of Psychiatric Research*, **12**, 189–198.

15 Tuokko, H., Hadjistavropoulos, T., Miller, J.A. & Beattie, B.L. (1992) The clock test: A sensitive measure to differentiate normal elderly from those with Alzheimer's disease. *Journal of the American Geriatrics Society*, **40**, 579–584.

16 Reisberg, B., Ferris, S.H., DeLeon, M.J. & Crook, T. (1982) The Global Deterioration Scale (GDS): an instrument for the assessment of primary degenerative dementia. *American Journal of Psychiatry*, **139**, 1136–1139.

17 Lawton, M.P. & Brody, E.M. (1969) Assessment of older people: self-maintaining and instrumental activities of daily living. *Gerontologist*, **9**, 179–186.

18 Katz, S., Ford, A.B., Moskowitz, R.W., Jackson, B.A. & Jaffe, M.W. (1963) Studies of illness in the aged. The index of the ADL: a standardized measure of biological and psychosocial functioning. Journal of the American Medical Association, **185**, 914–919.

19 Qui, C., De Ronchi, D. & Fratiglioni, L. (2007) The epidemiology of the dementias: an update. *Current Opinion in Psychiatry*, **20**, 380–385.

20 Kovach, C.R. (1997) *Late-stage dementia care*. Taylor & Francis, USA.

21 Volicer, L. & Hurley, A.C. (2003) Management of behavioral symptoms in progressive degenerative dementias. *Journals of Gerontology, Series A: Biological Sciences and Medical Sciences*, **58**. M837–M845.

22 Ship, J.A. (1992) Oral health of patients with Alzheimer's disease. *Journal of the American Dental Association*, **123**, 53–58.

23 Jones, J.A., Lavellee, N., Alman, J., Sinclair, C. & Garcia, R.L. (1993) Caries incidence in patients with dementia. *Gerodontics*, **10**(2), 76–82.

24 Lin, C.Y., Jones, D.B., Godwin, K., Godwin, R.K., Knebl, J.A. & Niessen, L. (1999) Oral health assessment by nursing facility staff of Alzheimer's patients in a long-term care facility. *Special Care in Dentistry*, **19**(2), 64–71.

25 Ellefsen, B., Holm-Pedersen, P., Morse, D.E., Schroll, M., Andersen, B.B. & Waldemar, G. (2008) Caries prevalence in older persons with and without dementia. *Journal of the American Geriatrics Society*, **56**, 59–67.

26 Ship, J.A., De Carli, C., Friedland, R.P. & Baum, B.J. (1990) Diminished submandibular salivary flow in dementia of the Alzheimer type. *Journal of Gerontology*, **45**(2), M61–M66.
27 Ship, J.A. & Puckett, S.A. (1994) Longitudinal study on oral health in subjects with Alzheimer's disease. *Journal of the American Geriatrics Society*, **42**, 57–63.
28 Warren, J.J., Chalmers, J.M., Levy, S.M., Blanco, V.L. & Ettinger, R.L. (1997) Oral health of persons with and without dementia attending a geriatric clinic. *Special Care in Dentistry*, **17**(2), 47–53.
29 Adam, H. & Preston, A.J. (2006) The oral health of individuals with dementia in nursing homes. *Gerodontology*, **23**, 99–105.
30 Rejnefelt, I., Andersson, P. & Renvert, S. (2006) Oral health status in individuals with dementia living in special facilities. *International Journal of Dental Hygiene*, **4**, 67–71.
31 Akiyama, S., Imanishi, H., Yasufuku, Y., Marukawa, Y., Minami, I., Kato, K., Mihara, J. & Morisaki, I. (1993) Dental findings of the elderly with or without senile dementia at a special nursing home. *Journal of Osaka University Dental School*, **33**, 21–26
32 Chalmers, J.M., Carter, K.D. & Spencer, A.J. (2002) Caries incidence and increments in community-living older adults with and without dementia. *Gerodontology*, **19**(2), 80–94.
33 Ellefsen, B., Holm-Pedersen, P., Morse, D.E., Schroll, M., Andersen, B.B. & Waldemar, G. (2009) Assessing caries increments in elderly patients with and without dementia. *Journal of the American Dental Association*, **140**, 1392–1400.
34 Yellowitz, J.A. (2005) Cognitive function, aging, and ethical decisions: recognizing change. *Dental Clinics of North America*, **49**, 389–410.
35 Henry, R.G. & Smith, B.J. (2009) Managing older patients who have neurologic disease: Alzheimer disease and cerebrovascular accident. *Dental Clinics of North America*, **53**, 269–294.
36 Chalmers, J.M. (2006) Minimal intervention dentistry: part 1. Strategies for addressing the new caries challenge in older patients. *Journal of the Canadian Dental Association*, **72**(5), 427–433.
37 Chalmers, J.M. (2006) Minimal intervention dentistry: part 2. Strategies for addressing restorative challenges in older patients. *Journal of the Canadian Dental Association*, **72**(5), 435–440.
38 Ghezzi, E.M., Chavez, E.M. & Ship, J.A. (2000) General anaesthesia protocol for the dental patient: emphasis for older adults. *Special Care in Dentistry*, **20**(3), 81–108.
39 World Health Organization. *WHO Definition of Palliative Care*, 10th edn, p. 560, Webster' Collegiate Dictionary, Merriam-Webster, Inc. 197, Springfield, MA.
40 Ettinger, R.L. (2012) The role of the dentist in geriatric palliative care. *Journal of the American Geriatrics Society*, **60**, 367–368.
41 Wiseman, M.A. (2006) The treatment of oral problems in the palliative patient. *Journal of the Canadian Dental Association*, **72**(5), 453–458.
42 Scully, C. & Ettinger, R.L. (2007) The influence of systemic diseases on oral health care in older adults. *Journal of the American Dental Association*, **138**, 7s–14s.
43 Ram, S., Kumar, S. & Navazesh, M. (2011) Management of xerostomia and salivary gland hypofunction. *Journal of the California Dental Association*, **39**, 656–659.
44 Henderson, A.S. and Jorm, A.F. (1998) *Dementia in Australia. Aged and Community Care Service Development and Evaluation Reports Number 35.* Aged and Community Care Division, Department of Health and Family Services, AGPS, Canberra.
45 Hallberg, I.R., Holst, G., Nordmark, A. & Edberg, A. (1995) Cooperation during morning care between nurses and severely demented institutionalized patients. *Clinical Nursing Research*, **4**(1), 78–104.
46 Shuman, S. & Bebeau, M. (1996) Ethical Issues in Nursing Home Care: Practice Guidelines for Difficult Situations. *Special Care in Dentistry*, **16**, 170–176.
47 Ettinger, R.L. (2006) Rational dental care: part 1. Has the concept changed in 20 years? *Journal of the Canadian Dental Association*, **72**(5), 441–445.

Index

figures are in *italics*; **tables/boxes** are in **bold**

A

acetaminophen (paracetamol), 92, 95, 99, 270, 275
acidulated phosphate fluoride (AFP), 195
actinic cheilitis (solar cheilitis), 72
Actinic elastosis of lower lip, 235
Actinomyces gerencseriae, 186
Actinomyces Israelii, 186
Active coronal/root caries in mandibular anterior teeth, 74
activities of daily living (ADL), 64, 70, 121–122, 315
acupuncture (salivary stimulation), 251
adaptation
 aging, 56
 response, 13
 theories, 7
Addison's disease, 72, 94
ADP antagonist platelet inhibitor, 257–258
adrenal gland disorders
 dental management, 94
 hyperadrenocortism (Cushing's disease), 17, 21, 94
 hypoadrenocortism (Addison's disease), 72, 94
 patients taking steroids, 94–95
adverse drug reactions (ADRs), 69, 145–146, 150, 152
Adverse drug reactions (ADRs)
 'Dental drugs', 150
 Signs, 69
 Types, 145
affective disorders
 bipolar disorders, 104
 depression, 103–104
 oral health, 112
African Americans (US), 55
age/disease interactions, 62
aged tooth clinical challenges
 operative dental procedures, 203–204
 pulp breakdown and old teeth, 204
 pulp symptoms/reaction patterns, 202–203
 root canal treatment, 204–207
age-related macular degeneration (AMD), 29
age-related changes
 age-related physiological changes, 61–62
 teeth and oral mucosa, 12
aging and periodontal disease
 epidemiology, 212–213
 periodontal inflammation, systemic diseases and aging, 218
 risk indicators/population, 213–215
 susceptibility, 215–218
alcohol
 dementia, 112
 mouth cancer, 158
 oral cancer, 136, 236
 sugars, 138
 tooth wear, 139
alendronate *see* bisphosphonate
allergy
 dental management, 82–83
 overview, 82
aloe vera, 251
Alveolar bone loss prevention, 160
alveolar ridge, 75, 142
Alzheimer's disease (AD)
 communication, 34
 dementia, 106–112
 depression, 103
 gingival plaque, 351
 neurological/neuromuscular disorders, 96
 oral disease, 351
 treatment plans, 176
 WHO classification, 346
American Academy of Orthopaedic Surgeons (AAOS), 99, 100
American Association for Retired Persons (AARP), 47, 57
American Dental Association (ADA), 99, 100, 116, 167
American Heart Association (AHA), 88–89
American Society of Anesthesiologists (ASA), 167–168, 256
amifostine, 252
amyloid precursor protein, 107
anesthetic agents
 intravenous sedation, 256–257
 nitrous oxide, 256
 oral sedation, 256
Anderson, Ferguson, 61
anethole trihione, 252
anetholetrilone, 252
angina, 271
angular cheilitis, 113, 228, 251
anticoagulant therapy
 ADP anticoagulant platelet inhibitor, 257–258
 cyclooxygenase inhibitors, 257
 warfarin, 257
antihistamines, 256
aphasia, 345
Appletree dental truck, 330
apraxia, 345
Arthritis and oral hygiene/denture insertion, 72
'artificial salivas', 251
Assessment tools for oral examination, 76
asthma
 dental management, 97–98
 overview, 97
Atrophic mandibular posterior ridge, 75
attrition (occlusal wear), 73–74
Attrition (occlusal wear), 74
atypical presentation of disease, 62
auditory function
 presbycusis, 29
 tinnitus, 30
Average fees for dental services, 319
Avlund Scales *see* Physical Activities of Daily Living

B

Baby Boomer generation, 41, 166
bacteraemia from dental procedures
 angina, 90
 arrhythmias, 90–91
 cardiac pacemakers, 90
 congestive heart failure, 90
 coronary artery bypass graft, 89–90
 coronary stents, 90
 heart transplantation, 90
 hypertension, 91
 myocardial infarction, 89
basal metabolic rate, 9
basic periodontal examination (BPE), 277–279
Behavioural problems in adult with dementia (causes), 350
Benign mucous membrane pemphigoid-bulla, 230
benign mucous membrane permphigoid, 229
bidi smoking (India), 233–234
Bidi Smoking and Oral Leukoplakia in Mumbai, India, 234

Textbook of Geriatric Dentistry, Third Edition. Edited by Poul Holm-Pedersen, Angus W. G. Walls and Jonathan A. Ship.

biology/physiology and aging
cells - molecular mechanisms, 8–9
cells - renewal and telomere loss theory, 10–11
immunological changes, 13–14
mitochondria, 10
oral environment, 12–13
organ systems, 12
oxidative stress theory, 9–10
salivary glands and secretion, 12–13
biology/physiology and aging
somatic mutation and DNA damage theories, 9–10
what is aging and why does it occur?, 7–8
biopsies
fine needle aspiration biopsy, 263
techniques, 262–263
Biopsy technique, 262
Bireen, James E., 39
bisphosphonate associated osteonecrosis (BON), 268
Bisphosphonate induced osteonecrosis of jaw, 358
bisphosphonates (alendronate, risedronate, ibandronate)
mechanism of action, 17–18
osteonecrosis, 147, 258
osteopenia/osteoporosis in men, 22
osteoporosis, 99, 268
root canal treatment, 204
bleeding disorders
coagulapathies of interest to dentistry, 83–84
common medicines that predispose to bleeding, 84
dental management, 84
overview, 83
bleeding and medications, 84
Blood pressure for adults (classification/management), 91
Body composition/physiological function and macro/micro nutrition, 131
Bone grafts, 261
bone loss *see* bone and muscle (aging); osteopenia
bone mineral density (BMD), 17, 18, 20–21
'bone multicellular unit', 18
bone and muscle (aging)
bone loss, 18
bone loss in craniofacial skeleton, 22
bone remodelling, 18–19
cardiac and smooth muscle loss, 23–24
immobilization and muscle/bone loss, 24
mineral metabolism and bone, 19–20
molecular mediators of remodelling, 19
osteopenea/osteoporosis, 18, 20–22
sarcopenia, 22–23, 24
summary, 17–18
bromhexine, 252
Buccal mucosa (dessicated), 248
burning mouth syndrome (BMS), 158, 238–239, 266, 272–273
Bur and root canal chamber, 205
Butler, Robert, 40

C
Caenorhabditis elegans, 8
'calcified canals', 207
calcitonin gene-related peptide (CGRP), 265
calcitrol, 20
calcium and bone/muscle loss, 17, 19
Cancer
chemotherapy, 87
head/neck radiotherapy, 85
cancer
overview, 84–85
radiation therapy, 85–86
see also oral cancer
Candida albicans, 155, 228, 229
Candida hyphae, 228
Candida sp., 155, 156, 157, 162, 233
candidiasis, 248–249
candidosis, 73, 227–228, 340, 357
cantilever bridges, 291
Cardiac conditions and endocarditis - prophylaxis with dental treatment, 88
cardiovascular (CVD) disorders
bacteraemia from dental treatment risk assessment, 89–91
nutrition and oral health, 135–136
other considerations, 91
overview, 88–89
caries
caries, 73–74
coronal, 183
operative dental procedures, 203–204
peridontal disease, 139, 186
prevention, 191–196
screening, 277–279
Caries Associated with Restorations (CARs), 181
caries (detection tools)
DIAGNOdent, 190
electronic caries monitor, 190–191
quantitative laser fluorescence, 190
caries (diagnosis)
location of lesions, 189–190
plaque, 189
root caries description, 184, 189
visual/radiographical examination, 189
caries (epidemiological studies)
numbers of teeth, 182
restorations, 182–183
surfaces at risk, 182
caries (identification/reduction of risk)
bacteria, 191–193
chemical intervention, 193
diet, 193
genetic modification of bacteria, 193
oral hygiene, 193
vaccination, 193
caries management by risk assessment (CAMBRA), 117
caries (nutrition/oral health), 137–139
alcohol, 138
erosive or acid-mediated dissolution of tooth tissue, 139
periodontal disease, 139
smoking, 138–139
sugars, 137–138

caries (older persons)
clinical appearance of root caries, 187–188
coronal caries, 183–184
detection tools, 190–191
diagnosis, 189–190
diet, 187, 193–196
epidemiology, 181–182, 182–184
fluoride, 187
histopathology of root caries and pulp dentine, 188–189
identification/reduction of risk, 191–193
introduction, 181
lesions, 188
operative management, 196–197
oral hygiene, 194–195
prevention, 191–192
risk factors, 185–187
root caries, 184–185
saliva, 187
summary, 197
caries (oral hygiene)
fluoride, 195–196
mechanical, 194–195
Caries prevalence in older populations, 182
caries (risk factors)
caries history, 185
periodontal disease, 186
plaque and microflora, 186–187
tissues exposed, 185
Caries risk in older populations, 183
cataracts, 29
cell-mediated response, 13
cell renewal and telomere loss theory, 10–11
Cellular damage and aging, 11
cerebral vascular disease
dental management, 92
overview, 91
cerebrovascular accident (CVA), 71, 91
cevimeline, 251, 338, 358
C. glabrata, 157
chat rooms, 52
Chemical plaque control, 156
chemotherapy (cancer)
oral complications, 87–88
overview, 86
patient assessment, 86–87
chewing
comfort, 280
foods choice, 139–141
China and social supports/family relations, 49
chlorhexidine (CHX), 156, 193, 196, 336–337
cholesterol, 135–6
Chronic impairments/habits in persons aged 65+, 6
Chronic Obstructive Pulmonary Disease (COPD), 98
C. krusei, 157
clarithromycin, 150
Classification of Behavioural and Mental Disorders (WHO), 346
Clinical variables and quality of life, 302
clinical assessment of elderly patients
conclusions, 78
geriatric medicine principles, 61–65
introduction, 61

patient assessment, 66–78
patient behaviour, 65
clinical management of cognitively impaired older adult/terminally ill patient
cognitively impaired older adult, 345–354
essential concepts, 359
terminally ill patients, 355–359
Clinical radiographic examination of head/neck (cancer patients), 85
clotrimazole, 86
cognitively impaired older adults
dementia care, 348–349
dementia diagnosis, 347
dementia treatment, 347–348
extent/severity of oral diseases/conditions, 350–351
rational dental care for dementia patients, 353–354
restraint, consent, legal guardians and ethical issues with dementia patients, 352–353
treatment planning/dental care and general anesthesia for dementia patients, 354–355
what is dementia?, 345–347
who has dementia?, 347
cognitive processes (aging)
constancy/change, 43
coping mechanisms, 44
decision-making and reasoning, 42–43
intellectual function, 41–42
memory, 42
personality/adjustment, 43
stress/coping, 43–44
Common chronic impairments/habits in persons aged 65+, 62
Common co-existing conditions in institutionalized elderly, 63
Communication techniques during dental examination of cognitively impaired adult, 350
Composite aged tooth, 202
Computer and PDA drug information software, 152
confusion and delirium (dementia)
Alzheimer's disease, 106–108
ethanol abuse, 111–112
frontotemporal, 110
Lewy bodies/Parkinsonism, 110–111
normal pressure hydrocephalus, 111
secondary to diverse physiological disturbances, 112
vascular, 108–110, 346
congestive heart failure (CHF), 90
consulting dentist, 339–340
coping (aging), 56
coronal caries, 183–184
Coronal dentine-pulp interface, 199
Coronal pulp, 202
Coronal/root caries, 184
coronary artery bypass graft (CABG), 89–90
coronary artery disease (CAD), 90
C-reactive protein (CRP), 271
Creutzfeld–Jakob disease, 111, 345–6
Cushing's disease, 17, 21, 94
cyclooxygenase (COX) inhibitors, 257

D

degenerative neuromuscular disorders
dental management, 97
motor neuron disease, 97
multiple sclerosis, 97
deletions (DNA), 8
dementia
care givers communication, 34–35
communication with patients, 34
orofacial pain in older adults, 266
see also cognitively impaired older adults; confusion and delirium
Dementia (geriatric minimal intervention), 353
Dementia and oral disease in older adult, 351
Dementia treatment (modifying factors), 353
demography (expanding elderly population)
individual aging/population aging, 3
introduction, 1
population aging, 1–3
population aging/geriatric dentistry, 3–4
Dental care
ASA classification, 168
elderly patients (planning/delivery), 166
dental caries *see* caries
dental hygienists, 161, 162, 320, 339
Dental hygienists, 161, 162
dental practitioner (sensory/cognitive decline in patients)
cognitive, 32–33
visual/auditory, 31–32
Dental procedures (AHA)
endocarditis prophylaxis, 88
regimens, 89
dental residency programmes, 320
Dental services utilization, 36
Dental Treatment of Homebound Persons, Kentucky, US, 332–333
Dentine-pulp complex responses to injury
aging pulp tissue, 201
cementum changes, 202
internal calcification of pulp, 201–202
tertiary dentine deposition, 200–201
dentoalveolar surgery in elderly patients
extractions, 259
planning, 258
preprosthetic surgery, 258–259
Denture irrigation hyperplasia prevalence, 230
dentures
case studies, 177–179
dementia patients, 113
hygiene, 161, 250, 298–299
'neutral zone', 174, 295
overlay, 175
plaque control, 298–299
recall, maintenance and repair, 296
removable partial, 140, 175, 290
saliva, 296
xerostomia, 295
Dentures
duplication technique, 295
labelling, 294
Denture stomatitis prevalence, 229
desire to look attractive, 317
diabetes mellitus
dehydration, 93
dental management, 93
history, 92
hyperglycemia, 92–93
hypoglycemia, 92–93
nutrition and oral health, 135
obesity, 134
overview, 92–93
salivary gland, 93
type I, II, 135
xerostomia, 93
Diagnostic and Statistical Manual of Mental Disorders Fourth Edition (DSM-IV), 345
Dietary Intake
CVD risk, 135
Nutrients and dental status, 138
diet (caries)
chewing efficiency, 194
frequency of sugars intake, 187, 193
malnourishment, 194
starches, 194
sugars replacement, 193–194
diphenylhydramine (Benadryl©), 256
Directors of Nursing (DONs), 327
disability in old age - oral health
conclusions, 128
consequences, 128
disability pathway, 119–121
disablement process, 119
functional ability in older populations, 122–123
gender differences, 124–125
measurement, 121–122
oral disability pathway, 125–127
risk factors, 121
selection due to mortality, 123–124
disability pathway
disability, 120–121
functional limitations, 120
impairments, 120
pathology, 119
Disablement process, 120, 121
disease chronicity, 62
disease-modifying anti-rheumatic drugs (DMARDS), 98, 99
disease-related changes, 61–62
Disposable soma theory, 8
DMF (Decayed, Missing, Filled), 182
DMFS (Decayed, Missing, Filled, Surface), 182
DMFT (Decayed, Missing, Filled, Tooth), 182
DNA
deletions, 8
drosophila melangaster, 9
insertions, 8
mitochondria (mDNA), 10
point mutations, 8
somatic mutation/damage theories, 9–10
drug abuse and addiction
alcoholism, 92
dental management, 92

drug abuse and addiction (*continued*)
- history and physical findings, 92
- overview, 91–92

Drugs
- **Adverse reactions**, 150
- **Internet based websites**, 151
- **Oral health/management**, 147
- **Reference text books**, 151

Dry mouth treatments in elderly patients, 250
dual X-ray absorptiometry (DXA, DEXA), 18, 20, 22

E

Edentulism rates in US, 313
edentulous patient (complete dentures)
- description, 294–295
- immediate, 293–294
- oldest old, 295–296

Edentulous patients (pre/post treatment) (OHIP), 308
Educational attainment by age cohort, 35
Elder-friendly communities concept, 47–48, 57
Elderly population of the world, 324
electrical stimulation (saliva), 251
Electric toothbrushes, 161
electronic caries monitor (ECM), 190–191
endocrine disorders
- adrenal gland, 94–95
- diabetes mellitus, 92–93
- thyroid gland, 93–94

Endodontic file and root canal chamber, 205
endodontic therapy, 172
Energy intakes, 133
erythrocyte sedimentation rate (ESR), 271
erythromycin, 150
erythroplakia, 234–235
Ethics/Conduct code, 169
executive functioning (aging), 42
Experimental gingivitis, 215
Extension Bridge for abutment teeth, 291
extraoral clinical examination
- breath, 72
- ears, 72
- eyes, 71
- facial form, 70–71
- hair, 71
- hands, 71
- lymph nodes, 72
- neck, 72
- sinuses, 72
- skin, 71
- temporomandibular joint/mastication muscles, 72

F

Facial symmetry, 70
Fatigue in daily activities, 123
Fatigued/not fatigued 70 year old women with functional decline, 124
filial piety belief, 50
fine needle aspiration biopsy (FNAB), 263
flavour enhancers and food, 142
Florida Dental Care Study, 316
Fluid-attenuation inversion recovery images (FLAIR), 109
fluoride
- caries in older persons, 187
- gels, pastes and rinses, 195–196
- milk, 196
- preventive/non-operative strategies, 196
- preventive oral health care for elderly people, 156–157
- rice, 196
- toothpaste, 336
- treatment planning, 171
- water, 195

fluoride (preventive/non-operative strategies)
- casein phosphopeptide-amorphous calcium phosphate, 196
- chlorhexidine, 196
- ozone, 196

Food and Drug Administration (FDA), US, 152, 251, 273
foods
- texture, 142
- *see also* nutrition; oral health and foods choice

'frailty' phenotype, 17
free radicals, 9
Freud, Sigmund, 40
functional loss (older people), 64
Functional presentation of illness, 64

G

Gastro Esophageal Reflux Disease, 139
General Anesthesia (dental treatment planning guidelines), 356
general anesthesia (GA), 354–355
Geriatric assessment dimensions, 67
Geriatric medicine
- *assessment*, 67
- *principles*, 61

geriatric medicine principles
- age/disease interactions, 62
- age-related physiological changes, 61–62
- atypical presentation of disease, 62
- disease chronicity, 62
- functional loss, 64
- function and disease, 64–65
- multiple pathology, 62–64
- polypharmacy, 64

Geriatric Minimal Intervention Dentistry (GMID), 353
Geriatric mobile unit and dental office, 335
giant cell arteritis (GCA), 270–271
Gingiva/clean teeth young/old comparison, 216
Gingiva mestastasis from breast carcinoma, 239
gingivitis/periodontitis
- etiology, 211
- periodontal disease pathogenesis, 211–212

Glass ionomer, 172, 177, 197
glass ionomer cements (GICs), 197
Glass Ionomer (Ketac Molar™) and carious lesions, 177
glaucoma, 29
glossodynia (painful tongue), 230
glossopyrosis (burning tongue), 230
Glostrup Aging Studies (Denmark), 122, 126
Graves' disease (thyroid), 93

H

Handbook of Aging and the Individual, 39
Harman, Denham, 9
Hashimoto's thyroiditis, 93
'Hayflick limit' (telomere shortening), 11
head and neck cancer (HNC), 274
Headrests, 333
Health effects of drugs in affective disorders, 115–116
Health Information Survey, 1984, US, 141
health promotion, 319
Health-related quality of life measures, 304–305
herpes zoster, 273
high density lipoprotein (HDL), 135
Hip fracture (12 month survival), 21
histopathology of root caries and pulp dentine
- arrested root caries, 189
- cementum, 188–189
- initial/advanced root dentine caries, 189

history taking
- family history, 82
- past medical history, 81–82
- social history, 82
- systems review, 82

hormone replacement therapy (HRT), 22
hospice, 325
Hospital readmissions (nutrient supplements/controls), 132
humoral response, 13
Hutchinson–Gilford progeria syndrome (HGPS), 12
Hydra and senescence, 10
hydrazine (Vistaril©), 256
hydrocortisone, 94–5
hyperbaric oxygen (HBO), 86
hypertension, 91
'idiopathic osteoporosis', 21

I

immunological changes, 13–14
Implant-retained lower overdenture, 178
implants, 176, 179
Implants
- *Mandibular*, 260
- **Placement indications**, 260
- *Retained overdenture*, 260

implants in elderly patients
- atrophic mandible/dental mental nerve compression, 262
- bone grafting, 261
- denture-induced hyperplasia, 262
- description, 259–260
- fraenectomy, 261–262
- maxillary tuberosity reduction, 262
- partially dentate patients, 260–261
- vestibuloplasty, 262

Implants for overdentures, 298
innate immune response, 13
insertions (DNA), 8
Institutionalized elderly conditions, 63
instrumental activities of daily living (IADL), 64, 70, 122
intensity modulated radiotherapy (IMRT), 252
Interacting dimensions of geriatric assessment, 67

Interdental spaces, 290
interdisciplinary team
consulting dentist, 339–340
dental hygienist, 339
dietician, 339
patient, 339
pharmacist, 339
physician, 339
social worker, 339
intergenerational transfers (resources), 51
Internet, 51
Interpersonal communication, 28
Interventions for prevention of behavioural problems (dementia), 349
intraoral and perioral soft/hard tissue examination
alveolar ridge, 75
occlusion, 75–76
periodontium, 74–75
soft tissue/dry mouth, 72–73
tooth structure loss, caries and restorations, 73–74
Ivoclar (Lactobilli/Strep Mutans), 192

J
Japan
society, 49
Sugar consumption/dental caries in children, 137
teledentistry, 330
Jung, Carl, 40

K
ketoconazole, 150

L
laboratory testing, 77
Laclede Oral Balance products, 338
Lactobacilli, 172, 186, 192
late-life delusional/paranoid psychoses, 105–106
learning and memory
cognitive processes, 42
perceptual speed, 30
secondary memory, 30–31
"leisure" term, 54
leukoariosis, 109
leukoplakia, 231–234
Leukoplakia, 231–233
lichen planus, 228
lifespan perspective of aging, 40
Lip cancer incidence in Denmark, 237
liver disease
dental management, 95
hepatitis A, B, C, D, 95
post-liver transplant, 95
'*Long Teeth*', 290
long-term facility care (LTC), 160, 314
lorazepam (Ativan©), 256
Low haematological intake in older people, 134
Low income elders' reasons for not using dental services, 316
Lower Reference Nutrient Intake (LRNI), 133
Lubben Social Network Scale, 48–49
lymphoma, 247
Lymphoma (palate), 239

M
magnetic resonance imaging (MRI), 109, 271
Malaligned occlusion/fractured teeth, 76
Mandibular implants, 260
Manual dexterity, 290
Maxillary molar lingual recession, 75
Maxillary sinuses and bone atrophy, 259
M-CSF (macrophage-colony stimulating factor), 19
Mechanical plaque removal, 221
Medicaid, 319
medical examination/assessment
allergies, 69
cognitive/mental status, 70
communication, 66–67
description, 67–70
diet history, 69
functional assessment, 70
ID (identification), 67
laboratory assessment, 69–70
medications, 68–69
physical examination, 69
social history, 69
vital signs, 69
medical examination/assessment (history), 67
past, 67–68
present illness, 67
taking, 66
medical issues in dental care of older adults
elderly patients, 81
history taking, 81–82
medical history, 81
medical management of surgical comorbidities
anticoagulant therapy, 257–258
biopsies, 262–263
bisphosphonate therapy, 254
dental implants in elderly patients, 259–262
dentoalveolar surgery in elderly patients, 258–259
key points, 263
mucosal fragility/impaired healing, 258
medical problems (oral health care)
allergy, 82–83
bleeding disorders, 83–84
cancer, 84–88
cardiovascular disorders, 88–91
cerebral vascular disease, 91
drug abuse and addiction, 91–92
endocrine disorders, 92–93
liver disease, 95
neurological/neuromuscular disorders, 96–97
pulmonary diseases, 97–98
renal disorders, 95–96
rheumatological diseases, osteoarthritis, osteoporosis and prosthetic joints, 98–100
Medicare Current Beneficiary Survey (MCBS), 314
Medicare (health insurance), 40
Medication non-compliance in elderly patients, 153
Medications review, 146
medicines that predispose to bleeding
aspirin, 84
clopidogrel (Plavix™), 84
dabigatran (Pradaxa™), 84
drug interactions, 84
heparin, low molecular weight heparins, 84
warfarin, 84
Medigap (insurance), 314
memory *see* learning and memory
Men/women (65+) with different diseases, 125
Men/women with/without caries and functional abilities, 127
Mesiodistal fracture, 203
metronidazole, 150
mild cognitive impairment (MCI), 107
Mineral Trioxide Aggregate, 207
Mini-Mental State Examination (MMSE), 70–71
Min-Mental State Examination (MMSE), 71
MI paste (Tooth Mousse), 338, 340
mitochondria
aging, 10
DNA, 10
Mob-H (Mobility–Help) scale, 122–123
mobile dental units, 331–332
Mobility and number of teeth, chewing and regular use of dentist, 126
Mob-T (Mobility–Tiredness) scale, 122–123
Mortality rates (ASA), 256
mucocutaneous diseases
benign mucous membrane pemphigoid, 229–230
denture irritation hyperplasia, 230
lichen planus, 229
mucosal-associated B cell (MALT) lymphomas, 247
mucosa
disease treatment, 158
disorders and medications, 147
infections, 155
inflammatory disease, 134, 156, 227
lesions prevalence, 227
multidrug-resistance (MDR) forms, 98
multiple pathology, 72
multiple sclerosis, 97
muscle loss *see* sarcopenia
Muscle mass and age, 132
myocardial infarction (MI), 89
myosin heavy chains (MyHCs), 24

N
National Cancer Institute, US, 274
National Diet and Nutrition Survey for people aged 65+, UK, 133
National Health Interview Survey (NHIS), 311, 313
National Health and Nutrition and Examination Survey (NHANES) III, US, 135, 141
National Institute of Aging, US, 0
National Survey of Oral Health, 1985–6, US, 212
Natural products and dental management, 147

nervous system diseases, burning mouth syndrome, 230–231
neurological/neuromuscular disorders
 Alzheimer's disease, 96
 degenerative neuromuscular disorders, 97
 dementia, 96
 dental management, 97
 medical history, 96
 motor neurone disease, 97
 Parkinson's disease, 96
 seizures/epilepsy, 96–97
Neuropathic pain, 272
'Neutral zone' (dentures), 174, 295
Niue (Polynesia) and older people status, 50
non-Hodgkin's lymphoma (NHL), 239–240
non-milk extrinsic sugars (NMES), 138
NSAIDS (non-steroidal anti-inflammatory drugs), 99, 150, 257, 269, 270, 275
nurse aides (NAs), 335
Nutrients intake in 65+ adults (dental status), 138
nutrition and oral health for older persons
 age requirements, 132–134
 dental caries, 137–139
 foods choice, 139–140
 introduction, 131–132
 masticatory efficiency, 140–141
 oral mucosa, 136
 periodontal disease, 139
 summary, 142
 systemic disease etiology, 134–136
 taste and smell, 141–142
 texture of foods, 142
 see also vitamins
nutrition and oral health for older persons (age requirements)
 energy, 132
 micronutrients intakes, 133–134
 physiological function, 134
 protein intake, 133

O

obesity and nutrition (oral health)
 CVD, 134
 Diabetes, 134
 hypertension, 134
 stroke, 134
occlusion, 75–76
oestrogen deficiency, 17
older adults' use of dental services
 best predictors of utilization, 317–318
 demographic variables, 311–313
 dental attitudes, 316
 dental/medical insurance, 314
 dental provider characteristics (help/hinder), 318
 dentition/health status, 314–315
 education/income, 313–314
 hope for the future, 318–319
 introduction/definitions, 311
 physical access/mobility, 315
 psychosocial variables as barriers/enablers, 315–316, 317
 racial/ethnic differences, 313
 research to improve dental service utilization, 319–320
 residence, 314
 social support, 316–317
Older people and micronutrients intakes, 133
Olovnikov, Alexei, 11
operative dental procedures
 caries management, 203–204
 pulp capping and pulpotomy, 204
Oral cancer, 236, 238–239
oral cancer
 alcohol, 236
 clinical features, 236–237
 diagnosis/referral, 237–238
 epidemiology/etiology, 236
 nutrition, 135
 prevention, 158–159
 tobacco, 236
 tongue, 236
Oral Cancer incidence in men, 237
Oral cancer prevention, 159
Oral conditions in patients
 affective disorders, 112
 dementia, 113
 psychotic disorders, 113
Oral disability pathway, 126
Oral disease prevention problems, 161
Oral-facial disorders medication (administration/prescribing), 149
oral health care programmes for homebound people, nursing home residents and elderly inpatients
 epidemiology, 323–324
 homebound people, 324–325
 hospice, 325–326
 institutionalized people, 326
 interdisciplinary team, 338–339
 introduction, 323
 oral health status/needs, 326–327
 population definition, 323
 preventive programmes, 335–338
 programmes, 327–335
 summary, 340–341
Oral health - conceptual model for measurement, 303
oral health and foods choice
 chewing efficiency, digestion and foods choice, 139–140
 dietary change prevention, 141
 masticatory efficiency, 140
 masticatory efficiency and digestion, 140–141
Oral Health Impact Profile (OHIP), 306–308
Oral health improvement for elderly patients (model), 162
oral health in patients with psychiatric disorders
 affective disorders, 112–113
 psychotic disorders, 113
Oral health measurement (model), 303
oral health programmes
 1. transfer to dental office/practice, 327–329
 2. on-site dental programmes, 329–330
 3. teledentistry, 330
 4. mobile dental vans, 330
 5. portable dentistry interventions, 331–333
 6. hospital-based/dental school-based mobile programmes, 333–335
oral health-related quality of life
 clinical intervention studies, 307–308
 descriptive population studies, 306–307
 health/disease models, 301–302
 health status measurement, 305–306
 health status measures, 304–305
 older people, 302
 oral health status measurement, 306
 subjective appraisal of oral health (qualitative methodology), 203–204
 summary/future, 08–309
 theoretical framework for measurement, 302–303
 uses to date/remaining problems, 306
 what is quality of life?, 301
Oral hygiene care protocols for older adults, 337
oral hygiene (caries)
 fluoride, 195–196
 mechanical, 194–195
Oral hygiene in patient with dementia, 156
Oral/intravenous sedation medication, 256
oral/maxillofacial surgery for geriatric patients
 anesthesia, 255
 introduction, 255
 local anesthesia, 255–256
 medical management of surgical comorbidities, 257–258
 sedation/general anesthesia, 256–257
oral mucosa
 alcohol, 136
 iron, vitamin B_{12} and folate, 136
 prevalence, 227
 smoking, 136
oral mucosa (common diseases - infectious origin)
 angular cheilitis, 228–229
 candidosis, 227–228
 denture stomatitis, 228
oral rehabilitation in elderly patients
 caries (screening), 277
 conventional/implant born reconstruction, 283–284
 dental prostheses efficiency, 296
 edentulous patients, 293–295
 implant placement, 297–298
 implant-supported overdentures, 296–297
 masticatory function/chewing ability, 297
 opportunistic infections, 277
 overdentures, 292–293
 partially dentate patients reconstruction, 282–283
 periodontal disease (screening), 277–279
 plaque control and denture hygiene, 298–299
 pretherapeutic single tooth prognosis, 279
 recall, maintenance and repair, 296
 reduced dentition, 292
 removable dental prosthesis, 287–290
 subjective chewing therapy, 280–281
 teeth replacement with acid-etched composite-bonded bridges, 291–292

treatment goals, 279–282
treatment planning, 282–283, 284–287
oral sequelae of head/neck radiotherapy
infections, 86
mucositis, 85
osteoradionecrosis (ORN), 86
taste loss, 86
xerostomia, 86
Oral side effects of drug classes, 148
Oral specific measures of health, 306
Oral symptoms enquiries, 68
organ systems, 12
Orofacial pain in older adults, 266–267
orofacial pain in older adults
age-related change in pain perception/reporting, 265
burning mouth syndrome, 272–273
chronic trigeminal neuropathy/non-odontogenic toothache, 273–274
common causes, 266–268
dementia, 266
dentofacial pain, 268–269
giant cell arteritis, 270–271
headache, 270
head/neck cancer, 274
neuropathic pain, 271
pain management in older patients, 274–275
postherpetic neuralgia, 273
reaction/adaptation to pain in older adults, 265–266
referred cardiac pain, 271
salivary disorders, 269
temporomandibular disorders, 269
treatment, 266
trigeminal neuralgia, 272
osteoarthritis (OA), 99
Osteoclast development regulation, 19
osteomyelitis, 268
osteonecrosis of the jaw (ONJ), 268
osteopenia/osteoporosis
definition, 18
men, 20–22
osteoporosis
dental management, 99
overview, 99
WHO definition, 159
osteoprotegerin (OPG), 19
osteoradionecrosis (ORN), 86
over-the-counter (OTC) products/medications, 146, 338
oxidative stress theory (aging), 9–10

P
pain management in older patients, 274–275
Palliative care (oral conditions), 357
parathyroid hormone (PTH), 17, 20
Parathyroid hormone (PTH) and bone loss, 20
Parkinson's disease, 96, 108, 110–111, 142, 159, 295
pathology/treatment of gingivitis/periodontitis in aging individuals
aging/periodontal disease, 212–218
conclusions, 223
gingivitis/peridontitis, 211–212
maintenance, 223
periodontal treatment and prophylaxis, 219–221, 221–223
prognosis, 218–219
pathology/treatment of oral mucosal diseases
clinical/histological changes in aging oral mucosa, 226–227
common diseases, 227–229
monocutaneous diseases, 229–230
nervous system, 230–231
oral cancer, 236–239
other malignancies, 239–240
periodontal aspects of normal oral mucosa, 225–226
premalignant lesions, 231–235
solar lip damage, 235–236
pathology/treatment of pulp disease
aged tooth clinical challenges, 202–207
age-related changes in dentine/pulp complex, 199
conclusions, 207
dentine/pulp complex responses to injury, 200–202
introduction, 199
operative dental procedures, 203–204
physiological age-changes, 199–200
patient assessment
diagnostic aids, 76–77
differential, 78
examination/assessment, 70–72
intraoral and perioral soft/hard tissue examination, 72–73
medical examination/assessment, 66–70
oral examination/assessment, 70–76
plan, 78
prosthetics, 77–78
patient behaviour
illness severity, 65
under-reporting of symptoms/disease, 65
Pearl, Raymond, 9
Peridontally compromised molar (root canal treatment), 204
Periodontal breakdown, 222
periodontal disease
aging, 212–215
care, 172, 175–176
caries, 139, 186
gingivitis/periodontitis, 211–212
screening, 277–279
susceptibility, 215–218
periodontal screening record (PSR), 277
Periodontal treatment, 220
periodontium, 74–75
pharmacology and aging
conclusions, 152–153
introduction, 145–146
medical conditions and dental care, 146
medication as indicator of medical conditions, 146
medications and dental prescribing, 159–150
non-compliance to medication, 152
oral side effects of medications, 147–148
pharmacodynamics and dental management, 148–152
Physical Activities of Daily Living (PADL, Avlund Scales), 122
physiological age-changes
physiological changes in pulp, 200
physiological peritubular dentine, 200
secondary dentine deposition, 200
tooth formation, 199–200
pilocarpine, 251, 338, 358
plaque
control and dental hygiene (dentures), 298–299
prevention, 155
plaque and microflora
gingival architecture, 186
oral hygiene, 186
partial denture, 186
visual acuity, 186–187
Plasminogen Activator Inhibitor, 1, 134
point mutations (DNA), 8
polymyalgia rheumatica (PMR), 270
polypharmacy, 64, 252
Poor oral hygiene cycles in nursing homes, 336
Portable Chairs, 333
Portable dental equipment, 334
Portable units, 331
positron emission tomography (PET), 271
postherpetic neuralgia (PHN), 273
premalignancy lesions
erythoplakia, 234
leukoplakia, 231–232
verrucous hyperplasia, 234–235
preventive oral health care for elderly people
barriers, 160–161
bone loss, 159–160
cancer, 158–159
cavity, 155
chemical plaque control, 156
dental erosion, 157
examples, 161–162
fluorides, 156–157
geriatric services, 162–163
healthier lifestyle, 162
mechanical cleaning, 156
mucosal diseases, 157–158
plaque induced diseases, 155
services planning, 160
temporomandibular dysfuction/myofascial pain, 160
xerostomia and burning mouth, 158
'primary osteoporosis', 18, 21
primary (working) memory, 30
Principle of Ethics/Code of Professional Conduct (ADA), 352
Private practitioner reports of older people in practice, 319–320
Professional Code of ethics/conduct, 169
Proportion of men/women with good functional ability, 122
prosthetic joints
dental management, 100
history, 99–100
overview, 99

Pseudomembraneous candidiasis
head/neck cancer, 249
palate, 72
pseudomembranous lesions, 228
psychiatric disorders in old age (implications for dental practitioners)
affective disorders, 109–110
anxiety disorders, 104–105
confusion and delirium, 106–112
dental management, 114–117
introduction, 109
late-life delusional/paranoid psychoses, 105–106
oral health in patients, 112–114
risk factors/indicators for oral disease, 114
Psychiatric patients (treatment), 114
psychology (aging)
ageism, 41
background, 39
cognitive processes, 41–44
conclusions, 44
history, 39
insights for clinicians, 44
lifespan/life course, 40–41
psychosocial variables as barriers/enablers
dental attitudes, 316
perceived versus normative needs, 315–316
social support, 316–317
pulmonary disease
asthma, 97–98
chronic obstructive pulmonary disease, 98
pulmonary tuberculosis, 98
pulp assessment, 77
Pulp (old/young) following trauma, 203
Pulp stones removal, 206
purified protein derivative (PPD), 98

Q
Quality of life
Clinical variables, 302
Dimensions, 305
Health-related measures, 304

R
radiation therapy (RT) for cancer, 85–86, 274
radiographic assessment, 76
Radiograph (periapical pathology), 77
radiographs, 76–77
raloxifene, 18
RANKL (nuclear factor kappa B ligand), 19
reactive oxygen species (ROS), 139
Recaldent CPP-ACP mouth crème, 338
reciprocity concept, 48
Reference Nutrient Intake (RFI), 133
Removable partial denture (s) (RPD), 290, 291
removable partial denture (s) (RPD), 140, 290, 291, 304
renal disorders
dental management, 96
overview, 95–96
renal transplants, 96
Renal/hepatic function guidelines, 149
Residential setting and caries rate, 315
respiratory quotients (RQ), 9
Restraint guidelines, 352
Retained teeth/Quality of Life - Australia/UK (OHIP), 307
rheumatoid arthritis (RA), 269
dental management, 99
overview, 98
rheumatological diseases, osteoarthritis, osteoporosis and prosthetic joints
osteoarthritis, 99
osteoporosis, 99
prosthetic joints, 99–100
rheumatoid arthritis, 98–99
risedronate *see* bisphosphonate
Risk factors for poor oral health (psychiatric conditions), 114
root canal treatment
canal enlargement, 207
canal identification, 205–206
canal negotiation/enlargement, 206–207
elective treatment, 204
pulp chamber access, 205
treatment, 204, 207
root caries, 173, 184–185
Root caries
Severity, 173
Treatment, 173
Root caries activity in older adults, 191
Root Caries Index, 182, 185
Root Caries Index, 185
Root surface decay on buccal mucosa margins, 249

S
saliva
caries, 187
dentures, 296
dysfunction, 336
flow, 158
formation, 245–246
glands/aging, 246–247
glands and secretion, 12–13
hypofunction, 86, 147
interdental spaces, 290
secretion, 245
substitutes/buffers, 338
taste, 36, 141
Saliva-check mutans kit, 192
Salivary flow and xerostomia treatment, 158
salivary functions/disorders in older adults
clinical evaluation, 247–248
clinical examination, 246
etiology of salivary hypofunction, 247
introduction, 245
orofacial pain, 269
past/present medical history, 248
preventive therapies, 250
saliva formation, 245–246
salivary stimulation, 251
serological evaluation, 249–250
symptomatic treatment, 250–251
systemic disorders, 252
systemic stimulation, 251
treatment strategies, 250
see also Sjögren's syndrome; xerostomia
salivary gland
biopsy, 249
hypofunction, 147, 337
imaging, 248–249
Sjögren's syndrome, 247
Salivary gland ducts (histologic organization), 246
Salivary hypofunction, 246
Salivary hypofunction
Medications, 246
Older adults, 246
Salivary problems (questions), 73
sarcopenia (muscle loss), 22–23, 24
Saunders, Cicely, 325
Secondary dentine deposition, 200
secondary (long-term) memory, 30–31
'secondary osteoporosis', 21
sedation/general anesthesia
anesthetic agents, 256
intravenous sedation, 256–257
selective oestrogen receptor modulators (SERMs), 17–18, 19
self-concept, 317
self-efficacy, 317
sensory changes and communications in practitioner-aged patient relationship
aging, 28–29
auditory function, 29–30
communications, 28
conclusions, 37
cultural differences/competences, 35–36
dementia, 34, 34–35
dental care system, 35–36
dental communication, 27–28
dental practitioner, 31–33
introduction, 27
memory and learning, 30–31
nonverbal communication, 33–34
oral-sensory functions, 36–37
sensory changes, 28–29
visual function, 29–30
Sensory and cognitive decline in older patients, 33
sertraline, 110
Severely worn prostheses and shift in mandibular position, 78
shortened dental arch, 280–282
Sjögren's syndrome (SS)
autoimmune disease, 246, 247, 249
cevimeline, 251
diagnosis, 250
dryness of mouth, 65, 73, 247
etiology, 247
facial form, 70
lymphoma, 247
pharmacotherapy, 158
pilocarpine, 251
rheumatoid arthritis, 99, 251–2, 269
salivary gland, 247–249
scintigraphy, 249
systemic disorders, 252
smell identification, 37
smoking, 138, 139
Social Security Act 1935, US, 312
society and environment (aging)
community resources, 56–57
intergenerational assistance, 51

introduction, 47
leisure roles, 54
older adults in community, 47–48
retirement as time of productivity, 53–54
role changes, 56
role changes/productivity, 52–53
social networks/support, 48–49
social supports/family relations in traditional cultures, 48–51
social supports interventions, 51–52
voluntary associations/volunteers, 55
volunteering, 55–56
Socioeconomic events and dentistry, 312
sodium lauryl sulphate (SLS), 336
solar lip damage, 235–236
somatic mutation and DNA damage theories (aging), 9–10
Splinting saves teeth, 174
squamous cell carcinoma (SCC), 159, 236, 237
'staying busy' in old age, 52
Strep mutans, 186, 192
Streptococcus anginosus, 186
Streptococcus mutans, 172
sugars
alcohol, 138
diet, 137
frequency/quantity intake, 137–138
importance, 138
medicines, 138
Sugar (sucrose) consumption and dental caries in Japanese children, 137
Survival probability after fracture, 21
systemic disease etiology
cardiovascular disease, 135–136
diabetes mellitus, 135
obesity, 134–135
oral cancer, 135

T
taste
function, 36
loss, 86
saliva, 36, 141
types, 142
unami (savoury), 142
taste and smell (aging)
smell perception, 142
taste perception, 141–142, 148
T-cell receptor, 13
Teeth positioning in neutral zone, 175
telomere shortening, 13
temporomandibular dysfunction (TMD), 160, 266, 269
temporomandibular joint (TMJ), 269–270, 274
tension type headache (TTHA), 270
terminally ill patients
oral conditions in palliative care, 356–359
Oral problems (prevalence), 325
What is palliative oral care?, 355–356
Terminally ill patients (care), 356
Tertiary dentine deposition, 201
texture of foods, 142
Thigh muscle scan, 23
thyroid gland disorders
dental management, 93
hyperthyroidism, 93
hypothyroidism, 93–94
tinnitus, 30
tobacco
leukoplakia, 232
oral cancer, 236
tongue
burning, 230
cancer, 236
colour, 170
dorsum (dry/depapillated), 248
painful, 230
tooth
wear and alcohol, 139
see also aged tooth clinical challenges
Topical anesthetics for mucositis pain, 86
transfer to dental office/practice
appointment times, 328–329
communications, 329
continence, 328
legal/ethical issues, 329
person's activity level, 328
transferability, 328
transient ischaemic attack (TIA), 91
Transportability of long-term care residents, 328
Treatment planning
Dementia, 353
General Anesthesia, 356
Implants, 283–7
Phases, 171
treatment planning for geriatric patients
accurate data/diagnosis, 169–171
conclusions, 179
dental practice, 165
ethics, 167–168
evidence to evaluate alternatives, 169
fundamentals, 167
geriatric plans, 176–179
implants, 176
introduction, 165
periodontal care, 175–176
plan, 171–172
prosthodontic care, 174
treatment, 172, 172–173
who are geriatric patients?, 165–167
triazolam (Halcion©), 256
tricyclic antidepressants (TCAs), 273–274, 275
trigeminal neuralgia (TN), 272, 273–274

U
unami (savoury taste), 142
underreporting of symptoms/disease, 65

V
vascular dementia, 108–110, 346
varicella zoster virus (VZV), 273
Verbal communication disorders associated with dementia, 34
verrucous hyperplasia, 234–235
Verrucous hyperplasia, 234–235
Vertebral fracture and age, 21
Visiting Nurse Association, 333
Visual Analogue Scales (VAS), 307
visual function
accommodation, 29
colour, depth/distance perception, 29
light/dark adaptation, 29
vitamins
B_{12}, 61, 131, 133, 134
C, 133, 134, 138
D, 17, 19–21, 131, 133, 134
E, 251

W
warfarin
alcoholism, 92
anticoagulation, 89, 91, 96, 150, 257
artificial heart valves, 88
atrial fibrillation, 70
bleeding disorders, 83–4
medications, 82
Watch-winding motion for root canal negotiation, 207
wear and tear theory of aging, 7
wound healing, 226
Why survive: Being old in America, 40
World Health Organization (WHO)
Alzheimer's disease classification, 346
edentulism (disability/handicap), 117, 296
impairment, disability and handicap classification, 303
men/women oral health strategies, 160–161
osteoporosis, 159
preventive services for elderly people, 160

X
xerostomia (dry mouth)
anti-seizure medications, 97
dementia, 113
dentures, 295
diabetes, 93
hypertension, 91
medications, 147
nocturnal, 252
prevention, 158, 336
radiotherapy, 86
rheumatoid arthritis, 99
salivary gland hypofunction, 248, 337
salivary stimulation, 251
Xerostomia inventory (XI), 338

Printed and bound by CPI Group (UK) Ltd, Croydon, CR0 4YY

16/04/2025

14658835-0001